Disorders of Thrombosis and Hemostasis in Pregnancy

Hannah Cohen • Patrick O'Brien
Editors

Disorders of Thrombosis and Hemostasis in Pregnancy

A Guide to Management

Second Edition

Springer

Editors
Hannah Cohen
Department of Haematology
University College London Hospitals
NHS Foundation Trust
London
UK

Patrick O'Brien
Institute for Women's Health
University College London Hospitals
NHS Foundation Trust
London
UK

ISBN 978-3-319-34245-0 ISBN 978-3-319-15120-5 (eBook)
DOI 10.1007/978-3-319-15120-5

Springer Cham Heidelberg New York Dordrecht London

Softcover reprint of the hardcover 2nd edition 2015

Printed on acid-free paper

Springer is part of Springer Science+Business Media (www.springer.com)

Preface to the Second Edition

The first edition of this book quickly established itself as an invaluable resource for those caring for women during pregnancy and fertility treatment. This second edition expands its scope, including new chapters on anticoagulants and antiplatelet agents, cerebrovascular disease, pre-eclampsia, obstetric haemorrhage, thrombotic microangiopathies, paroxysmal nocturnal haemoglobinuria and analgesia and anaesthesia in women with haemostatic or thrombotic disorders in pregnancy. It also updates the previous content with the most recent research evidence. The book provides a contemporary and comprehensive guide to the management of haematological disorders in pregnancy. It covers a wide range of important clinical disorders that are associated with a potentially significant risk of morbidity and mortality in both the mother and the baby. The focus in each chapter is on authoritative, practical clinical advice, in the context of the available scientific evidence, on the management of women with both common and rare disorders of thrombosis and haemostasis in pregnancy. Included also are disorders where the management of thrombotic aspects are highly relevant, such as cardiac disorders, haemoglobinopathies and assisted conception. In addition, chapters include key learning points, and, when called for, case studies that highlight the pertinent clinical aspects of the topics covered. It is well recognized that in this population, many recommendations are based on observational studies and extrapolation from other populations rather than on appropriately designed clinical trials, and this is reflected in some degree of variation in the opinions expressed in different chapters. The approach is multidisciplinary – the authorship brings together wide-ranging expertise in haematology, obstetrics and gynaecology, obstetric medicine, cardiology, neonatology and assisted conception, resulting in a unique and clinically indispensable resource. This book will therefore be of interest and value to all those involved in the management of women with disorders of thrombosis and haemostasis in pregnancy and fertility treatment – haematologists, obstetricians and gynaecologists, midwives and obstetric and general physicians as well as neonatologists at both consultant and trainee level.

London, UK — Hannah Cohen, MB ChB, MD, FRCP, FRCPath
London, UK — Patrick O'Brien, MBBCh, FRCOG, FICOG, FFSRH

Contents

Contributors

Deepa Jayakody Arachchillage, MBBS, MRCP, FRCPath Department of Haematology, University College London Hospitals NHS Foundation Trust, London, UK

Trevor Baglin, MA, MB ChB, PhD, FRCP, FRCPath Department of Haematology, Addenbrooke's Hospital, Cambridge University Hospitals NHS Foundation Trust, Cambridge, UK

Rory Bell, MBBS, FRCA Department of Anaesthesia, University College London Hospitals NHS Foundation Trust, London, UK

Louise Bowles, MBBS, BSc, MRCP, FRCPath Department of Clinical Haematology, The Royal London Hospital, London, UK

Amanda Clark, BSc, MBBS, FRCPath Department of Haematology, Bristol Haematology and Oncology Centre, University Hospitals Bristol NHS Foundation Trust, Bristol, UK

Katherine Clesham, MB ChB, MRCP, FRCPath Department of Haematology, University College London Hospitals NHS Foundation Trust, London, UK

Hannah Cohen, MB ChB, MD, FCRP, FRCPath Department of Haematology, University College London Hospitals NHS Foundation Trust, London, UK

Nichola Cooper, MB ChB, MA, MD, FRCP, FRCPath Department of Haematology, Faculty of Medicine, Hammersmith Hospital, Imperial College Healthcare NHS Trust, London, UK

Anna E. Curley, MB ChB, MRCP, MD, LLB Neonatal Intensive Care Unit, Cambridge University Hospitals NHS Trust, Cambridge, UK

Charlie Davie, MB ChB, MD, FRCP Department of Clinical Neurosciences, The Royal Free Hampstead NHS Trust, London, UK

Anja B. Drebes, MB ChB, MRCP, FRCPath Katharine Dormandy Haemophilia Centre and Thrombosis Unit, The Royal Free Hospital, Royal Free NHS Foundation Trust, London, UK

Maria Efthymiou, BSc, MSc, PhD Haemostasis Research Unit, Department of Haematology, University College London Hospitals NHS Foundation Trust, London, UK

Asma A. Eissa, MBBS, MRCOG, MD Department of Obstetrics and Gynaecology, The Royal Free Hospital, Royal Free London NHS Foundation Trust, London, UK

A. Lola Emanuel-Kole, MBBS, FRCA Department of Anaesthesia, The Royal Free Hospital NHS Foundation Trust, London, UK

Charlotte J. Frise, BM BCh, MA, MRCP Acute General Medicine, John Radcliffe Hospital, Oxford University Hospitals NHS Trust, Headington, Oxford, UK

Chris Gardiner, MSc, PhD Nuffield Department of Obstetrics and Gynaecology, Level 3, Women's Centre, John Radcliffe Hospital, University of Oxford, Oxford University Hospitals NHS Foundation Trust, Oxford, Oxfordshire, UK

Carolyn Gates, BPharm (Hons), MSc, MRPharmS Pharmacy Department, University College London Hospitals NHS Foundation Trust, London, UK

Claire N. Harrison, MB ChB, DM, FRCP, FRCPath Department of Haematology, Guy's Hospital, Guy's and St. Thomas' NHS Foundation Trust, London, UK

Anna S. Herrey, MB ChB, MD, PhD, MRCP Department of Cardiology, The Heart Hospital, University College London Hospitals NHS Foundation Trust, London, UK

Peter Hillmen, MB ChB, PhD, FRCP, FRCPath Department of Haematology, St James's University Hospital NHS Trust, Leeds, UK

Joanna Howard, MBBS, MRCP, FRCPath Department of Haematology, Guy's Hospital, Guy's and St Thomas' NHS Foundation Trust, London, UK

Rezan A. Kadir, MB ChB, MRCOG FRCS(Ed), MD Department of Obstetrics and Gynaecology, Royal Free Hospital, Royal Free London NHS Foundation Trust, London, UK

Asma Khalil, MB BCh, MD, MRCOG, MSc, DFSRH Department of Obstetrics and Gynaecology, St. George's Hospital, St George's Healthcare NHS Trust, Tooting, London, UK

Irfana Koita-Kazi, MB ChB, MRCOG The Centre for Reproductive and Genetic Health, Eastman Dental Hospital, London, UK

Michael Laffan, MB ChB, DM, FRCP, FRCPath Faculty of Medicine, Centre for Haematology, Hammersmith Hospital, Imperial College Healthcare NHS Trust, London, UK

Christine A. Lee, MB ChB, MA, MD, DSc, FRCP, FRCPath Department of Haemophilia, University of London, London, UK

Peter K. MacCallum, MB ChB, MD, FRCP, FRCPath Wolfson Institute of Preventive Medicine, Barts Health NHS Trust, Barts and The London School of Medicine and Dentistry, London, UK

Lucy H. Mackillop, BM BCh, MA, FRCP Nuffield Department of Obstetrics and Gynaecology, Women's Center, John Radcliffe Hospital, Oxford University Hospitals NHS Trust, Headington, Oxford, UK

Fiona Maguire, BPharm (Hons), ClinDipPharm, MRPharmS Pharmacy Department, University College London Hospitals NHS Foundation Trust, London, UK

Marzia Menegatti, PhD Angelo Bianchi Bonomi, Hemophilia and Thrombosis Center, Fondazione IRCCS Ca' Granda Ospedale Maggiore Policlinico, Milan, Italy

Department of Pathophysiology and Transplantation, Università degli Studi di Milano and Luigi Villa Foundation, Milan, Italy

Carolyn M. Millar, MB ChB, MD, FRCP, FRCPath Faculty of Medicine, Centre for Haematology, Hammersmith Hospital, Imperial College Healthcare NHS Trust, London, UK

Andrew D. Mumford, MB ChB, PhD, FRCPath School of Cellular and Molecular Medicine, University of Bristol, Bristol Royal Infirmary, Bristol, UK

Catherine Nelson-Piercy, MBBS, MA, FRCP, FRCOG Women's Health Academic Centre, Guy's & St Thomas' Foundation Trust and Imperial College Healthcare Trust, St Thomas' Hospital, London, UK

Patrick O'Brien, MBBCh, FRCOG, FICOG, FFSRH Institute of Women's Health, University College London Hospitals NHS Foundation Trust, London, UK

Pranav P. Pandya, BSc, MBBS, MD, FRCOG Fetal Medicine Unit, University College London Hospitals NHS Foundation Trust, London, UK

Donald Peebles, MA, MD, FRCOG Institute for Women's Health, University College London Hospitals NHS Foundation Trust, London, UK

Flora Peyvandi, MD, PhD Angelo Bianchi Bonomi, Hemophilia and Thrombosis Center, Fondazione IRCCS Ca' Granda Ospedale Maggiore Policlinico, Milan, Italy

Department of Pathophysiology and Transplantation, Università degli Studi di Milano and Luigi Villa Foundation, Milan, Italy

Sathana Ponnampalam, MB ChB Department of Obstetrics and Gynaecology, National Women's Hospital, Auckland, New Zealand

John Porter, MB ChB, MA, MD, FRCP, FRCPath Department of Haematology, University College London Hospitals NHS Foundation Trust, London, UK

Raj Rai, MB ChB, MD, MRCOG Department of Obstetrics and Gynaecology, Imperial College Healthcare NHS Trust, St Mary's Hospital, Mint Wing, Imperial College Hospitals NHS Trust, London, UK

Lesley Regan, MB ChB, MD, FRCOG Department of Obstetrics and Gynaecology, Imperial College Healthcare NHS Trust, St Mary's Hospital, Mint Wing, London, UK

Susan E. Robinson, MB ChB, MRCP, FRCPath, MDRes Department of Haematology, Guy's Hospital, Guy's and St. Thomas' NHS Foundation Trust, London, UK

Marie Scully, MB ChB, BSc (Hons), MD, MRCP, FRCPath Thrombotic Microangiopathy, Department of Haematology, University College London Hospitals NHS Foundation Trust, London, UK

Paul Serhal, MB ChB, MRCOG The Centre for Reproductive and Genetic Health, Eastman Dental Hospital, London, UK

Simona Maria Siboni, MD, PhD Angelo Bianchi Bonomi, Hemophilia and Thrombosis Center, Fondazione IRCCS Ca' Granda Ospedale Maggiore Policlinico, Milan, Italy

Simon Stanworth, BM BCh, BA, DPhil, MRCP NHS Blood and Transplant, John Radcliffe Hospital, Oxford University Hospitals NHS Foundation Trust, Oxford, UK

Stavroula Tsiara, MB ChB, MD, PhD, FRCP Department of Internal Medicine, University Hospital of Ioannina, Ioannina, Greece

Susan M. Tuck, MB ChB, MD, MRCGP, FRCOG The Royal Free Hospital, Royal Free London NHS Foundation Trust, London, UK

Manu Vatish, MB BChir, MA, DPhil, MRCOG Nuffield Department of Obstetrics and Gynaecology, Level 3, Women's Centre, John Radcliffe Hospital, University of Oxford, Oxford University Hospitals NHS Foundation Trust, Oxford, Oxfordshire, UK

Sukrutha Veerareddy, BSc, MBBS, MRCOG, PhD Women's Health Services, Queen Elizabeth Hospital, Lewisham and Greenwich NHS Trust, London, UK

Vidheya Venkatesh, MB ChB, MRCP, MPhil Neonatal Intensive Care Unit, Cambridge University Hospitals NHS Trust, Cambridge, UK

Fiona Walker, MB ChB, BM(Hons), FRCP, FESC Department of Cardiology, The Heart Hospital, University College London Hospitals NHS Foundation Trust, London, UK

Sasha Wilson, RGN Haematology/Blood Transfusion, University College London Hospitals NHS Foundation Trust, London, UK

1 Hemostatic Changes in Normal Pregnancy

Carolyn M. Millar and Michael Laffan

Abstract

Hemostasis represents a balance between pro- and anti-coagulant processes, with variations in this balance determining the net outcome. Significant physiological changes during pregnancy result in a hypercoagulable and hypofibrinolytic state that serves to protect the mother from bleeding complications at the time of placental separation. This chapter describes the effects of pregnancy on parameters of primary hemostasis, coagulation factors, anticoagulant pathways and the fibrinolytic system.

Keywords

Hemostasis • Physiological • Pregnancy • Hypercoagulability • Hypofibrinolysis

1.1 Introduction

Under normal conditions, blood flows within the vascular system, transporting oxygen, nutrients, and hormonal information around the body and removing metabolic waste. The confinement of circulating blood to the vascular bed and maintenance of blood fluidity are dependent upon a complex hemostatic system that involves interaction between the vasculature, platelets, coagulation factors, and the fibrinolytic system. Such interaction enables the stimulation of coagulation following injury, limits the extent of the response to the area of injury, and initiates the eventual breakdown of the clot as part of the process of healing. Thus, hemostasis may be viewed as a delicate balance between the pro- and anticoagulant processes, with variations in this balance determining the net outcome.

As well as a significant expansion in plasma volume, normal pregnancy is accompanied by major changes in the maternal hemostatic system, most likely mediated by hormonal influences, the net effect of which is to create a state of hypercoagulability and hypofibrinolysis. Together with the stemming of placental blood flow by myometrial contraction, these changes

C.M. Millar, MB ChB, MD, FRCP, FRCPath (✉)
M. Laffan, MB ChB, DM, FRCP, FRCPath
Centre for Haematology, Faculty of Medicine, Hammersmith Campus, Imperial College, London W12 0NN, UK
e-mail: c.millar@imperial.ac.uk; m.laffan@imperial.ac.uk

H. Cohen, P. O'Brien (eds.), *Disorders of Thrombosis and Hemostasis in Pregnancy: A Guide to Management*, DOI 10.1007/978-3-319-15120-5_1,

protect the mother from bleeding complications at the time of delivery. However, potentiation of the coagulation system also confers an increased risk of venous thromboembolism (VTE) and disseminated intravascular coagulation (DIC), leading causes of morbidity and mortality in pregnancy and the postpartum period.

In order to understand the physiological effects of pregnancy on the hemostatic system, an appreciation of hemostasis in the nonpregnant individual is required. Thus, while this chapter will focus on the hemostatic changes during pregnancy, each will be discussed in the context of normal hemostatic processes. It should be borne in mind that although these will be covered individually, they should not be considered to act in isolation. Furthermore, caution needs to be exercised when interpreting data obtained from studies in pregnancy. Data reported from these studies are often conflicting, and the study design and methods by which data are analyzed and reported require careful consideration. For example, it is generally preferable to obtain serial measurements from women throughout pregnancy rather than a set of cross-sectional data from different groups. This will allow the detection of subgroups and effects of starting (pre- or early pregnancy) values although it may be possible to derive reference ranges from cross-sectional studies providing the sample size is sufficiently large. Nonetheless, the reader should be aware that individual cases may deviate from the pooled data.

1.2 Primary Hemostasis

1.2.1 Platelets

Platelets are produced in the bone marrow by megakaryocytes and have a circulating life span of approximately 10 days. Following vascular injury, platelets adhere to the subendothelium, either directly to collagen via glycoprotein (GP) IaIIa and GPVI or indirectly via von Willebrand factor (VWF) and GPIb. Adhesion initiates platelet activation, with release of granular contents, notably ADP, and the synthesis of thromboxane A2. These factors have a positive feedback effect and activate more platelets, which are captured by VWF also released from platelet granules. Platelet activation is completed by a platelet shape change and a conformational change in the GPIIbIIIa receptor resulting in platelet aggregates held together by VWF and fibrinogen. These effects are normally counterbalanced by the active flow of blood and the endothelial production of prostacyclin, nitric oxide, and ADPase, which suppress platelet activation and prevent inappropriate platelet aggregation.

During pregnancy, there is a physiological decrease in the maternal platelet count of approximately 10 % [1–4]. While the resultant platelet count at term is usually maintained within the normal range, the prevalence of gestational thrombocytopenia, as defined by a platelet count of less than $150 \times 10^9\ L^{-1}$, has been shown to range between 5 and 12 % in population-based studies [4–6]. Subsequently, the platelet count has been shown to rise on days 2–5 postpartum [7]. The degree of thrombocytopenia is mild in most cases of gestational thrombocytopenia, with platelet counts of greater than $115 \times 10^9\ L^{-1}$ reported in more than 80 % of cases, but a level down to $80 \times 10^9\ L^{-1}$ is regarded as normal [4]. Factors such as hemodilution and accelerated platelet clearance that may contribute to the fall in platelet count have not been well defined. Earlier studies do not consistently show reduced platelet survival in pregnancy [8, 9], and means of directly assessing platelet lifespan are limited in pregnant women. It is possible that the increase in platelet volume reported in conjunction with falling platelet counts in the third trimester indicates a state of increased platelet destruction [10, 11]. Moreover, while enhanced platelet activation has been demonstrated in pregnancies complicated by hypertension or preeclampsia, it is less clear whether this occurs in normal pregnancy. Spontaneous platelet aggregation, increased platelet reactivity to arachidonic acid, and, more recently, increased platelet activation and adhesion have been variously demonstrated in normotensive pregnant women [12–14]. Increased numbers of circulating platelet aggregates and a rise in levels of β-thromboglobulin, platelet factor 4, and thromboxane B2 (the stable product of thromboxane A2) have also been reported, all suggestive of enhanced platelet reactivity [15–17]. Thus, there is some evidence of increased platelet activation in uncomplicated pregnancies, but it is not clear to what extent this contributes to the fall in platelet count. Some increased activation would be consistent with other evidence for coagulation activation that is exaggerated in preeclampsia. Platelet aggregation has been shown to return to normal by 6 weeks postpartum [12, 13].

1.2.2 Von Willebrand Factor

Von Willebrand factor is a multimeric glycoprotein synthesized by endothelial cells and megakaryocytes that mediates the adhesion of platelet to sites of injury and promotes platelet-platelet aggregation. In addition to its adhesive properties, VWF is a specific carrier for factor VIII (FVIII), and the VWF/FVIII complex usually circulates with a molar ratio of FVIII to VWF monomer of 1:50 (although this is defined as a ratio of 1 in units/dL). Levels of maternal VWF rise progressively with advancing gestational age, increasing early in the first trimester of pregnancy and continuing to increase thereafter [1, 18, 19]. By the time of delivery, levels of VWF may have reached double or more those of the nonpregnant state, falling rapidly following delivery and returning to baseline non-pregnant values within a few weeks [2, 18–21]. Factor VIII levels also increase progressively throughout pregnancy [2, 18, 19, 22], rising early in the first trimester and returning to near-normal values by around 8 weeks postpartum [22]. The increase in FVIII has been shown in some studies to parallel the rise in VWF levels, thus maintaining the VWF:Ag/FVIII ratio close to normal [18, 19, 23]. Other studies have demonstrated an increase in this ratio, in particular during the third trimester of pregnancy [2, 20, 21, 24, 25], reflecting a relatively greater rise in VWF levels with advancing gestation. This discrepancy may reflect variation in the degree of endothelial perturbation, as it is recognized that the rise in VWF levels is greater in conditions associated with endothelial cell damage such as preeclampsia [24, 25]. The functional activity of VWF is determined by its multimeric size, which is regulated by the protease ADAMTS13. Studies of ADAMTS13 during pregnancy have shown a mild progressive decrease in its activity from early in the second trimester until the first or second postpartum day [26, 27], and discrepancies between ADAMTS13 antigen and activity have been reported in pregnancy in older mothers [28]. A reduction in ADAMTS13 activity would be consistent with a reported disproportionate increase in large VWF multimers in the third trimester [24] and an increase in the specific functional activity of VWF, although this finding is not consistently reported [19, 21].

1.2.3 Hematocrit

Hematocrit also plays a role in primary hemostasis by influencing blood viscosity and platelet adhesion. However, as with the decreased platelet count, any decrease in platelet adhesion that may result from a reduction in hematocrit appears to be outweighed by the increase in VWF levels. This is discussed further when we consider global measures of primary hemostatic function.

1.3 Coagulation System

Blood coagulation pathways center on the generation of thrombin [29], which cleaves fibrinogen to generate fibrin, the structural scaffold that stabilizes platelet aggregates at sites of vascular injury [30].

1.3.1 Initiation of Coagulation

The extrinsic or tissue factor (TF)-dependent pathway of coagulation represents the major route by which thrombin generation is initiated in response to vessel damage. TF is an integral membrane protein and is the only procoagulant factor that does not require proteolytic activation. TF is primarily located at extravascular sites that are not usually exposed to the blood under normal physiological conditions [31]. As a result, the blood only encounters TF-presenting cells thus activating the extrinsic pathway, at sites of vascular injury. This dogma has been challenged by the identification of microparticle-associated TF and an alternatively transcribed, soluble TF molecule in blood, both of which have been implicated in the development of thrombosis [32, 33].

As well as being the principal initiator of coagulation, TF is essential for other cellular processes including implantation, embryogenesis, and angiogenesis [34]. The decidua and placenta are both rich sources of TF, with high levels of expression on syncytiotrophoblasts, while tissue factor pathway inhibitor (TFPI) is expressed in human umbilical vein endothelial cells [35]. Progesterone has been shown to upregulate TF gene expression by decidualized endometrial stromal cells, principally mediated by the promoter-specific transcription factor Sp1 [36]. This may be relevant in reducing postimplantation hemorrhage, although few studies have addressed the role of TF and TFPI in the pathogenesis of gestational complications [37].

1.3.2 Overview of Coagulation and Its Regulation

Following the exposure of TF-presenting cells to the blood, TF comes into contact with factor VII (FVII), a fraction (~1 %) of which circulates in its active form, FVIIa. TF binds both FVII and FVIIa with high affinity. The trace amount of TF-FVIIa that forms is enough to activate factor X (FX) both directly (extrinsic pathway) and indirectly via activation of factor IX (FIX) [38, 39]. However, FXa production by this route is rapidly terminated by the action of TFPI which binds FXa and VIIa forming an inactive TF-VIIa-Xa-TFPI complex. The limited quantities of FXa that are generated via this route facilitate the inefficient conversion of trace quantities of prothrombin to thrombin [40, 41]. The low concentrations of thrombin that arise mediate the feedback activation of the cofactors FVIII and factor V (FV). Binding of FIXa to FVIIIa forming the intrinsic tenase activates further FX thus bypassing the reliance upon TF-FVIIa as a source of FXa generation. The subsequent assembly of FXa and FVa on activated platelets (prothrombinase) leads to a rapid burst in thrombin generation at the site of vessel damage. Binding of the intrinsic tenase and prothrombinase complexes to the phospholipid surfaces expressed by platelets is mediated by calcium ions bound to the terminal gamma-carboxy residues on FXa and FIXa. Gamma-carboxylation of glutamic acid residues on FIX and FX as well as prothrombin and FVII requires vitamin K.

Fibrin is produced by proteolytic cleavage of fibrinogen by thrombin with the release of fibrinopeptides A and B and precipitation of insoluble fibrin monomer followed by polymerization and cross-linkage by factor XIII (FXIII). Thrombin has many functions that influence both coagulation and the vascular system; in addition to cleaving fibrinogen to produce fibrin and activating FVIII and FV as described above, other procoagulant functions of thrombin include the activation of platelets, factor XI (FXI), FXIII, and thrombin-activatable fibrinolysis inhibitor (TAFI).

1.3.3 Effect of Pregnancy on Coagulation Factors

As already discussed, normal pregnancy is accompanied by a rise in the plasma concentration of FVIII, which is likely to be secondary, at least in part, to increased VWF levels. Pregnancy also results in substantial progressive increases in the plasma concentrations of FVII [2, 42, 43] and fibrinogen [2, 3, 22, 42]. The increase in FVII levels appears to be greatest in the second trimester of pregnancy, with rises of around 50 % observed by the early third trimester [2, 42]. FVII levels fall sharply after delivery [2]. By term, levels of fibrinogen may reach double their prepregnancy values, and fall more slowly following delivery, returning to basal levels within 5 weeks post-partum [2, 3, 42]. A modest gradual increase in the plasma concentration of FX is apparent until around 30 weeks' gestation, following which there are reports of both a persistent elevation and a mild fall in levels through the remainder of pregnancy [2, 19, 20, 42]. Levels of prothrombin and FV remain unchanged throughout pregnancy [2, 19, 42, 44]. Data available regarding the effect of pregnancy on plasma concentrations of FIX and FXI are variable; several early studies reported a steady increase in FIX levels with advancing gestation [45–47], but no significant effect on FIX levels was shown in a subsequent cross-sectional study [19]. A longitudinal study has confirmed the earlier findings, demonstrating FIX levels at delivery to be above the non-pregnant upper reference value in approximately 50 % of women, with a further rise during the early puerperal period [42]. The finding of a prolonged activated partial thromboplastin time (APTT) at term not infrequently results in the incidental finding of reduced FXI levels, which subsequently normalize in the months following delivery. Indeed, a progressive decrease in FXI levels throughout pregnancy has been found in several studies, reaching a nadir at term [20, 48, 49]. There are also reports of unchanged FXI levels in pregnancy, although these studies report grouped data and may not detect individual trends [19, 42].

It has been shown that, following an initial early increase, FXIII levels have been shown to gradually fall throughout pregnancy, reaching levels around half nonpregnant values by term [50]. The significance of this is not clear because the minimum hemostatic level of FXIII is not established although some studies suggest that this might be low enough to increase the risk of bleeding.

There is considerable interindividual variation in the extent to which plasma levels of coagulation factors change with advancing gestational age. It is likely that some of the reduction is due to dilution caused by the progressive increase in plasma volume until around the 32nd week of gestation. However, as the plasma volume expands by approximately 50 %, increased synthesis is necessary to maintain clotting factor concentrations at equivalent nonpregnant values. This is most likely to be mediated by hormonal factors. Altered transcriptional activity in the presence of estrogenic factors has been demonstrated for some coagulation factors, with the identification of estrogen response elements in gene promoter regions [51]. Estrogen levels increase as pregnancy progresses; however, as with other placentally derived hormones, levels vary significantly between individuals [52].

1.4 Anticoagulant Pathways

The hemostatic response is confined to the site of injury by the action of inhibitory pathways preventing spontaneous activation of coagulation and generalized thrombosis. As already discussed, TFPI is the principal inhibitor of TF-mediated coagulation [53] and acts by binding and inhibiting FXa [54]. The resultant TFPI-FXa complex acts in a negative feedback loop through the binding and inactivation of TF-FVIIa [55] and in this way switches off the initiating procoagulant stimulus. This ensures that a small procoagulant stimulus does not elicit uncontrolled generation of thrombin. In addition to TFPI, the normal hemostatic response is regulated by anti-thrombin and the protein C–protein S pathway. Together, these pathways modulate the generation and activity of thrombin and are critical for appropriate and controlled hemostatic plug formation.

1.4.1 Antithrombin

The half-life of thrombin in plasma is around 14 s. This is mainly due to the inhibitory action of antithrombin (previously designated antithrombin III), a plasma-borne serine protease inhibitor synthesized in the liver. Although antithrombin inactivates several protease substrates of the coagulation system, its main physiological targets are thrombin and FXa, and it is through the inhibition of these serine proteases that antithrombin exerts its anticoagulant function. These interactions are enhanced by the action of heparan sulfate proteoglycans, as well as exogenously administered heparins, on the surface of endothelial cells. The activity of antithrombin is reduced in liver disease and hypercoagulable states including DIC. However, there is little variation in the plasma concentration of antithrombin both during healthy pregnancy and following delivery [2, 3, 19, 20, 42, 56]. In contrast, modest effects on the thrombin inhibitors α_2-macroglobulin and heparin cofactor II (HCII) are found; the plasma concentration of α_2-macroglobulin is reduced and HCII activity increased in normal pregnancy [2, 57, 58], while HCII activity is reduced in pregnancies complicated by hypertension and preeclampsia [59].

1.4.2 Protein C and Protein S

Thrombin generation is also downregulated by the anticoagulant activities of protein C and its cofactor protein S, both vitamin K-dependent glycoproteins that are synthesized mainly in the liver. Protein C is activated by thrombin bound to thrombomodulin (TM), an integral membrane protein expressed on the surface of endothelial cells. This activation process is enhanced by a second endothelial cell surface protein, the endothelial cell protein C receptor (EPCR). Both the TM and EPCR receptors are also expressed by placental trophoblasts. Aided by protein S, activated protein C (APC) catalyzes the inactivation of FVIIIa and FVa [60], thereby limiting further generation of thrombin. As the intact endothelium (i.e., adjacent to the site of vascular injury) normally expresses TM [61], thrombin diffusing away from the site of injury can bind to TM and its activity "switched" to impart an anticoagulant function [62]. Thus, the action of thrombin can be modulated depending on its location relative to the thrombus. In addition to its cofactor-mediated anticoagulant function, protein S has been shown to exhibit anticoagulant properties in the absence of APC, including cofactor activity for TFPI [63, 64].

Protein S circulates in plasma in two forms. Approximately 60 % is bound to complement 4b-binding protein (C4BP), a regulatory protein of the classical pathway of the complement system [65, 66], while the remaining 40 % is free. While it was previously thought that only protein S in its free form was active, APC cofactor activity for FVa and FVIIIa inactivation has now also been claimed for C4BP-bound protein S, albeit to a lesser degree than the activity of free protein S [67, 68]. Similarly, while TFPI cofactor activity has been suggested for bound protein S [63], recent data suggest that this is less potent than that of free protein S [69]. The implications of these recent findings for pregnancy-associated hemostasis remain to be clarified.

A decrease in the plasma concentration of protein S has been reported during both pregnancy and the puerperium, frequently to levels comparable to protein S-deficient heterozygotes. Two early cross-sectional studies showed plasma levels of both total and free protein S to be reduced in pregnancy, irrespective of whether the free protein S fraction was measured by an immunological or a functional method [70, 71]. The latter study showed more pronounced reductions in free protein S compared to total protein S that may be explained by the parallel increase in C4BP concentration; no change in C4BP was demonstrated in the former. Furthermore, concordant reductions in total and free protein S levels with no increase in C4BP have been found in women taking the combined oral contraceptive pill [71]. Together, these findings suggest that the reduction in protein S activity in pregnancy may not be wholly attributable to alterations in the free/bound protein S equilibrium. Similarly, progressive reductions throughout pregnancy in the plasma concentrations of both free and total protein S have subsequently been reported, with greater relative decreases in the free fraction [3, 19, 42]. The majority of studies report that the decrease in protein S levels begins early in the first trimester, with most reduction having occurred by the end of the second trimester [3, 19, 22, 42, 71]. A cross-sectional study demonstrated a significant decrease in the levels of free protein S from the 10th week of gestation, and total protein S levels from the 20th week, with no significant increase in C4BP at term compared to nonpregnant samples [72]. Total protein S has been shown to return to prepregnancy levels by the end of the first week postpartum [71], while levels of free protein S remain below the normal range in 15 % of women at 8 weeks postpartum [3, 22]; this should be considered when evaluating the results of thrombophilic tests.

It is possible that some of the discrepancies in findings are attributable to assay variability; however, the underlying mechanism for the decrease in protein S levels in pregnancy remains unclear. A dilution effect could account for some of the findings but would not explain the reduction in protein S levels associated with the combined oral contraceptive pill. Similarly, the reduction in free protein S levels may not be wholly attributable to increased C4BP levels, as has been the widely held view to date. Estrogen response elements have also been identified in the protein S gene promoter, which may alter the transcription activity of protein S, and this seems to offer the most likely explanation.

Unlike protein S, neither the concentration nor functional activity of protein C has been shown to be significantly affected by gestation [18, 19, 73]. Some minor variations in protein C activity have been demonstrated with a peak in levels in the second trimester; however, all values remained within the normal range [3, 18, 71]. Elevated protein C levels and activity have been reported in the early puerperal period with mean levels equivalent to nonpregnant upper reference values [19, 42, 74].

In addition to their anticoagulant activities, protein C and protein S appear to have other physiological effects including cellular protective, anti-inflammatory, and anti-apoptotic properties. Immunohistochemical analysis has recently demonstrated the deposition of protein S in damaged villi at the fetal-maternal interface, suggesting its involvement in the protection or restoration of damaged placental trophoblasts [72]. It is possible that protein S consumption at the fetal-maternal interface could contribute toward the observed reduction in its levels in pregnancy. Low levels of anti-protein S and anti-protein C antibodies have recently been shown in a cross-sectional study of healthy pregnant women, the significance of which is not known [75]. Plasma levels of anti-protein C antibodies were shown to decrease with advancing gestational age and were no longer detectable by the third trimester [75].

Measurable levels of soluble TM are found in plasma and are likely to derive from the proteolysis of endothelial cell TM. As well as being a potential marker of preeclampsia, TM levels have been shown to increase gradually during normal pregnancy and fall postpartum rapidly [76, 77].

1.5 Fibrinolytic System

The principal fibrinolytic enzyme is plasmin, which circulates in its inactive zymogen form, plasminogen. The activation of plasmin is mediated by two types of plasminogen activator: tissue type and urokinase type. Tissue plasminogen activator (tPA) is released into the blood by endothelium in its active form but does not activate plasminogen until they are brought together when they bind to fibrin. Plasmin is inhibited both directly by plasmin inhibitor (α_2-antiplasmin) and α_2-macroglobulin and indirectly by plasminogen activator inhibitor-1 (PAI-1) produced by endothelial cells and platelets. Plasmin activation is reduced by TAFI, which removes the terminal lysine residues from fibrin, to which tPA and plasminogen bind.

It has been a long-held view that maternal plasma fibrinolytic activity decreases in pregnancy, which has been attributed, at least in part, to the production of a plasminogen inhibitor by the placenta known as plasminogen activator inhibitor-2 (PAI-2) [2, 78, 79]. The decreased fibrinolytic activity reported by many of these studies is based on fibrin plate and clot lysis analyses of euglobuin fractions (which contain factors important in fibrinolysis: plasminogen, plasminogen activators (primarily tPA) and fibrinogen), although it is unclear how accurately these reflect the blood fibrinolytic capacity in pregnancy. In addition to PAI-2, the placenta and decidua are sources of PAI-1, levels of which have been shown to rise progressively throughout pregnancy, reaching at least fivefold basal values by term [1, 3, 22, 79]. The decidual expression of PAI-1 appears to be regulated by progesterone by similar mechanisms to those described for TF [80]. Circulating tPA antigen levels have been shown to remain constant or rise during pregnancy [76, 79, 81–83], and the increase in PAI-1 and PAI-2 leads to a decrease in the release of endothelial tPA [84] and its measurable activity [22, 79]. A rise in levels of urokinase-type plasminogen activator (uPA) antigen, which also appears to derive from the placenta, has also been demonstrated [83, 85]. Fibrinolytic activity may be further depressed in pregnancy by increased thrombin generation leading to an increase in TAFI activity [86–89]. A slight initial rise in α_2-macroglobulin levels followed by a steady fall throughout pregnancy and the postpartum period has been reported [2]. Levels of plasminogen and plasmin inhibitor appear to remain largely unchanged throughout pregnancy [83, 90]. A brisk fall in PAI-1 and rise in tPA activity immediately following delivery result in a rapid increase in fibrinolytic activity and a return to non-pregnant values within 3–5 days [2, 79, 83]. However, high levels of PAI-2 antigen persist for a further few days [83].

Despite the decrease in fibrinolytic activity, levels of fibrin degradation products including D-dimers have been shown to rise with advancing gestational age [3, 22, 42], but these reflect the enhanced coagulation activation in pregnancy. D-dimer concentrations rise above the level used for exclusion of VTE in over one quarter of women by the second trimester of pregnancy and in nearly all women by term [42], confounding their use in diagnosis. Levels peak at the first postpartum day and may take several weeks to return to normal [3, 22, 42]. Other measures that reflect increased in vivo thrombin generation or fibrin formation include the prothrombin fragment 1.2 (PF1.2), thrombin-antithrombin complexes (TAT), and soluble fibrin polymer, all of which have been shown to increase during pregnancy [1, 3, 22, 91, 92].

1.6 Measures of Coagulation

1.6.1 Measures of Primary Hemostasis

The bleeding time is shortened in pregnant women [46], although its use in the evaluation of primary hemostasis has been largely abandoned or superseded by the platelet function analyzer (PFA-100TM). The PFA-100 may be sensitive to quantitative and qualitative defects in platelets and VWF. The progressive shortening in PFA-100 closure times observed with advancing gestation mostly reflects the physiological rises in VWF levels.

1.6.2 Standard Coagulation Tests

The prothrombin time (PT), APTT and thrombin time (TT) may be normal or decreased in pregnancy with some variation in results according to the method and reagents used [3, 42, 46, 93]. While these findings may reflect some rises in procoagulant levels, standard coagulation tests are limited in their ability to reflect the overall coagulation potential of plasma.

1.6.3 Global Assays of Coagulation

The in vitro analysis of coagulation is facilitated by the use of global measures of hemostasis, which include thromboelastography (TEG) and rotational thromboelastometry (RoTEM). These assays take into consideration the activity of platelets and all plasma proteins relevant to coagulation and therefore may provide a useful overall measure of thrombotic and hemorrhagic risk. TEG and RoTEM monitor hemostasis as a whole dynamic process, determining the kinetics of clot formation and growth as well as the strength and stability of the formed clot. These tests can be performed at the patient's bedside and are widely used in obstetric practice to provide an early and reliable assessment of coagulation problems associated with postpartum hemorrhage. The hypercoagulable state of pregnancy affects a number of the parameters recorded in the TEG and RoTEM profiles, resulting in shortening of the time for clot formation to reach a defined amplitude (*k* time and clot formation time [CFT], respectively), an increase in the clot amplitude early in clot formation, and an increase in maximum amplitude (MA) of the TEG tracing and its RoTEM equivalent, the maximum clot firmness (MCF) [46, 93, 94]. These findings are all consistent with increased concentrations of coagulation initiators (FVIIa-TF) and procoagulant factors, resulting in increased generation of thrombin. The shortened CFT and increased MCF are apparent in the first trimester, with the greatest changes occurring during the second trimester and persisting into the third trimester [93]. Shortening of the time from the start of measurement until the start of clot formation has been demonstrated by TEG (*r* time) [94]; however, surprisingly the equivalent measurement by RoTEM (clotting time, CT) has been shown not to be affected by pregnancy [93]. No effects on fibrinolytic parameters have been reported [93].

1.6.4 APC Resistance

The procoagulant state in pregnancy is also demonstrated in vitro as a poor anticoagulant response of plasma to APC, known as APC resistance (APCR) [95]. APCR is usually demonstrated by a reduction in the ratio of APTT in the presence and absence of added APC, known as the classic APC-sensitivity ratio (APC-SR). APCR mostly results from a mutation at an APC cleavage site in FV, R506Q, widely known as factor V Leiden [96], although it may be acquired in the presence of antiphospholipid antibodies [97] or other factors affecting the APTT such as high levels of FVIII or FIX [98, 99]. APCR is found to be increased in as many as 60 % of pregnancies, as well in users of oral contraceptives and hormone replacement therapy [22, 99–101]. While it is likely that increased FVIII and FIX levels contribute to the acquired APCR in pregnancy [19], correlation between these variables has not been consistently reported [19, 22, 102, 103].

The physiological significance of acquired APCR in pregnancy is not clear; APCR has been shown to be associated with an increased risk of preeclampsia; however, it is not routinely assessed in pregnant women [104].

1.7 Hemostasis in the Uteroplacental Circulation

The placenta is a highly vascularized organ functioning as the interface between fetal blood, which is confined to the villous blood vessels, and maternal blood, which flows in decidual arteries and washes the intervillous spaces in contact with syncytiotrophoblasts. Placental separation at birth presents a significant hemostatic challenge, and the interruption of blood flow to the placental site achieved by the combined effects of myometrial contraction and thrombotic occlusion of the sheared maternal vessels is balanced against maintaining the fluidity of maternal blood at the fetal-maternal interface. A detailed description of the physiological adaptation of the uteroplacental vasculature facilitating increased blood flow is beyond the scope of this book, and our understanding of hemostasis in the uteroplacental circulation is hampered by extremely limited available data. A transitory shortening of whole blood clotting time and pronounced increase in FVIII activity during placental separation have previously been demonstrated in blood samples obtained from the uterine vein [105]. Uterine venous samples have also demonstrated higher levels of fibrinolytic activity when compared to peripheral blood both during and immediately following placental separation [105]. Levels of TAT complexes, soluble fibrin polymer, D-dimers, and plasmin-α_2-antiplasmin complexes have all been shown to be higher in the uterine than peripheral maternal circulations [106].

1.8 Microparticles

Microparticles (MP) are formed by cytoskeleton structural rearrangements and are shed from cell membranes upon activation or apoptosis. MPs may be produced by all cell types; however, those derived from platelets, monocytes, and endothelial cells have been implicated in a number of prothrombotic disorders. MPs influence hemostasis by a variety of mechanisms, including increased TF and platelet activation, provision of a catalytic surface for assembly of intrinsic tenase and prothrombinase complexes, and endothelial activation resulting in increased VWF expression. Normal pregnancy is characterized by increased levels of platelet- and endothelial-derived MPs [107]; however, their relevance in gestational complications remains unclear. MPs are also produced during syncytiotrophoblast differentiation (often called STBMs) and are detectable in normal pregnancies by the second trimester, their numbers significantly increasing in the third trimester. STBMs interact with immune and endothelial cells and may contribute to the systemic maternal inflammatory reaction associated with pregnancy. This reaction is exaggerated in preeclampsia, in which higher levels of circulating STBMs have been demonstrated [108].

1.9 Summary

Hemorrhage remains a leading cause of maternal morbidity and mortality worldwide. The hypercoagulable state of pregnancy confers some degree of protection from hemorrhage during implantation and placental separation at delivery. However, this in turn predisposes women to VTE, which is once again the leading cause of direct maternal death in the UK [109]. Furthermore, the hypercoagulable state may contribute toward many complications of pregnancy including placental abruption and preeclampsia. The change in the balance of hemostasis during pregnancy results from some major physiological changes which have been described here. It is important that these are not confused with similar changes outside pregnancy when their significance is quite different.

Key Learning Points

- Pregnancy is associated with a significant overall increase in the activity and potential of the hemostatic system.
- Pregnancy results in substantial rises in plasma levels of fibrinogen, VWF, FVII, and FVIII and modest rises in FIX and FX.
- Protein S and platelet levels fall during normal pregnancy.
- Levels of prothrombin, FV, antithrombin, and protein C do not vary significantly in pregnancy.
- The increase in coagulation activity may manifest in some standard laboratory tests such as D-dimer and APTT.
- Many of the coagulation changes take 6–8 weeks to return to normal after delivery.

References

1. Cadroy Y, Grandjean H, Pichon J, et al. Evaluation of six markers of haemostatic system in normal pregnancy and pregnancy complicated by hypertension or pre-eclampsia. Br J Obstet Gynaecol. 1993; 100:416–20.
2. Stirling Y, Woolf L, North WR, Seghatchian MJ, Meade TW. Haemostasis in normal pregnancy. Thromb Haemost. 1984;52:176–82.
3. Bremme K, Ostlund E, Almqvist I, Heinonen K, Blomback M. Enhanced thrombin generation and fibrinolytic activity in normal pregnancy and the puerperium. Obstet Gynecol. 1992;80:132–7.
4. Boehlen F, Hohlfeld P, Extermann P, Perneger TV, de Moerloose P. Platelet count at term pregnancy: a reappraisal of the threshold. Obstet Gynecol. 2000; 95:29–33.
5. Burrows RF, Kelton JG. Fetal thrombocytopenia and its relation to maternal thrombocytopenia. N Engl J Med. 1993;329:1463–6.
6. Sainio S, Kekomaki R, Riikonen S, Teramo K. Maternal thrombocytopenia at term: a population-based study. Acta Obstet Gynecol Scand. 2000;79: 744–9.
7. Dahlstrom BL, Nesheim BI. Post partum platelet count in maternal blood. Acta Obstet Gynecol Scand. 1994;73:695–7.
8. Wallenburg HC, van Kessel PH. Platelet lifespan in normal pregnancy as determined by a nonradioisotopic technique. Br J Obstet Gynaecol. 1978;85:33–6.
9. Rakoczi I, Tallian F, Bagdany S, Gati I. Platelet lifespan in normal pregnancy and pre-eclampsia as determined by a non-radioisotope technique. Thromb Res. 1979;15:553–6.
10. Fay RA, Hughes AO, Farron NT. Platelets in pregnancy: hyperdestruction in pregnancy. Obstet Gynecol. 1983;61:238–40.
11. Sill PR, Lind T, Walker W. Platelet values during normal pregnancy. Br J Obstet Gynaecol. 1985;92:480–3.
12. Burgess-Wilson ME, Morrison R, Heptinstall S. Spontaneous platelet aggregation in heparinised blood during pregnancy. Thromb Res. 1986;41:385–93.
13. Morrison R, Crawford J, MacPherson M, Heptinstall S. Platelet behaviour in normal pregnancy, pregnancy complicated by essential hypertension and pregnancy-induced hypertension. Thromb Haemost. 1985;54:607–11.
14. Karalis I, Nadar SK, Al Yemeni E, Blann AD, Lip GY. Platelet activation in pregnancy-induced hypertension. Thromb Res. 2005;116:377–83.
15. O'Brien WF, Saba HI, Knuppel RA, Scerbo JC, Cohen GR. Alterations in platelet concentration and aggregation in normal pregnancy and preeclampsia. Am J Obstet Gynecol. 1986;155:486–90.
16. Fitzgerald DJ, Mayo G, Catella F, Entman SS, FitzGerald GA. Increased thromboxane biosynthesis in normal pregnancy is mainly derived from platelets. Am J Obstet Gynecol. 1987;157:325–30.

17. Douglas JT, Lowe GD, Forbes CD, Prentice CR. Beta-thromboglobulin and platelet counts – effect of malignancy, infection, age and obesity. Thromb Res. 1982;25:459–64.
18. Mahieu B, Jacobs N, Mahieu S, et al. Haemostatic changes and acquired activated protein C resistance in normal pregnancy. Blood Coagul Fibrinolysis. 2007;18:685–8.
19. Clark P, Brennand J, Conkie JA, McCall F, Greer IA, Walker ID. Activated protein C sensitivity, protein C, protein S and coagulation in normal pregnancy. Thromb Haemost. 1998;79:1166–70.
20. Hellgren M, Blomback M. Studies on blood coagulation and fibrinolysis in pregnancy, during delivery and in the puerperium. I. Normal condition. Gynecol Obstet Invest. 1981;12:141–54.
21. Sanchez-Luceros A, Meschengieser SS, Marchese C, et al. Factor VIII and von Willebrand factor changes during normal pregnancy and puerperium. Blood Coagul Fibrinolysis. 2003;14:647–51.
22. Kjellberg U, Andersson NE, Rosen S, Tengborn L, Hellgren M. APC resistance and other haemostatic variables during pregnancy and puerperium. Thromb Haemost. 1999;81:527–31.
23. Sie P, Caron C, Azam J, et al. Reassessment of von Willebrand factor (VWF), VWF propeptide, factor VIII:C and plasminogen activator inhibitors 1 and 2 during normal pregnancy. Br J Haematol. 2003;121:897–903.
24. Brenner B, Zwang E, Bronshtein M, Seligsohn U. von Willebrand factor multimer patterns in pregnancy-induced hypertension. Thromb Haemost. 1989;62:715–7.
25. Bergmann F, Rotmensch S, Rosenzweig B, How H, Chediak J. The role of von Willebrand factor in preeclampsia. Thromb Haemost. 1991;66:525–8.
26. Sanchez-Luceros A, Farias CE, Amaral MM, et al. von Willebrand factor-cleaving protease (ADAMTS13) activity in normal non-pregnant women, pregnant and post-delivery women. Thromb Haemost. 2004;92:1320–6.
27. Mannucci PM, Canciani MT, Forza I, Lussana F, Lattuada A, Rossi E. Changes in health and disease of the metalloprotease that cleaves von Willebrand factor. Blood. 2001;98:2730–5.
28. Feys HB, Deckmyn H, Vanhoorelbeke K. ADAMTS13 in health and disease. Acta Haematol. 2009;121:183–5.
29. Mann KG. Thrombin formation. Chest. 2003;124:4S–10.
30. Savage B, Cattaneo M, Ruggeri ZM. Mechanisms of platelet aggregation. Curr Opin Hematol. 2001;8:270–6.
31. Wilcox JN, Smith KM, Schwartz SM, Gordon D. Localization of tissue factor in the normal vessel wall and in the atherosclerotic plaque. Proc Natl Acad Sci U S A. 1989;86:2839–43.
32. Bogdanov VY, Balasubramanian V, Hathcock J, Vele O, Lieb M, Nemerson Y. Alternatively spliced human tissue factor: a circulating, soluble, thrombogenic protein. Nat Med. 2003;9:458–62.
33. Falati S, Liu Q, Gross P, et al. Accumulation of tissue factor into developing thrombi in vivo is dependent upon microparticle P-selectin glycoprotein ligand 1 and platelet P-selectin. J Exp Med. 2003;197:1585–98.
34. Mackman N. Role of tissue factor in hemostasis, thrombosis, and vascular development. Arterioscler Thromb Vasc Biol. 2004;24:1015–22.
35. Aharon A, Brenner B, Katz T, Miyagi Y, Lanir N. Tissue factor and tissue factor pathway inhibitor levels in trophoblast cells: implications for placental hemostasis. Thromb Haemost. 2004;92:776–86.
36. Krikun G, Schatz F, Mackman N, Guller S, Demopoulos R, Lockwood CJ. Regulation of tissue factor gene expression in human endometrium by transcription factors Sp1 and Sp3. Mol Endocrinol. 2000;14:393–400.
37. Dusse LM, Carvalho MG, Cooper AJ, Lwaleed BA. Tissue factor and tissue factor pathway inhibitor: a potential role in pregnancy and obstetric vascular complications? Clin Chim Acta. 2006;372:43–6.
38. Morrison SA, Jesty J. Tissue factor-dependent activation of tritium-labeled factor IX and factor X in human plasma. Blood. 1984;63:1338–47.
39. Osterud B, Rapaport SI. Activation of factor IX by the reaction product of tissue factor and factor VII: additional pathway for initiating blood coagulation. Proc Natl Acad Sci U S A. 1977;74:5260–4.
40. Esmon CT, Owen WG, Jackson CM. The conversion of prothrombin to thrombin. V. The activation of prothrombin by factor Xa in the presence of phospholipid. J Biol Chem. 1974;249:7798–807.
41. Dahlback B, Stenflo J. The activation of prothrombin by platelet-bound factor Xa. Eur J Biochem. 1980;104:549–57.
42. Szecsi PB, Jorgensen M, Klajnbard A, Andersen MR, Colov NP, Stender S. Haemostatic reference intervals in pregnancy. Thromb Haemost. 2010;103:718–27.
43. Dalaker K, Prydz H. The coagulation factor VII in pregnancy. Br J Haematol. 1984;56:233–41.
44. Nilsson IM, Kullander S. Coagulation and fibrinolytic studies during pregnancy. Acta Obstet Gynecol Scand. 1967;46:273–85.
45. Todd ME, Thompson Jr JH, Bowie EJ, Owen Jr CA. Changes in blood coagulation during pregnancy. Mayo Clin Proc. 1965;40:370–83.
46. Beller FK, Ebert C. The coagulation and fibrinolytic enzyme system in pregnancy and in the puerperium. Eur J Obstet Gynecol Reprod Biol. 1982;13:177–97.
47. Fresh JW, Ferguson JH, Lewis JH. Blood-clotting studies in parturient women and the newborn. Obstet Gynecol. 1956;7:117–27.
48. Phillips LL, Rosano L, Skrodelis V. Changes in factor XI (plasma thromboplastin antecedent) levels during pregnancy. Am J Obstet Gynecol. 1973;116:1114–6.
49. Nossel HL, Lanzkowsky P, Levy S, Mibashan RS, Hansen JD. A study of coagulation factor levels in women during labour and in their newborn infants. Thromb Diath Haemorrh. 1966;16:185–97.

50. Persson BL, Stenberg P, Holmberg L, Astedt B. Transamidating enzymes in maternal plasma and placenta in human pregnancies complicated by intrauterine growth retardation. J Dev Physiol. 1980;2:37–46.
51. Di Bitondo R, Hall AJ, Peake IR, Iacoviello L, Winship PR. Oestrogenic repression of human coagulation factor VII expression mediated through an oestrogen response element sequence motif in the promoter region. Hum Mol Genet. 2002;11:723–31.
52. Smith R, Smith JI, Shen X, et al. Patterns of plasma corticotropin-releasing hormone, progesterone, estradiol, and estriol change and the onset of human labor. J Clin Endocrinol Metab. 2009;94:2066–74.
53. Bajaj MS, Birktoft JJ, Steer SA, Bajaj SP. Structure and biology of tissue factor pathway inhibitor. Thromb Haemost. 2001;86:959–72.
54. Huang ZF, Wun TC, Broze Jr GJ. Kinetics of factor Xa inhibition by tissue factor pathway inhibitor. J Biol Chem. 1993;268:26950–5.
55. Broze Jr GJ, Warren LA, Novotny WF, Higuchi DA, Girard JJ, Miletich JP. The lipoprotein-associated coagulation inhibitor that inhibits the factor VII-tissue factor complex also inhibits factor Xa: insight into its possible mechanism of action. Blood. 1988;71:335–43.
56. Weiner CP, Brandt J. Plasma antithrombin III activity in normal pregnancy. Obstet Gynecol. 1980;56:601–3.
57. Massouh M, Jatoi A, Gordon EM, Ratnoff OD. Heparin cofactor II activity in plasma during pregnancy and oral contraceptive use. J Lab Clin Med. 1989;114:697–9.
58. Uchikova EH, Ledjev II. Changes in haemostasis during normal pregnancy. Eur J Obstet Gynecol Reprod Biol. 2005;119:185–8.
59. Bellart J, Gilabert R, Cabero L, Fontcuberta J, Monasterio J, Miralles RM. Heparin cofactor II: a new marker for pre-eclampsia. Blood Coagul Fibrinolysis. 1998;9:205–8.
60. Esmon CT. The protein C pathway. Chest. 2003;124: 26S–32.
61. Maruyama I, Bell CE, Majerus PW. Thrombomodulin is found on endothelium of arteries, veins, capillaries, and lymphatics, and on syncytiotrophoblast of human placenta. J Cell Biol. 1985;101:363–71.
62. Esmon CT, Esmon NL, Harris KW. Complex formation between thrombin and thrombomodulin inhibits both thrombin-catalyzed fibrin formation and factor V activation. J Biol Chem. 1982;257:7944–7.
63. Hackeng TM, Sere KM, Tans G, Rosing J. Protein S stimulates inhibition of the tissue factor pathway by tissue factor pathway inhibitor. Proc Natl Acad Sci U S A. 2006;103:3106–11.
64. Hackeng TM, van't Veer C, Meijers JC, Bouma BN. Human protein S inhibits prothrombinase complex activity on endothelial cells and platelets via direct interactions with factors Va and Xa. J Biol Chem. 1994;269:21051–8.
65. van de Poel RH, Meijers JC, Bouma BN. The interaction between anticoagulant protein S and complement regulatory C4b-binding protein (C4BP). Trends Cardiovasc Med. 2000;10:71–6.
66. Dahlback B. Inhibition of protein Ca cofactor function of human and bovine protein S by C4b-binding protein. J Biol Chem. 1986;261:12022–7.
67. Maurissen LF, Thomassen MC, Nicolaes GA, et al. Re-evaluation of the role of the protein S-C4b binding protein complex in activated protein C-catalyzed factor Va-inactivation. Blood. 2008;111:3034–41.
68. van de Poel RH, Meijers JC, Bouma BN. C4b-binding protein inhibits the factor V-dependent but not the factor V-independent cofactor activity of protein S in the activated protein C-mediated inactivation of factor VIIIa. Thromb Haemost. 2001;85:761–5.
69. Maurissen LFA, Castoldi E, Simioni P, Rosing J, Hackeng TM. Thrombin generation-based assays to measure the activity of the TFPI-protein S pathway in plasma from normal and protein S-deficient individuals. J Thromb Haemost. 2010;8:750–8.
70. Comp PC, Thurnau GR, Welsh J, Esmon CT. Functional and immunologic protein S levels are decreased during pregnancy. Blood. 1986;68:881–5.
71. Malm J, Laurell M, Dahlback B. Changes in the plasma levels of vitamin K-dependent proteins C and S and of C4b-binding protein during pregnancy and oral contraception. Br J Haematol. 1988;68: 437–43.
72. Matsumoto M, Tachibana D, Nobeyama H, et al. Protein S deposition at placenta: a possible role of protein S other than anticoagulation. Blood Coagul Fibrinolysis. 2008;19:653–6.
73. Faught W, Garner P, Jones G, Ivey B. Changes in protein C and protein S levels in normal pregnancy. Am J Obstet Gynecol. 1995;172:147–50.
74. Mannucci PM, Vigano S, Bottasso B, et al. Protein C antigen during pregnancy, delivery and puerperium. Thromb Haemost. 1984;52:217.
75. Torricelli M, Sabatini L, Florio P, et al. Levels of antibodies against protein C and protein S in pregnancy and in preeclampsia. J Matern Fetal Neonatal Med. 2009;22:993–9.
76. de Moerloose P, Mermillod N, Amiral J, Reber G. Thrombomodulin levels during normal pregnancy, at delivery and in the postpartum: comparison with tissue-type plasminogen activator and plasminogen activator inhibitor-1. Thromb Haemost. 1998;79:554–6.
77. Boffa MC, Valsecchi L, Fausto A, et al. Predictive value of plasma thrombomodulin in preeclampsia and gestational hypertension. Thromb Haemost. 1998;79:1092–5.
78. Astedt B, Hagerstrand I, Lecander I. Cellular localisation in placenta of placental type plasminogen activator inhibitor. Thromb Haemost. 1986;56:63–5.
79. Wright JG, Cooper P, Astedt B, et al. Fibrinolysis during normal human pregnancy: complex interrelationships between plasma levels of tissue plasminogen activator and inhibitors and the euglobulin clot lysis time. Br J Haematol. 1988;69:253–8.
80. Lockwood CJ. Regulation of plasminogen activator inhibitor 1 expression by interaction of epidermal growth factor with progestin during decidualization of human endometrial stromal cells. Am J Obstet Gynecol. 2001;184:798–804; discussion –5.
81. Halligan A, Bonnar J, Sheppard B, Darling M, Walshe J. Haemostatic, fibrinolytic and endothelial variables in normal pregnancies and pre-eclampsia. Br J Obstet Gynaecol. 1994;101:488–92.

82. Cerneca F, Ricci G, Simeone R, Malisano M, Alberico S, Guaschino S. Coagulation and fibrinolysis changes in normal pregnancy. Increased levels of procoagulants and reduced levels of inhibitors during pregnancy induce a hypercoagulable state, combined with a reactive fibrinolysis. Eur J Obstet Gynecol Reprod Biol. 1997;73:31–6.
83. Kruithof EK, Tran-Thang C, Gudinchet A, et al. Fibrinolysis in pregnancy: a study of plasminogen activator inhibitors. Blood. 1987;69:460–6.
84. Robb AO, Mills NL, Din JN, et al. Acute endothelial tissue plasminogen activator release in pregnancy. J Thromb Haemost. 2009;7:138–42.
85. Shimada H, Takashima E, Soma M, et al. Source of increased plasminogen activators during pregnancy and puerperium. Thromb Res. 1989;54:91–8.
86. Mousa HA, Downey C, Alfirevic Z, Toh CH. Thrombin activatable fibrinolysis inhibitor and its fibrinolytic effect in normal pregnancy. Thromb Haemost. 2004;92:1025–31.
87. Ku DH, Arkel YS, Paidas MP, Lockwood CJ. Circulating levels of inflammatory cytokines (IL-1 beta and TNF-alpha), resistance to activated protein C, thrombin and fibrin generation in uncomplicated pregnancies. Thromb Haemost. 2003;90:1074–9.
88. Chabloz P, Reber G, Boehlen F, Hohlfeld P, de Moerloose P. TAFI antigen and D-dimer levels during normal pregnancy and at delivery. Br J Haematol. 2001;115:150–2.
89. Watanabe T, Minakami H, Sakata Y, Matsubara S, Sato I, Suzuki M. Changes in activity of plasma thrombin activatable fibrinolysis inhibitor in pregnancy. Gynecol Obstet Invest. 2004;58:19–21.
90. Chen J, Fu X, Wang Y, et al. Oxidative modification of von Willebrand factor by neutrophil oxidants inhibits its cleavage by ADAMTS13. Blood. 2010; 115:706–12.
91. Rosen T, Kuczynski E, O'Neill LM, Funai EF, Lockwood CJ. Plasma levels of thrombin-antithrombin complexes predict preterm premature rupture of the fetal membranes. J Matern Fetal Med. 2001;10:297–300.
92. Comeglio P, Fedi S, Liotta AA, et al. Blood clotting activation during normal pregnancy. Thromb Res. 1996;84:199–202.
93. Huissoud C, Carrabin N, Benchaib M, et al. Coagulation assessment by rotation thromboelastometry in normal pregnancy. Thromb Haemost. 2009;101:755–61.
94. Steer PL, Krantz HB. Thromboelastography and Sonoclot analysis in the healthy parturient. J Clin Anesth. 1993;5:419–24.
95. Dahlback B, Carlsson M, Svensson PJ. Familial thrombophilia due to a previously unrecognized mechanism characterized by poor anticoagulant response to activated protein C: prediction of a cofactor to activated protein C. Proc Natl Acad Sci U S A. 1993;90:1004–8.
96. Bertina RM, Koeleman BP, Koster T, et al. Mutation in blood coagulation factor V associated with resistance to activated protein C. Nature. 1994;369:64–7.
97. Bokarewa MI, Bremme K, Falk G, Sten-Linder M, Egberg N, Blomback M. Studies on phospholipid antibodies, APC-resistance and associated mutation in the coagulation factor V gene. Thromb Res. 1995;78:193–200.
98. Laffan MA, Manning R. The influence of factor VIII on measurement of activated protein C resistance. Blood Coagul Fibrinolysis. 1996;7:761–5.
99. Lowe GD, Rumley A, Woodward M, Reid E, Rumley J. Activated protein C resistance and the FV:R506Q mutation in a random population sample–associations with cardiovascular risk factors and coagulation variables. Thromb Haemost. 1999;81:918–24.
100. Kemmeren JM, Algra A, Meijers JC, et al. Effect of second- and third-generation oral contraceptives on the protein C system in the absence or presence of the factor VLeiden mutation: a randomized trial. Blood. 2004;103:927–33.
101. Mathonnet F, de Mazancourt P, Bastenaire B, et al. Activated protein C sensitivity ratio in pregnant women at delivery. Br J Haematol. 1996;92:244–6.
102. Cumming AM, Tait RC, Fildes S, Yoong A, Keeney S, Hay CR. Development of resistance to activated protein C during pregnancy. Br J Haematol. 1995;90:725–7.
103. Bokarewa MI, Wramsby M, Bremme K, Blomback M. Variability of the response to activated protein C during normal pregnancy. Blood Coagul Fibrinolysis. 1997;8:239–44.
104. Clark P, Sattar N, Walker ID, Greer IA. The Glasgow outcome, APCR and lipid (GOAL) pregnancy study: significance of pregnancy associated activated protein C resistance. Thromb Haemost. 2001;85:30–5.
105. Bonnar J, Prentice CR, McNicol GP, Douglas AS. Haemostatic mechanism in the uterine circulation during placental separation. Br Med J. 1970;2:564–7.
106. Higgins JR, Walshe JJ, Darling MR, Norris L, Bonnar J. Hemostasis in the uteroplacental and peripheral circulations in normotensive and pre-eclamptic pregnancies. Am J Obstet Gynecol. 1998;179:520–6.
107. Bretelle F, Sabatier F, Desprez D, et al. Circulating microparticles: a marker of procoagulant state in normal pregnancy and pregnancy complicated by preeclampsia or intrauterine growth restriction. Thromb Haemost. 2003;89:486–92.
108. Germain SJ, Sacks GP, Sooranna SR, Sargent IL, Redman CW. Systemic inflammatory priming in normal pregnancy and preeclampsia: the role of circulating syncytiotrophoblast microparticles. J Immunol. 2007;178:5949–56.
109. Knight M, Kenyon S, Brocklehurst P, Neilson J, Shakespeare J, Kurinczuk JJ (Eds.) on behalf of MBRRACE-UK. Saving Lives, Improving Mothers' Care - Lessons learned to inform future maternity care from the UK and Ireland Confidential Enquiries into Maternal Deaths and Morbidity 2009–12. Oxford: National Perinatal Epidemiology Unit, University of Oxford 2014.

2 Anticoagulants and Antiplatelet Agents in Pregnancy

Anja B. Drebes, Carolyn Gates, and Fiona Maguire

Abstract

Management of anticoagulant or antiplatelet therapy in pregnant women is challenging because of a paucity of data on its efficacy and safety during pregnancy. Current recommendations are based largely on extrapolation of data from non-pregnant patients, and case reports and case series of pregnant women. The treating physician has to consider the potential complications for both mother and fetus, and the possible impact of the frequently altered pharmacokinetics and pharmacodynamics of anticoagulants during pregnancy. Decision making should also be informed by the values and preferences of the pregnant woman. Here we collate and discuss current information and consensus guidance on the safety and efficacy of anticoagulants and several antiplatelet agents during pregnancy and lactation, providing a tool to aid management.

Keywords

Pregnancy • Anticoagulation • Antiplatelet therapy • Low-molecular-weight heparin • Aspirin • Pharmacokinetics • Safety • Efficacy • Dosing • Monitoring • Obstetric thromboprophylaxis • Warfarin embryopathy

A.B. Drebes, MB ChB, MRCP, FRCPath (✉)
Katharine Dormandy Haemophilia Centre and Thrombosis Unit, Royal Free London NHS Foundation Trust, Pond Street, London NW3 2QG, UK
e-mail: a.drebes@nhs.net

C. Gates, MB ChB, BPharm (Hons), MSc, MRPharmS
F. Maguire, BPharm (Hons), ClinDipPharm, MRPharmS
Pharmacy Department, University College London Hospitals NHS Foundation Trust, London NW1 2PG, UK
e-mail: carolyn.gates@uclh.nhs.uk; fiona.maguire@uclh.nhs.uk

2.1 Introduction

In pregnancy, anticoagulants are used primarily for the prevention and treatment of systemic venous and arterial thromboembolism. Other areas of use include the prevention of recurrent pregnancy loss in patients with antiphospholipid syndrome and, more controversially, the prevention of recurrent pregnancy loss and late placenta-mediated obstetric complications of other aetiology. There is a general paucity of data regarding the efficacy of anticoagulants during

H. Cohen, P. O'Brien (eds.), *Disorders of Thrombosis and Hemostasis in Pregnancy: A Guide to Management*, DOI 10.1007/978-3-319-15120-5_2, © Springer-Verlag London 2015

pregnancy and recommendations are based largely on extrapolation of data from non-pregnant patients and case reports and case series of pregnant women. There are many challenges associated with the use of anticoagulant therapy in pregnancy. The potential complications for both mother and fetus have to be considered, as does the possible impact of the frequently altered pharmacokinetics and pharmacodynamics of anticoagulants during pregnancy. This chapter discusses the main anticoagulants and antiplatelet agents currently available, and the special considerations required for their safe use in pregnancy and during breastfeeding.

2.2 Hemostatic Mechanism

The normal hemostatic mechanism is described in detail in Chap. 1. The coagulation system is a finely balanced network of interacting procoagulant and anticoagulant factors (Fig. 2.1). The first step in its

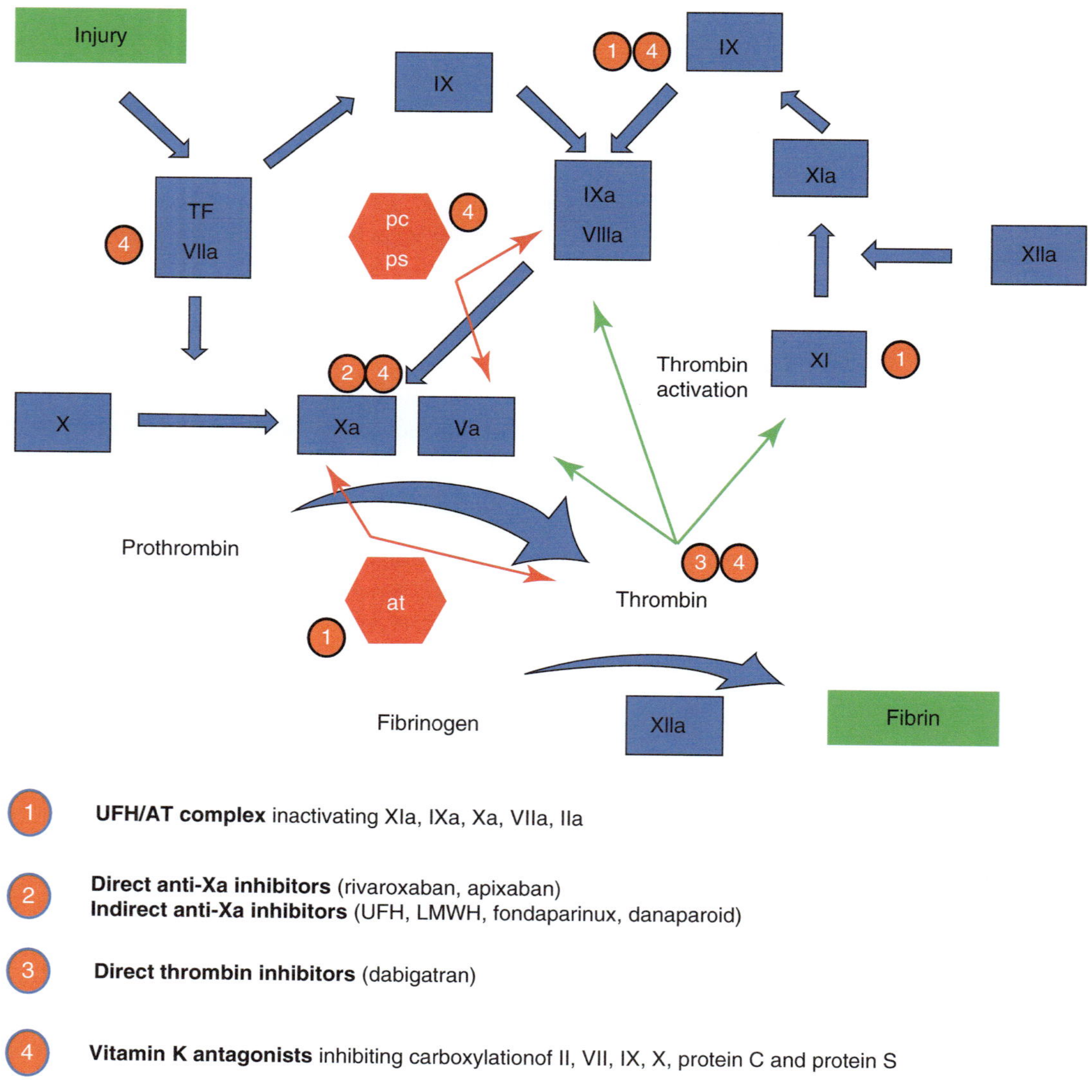

Fig. 2.1 Coagulation mechanism and targets for action of different anticoagulants. *UFH* unfractionated heparin, *AT* antithrombin, *LMWH* low-molecular-weight heparin

activation is usually the exposure of tissue factor at a site of vascular injury, which leads to the binding and activation of factor VII. The tissue factor/VIIa complex then activates factor X but also factor IX, which leads to amplification of the coagulation response. In the presence of factor Va and calcium, activated factor X cleaves prothrombin, and the resulting thrombin converts fibrinogen to fibrin. The fibrin clot is stabilised by cross-linking, catalysed by factor XIII.

The amount of activated factor X is further enhanced by the simultaneous formation of factor IXa which, in the presence of factor VIIIa and calcium, also leads to activation of factor X. The tissue factor/VIIa complex is inhibited by circulating tissue factor pathway inhibitor (TFPI), but fibrin generation continues due to the back-activation of factor IX, V and VIII by thrombin.

Antithrombin regulates coagulation by irreversibly binding to the active serine site of thrombin (factor IIa) and other activated clotting factors including Xa, IXa, XIa and XIIa. In the absence of heparin, the rate of inactivation is slow. Heparin-like glycosaminoglycans such as heparan sulphate are expressed on the surface of endothelial cells. Once heparan sulphate binds to a lysine residue on the antithrombin molecule, a conformational change occurs at the arginine reactive centre resulting in a marked increase in activity.

Thrombomodulin is expressed on endothelial cells and platelets. Thrombomodulin binds thrombin, and the thrombin-thrombomodulin complex is a potent activator of protein C. Protein C and protein S are both vitamin-K dependent plasma proteins. In its activated form protein C, together with protein S as a cofactor, then inactivates factors Va and VIIIa. In addition, protein C possesses profibrinolytic activity that results from neutralisation of plasminogen activator inhibitor-1 (PAI-1) activity.

Older anticoagulants such as unfractionated heparin (UFH), low-molecular-weight heparin (LMWH) and warfarin, and other vitamin K antagonists (VKA), act on a number of targets whereas the newer agents (e.g. direct thrombin inhibitors, anti-Xa inhibitors) have been designed to have highly specific targets within the coagulation mechanism (Fig. 2.1).

2.3 Parenteral Anticoagulants

2.3.1 Unfractionated Heparin (UFH)

Heparin is a negatively charged, sulphated glycosaminoglycan, which exerts its anticoagulant effect primarily by activating antithrombin. Only one third of the heparin chains contain the critical pentasaccharide sequence, which allows for high-affinity binding to antithrombin. At therapeutic concentrations the remaining two thirds have minimal anticoagulant activity [1]. The binding of heparin to antithrombin induces the conformational change in the reactive site of antithrombin, which leads to rapid inhibition of the procoagulant activity of thrombin and factors IXa, Xa, XIa and XIIa. The average length of the heparin chains in unfractionated heparin (UFH) preparations is 45 saccharide units, with the molecular weight ranging from 3,000 to 30,000 Da (mean 15,000 Da). Only heparin chains of 18 saccharide units or longer are of sufficient length to simultaneously bind to antithrombin and thrombin, which is required to catalyse the inhibition of thrombin. The inhibition of thrombin is particularly important as it prevents fibrin formation but also thrombin-induced activation of platelets and factors V, VIII and XI. In contrast, the inhibition of factor Xa can be achieved with shorter heparin chains containing the pentasaccharide sequence [1].

2.3.1.1 Pharmacokinetics of UFH

Heparin is poorly absorbed from the gastrointestinal tract and must be administered parenterally, either by continuous intravenous infusion or subcutaneous injection [2]. The bioavailability of UFH after subcutaneous administration is poor and variable (20–30 %) [3, 4] and its use has largely been superseded in clinical practice by subcutaneous low-molecular-weight heparins (LMWHs).

UFH has complex pharmacokinetics, resulting in a nonlinear anticoagulant response at therapeutic doses, with both the intensity and duration of anticoagulant effect rising disproportionately with increasing doses [5, 6]. There is also wide inter-patient variation in the response to UFH and the adequate dose must be determined on each occasion.

Once UFH reaches the bloodstream, it binds to many plasma proteins as well as to endothelial cells and macrophages [7, 8] which contributes to the inter-individual variability of its anticoagulant effect. It is cleared through a combination of a rapid saturable mechanism and a slower, non-saturable, renal mechanism [5, 6, 9].

2.3.1.2 Safety and Efficacy of UFH in Pregnancy

Several studies have found that UFH does not cross the placenta [10, 11] and therefore lacks the potential to cause fetal bleeding or teratogenicity [12]. Ginsberg et al. [13] examined 186 reports describing fetal/infant outcomes in 1,325 pregnancies associated with anticoagulant therapy. They found that pregnancy outcomes in UFH-treated women were similar to those in the normal population. This was after exclusion of pregnancies in which women had comorbid conditions independently associated with adverse outcomes. A retrospective cohort study of 100 pregnancies in 77 women who received UFH for the prevention or treatment of venous thromboembolism (VTE) (98 pregnancies) or prosthetic heart valves (2 pregnancies) also noted that the rates of prematurity, miscarriage, stillbirth, neonatal death and congenital abnormalities were similar to those in the normal population. There were two bleeding episodes and no symptomatic thrombotic episodes. The authors concluded that maternal UFH therapy is safe for the fetus [13].

Therapeutic anticoagulation with UFH requires a continuous intravenous infusion with regular monitoring of the activated thromboplastin time (APTT) ratio and resultant dose changes in accordance with local nomograms. Twice daily subcutaneous injections have also been advocated; however, Hull et al. [3] showed in a randomised double-blind trial that intermittent subcutaneous heparin was inferior to continuous intravenous heparin infusion in preventing recurrence of VTE in non-pregnant patients with an acute proximal DVT. The need for labour intensive monitoring, coupled with its variable pharmacokinetics, has largely relegated the use of intravenous UFH to specific clinical situations, where a faster 'on-off' anticoagulant effect is required in preference to the longer acting LMWH. Intravenous UFH is advisable in the context of massive pulmonary thromboembolism with cardiovascular compromise where thrombolysis or thrombectomy might be required [14].

Non-hemorrhagic side-effects of UFH such as heparin-induced thrombocytopenia (HIT) and heparin-induced osteoporosis will be discussed in more detail later in this chapter.

2.3.1.3 Use in Lactation

UFH does not pass into breast milk due to its high molecular weight and its strong negative charge [12, 15].

2.3.2 Low-Molecular-Weight Heparins

LMWHs are fragments of UFH produced by either chemical or enzymatic depolymerisation. The resulting heparin chains are approximately 15 saccharide units in length and have a mean molecular weight of 4,000–5,000 Da. Like UFH, LMWHs exert their anticoagulant effect through the catalysis of antithrombin activity, but the chain length of most of the fragments is too short to achieve inhibition of thrombin (IIa) [16]. On the other hand, factor Xa inhibition does not depend on chain length and is unaffected. This explains why UFH has an equivalent inhibitory effect on Factor Xa and thrombin whilst LMWHs possess proportionately greater anti-Xa than anti-IIa activity (2:1 to 4:1) [6, 16]. There is, however, no evidence that this difference impacts on clinical outcomes [6].

2.3.2.1 Pharmacokinetics of LMWHs

LMWHs have a more favourable pharmacokinetic profile compared to UFH. Their lower affinity for plasma proteins and cells leads to a more predictable dose-response relationship [17], longer plasma half-life [18, 19] and lower incidence of side-effects. Table 2.1 summarises key pharmacokinetic parameters for commonly used LMWHs: dalteparin (Fragmin; Pfizer) [20]; enoxaparin (Clexane; Sanofi-Aventis) [22] and tinzaparin (Innohep; Leo-Laboratories) [16, 21, 23–25].

Table 2.1 Comparison of key pharmacokinetic parameters for commonly used LMWHs

LMWH	Mean molecular weight (Da)	Bioavailability (post SC)	T_{max} plasma anti-Xa (post SC)	Plasma T1/2 (post SC)	Anti-Xa/anti-IIa ratio
Dalteparin [20]	4,000–6,000	87 %	3–4 h [21]	3.5–4 h	2.7 [16]
Enoxaparin [22]	4,500	~100 % [23]	1–4 h	4–5 h	3.8 [16]
Tinzaparin [24]	6,500 [25]	90 %	4–6 h	90 min	1.9 [16]

After a subcutaneous injection, the bioavailability of UFH is only around 20–30 % whilst the bioavailability of LMWHs depends on the product used but is generally around 90 % or more (Table 2.1) [26]. This means that therapeutic treatment levels can be achieved with once or twice daily subcutaneous dosing, rather than a continuous intravenous infusion as is required for anticoagulation with UFH.

With LMWH, peak anti-Xa levels are achieved 3–5 h after subcutaneous administration. LMWHs are eliminated by a non-saturable renal mechanism [27], with an elimination half-life of approximately 3–6 h after a subcutaneous injection that is independent of dose [26].

In the non-pregnant state, the dose for therapeutic anticoagulation in patients with a normal body mass index (BMI) is usually based on the actual body weight and administered every 24 h without the need for any specific monitoring. For patients with extreme BMIs at either end of the spectrum, anti-Xa monitoring should be considered; in very obese patients a twice daily dosing regimen is sometimes used.

LMWHs can accumulate in renal failure, leading to concerns about an increased bleeding risk especially when therapeutic doses are administered. If LMWH is used in patients with an estimated creatinine clearance of less than 30 mL/min (less than 20 mL/min with tinzaparin), an empirical dose reduction is recommended (limited data available) and concurrent monitoring of anti-Xa activity should be considered [6].

2.3.2.2 Dosing and Monitoring of LMWHs During Pregnancy

Physiological changes during pregnancy lead to a marked increase in the glomerular filtration rate (GFR). Studies of healthy pregnant women found a 40–65 % rise in the GFR by the end of the first trimester [28], which is maintained for most of the pregnancy [29], then decreases during the last 4–6 weeks before term [29, 30]. In addition, the volume of distribution is increased in pregnancy due to a 35–45 % increase in plasma volume together with a variable degree of weight gain. These changes, along with the production of placental heparinase, might all affect the pharmacokinetics of heparin in pregnancy.

Both Casele et al. [31] and Blomback et al. [32] investigated pregnant women on a fixed prophylactic dose of LMWH (enoxaparin 40 mg once daily and dalteparin 5,000 units once daily, respectively) and found that the clearance of LMWH was increased during pregnancy.

In a study by Lebaudy et al. [33], the pharmacokinetics of prophylactic dose enoxaparin were examined in 75 pregnant and 38 non-pregnant women. In accordance with the physiological changes in pregnancy, the clearance of the drug was higher throughout pregnancy compared with clearance in non-pregnant women. The volume of distribution changed according to the increase in body weight, with an additional 41 % increase in the last trimester of pregnancy, which occurred independent of changes in body weight.

Notwithstanding these findings, prophylactic dose LMWH is generally prescribed once daily. However, a twice daily weight-based dosing regimen would seem preferable when therapeutic anticoagulation is required, and this is in line with UK RCOG recommendations [14]. Advice on dosing for various clinical indications is detailed in individual chapters.

Controversy also exists around the question of whether monitoring with anti-Xa levels and dose adjustments are required in pregnancy, particularly for therapeutic anticoagulation. The RCOG guidelines on the management of VTE in pregnancy state that "routine measurement of peak anti-Xa activity for patients on LMWH for treatment of acute VTE in pregnancy is not recommended except in women at extremes of body weight (less than 50 kg or more than 90 kg) or with other complicating factors, such as renal impairment or recurrent VTE" [14]. The American College of Chest Physicians (ACCP) 2012 guidelines state that monitoring of anti-Xa levels may be advisable when treatment doses of LMWH are given during pregnancy [6].

The study by Rodie et al. [34] is often quoted in support of the notion that anti-Xa monitoring is not required during pregnancy. This case series comprised 33 pregnant women receiving therapeutic dose enoxaparin 1 mg/kg subcutaneously (sc) twice daily based on their early pregnancy weight for treatment of VTE. Peak anti-Xa levels taken 3 h after administration of enoxaparin remained within the therapeutic range, defined in this study as 0.44–1.0 IU/mL, throughout pregnancy. Three women required a dose reduction because peak anti-Xa levels were above the therapeutic range (1.2, 1.2 and 1.1 IU/mL). No woman had a further thromboembolic event. Of note, trough anti-Xa levels were not measured in this study.

In contrast, Jacobsen et al. [35] reported on 20 pregnant women treated with therapeutic dose dalteparin. Thirteen women were commenced on a conventional dose of 100 IU/kg sc twice daily and nine women required a dose escalation to reach the target peak anti-Xa activity of 0.5–1.0 IU/mL. Stable target anti-Xa levels were achieved after dose adjustments to a median of 113 IU/kg bd (range 105–125 IU/kg bd). Six women initially started with higher doses of dalteparin, median 112 IU/kg bd (range 105–125 IU/kg bd) and target anti-Xa levels were achieved in all six women. Only one woman required a dose reduction but her starting dose was significantly higher at 133 IU/kg bd. No recurrence of VTE was reported. Based on their findings the authors suggested that pregnant women should receive a 10–20 % higher dose of dalteparin than non-pregnant patients from the outset, which should then be adjusted on a regular basis according to weight gain.

Similar observations were made by Barbour et al. [36] who reported on 13 pregnant women who received therapeutic dose dalteparin at a regular dose of 100 IU/kg sc twice a day. With this dose, therapeutic peak levels of anticoagulation (anti-Xa level 0.5–1.0 IU/mL) were achieved in only 54 % of women at the start of treatment and by the third trimester this had dropped to 12 %. Despite twice daily dosing very few patients achieved trough levels within the therapeutic range. Even in patients with high therapeutic peak anti-Xa levels, trough levels were in the therapeutic range only 15 % of the time.

More recently, Friedrich and Hameed [37] reported on 15 pregnant women who were treated with subcutaneous enoxaparin 1 mg/kg ± 20 % twice a day. All peak anti-Xa levels (3–4 h after injection) were within the therapeutic range as reported by Rodie et al. [34]. However, 20 % of the 8-h and 73 % of the trough levels were reported to be subtherapeutic.

It remains unclear whether these short periods of what is considered to be subtherapeutic anti-Xa levels are significant but there is some concern that anticoagulation failure might occur as a result. Nevertheless, no further venous thromboembolic events were reported in any of the above studies but the numbers were too small to detect such differences with statistical validity.

It should be noted that, whilst recognising its limitations, the anti-Xa assay is the most informative assay available for monitoring of LMWH therapy [38, 39]. Inter-assay variability of results is high [38] and data to support the association between the clinical efficacy of LMWH and peak anti-Xa levels are limited [40]. In clinical trials evaluating the efficacy of LMWHs in non-pregnant patients, dosing was weight-based and not guided by target anti-Xa levels, but dosing data for special populations are lacking.

The International Society of Thromb Haemost (ISTH) Control of Anticoagulation Subcommittee of the ISTH Standardisation Committee stated in 2002: "Use of anti-Xa assays may provide some clue to the pharmacokinetics of LMWH when used to treat thrombosis in those in whom standard or weight adjusted dosing is likely to be unreliable, especially subjects with severe renal failure, the obese, the pregnant, neonates and infants" [41].

2.3.2.3 Safety and Efficacy of LMWH in Pregnancy

There is a paucity of data regarding the efficacy of LMWHs in pregnancy and recommendations are based largely on extrapolation of data from non-pregnant patients as well as case reports and case series from pregnant patients. Several large clinical trials in non-pregnant patients showed that LMWH is at least as effective and safe as UFH for the treatment of patients with acute DVT and PE [42, 43], and for the prevention of DVT in patients who undergo surgery [44]. There are also studies in non-pregnant patients showing that long-term LMWH (and UFH) is as effective and safe as warfarin for the prevention of recurrent VTE [45–47].

In 2005, Greer and Nelson-Piercy published a systematic review on the safety and efficacy of LMWH for thromboprophylaxis and treatment of VTE in pregnancy [48]. Sixty-four studies reporting on 2, 777 pregnancies were included in the analysis. The risk of VTE recurrence using treatment dose LMWH was reported as 1.15 %, which compares favourably with recurrence rates of 5–8 % in non-pregnant patients treated with LMWH or UFH followed by warfarin. LMWH was also shown to have a reduced risk of bleeding when compared to UFH. In 55 of 2,777 (1.98 %) pregnancies, significant bleeding occurred of which 12 (0.43 %) were antenatal bleeding complications, 17 (0.61 %) were wound hematomas and 26 (0.94 %) were postpartum hemorrhage (PPH; blood loss >500 ml). In most cases of PPH a primary obstetric cause was identified. This compares favourably with the estimated risk of PPH after vaginal delivery of 4 % in the general population and a rate of massive PPH (blood loss >1,500 mL) of 0.7 % from one prospective study of women not receiving LMWH [49]. There was a reported rate of 1.8 % of skin reactions, no reports of heparin-induced thrombocytopenia and a low rate of heparin-induced osteoporosis (0.04 %). The authors concluded that LMWH is both safe and effective to prevent or treat VTE in pregnancy.

There is no evidence in the literature to suggest that placental transfer of LMWH occurs during pregnancy. No anti-Xa activity was detected when fetal blood samples or cord blood of women receiving LMWH during the second and third trimesters of pregnancy were tested [11, 50, 51]. LMWH therefore lacks the potential to cause fetal bleeding or teratogenicity. It should however be noted that several multidose formulations of LMWH contain benzyl alcohol as a preservative. These should be avoided in pregnancy because benzyl alcohol can cross the placenta and has been associated with fatal "gasping" syndrome in premature neonates [52].

2.3.2.4 Use in Breastfeeding

There are limited data available regarding the excretion of LMWH into human breast milk. Richter et al. [53] reported on 15 women receiving 2,500 IU of dalteparin daily as thromboprophylaxis after Cesarean section. Low anti-Xa activity was detected in the breast milk of 11 women. The oral absorption of LMWH is, however, extremely low as it is inactivated in the gastrointestinal tract so the risk to a breastfeeding infant from these drugs is negligible [15].

2.3.3 Fondaparinux

Fondaparinux [54] is a synthetic analogue of the heparin pentasaccharide sequence required for antithrombin binding and was the first of a new class of selective factor Xa inhibitors. It has a molecular weight of 1,728 Da and high affinity for antithrombin. Its specific anti-Xa activity is seven times higher than that of LMWH [55]. After binding to antithrombin, a conformational change occurs which significantly increases the ability of antithrombin to covalently bind to factor Xa. Fondaparinux is then released and available to activate further antithrombin molecules. The saccharide chain of fondaparinux is too short to bridge the distance between antithrombin and thrombin, so it does not have any inhibitory effect on thrombin [55].

2.3.3.1 Pharmacokinetics of Fondaparinux

After subcutaneous dosing, fondaparinux is completely and rapidly absorbed (absolute bioavailability 100 %), reaching peak levels approximately 2 h after administration. There is negligible binding to plasma proteins or red cells. Fondaparinux is not metabolised and there is no formation of active metabolites. The elimination half-life ($t_{1/2}$) is approximately 17–21 h. Approximately 64–77 % of the drug is renally excreted as unchanged compound. It is contraindicated in severe renal impairment (creatinine clearance less than 30 mL/min) and should be used with caution in women weighing less than 50 kg or with moderate renal impairment [54].

Fondaparinux is usually administered as a once daily subcutaneous injection, without the need for anticoagulant monitoring in most situations. For venous thromboprophylaxis a dose of 2.5 mg is recommended and the treatment dose is based on body weight [54].

2.3.3.2 Use in Pregnancy

In an ex vivo model with the use of dually perfused human cotyledon, no placental transfer of fondaparinux was observed [56]. Dempfle [57] reported on five pregnant women who were treated with fondaparinux at a dose of 2.5 mg once a day because they had severe cutaneous allergic reactions to LMWH. In four patients, the anti-Xa activity was elevated in the cord blood sample and the concentration of fondaparinux was approximately 1/10 of the level in the maternal plasma [57]. The concentration of fondaparinux detected in the cord blood was well below the concentration required for effective anticoagulation and no adverse effects were noted in the newborns.

Winger and Reed [58] reported in a retrospective study on the use of fondaparinux (2.5 mg sc once daily) in 29 pregnancies. Safety and efficacy outcomes were compared with the results from 98 pregnancies treated with enoxaparin (30 mg sc twice daily) over the same time period. The decision regarding which anticoagulant to use was based mainly on physician's choice. The women had a history of miscarriage and/or infertility and the anticoagulant was commenced on day 6 of the conception cycle. The pregnancy success rate was similar in the two groups. Treatment was well tolerated and no severe bleeding complications or serious allergic reactions were observed [58].

Knol et al. [59] recently published a report on ten pregnant women who were switched from LMWH to fondaparinux due to hypersensitivity skin reactions to LMWH. The data were collected as part of a prospective cohort study and no increase in bleeding, thromboembolic complications or fetal abnormalities were noted in relation to the use of fondaparinux.

In view of the limited data, the ACCP recommends in its 2012 guidelines that the use of fondaparinux in pregnancy should be reserved for women with heparin-induced thrombocytopenia (HIT) or a history of HIT who cannot receive danaparoid [60]. To date no embryo/fetal harm has been reported with the use of fondaparinux in pregnancy and it should not be withheld if clinically indicated [15].

2.3.3.3 Use in Breastfeeding

Fondaparinux has been shown to pass into the milk of lactating rats; therefore transfer into human milk is possible [54]. However, oral absorption by the infant is unlikely, so the potential for harm in the breastfeeding infant is considered negligible [15].

2.3.3.4 Other Non-hemorrhagic Side-Effects

Other non-hemorrhagic side-effects are very uncommon and include skin reactions that can progress to necrosis, alopecia and hypersensitivity.

2.3.4 Heparin-Induced Thrombocytopenia

Heparin-induced thrombocytopenia (HIT) is an antibody-mediated adverse effect of heparin that is strongly associated with arterial as well as venous thrombosis and can lead to life-threatening complications if not diagnosed early. The pathophysiological basis of HIT is the development of IgG antibodies to a complex of platelet factor four (PF4) and heparin that leads to intravascular platelet activation [61]. PF4 forms tetramers, which allow for the interaction with heparin. The binding of heparin to PF4 leads to a conformational change and this is thought to stimulate antibody formation [62]. The ability to induce conformational change depends on the chain length and degree of sulphation of the glycosaminoglycan, which explains the difference in incidence of HIT observed with different heparins [63].

The frequency of HIT among patients exposed to heparin is highly variable and is influenced by the heparin preparation used, duration of heparin exposure and patient population [60]. For patients receiving UFH in therapeutic doses, the risk of HIT has been estimated at 1 % at most [64]. For obstetric patients receiving prophylactic dose UFH, the incidence of HIT is considered to be infrequent (0.1–1 %), whilst for those receiving only LMWH or Fondaparinux, the risk of HIT is considered rare (<0.1 %) [60].

The RCOG guidelines [14] recommend that platelet monitoring for HIT is not required for obstetric patients receiving LMWH unless they have also received UFH. The ACCP [60] and British Committee for Standards in Haematology (BCSH) guidelines [63] concur with this approach. If acute or subacute HIT is strongly suspected or confirmed then heparin (UFH/LMWH) should be discontinued and therapeutic anticoagulation with an alternative non-heparin anticoagulant is required. The data to guide the choice of an alternative anticoagulant are of poor quality. The ACCP guidelines suggest danaparoid over other non-heparin anticoagulants, with the use of fondaparinux only if danaparoid is not available [60]. The BCSH guidelines concur with this [63]. In patients with a past history of HIT who require thromboprophylaxis, the limited available evidence suggests that the longer the re-exposure to heparin, the higher the likelihood of re-emergence of HIT antibodies and thus the potential for acute HIT. Therefore, in pregnancy where generally prolonged thromboprophylactic anticoagulation is required, a non-heparin anticoagulant should be used. As 25 % of patients with HIT develop thrombosis before the platelet count falls, platelet count monitoring may not detect sensitisation.

2.3.5 Effect of Heparin on Bone Turnover

During pregnancy and lactation, significant changes occur in maternal calcium and bone metabolism. The daily transfer of calcium from mother to fetus in the first trimester is 2–3 mg/day whereas the rate at 35–36 weeks' gestation is estimated at 250 mg/day [65, 66]. Maternal absorption of calcium from the intestine increases significantly to meet the calcium requirements of the fetus. Maternal bone loss may occur in the last months of pregnancy when the fetal skeleton is rapidly mineralising. During lactation there is additional mobilisation of calcium from maternal bone which can lead to a transient loss of approximately 3–7 % of bone mineral density (BMD). This is rapidly regained after weaning [67]. The rate and extent of recovery is influenced by the duration of lactation and postpartum amenorrhea and differs by skeletal site, but recovery is thought to be complete for most women [65, 68].

The long-term use of UFH has been associated with an increased risk of bone loss and osteoporotic fractures [69–71]. This is particularly relevant in pregnancy, as this is one of the few times when long-term prophylaxis or treatment with heparin might be required. Muir et al. [72] demonstrated in a rat model of heparin-induced osteoporosis, that UFH and LMWH both cause a dose-dependent decrease in bone density by reducing the number and activity of osteoblasts, but only UFH was found to increase the number and activity of osteoclasts leading to increased bone resorption.

In vitro the inhibitory effect of LMWH on bone nodule formation was found to be six to eightfold lower than that of UFH [73]. Longer chain length and higher net negative charge of heparin appear to determine the extent of suppression of bone nodule formation [72, 74]. The effect of heparin on osteoblast activity correlated with molecular weight and was pentasaccharide-independent.

Rajgopal et al. [75] reviewed the published clinical trials on this subject and found that pregnant women who received UFH at a dose of 12,000–40,000 IU/day for 25–35 weeks were reported to have a 5 % [76] to 7 % [77] reduction in BMD compared to untreated controls. The reported symptomatic vertebral fracture rate as determined by radiography was 2.2–3.6 % with UFH [78, 79].

Several studies have investigated the effect of prophylactic doses of LMWH on BMD in pregnant women. Nelson-Piercy et al. [80] reported on 61 women receiving enoxaparin 20–40 mg/day for 7.5 months and 30 % had a significant reduction in BMD. Two studies conducted by Pettila et al. [79] and Carlin et al. [81] were unable to demonstrate a difference in the reduction of BMD between the treatment group (dalteparin 2,500–7,500 IU/day) and the control group (no treatment with heparin). In the randomised controlled substudy of the multicentre randomised TIPPS (Thrombophilia in Pregnancy Prophylaxis Study) trial, thrombophilic pregnant women were randomised to either dalteparin 5,000 IU once daily until 20 weeks followed by 5,000 IU twice daily, or to the control group. Thirty-three patients received a mean of 212 days of dalteparin in the intervention group and 29 patients received a mean of 38 days of postpartum thromboprophylaxis with dalteparin in the control group. There was no difference in the mean BMD at 6 weeks postpartum between the intervention group and the control group, suggesting that the use of long-term prophylaxis with dalteparin in pregnancy is not associated with a significant decrease in the mean BMD [82]. Greer and Nelson-Piercy [48] reviewed 64 reports on the use of LMWH for thromboprophylaxis and treatment of venous thrombosis in a total of 2,777 pregnancies. Only one case of osteoporotic fracture was reported in a woman receiving high doses of dalteparin (15,000 IU/day) for a total of 36 weeks (overall risk 0.04 %).

These data combined suggest that the reduction in BMD is more pronounced with UFH than with LMWH and that the risk for developing an osteoporotic fracture after long-term use of prophylactic dose LMWH in pregnancy is low, although data on therapeutic dose LMWH are limited.

In vitro studies comparing the effect of LMWH and fondaparinux on bone remodelling did not show any significant inhibitory effect of fondaparinux on osteoblast proliferation or activity [83, 84]. Clinical data supporting these findings, however, are lacking.

2.3.6 Danaparoid Sodium

Danaparoid [85] is a mixture of low molecular weight sulphated glycosaminoglycuronans derived from animal mucosa, comprising heparan sulphate (approx 84 %), dermatan sulphate (approx 12 %) and a minor amount of chondroitin sulphates A and C (approx 4 %) [85, 86]. It has a mean molecular weight of approximately 5,500 Da. Although often termed a low molecular weight 'heparinoid', it is free of heparin or heparin fragments and differs in chemical structure. Danaparoid has a high anti-Xa to anti-IIa activity ratio [86]. It exerts its anticoagulant effect primarily through inhibition of factor Xa in an antithrombin-dependent fashion [6], resulting in an effective inhibition of thrombin generation and thrombus formation [85].

2.3.6.1 Pharmacokinetics of Danaparoid

After subcutaneous administration, the absolute bioavailability of danaparoid approaches 100 % and the time to reach peak plasma anti-Xa activity levels is approximately 4–5 h [85]. Based on anti-Xa levels, its elimination half-life is approximately 25 h after subcutaneous or intravenous administration and is independent of the dose [85]. Steady-state levels of plasma anti-Xa activity are usually reached within 4–5 days of dosing.

Renal excretion is the main route of elimination, accounting for approximately 40–50 % of the total plasma clearance of anti-Xa activity following intravenous administration [87]. The manufacturer recommends that it should be used with caution in patients with moderately impaired renal and/or liver function with impaired hemostasis, and it should not be used in patients with severe renal impairment/hepatic function unless the patient has HIT and no alternative treatment is available [85].

Plasma anti-Xa activity is linearly related to the dose of danaparoid administered. Anti-Xa assays have been used to monitor danaparoid but whether these are useful is not clear. Expert opinion suggests that monitoring may be of value in patients with severe renal impairment and extremes of body weight (<55 and >90 kg) [63, 85, 88].

2.3.6.2 Efficacy and Safety in Pregnancy

In pregnancy the use of danaparoid is limited to women with current HIT, a past history of HIT or other forms of heparin intolerance. The in vitro cross-reactivity of danaparoid to HIT antibodies can be up to 50 % depending on the sensitivity of the assays used [89] but *in vivo* cross-reactivity is rare [90] and danaparoid remains one of the therapeutic options for the management of HIT within consensus guidelines [60, 63].

The evidence in the literature regarding the safety of danaparoid use in pregnancy is limited. Animal studies have not demonstrated any teratogenic effect or placental transfer [85, 91]. In a recent review of 91 pregnancies in 83 women treated with danaparoid, it was also concluded that none of the fetal adverse events that occurred were attributable to maternal danaparoid use [92]. Of note, there was an increase only in the premature birth rate. None of the six fetal cord blood samples or five breast milk samples obtained showed transfer of anti-Xa activity [92].

2.3.6.3 Use in Breastfeeding

Studies have not formally evaluated the use of danaparoid in lactation, but the molecule is large and should not be expected to pass into human milk. In addition, the drug will be inactivated in the human gastrointestinal tract so is unlikely to cause harm to a breastfeeding infant [15].

2.3.7 Lepirudin

Lepirudin is a direct, irreversible thrombin inhibitor with a molecular weight of approximately 7,000 Da, used in the treatment of HIT. There are only a small number of case reports describing a favourable outcome with its use in pregnant women [93–96]. However, data from animal studies suggests that placental transfer of lepirudin might occur [97, 98] and at present there is not enough evidence to evaluate the safety of its use in pregnancy. The ACCP guidelines therefore recommend its restriction to women with severe allergic reactions to heparin (including HIT) who cannot receive danaparoid [99]. It should be noted that the manufacturer ceased to supply Refludan® (Lepirudin) leading to the permanent discontinuation of Refludan® in the European Union from 1st April 2012. This decision was not related to any safety concerns.

2.3.8 Argatroban

Argatroban [100] is a synthetic inhibitor of thrombin and is derived from L-arginine. It exerts its anticoagulant effect by reversibly binding to the active site of thrombin. It is primarily indicated as an anticoagulant for the treatment of thrombosis in patients with HIT. Administration is by continuous infusion, and subsequent dose adjustments are based on APTT monitoring. The drug undergoes partial metabolism in the liver. The terminal elimination half-life is 39–51 min [100]. The published evidence of the use of argatroban in pregnancy is limited to a small number of case reports [101–103]. It is not known whether argatroban crosses the placenta, but one would expect some fetal exposure due to the low molecular weight (527), low metabolism and moderate serum binding of the drug [15]. The effect of argatroban on reproduction has been incompletely studied in animal experiments, as technical issues have limited systemic exposure [15, 100].

Information concerning the passage of argatroban into human milk is not available. In animal studies transfer into breast milk was demonstrated. Breast feeding is therefore not recommended during treatment [100, 104].

2.3.9 Reversal of Anticoagulant Effect

One advantage of UFH over LMWH is that its anticoagulant effect can be rapidly and completely reversed by the intravenous administration of protamine sulphate. However, severe hypotension and anaphylactoid reactions have been reported, particularly with large doses and rapid administration [6, 105]. When used at doses in excess of that required to neutralise anticoagulation, protamine sulphate may exert its own anticoagulant effect and cause bleeding complications [105].

Protamine sulphate only partially reverses the effects of LMWHs. It neutralises the anti-IIa activity (hence normalising the APTT and thrombin time) but only partly neutralises the anti-Xa activity [106]. In addition, the longer half-life of LMWH compared to UFH and the possibility of continued absorption from a subcutaneous depot, means that repeated doses of protamine may be required for up to 24 h after subcutaneous administration of LMWH [105].

There is no known pharmacological antidote to fondaparinux. In the event of severe bleeding, initiation of appropriate therapy such as surgical hemostasis, blood replacement, fresh plasma transfusion or plasmapheresis should be considered [54]. There are also no known pharmacological antidotes to danaparoid, argatroban or lepirudin. Management of bleeding should be through cessation of treatment and general hemostatic measures, with activation of the hospital's major hemorrhage protocol if appropriate.

2.4 Antiplatelet Agents

2.4.1 Aspirin

Aspirin (acetylsalicylic acid) irreversibly inactivates cyclooxygenase by acetylation. Cyclooxygenase is required for the synthesis of prostaglandins and thromboxane and exists in two isoforms COX-1 and COX-2. COX-1 is present in most cells and involved in the physiological production of prostaglandins. COX-2 is induced by cytokines, mitogens and endotoxins in inflammatory cells and is responsible for the production of prostaglandins during inflammatory processes.

Cyclooxygenase converts arachidonic acid to prostaglandin H_2, which is the precursor for the different prostanoids. Subsequent steps differ depending on cell type. Human platelets primarily produce thromboxane A2 leading to the induction of platelet aggregation and promotion of vasoconstriction [107].

On the other hand, vascular endothelial cells produce prostacyclin (PGI_2) via the COX-1 and, to a greater extent, the COX-2 pathways [108], leading to the inhibition of platelet aggregation and induction of vasodilation [107]. In the gastric mucosa the activation of COX-1 leads to the production of prostacyclin, which exerts a cytoprotective effect.

Aspirin blocks the COX channel by acetylation of a serine residue that prevents access of the substrate to the catalytic site of the enzyme [109]. Inhibition of the COX-1-dependent platelet function can be achieved with low-dose aspirin whilst high-dose aspirin inhibits both COX-1 and COX-2. The platelet inhibitory effect of aspirin lasts for the lifespan of the platelet [110–112], which is approximately 8–10 days in humans.

2.4.1.1 Pharmacokinetics of Aspirin

Aspirin is absorbed by passive diffusion of unionised drug in the stomach and upper small intestine and has a bioavailability of 40–50 % [113]. The plasma half-life of aspirin is approximately 20 min as it is rapidly converted to salicylate once absorbed. Both aspirin and salicylate are bound to serum albumin and are widely distributed (including to the synovial cavity, central nervous system and saliva). Both have pharmacological activity although only aspirin has an antiplatelet effect. Measurable inhibition of platelet function occurs within 60 min of oral intake [113]. Salicylate is eliminated mainly by hepatic metabolism but is also partly excreted unchanged in the urine (the amount depends on plasma concentration and urinary pH).

2.4.1.2 Aspirin—Other Points for Consideration

An expert consensus document on reducing the gastrointestinal (GI) risks associated with the use of antiplatelet agents and non-steroidal anti-inflammatory drugs (NSAIDs) acknowledged that the use of low-dose aspirin is associated with a two- to fourfold increase in the risk of upper gastrointestinal side-effects which is not reduced by the use of buffered or enteric-coated preparations [114]. Anecdotal reports of reduced dyspepsia with these products, however, have probably contributed to their continued uptake in clinical practice [115].

Whilst ranitidine is considered safe for use in pregnancy and breastfeeding [15], the level of acid suppression provided by traditional doses does not prevent most NSAID-related gastric ulcers [114]. There are few data on the use of ranitidine in conjunction with aspirin. If therapeutic or prophylactic gastroprotection is required, a proton pump inhibitor is the preferred option.

Based on findings from a large Swedish cohort study [116], the administration of omeprazole during pregnancy appears to pose little risk to the fetus. In a multicentre prospective controlled study, exposure to omeprazole, lansoprazole or pantoprazole in the first trimester of pregnancy did not cause any increase in the rate of major congenital malformations compared to the control group [117]. Case reports of women receiving omeprazole or pantoprazole during lactation report detection of traces of the drug in the breast milk but no adverse effects were seen in the infants [118, 119].

2.4.1.3 Use in Pregnancy

The use of low-dose aspirin in pregnancy is based on the suspected role of prostanoids in normal pregnancy physiology. An imbalance in prostanoids, with a deficiency in vasodilatory prostacyclin (PGI2) and/or dominance of vasoconstrictory thromboxane A2, was reported in women with a history of recurrent early miscarriage [120] and in women with late pregnancy complications such as intrauterine growth restriction and preeclampsia [121]. Thromboxane A2 overproduction was also found in pregnant women with systemic lupus erythematosus and detectable antiphospholipid antibodies [122]. Low dose aspirin (defined as 40–150 mg) predominantly inhibits COX-1, leading to a reduction in the synthesis of thromboxane A2 without affecting the synthesis of prostacyclin (PGI2). It thereby restores the ratio of the two substances to a more normal value in women with a history of these obstetric complications.

In the 1970s, aspirin was one of the most frequently ingested drugs in pregnancy with more than 50 % of pregnant women taking it [123]. Several large studies investigated the possible relationship between ingestion of aspirin in the first trimester and congenital defects. The Collaborative Perinatal Project monitored 50,282 mother-child pairs, 14,864 of whom used aspirin during the first trimester [124]. The investigators did not find any evidence to suggest that aspirin ingestion in conventional doses during pregnancy is associated with a teratogenic effect. Kozer et al. [125] conducted a meta-analysis of 22 previously published case-control studies and found no evidence of an overall increase in the risk of congenital malformations in relation to aspirin exposure during the first trimester.

In five case-control studies the risk of gastroschisis was reported to be increased (odds ratio 2.37; 95 % CI 1.44–3.88) but the authors commented that the results should be interpreted with caution due to the limitations of the studies involved [125]. Gastroschisis is a rare congenital abnormality occurring in 3–6 of every 100,000 births, and even in a large cohort study it is unlikely that the increased risk that was reported could be detected. In addition, most of the studies were observational and causality between aspirin use and congenital anomalies could not be established. Norgard et al. [126] used data from the Hungarian Case Control Surveillance of Congenital Abnormalities from 1980 to 1996 to examine the association between maternal aspirin use during the first trimester and neural tube defects, gastroschisis or cleft lip and palate in the fetus. Reporting malformed fetuses is compulsory in Hungary. Three thousand and four hundred and fifteen children with one of these congenital abnormalities were included in the study. Information on aspirin use was obtained from a questionnaire and, in order to offset potential recall bias, the control group comprised children with different congenital abnormalities. No increased risk was found for the selected congenital abnormalities in relation to maternal aspirin use.

In the CLASP study, 9,364 women at risk of preeclampsia or IUGR were randomised to receive either 60 mg of aspirin daily or placebo after the first trimester. A questionnaire-based follow-up of over 4,000 of the surviving children at 12 and 18 months of age did not reveal any statistically significant differences with regards to congenital malformation, motor deficit, developmental delay, respiratory problems or bleeding problems in the two cohorts [127].

Aspirin readily crosses the placenta [128]. The elimination of salicylate depends on renal and liver function, both of which are not yet fully developed in the neonate, leading to slower elimination and longer exposure to the drug [129]. Nöschel et al. [130] found an increase in the neonatal-maternal serum concentration ratio of salicylate of up to 1.5 beyond 4 h after intravenous administration of salicylate. The slower elimination of the drug in the neonate is compounded by a higher distribution volume [129]. Salicylate concentrations in the mother at delivery are therefore not an accurate reflection of the exposure in the neonate [129]. The reduction in the ability of the neonate to eliminate salicylate, however, appears to be of significance only in the context of maternal ingestion of high doses of aspirin.

Benigni et al. [131] investigated the effect of low-dose aspirin on fetal and maternal generation of thromboxane. Women at risk of pregnancy-induced hypertension were randomised to daily oral administration of aspirin 60 mg or placebo. They found that serum levels of thromboxane B2, a stable product of thromboxane A2, were almost completely inhibited in women taking low-dose aspirin whilst the synthesis of prostacyclin was not affected. Of note is that the neonatal platelet thromboxane B2 was only partially suppressed and no haemorrhagic complications were observed in the newborns.

Despite the significant inhibition of the production of thromboxane A2 achieved with low-dose aspirin, there has been no evidence of increased maternal bleeding complications in published studies in the context of low-dose aspirin in pregnancy. The reported bleeding times were statistically increased but not to clinically significant values [131, 132]. Concern about the potential risk of bleeding complications in relation to epidural anaesthesia in women taking regular low-dose aspirin in pregnancy has not been substantiated. Sibai et al. [133] reported 891 women who had received epidural anaesthesia during childbirth. During pregnancy 451 had been assigned to low-dose aspirin and 440 to placebo. A bleeding time was obtained in 303 women. The prolongation of the bleeding time in the women on aspirin was statistically significant but only 29 had a bleeding time ≥10 min and 6 had a bleeding time ≥15 min. 13 of the 29 and 2 of the 6 women had epidural anaesthesia. The increase in bleeding time was not associated with increased maternal blood loss during delivery or postpartum, nor was it associated with increased neonatal bleeding complications. No incidence of bleeding was observed in relation to the epidural anaesthesia in any of the 891 women. Regional (epidural or spinal) anaesthesia is not contraindicated in patients taking low-dose aspirin (75–150 mg daily) in isolation [134, 135].

Aspirin has tocolytic properties and, when administered in high doses near term (>3 g/day), it can delay the onset of labour and prolong the duration of labour [136]. High doses of aspirin may lead to early closure of the fetal ductus ateriosus in utero, resulting in persistent pulmonary hypertension of the newborn. In addition, Aspirin given in doses of 300 mg or more per day in the week before delivery may affect the haemostasis of mother and newborn and increase the risk of haemorrhage especially in premature infants [15]. It is therefore recommended that aspirin in analgesic doses is avoided during pregnancy [137]. However, low-dose aspirin (75–150 mg daily) is generally regarded as safe for the fetus during pregnancy.

2.4.1.4 Use in Breastfeeding

Aspirin passes into breast milk and can be absorbed by the infant. The use of aspirin in infants and children is implicated in Reye's syndrome, although the dose-response relationship is uncertain. For women taking low dose aspirin, the amount of drug passing into the breast milk and the risk to the infant is thought to be low [104, 123, 129]. The ACCP guidelines recommend that lactating women using low dose Aspirin (75 mg/day) for vascular indications should continue this medication if they wish to breastfeed [12].

Women taking higher doses of aspirin however, should avoid breastfeeding. Metabolic acidosis has been reported in one infant and there is a theoretical risk of impaired platelet function [137, 138].

2.4.2 Clopidogrel

Clopidogrel hydrogen sulphate is a pro-drug with a molecular weight of approximately 420 Da [139]. Metabolism by several CYP450 enzymes (CYP3A4, CYP2C19, CYP1A2 and CYP2B6) is required to produce the active metabolite that selectively inhibits ADP induced platelet aggregation [140]. Due to irreversible binding, exposed platelets are affected for the remainder of their lifespan (approximately 8–10 days), with recovery of normal platelet function occurring at a rate consistent with platelet turnover. Platelet aggregation induced by agonists other than ADP is also inhibited by blocking of the amplification of platelet activation by released ADP [140].

2.4.2.1 Pharmacokinetics of Clopidogrel

Clopidogrel is rapidly absorbed (at least 50 %) with mean peak plasma levels occurring approximately 45 min after a single dose. It has a half-life of approximately 6 h after a single dose, with an elimination half-life of 8 h for the main circulating metabolite after single and repeated administration [140].

2.4.2.2 Use in Pregnancy

In preclinical safety studies, clopidogrel was given to pregnant rats and rabbits; it was found to have no effect on fertility and was not teratogenic [140]. There have been no studies of transplacental passage but, given the relatively low molecular weight of clopidogrel, it would be expected to pass to the fetus [139]. No clinical trials have been conducted on the use of clopidogrel in pregnant women. A recent review summarises the findings from case reports published to date [141]. The authors identified a total of ten such reports. Three described exposure from the first trimester through to delivery [142–144]. In the other cases, clopidogrel was commenced at a later stage in pregnancy. One fetal death occurred at 26 weeks' gestation after the mother had undergone coronary artery bypass grafting [145]. One child was born at term with a permeable foramen ovale of 0.2 mm, restrictive interventricular muscle communication and moderate mitral insufficiency [143].

The published experience of the use of clopidogrel in pregnancy is limited and prevents a complete assessment of the risk. Briggs et al. [15] therefore suggest that treatment in pregnancy should not be withheld if the known benefits to a woman would appear to outweigh the unknown embryo-fetal risks.

2.4.2.3 Lactation

In animal studies clopidogrel has been shown to pass into the breast milk [140]. There have been no studies of the passage of clopidogrel into human breast milk but, given its low molecular weight, it would be expected to pass into milk and the effect on the infant is not known [15].

2.4.3 Dipyridamole

Dipyridamole [146], with a molecular weight of approximately 500 Da [139], is a pyrimidopyrimidine derivative with vasodilator and antiplatelet properties [147]. In the presence of dipyridamole, platelet aggregation in response to various stimuli such as PAF, collagen and ADP, is inhibited [146].

2.4.3.1 Pharmacokinetics of Dipyridamole

The absolute bioavailability of conventional dipyridamole tablets at steady state is approximately 60 % [146]. Peak plasma levels occur around 60 min after a tablet dose and approximately 2–3 h after the modified release formulation [146]. Dipyridamole is high lipophilic but does not cross the blood-brain barrier to a significant extent. Protein binding is approximately 97–99 %, primarily to alpha 1-acid glycoprotein and albumin. Metabolism is via hepatic glucuronidation and the majority of the metabolites (~95 %) undergo biliary excretion. Renal excretion of both the parent compound and its metabolites is low. The dominant half-life ranges from 2 to 3 h, with a prolonged terminal half-life of approximately 15 h [146].

2.4.3.2 Use in Pregnancy

Dipyridamole has very low placental transfer. There is inadequate evidence of safety in human pregnancy, but dipyridamole has been used for many years without any apparent adverse consequence [146]. Neither the animal nor the limited human pregnancy data available suggest that dipyridamole causes developmental toxicity [15].

2.4.3.3 Use in Breastfeeding

Dipyridamole is excreted into breast milk at levels approximately 6 % of the plasma concentration [146]. The effect on the nursing infant is unknown [15], although no untoward effects have been reported [104].

2.5 Oral Anticoagulants

2.5.1 Vitamin K Antagonists

The coagulation factors II, VII, IX and X undergo post-translational gamma carboxylation in the liver, which is a prerequisite for their procoagulant activity. This process is vitamin K dependent and requires the cyclical conversion of oxidised vitamin K to its reduced form, which then participates in the carboxylation of the coagulation factor precursors. Vitamin K antagonists (e.g. warfarin, acenocoumarol, phenprocoumon, phenindione) inhibit vitamin K oxide reductase, the enzyme responsible for the cyclical conversion of vitamin K. This results in the hepatic production of partially carboxylated and decarboxylated coagulation factors, with a 30–50 % reduction in their coagulant activity.

Warfarin sodium (molecular weight 330 Da) is the most common vitamin K antagonist in clinical use in the UK. It has a slow onset of action and a narrow therapeutic window. This, as well as its numerous drug and dietary interactions, and potential for variation of action with alcohol, intercurrent illness, exercise and smoking, necessitates frequent monitoring of the International Normalised Ratio (INR), which is inconvenient and costly. Over-anticoagulation with warfarin is associated with a risk of bleeding, and under-anticoagulation with thrombosis.

2.5.1.1 Use in Pregnancy

Vitamin K antagonists cross the placenta and can lead to spontaneous miscarriage, stillbirth, preterm birth, embryopathy and haemorrhagic complications in the fetus. Features of warfarin embryopathy include nasal hypoplasia due to failure of development of the nasal septum and epiphyseal stippling [148]. In addition, hypoplasia of the extremities, ocular abnormalities (i.e. optic atrophy, microphthalmia, blindness) and developmental delay may occur [148]. The critical period of exposure for embryopathy to occur appears to be between 6 and 12 weeks of gestation.

Vitamin K antagonists can also cause haemorrhagic fetal complications. The fetal liver is immature and levels of vitamin K dependent coagulation factors, which are normally low at birth, are further reduced by the maternal ingestion of a vitamin K antagonist and can significantly increase the risk of bleeding in the neonate around the time of delivery. ACCP guidelines recommend the use of LMWH over a vitamin K antagonist for the treatment of venous thrombosis in pregnancy [12]. For women on anticoagulation with a vitamin K antagonist prior to conception this should be substituted by LMWH early in pregnancy [12].

To further evaluate the frequency of warfarin induced adverse effects in pregnancy, Chan et al. [149] performed a systematic review of the literature investigating the fetal and maternal outcome in women with mechanical heart valves. 976 women with 1,234 pregnancies were included. The women were divided into four groups: (1) those who received oral anticoagulants throughout pregnancy, (2) those in whom vitamin K antagonists were replaced with heparin in the first trimester (from 6 to 12 weeks' gestation), (3) those who received heparin throughout pregnancy and (4) those who were not on any anticoagulant therapy. They found that continued exposure to vitamin K antagonists beyond 6 weeks' gestation was associated with warfarin embryopathy in 6.4 % of live births and the risk of fetal loss increased by 50 %. No case of warfarin embryopathy was observed in women who were switched to heparin before 6 weeks' gestation. The European Network of Teratology Information Services (ENTIS) prospectively collected data between 1988 and 2004 on 666 pregnant women exposed to vitamin K antagonists and compared this to data from a non-exposed control group (n = 1,094) [150]. Major birth defects were observed in 4.8 % of pregnancies exposed to vitamin K antagonists in the first trimester and 1.4 % in the control group (odds ratio (OR) 3.86; 95 % CI, 1.86–8.00). The miscarriage rate was significantly increased: 24.7 % versus 8.6 % (OR 3.78; 95 % CI 2.77–5.18; $p<0.001$). The strongest effect was found after exposure to phenprocoumon. Preterm birth was more frequent (16.0 % versus 7.6 %); mean gestational age at delivery and mean birthweight of term infants were lower compared to controls. Furthermore, there is evidence to suggest that warfarin embroyopathy is dose-dependent, with a higher incidence in women taking more than 5 mg of warfarin per day [151].

Exposure to vitamin K antagonists during any trimester of pregnancy may be linked with an increased risk of neurodevelopmental problems in the offspring. Chong et al. [152] reported no significant difference versus matched controls in physical and mental development in a study on 22 patients, whereas in a study comparing 274 school-age children with 231 matched controls, Wesseling et al. [153] concluded that prenatal exposure to coumarins is associated with an increased risk of minor neurological dysfunction and of a lower intelligence quotient (IQ). However, in the vast majority of children there was no clinically significant effect on growth or long-term development [152, 153].

2.5.1.2 Use in Breastfeeding

The use of warfarin and dicoumarol is considered compatible with breastfeeding [12, 137, 138]. There have been two reports investigating the use of warfarin in lactating women. Orme et al. [154] evaluated the excretion of warfarin into breast milk in 13 women treated with warfarin 5–12 mg per day. Warfarin was undetectable (<0.08 mmol/L) in all milk samples. Seven women elected to continue breastfeeding their infants. Warfarin was undetectable in plasma samples from all seven infants. In addition, all seven infants had normal prothrombin times. McKenna et al. [155] reported similar findings. Two women who required warfarin anticoagulation after delivery and their infants were followed, in one case for 56 days and in the other for 131 days. Both women elected to continue to breastfeed. At no time was warfarin detected in the milk of either mother nor were there any changes in prothrombin activity in either infant.

Phenindione and anisindione are less polar and more lipophilic and more likely to cross into the breast milk [156]. This appears to be dose-dependent but with doses of 50–75 mg the drug is usually detectable in breast milk [156] and should be avoided during breastfeeding due to the risk of hemorrhage in the infant [137].

2.5.2 The New Oral Anticoagulant Agents

The past decade has seen the exciting development of a number of non-vitamin K antagonist oral anticoagulants (direct thrombin inhibitors and direct anti-Xa inhibitors) (NOAC) or oral direct inhibitors (ODI) of coagulation, which offer several advantages over warfarin. These include reliable pharmacokinetics with a consistent anticoagulant response, fixed dosing with no need for routine anticoagulant monitoring and reduced drug and food interactions.

NOAC include dabigatran etexilate [157], a direct thrombin inhibitor, and rivaroxaban (Xarelto®; Bayer HealthCare AG) and apixaban (Eliquis®; Bristol-MyersSquibb-Pfizer), both direct factor Xa inhibitors. These agents are licensed by the European Medicines Agency and approved by the National Institute for Health and Care Excellence (NICE) in England and the US Food and Drug Administration (FDA) for the prevention of venous thromboembolism (VTE) in patients undergoing hip or knee replacement stroke or systemic embolization in patients with atrial fibrillation (AF).

NOAC have also undergone phase III trials for the treatment of acute DVT and PE and secondary prevention of VTE, and all three agents have now been licensed for these indications and approved by NICE and the FDA. It should be noted that clinical trials of therapeutic dose NOAC versus warfarin in patients with AF or VTE have used warfarin at a target INR of 2.5 (i.e. range 2.0–3.0) as the comparator. The RAPS (Rivaroxaban in AntiPhospholipid Syndrome (APS)) trial is assessing the use of rivaroxaban in thrombotic APS (http://www.controlled-trials.com/ISRCTN68222801). Further studies are required to elucidate the role of NOAC in APS-related stroke. In the Randomized, Phase II Study to Evaluate the Safety and Pharmacokinetics of Oral Dabigatran Etexilate in Patients after Heart Valve Replacement (RE-ALIGN) study, dabigatran (150–300 mg twice daily) was associated with increased rates of thromboembolic and bleeding complications, as compared with warfarin, thus showing no benefit but an excess risk [158].

2.5.2.1 Direct Thrombin Inhibitors (DTI)

After the withdrawal of ximelagatran in 2006 due to hepatic toxicity, dabigatran etexilate is currently the only licensed oral agent available in this class. It is a prodrug with a low molecular weight (724). Once absorbed, it is converted to its active moiety (dabigatran) by plasma esterases. In its active form, dabigatran is a potent, competitive, reversible direct thrombin inhibitor, that binds and inactivates both fibrin-bound and unbound thrombin, the final effector in blood coagulation [159–162].

2.5.2.2 Use in Pregnancy

Studies in animals have shown reproductive toxicity and the potential risk for humans is unknown [157]. There are currently no adequate data on the use of dabigatran etexilate in pregnant women so pregnancy should be avoided during treatment [157]. From a practical perspective, this implies that women of childbearing potential treated with dabigatran etexilate should be strongly advised to ensure adequate contraception and, in the event of unexpected pregnancy, require early review by a hematologist and obstetrician to discuss the potential implications and management. There is no evidence-based guidance on what to do when conception is planned. One approach in women taking a new oral anticoagulant would be to substitute with LMWH pre-conception.

2.5.2.3 Use in Breastfeeding

There are no clinical data of the effect of dabigatran on infants during breastfeeding and the manufacturer states that it should be discontinued during breastfeeding [157].

2.5.2.4 Factor Xa Inhibitors

Rivaroxaban (molecular weight 435) and apixaban (molecular weight 459) are both small molecules that reversibly and competitively inhibit factor Xa in a concentration dependent manner [163, 164]. They inhibit both prothrombinase-bound and thrombus-associated factor Xa [163, 164].

2.5.2.5 Use in Pregnancy

There are no adequate data on the use of rivaroxaban in pregnant women [165]. Animal studies have shown reproductive toxicity related to its pharmacological mode of action (e.g. hemorrhagic complications). Embryo/fetal toxicity (post-implantation loss, retarded/progressed ossification, hepatic multiple light coloured spots) and an increase in the incidence of common malformations, as well as placental changes, were observed at clinically relevant plasma concentrations. In the pre- and post-natal studies in rats, reduced viability of the offspring was observed at doses that were toxic to the dams.

Due to the potential reproductive toxicity, the intrinsic risk of bleeding and the evidence that rivaroxaban crosses the placenta, rivaroxaban is contraindicated in pregnancy. Practical advice to women of childbearing potential is as detailed above for dabigatran etexilate.

There are no data on the use of apixaban in pregnant women [166]. According to the manufacturer, animal studies did not indicate direct or indirect harmful effects with respect to reproductive toxicity [166]. Apixaban is not recommended during pregnancy.

2.5.2.6 Use in Breastfeeding

No data on the use of rivaroxaban or apixaban in breastfeeding women are available and data from animals indicate that rivaroxaban and apixaban are both secreted into breast milk. Therefore, rivaroxaban and apixaban are contraindicated during breastfeeding [165, 166].

2.6 Case Study

A 36 year old woman presented with a pulmonary embolism at 20 weeks' gestation in her second pregnancy. She was commenced on therapeutic anticoagulation with tinzaparin, but 45 min after administration of the first dose she had an allergic reaction with tingling of the lips, tongue and neck swelling. This was successfully treated with an antihistamine and hydrocortisone. She was then commenced on an intravenous infusion of UFH and subsequently switched to fondaparinux. She experienced severe pruritus in relation to fondaparinux. Other therapeutic options considered at this point were exposure to another LMWH with the risk of a severe allergic reaction or a switch to subcutaneous UFH at a therapeutic dose, or warfarinisation. In dialogue with the woman it was agreed to continue fondaparinux and the pruritus was managed with sparing use of a hydrocortisone cream.

For the delivery she was commenced on an intravenous infusion of UFH 24 h after the last dose of fondaparinux. This was discontinued 6 h before elective Cesarean section. In addition, her anti-Xa level was checked prior to the epidural anesthetic. The continuous infusion of UFH was recommenced 6 h after delivery. The dose was reduced by 25 %, no bolus was given and APTT monitoring was resumed. Warfarin was commenced on day 4 after delivery and continued for 8 weeks postpartum. A subsequent trial of enoxaparin with close observation was uneventful.

Key Learning Points

- Low-molecular-weight heparin (LMWH) is the agent of choice if therapeutic anticoagulation is required during pregnancy.
- Physiological changes in pregnancy are likely to affect pharmacokinetics and pharmacodynamics of LMWHs.
- Anti-Xa monitoring should be considered if LMWHs are used in women with an extreme BMI (at either end of the spectrum) or in women with renal failure (estimated creatinine clearance of less than 30 mL/min)
- The incidence of heparin-induced thrombocytopenia (HIT) in obstetric patients receiving thromboprophylaxis or therapeutic anticoagulation with LMWH is low. Platelet monitoring for HIT is not required unless women have also previously received unfractionated heparin (UFH).
- If HIT is strongly suspected or confirmed, then heparin (UFH/LMWH) should be discontinued and a non-cross reacting anticoagulant used—danaparoid where available and fondaparinux also considered.
- Vitamin K antagonists such as warfarin cross the placenta and can lead to spontaneous miscarriage, stillbirth, preterm birth, embryopathy and hemorrhagic complications in the fetus.
- Vitamin K antagonists should be substituted with a LMWH early in pregnancy, and certainly before 6 weeks' gestation, to prevent embryopathy.
- The use of warfarin is NOT a contraindication to breastfeeding.
- The non-vitamin K antagonist oral anticoagulants (dabigatran etixilate, rivaroxaban, apixaban) (NOAC) should not be used during pregnancy or breastfeeding. There is evidence of reproductive toxicity from animal studies for both dabigatran etixilate and rivaroxaban.

References

1. Hirsh J. Heparin. N Engl J Med. 1991;324(22):1565–74.
2. Windsor E, Freeman L. Investigation of routes of administration of heparin other than injection. Am J Med. 1964;37(3):408–16.
3. Hull RD, Raskob GE, Hirsh J, Jay RM, Leclerc JR, Geerts WH, et al. Continuous intravenous heparin compared with intermittent subcutaneous heparin in the initial treatment of proximal vein thrombosis. N Engl J Med. 1986;315(18):1109–14.
4. Pini M, Pattacini C, Quintavalla R, Poli T, Megha A, Tagliaferri A, et al. Subcutaneous vs intravenous heparin in the treatment of deep venous thrombosis—a randomized clinical-trial. Thromb Haemost. 1990;64(2):222–6.
5. De Swart CAM, Nijmeyer B, Roelofs JMM, Sixma JJ. Kinetics of intravenously administered heparin in normal humans. Blood. 1982;60(6):1251–8.
6. Garcia DA, Baglin T, Weitz JI, Samama MM, American College of Chest Physicians. Parenteral anticoagulants: Antithrombotic Therapy and Prevention of Thrombosis, 9th ed: American College of Chest Physicians Evidence-Based Clinical Practice Guidelines. Chest. 2012;141(2 Suppl):e24S–43.
7. Glimelius B, Busch C, Hook M. Binding of heparin on surface of cultured human endothelial cells. Thromb Res. 1978;12(5):773–82.
8. Mahadoo J, Hiebert L, Jaques LB. Vascular sequestration of heparin. Thromb Res. 1978;12(1):79–90.
9. Bjornsson TD, Wolfram KM, Kitchell BB. Heparin kinetics determined by 3 assay-methods. Clin Pharmacol Ther. 1982;31(1):104–13.
10. Flessa HC, Kapstrom AB, Glueck HI, Will JJ. Placental transport of heparin. Am J Obstet Gynecol. 1965;93(4):570–3.
11. Schneider D, Heilmann L, Harenberg J. Placental transfer of low-molecular heparin. Geburtshilfe Frauenheilkd. 1995;55(2):93–8.
12. Bates SM, Greer IA, Middeldorp S, Veenstra DL, Prabulos AM, Vandvik PO, American College of Chest Physicians. VTE, thrombophilia, antithrombotic therapy, and pregnancy: Antithrombotic Therapy and Prevention of Thrombosis, 9th ed: American College of Chest Physicians Evidence-Based Clinical Practice Guidelines. Chest. 2012;141(2 Suppl):e691S–736.
13. Ginsberg JS, Kowalchuk G, Hirsh J, Brilledwards P, Burrows R. Heparin-therapy during pregnancy—risks to the fetus and mother. Arch Intern Med. 1989;149(10):2233–6.
14. Royal College of Obstetricians and Gynaecologists. Reducing the risk of venous thromboembolism during pregnancy and the puerperium, Green-top guideline no 37a. London RCOG; 2015. https://www.rcog.org.uk/guidelines.
15. Briggs GG, Freeman RK, Yaffee SJ. Drugs in pregnancy and lactation: a reference guide to fetal and neonatal risk. 9th ed. Philadelphia: Wolters Kluwer/Lippincott Williams & Wilkins; 2011.
16. Weitz JI. Low-molecular-weight heparins. N Engl J Med. 1997;337(10):688–98.
17. Handeland GF, Abildgaard U, Holm HA, Arnesen KE. Dose adjusted heparin treatment of deep venous thrombosis—a comparison of unfractionated and low-molecular-weight heparin. Eur J Clin Pharmacol. 1990;39(2):107–12.
18. Harenberg J. Pharmacology of low-molecular-weight heparins. Semin Thromb Hemost. 1990;16(Suppl):12–8.
19. Bara L, Samama M. Pharmacokinetics of low-molecular-weight heparins. Acta Chir Scand Suppl. 1988;543:65–72.
20. Pfizer. Summary of product characteristics: Fragmin (dalteparin) 10,000 units/ml—treatment of VTE. The electronic medicines compendium. 2013. https://www.medicines.org.uk/emc/.
21. Dunn CJ, Jarvis B. Dalteparin—an update of its pharmacological properties and clinical efficacy in the prophylaxis and treatment of thromboembolic disease. Drugs. 2000;60(1):203–37.
22. Sanofi-Aventis. Summary of product characteristics: Clexane (enoxaparin) pre-filled syringes and Clexane multidose vial. The electronic medicines Compendium. 2014. https://www.medicines.org.uk/emc/.
23. Siddiqui MAA, Wagstaff AJ. Enoxaparin—a review of its use as thromboprophylaxis in acutely ill, non-surgical patients. Drugs. 2005;65(7):1025–36.
24. Leo-Laboratories. Summary of product characteristics: Innohep (tinzaparin) 20,000 IU/ml and InnohepSyringe 20,000 IU/ml. The electronic medicines compendium. 2015. https://www.medicines.org.uk/emc/.
25. Cheer SM, Dunn CJ, Foster R. Tinzaparin sodium—a review of its pharmacology and clinical use in the prophylaxis and treatment of thromboembolic disease. Drugs. 2004;64(13):1479–502.
26. Samama MM, Gerotziafas GT. Comparative pharmacokinetics of LMWHs. Semin Thromb Hemost. 2000;26:31–8.
27. Boneu B, Caranobe C, Sie P. Pharmacokinetics of heparin and low-molecular-weight heparin. Baillieres Clin Haematol. 1990;3(3):531–44.
28. Davison JM, Noble MCB. Serial changes in 24-hour creatinine clearance during normal menstrual cycles and the first trimester of pregnancy. Br J Obstet Gynaecol. 1981;88(1):10–7.
29. Anderson GD. Pregnancy-induced changes in pharmacokinetics—a mechanistic-based approach. Clin Pharmacokinet. 2005;44(10):989–1008.
30. Paaby P, Nielsen A, Mollerpetersen J, Raffn K. Cyclical changes in endogenous overnight creatinine clearance during the 3rd trimester of pregnancy. Acta Med Scand. 1988;223(5):459–68.
31. Casele HL, Laifer SA, Woelkers DA, Venkataramanan R. Changes in the pharmacokinetics of the low-molecular-weight heparin enoxaparin sodium during pregnancy. Am J Obstet Gynecol. 1999;181(5):1113–7.

32. Blomback M, Bremme K, Hellgren M, Lindberg H. A pharmacokinetic study of dalteparin (Fragmin (R)) during late pregnancy. Blood Coagul Fibrinolysis. 1998;9(4):343–50.
33. Lebaudy C, Hulot JS, Amoura Z, Costedoat-Chalumeau N, Serreau R, Ankri A, et al. Changes in enoxaparin pharmacokinetics during pregnancy and implications for antithrombotic therapeutic strategy. Clin Pharmacol Ther. 2008;84(3):370–7.
34. Rodie VA, Thomson AJ, Stewart FM, Quinn AJ, Walker ID, Greer IA. Low-molecular-weight heparin for the treatment of venous thromboembolism in pregnancy: a case series. BJOG. 2002;109(9): 1020–4.
35. Jacobsen AF, Qvigstad E, Sandset PM. Low-molecular-weight heparin (dalteparin) for the treatment of venous thromboembolism in pregnancy. BJOG. 2003;110(2):139–44.
36. Barbour LA, Oja JL, Schultz LK. A prospective trial that demonstrates that dalteparin requirements increase in pregnancy to maintain therapeutic levels of anticoagulation. Am J Obstet Gynecol. 2004;191(3):1024–9.
37. Friedrich E, Hameed AB. Fluctuations in anti-factor Xa levels with therapeutic enoxaparin anticoagulation in pregnancy. J Perinatol. 2010;30(4):253–7.
38. Kitchen S, Iampietro R, Woolley AM, Preston FE. Anti-Xa monitoring during treatment with low-molecular-weight heparin or danaparoid: inter-assay variability. Thromb Haemost. 1999;82(4):1289–93.
39. Baglin T, Barrowcliffe TW, Cohen A, Greaves M, British Committee for Standards in Haematology. Guidelines on the use and monitoring of heparin. Br J Haematol. 2006;133(1):19–34.
40. Levine MN, Planes A, Hirsh J, Goodyear M, Vochelle N, Gent M. The relationship between anti-factor Xa level and clinical outcome in patients receiving Enoxaparine low-molecular weight heparin to prevent deep-vein thrombosis after hip-replacement. Thromb Haemost. 1989;62(3):940–4.
41. Greaves M. Limitations of the laboratory monitoring of heparin therapy. Thromb Haemost. 2002;87(1): 163–4.
42. Dolovich LR, Ginsberg JS, Douketis JD, Holbrook AM, Cheah G. A meta-analysis comparing low-molecular-weight heparins with unfractionated heparin in the treatment of venous thromboembolism—examining some unanswered questions regarding location of treatment, product type, and dosing frequency. Arch Intern Med. 2000;160(2):181–8.
43. Gould MK, Dembitzer AD, Doyle RL, Hastie TJ, Garber AM. Low-molecular-weight heparins compared with unfractionated heparin for treatment of acute deep venous thrombosis—a meta-analysis of randomized, controlled trials. Ann Intern Med. 1999;130(10):800–9.
44. Nurmohamed MT, Rosendaal FR, Buller HR, Dekker E, Hommes DW, Vandenbroucke JP, et al. Low-molecular-weight heparin versus standard heparin in general and orthopedic surgery—a metaanalysis. Lancet. 1992;340(8812):152–6.
45. Lopaciuk S, Bielska-Falda H, Noszczyk W, Bielawiec M, Witkiewicz W, Filipecki S, et al. Low-molecular-weight heparin versus acenocoumarol in the secondary prophylaxis of deep vein thrombosis. Thromb Haemost. 1999;81(1):26–31.
46. van der Heijden JF, Prins MH, Buller HR. Low-molecular-weight heparins: are they interchangeable? Haemostasis. 2000;30:148–57.
47. Pini M, Aiello S, Manotti C, Pattacini C, Quintavalla R, Poli T, et al. Low-molecular-weight heparin versus warfarin in the prevention of recurrence after deep vein thrombosis. Thromb Haemost. 1994; 72(2):191–7.
48. Greer IA, Nelson-Piercy C. Low-molecular-weight heparins for thromboprophylaxis and treatment of venous thromboembolism in pregnancy: a systematic review of safety and efficacy. Blood. 2005;106(2):401–7.
49. Waterstone M, Bewley S, Wolfe C. Incidence and predictors of severe obstetric morbidity: case-control study. Br Med J. 2001;322(7294):1089–93.
50. Forestier F, Daffos F, Capellapavlovsky M. Low-molecular-weight heparin (PK-10169) does not cross the placenta during the 2nd trimester of pregnancy by direct fetal blood-sampling under ultrasound. Thromb Res. 1984;34(6):557–60.
51. Forestier F, Daffos F, Rainaut M, Toulemonde F. Low-molecular-weight heparin (CY216) does not cross the placenta during third trimester of pregnancy. Thromb Haemost. 1987;57(2):234.
52. Robertson AF. Reflections on errors in neonatology III. The "experienced" years, 1970 to 2000. J Perinatol. 2003;23:240–49.
53. Richter C, Sitzmann J, Lang P, Weitzel H, Huch A, Huch R. Excretion of low-molecular-weight heparin in human milk. Br J Clin Pharmacol. 2001;52(6): 708–10.
54. GlaxoSmithKline. Summary of product characteristics: Arixtra (fondaparinux) 2.5mg, 5mg, 7.5mg, 10mg solution for injection, pre-filled syringe. The electronic medicines Compendium. 2013. 12 June 2011.
55. Samama MM, Gerotziafas GT. Evaluation of the pharmacological properties, and clinical results of the synthetic pentasaccharide (fondaparinux). Thromb Res. 2003;109(1):1–11.
56. Lagrange F, Vergnes C, Brun JL, Paolucci F, Nadal T, Leng JJ, et al. Absence of placental transfer of pentasaccharide (Fondaparinux, Arixtra) in the dually perfused human cotyledon in vitro. Thromb Haemost. 2002;87(5):831–5.
57. Dempfle CEH. Minor transplacental passage of fondaparinux in vivo. N Engl J Med. 2004;350(18):1914–5.
58. Winger E, Reed J. Fondaparinux versus enoxaparin treatment in women with infertility or pregnancy loss. Haematologica. 2009;95:0455.
59. Knol HM, Schultinge L, Erwich J, Meijer K. Fondaparinux as an alternative anticoagulant therapy during pregnancy. J Thromb Haemost. 2010;8(8):1876–9.

60. Linkins LA, Dans AL, Moores LK, Bona R, Davidson BL, Schulman S, Crowther M, American College of Chest Physicians. Treatment and prevention of heparin-induced thrombocytopenia: Antithrombotic Therapy and Prevention of Thrombosis, 9th ed: American College of Chest Physicians Evidence-Based Clinical Practice Guidelines. Chest. 2012;141(2 Suppl):e495S–530.
61. Rauova L, Poncz M, McKenzie SE, Reilly MP, Arepally G, Weisel JW, et al. Ultralarge complexes of PF4 and heparin are central to the pathogenesis of heparin-induced thrombocytopenia. Blood. 2005; 105(1):131–8.
62. Horsewood P, Warkentin TE, Hayward CPM, Kelton JG. The epitope specificity of heparin-induced thrombocytopenia. Br J Haematol. 1996;95(1):161–7.
63. Watson H, Davidson S, Keeling D. Guidelines on the diagnosis and management of heparin-induced thrombocytopenia: second edition. Br J Haematol. 2012;159(5):528–40.
64. Martel N, Lee J, Wells PS. Risk for heparin-induced thrombocytopenia with unfractionated and low-molecular-weight heparin thromboprophylaxis: a meta-analysis. Blood. 2005;106(8):2710–5.
65. Kalkwarf HJ, Specker BL. Bone mineral changes during pregnancy and lactation. Endocrine. 2002; 17(1):49–53.
66. Koo WW, Walters JC, Esterlitz J, Levine RJ, Bush AJ, Sibai B. Maternal calcium supplementation and fetal bone mineralization. Obstet Gynecol. 1999;94(4):577–82.
67. Khastgir G, Studd J. Pregnancy-associated osteoporosis. Br J Obstet Gynaecol. 1994;101(10):836–8.
68. Khovidhunkit W, Epstein S. Osteoporosis in pregnancy. Osteoporos Int. 1996;6(5):345–54. 2.
69. Murphy MS, John PR, Mayer AD, Buckels JA, Kelly DA. Heparin therapy and bone fractures. Lancet. 1992;340(8827):1098.
70. Rupp WM, McCarthy HB, Rohde TD, Blackshear PJ, Goldenberg FJ, Buchwald H. Risk of osteoporosis in patients treated with long-term intravenous heparin therapy. Curr Surg. 1982;39(6):419–22.
71. Sackler JP, Liu L. Heparin-induced osteoporosis. Br J Radiol. 1973;46(547):548–50.
72. Muir JM, Hirsh J, Weitz JI, Andrew M, Young E, Shaughnessy SG. A histomorphometric comparison of the effects of heparin and low-molecular-weight heparin on cancellous bone in rats. Blood. 1997;89(9):3236–42.
73. Bhandari M, Hirsh J, Weitz JI, Young E, Venner TJ, Shaughnessy SG. The effects of standard and low-molecular-weight heparin on bone nodule formation in vitro. Thromb Haemost. 1998;80(3):413–7.
74. Shaughnessy SG, Young E, Deschamps P, Hirsh J. The effects of low-molecular-weight and standard heparin on calcium loss from fetal-rat calvaria. Blood. 1995;86(4):1368–73.
75. Rajgopal R, Bear M, Butcher MK, Shaughnessy SG. The effects of heparin and low-molecular-weight heparins on bone. Thromb Res. 2008;122(3):293–8.
76. Dahlman TC, Sjoberg HE, Ringertz H. Bone-mineral density during long-term prophylaxis with heparin in pregnancy. Am J Obstet Gynecol. 1994;170(5):1315–20.
77. Douketis JD, Ginsberg JS, Burrows RF, Duku EK, Webber CE, Brill-Edwards P. The effects of long-term heparin therapy during pregnancy on bone density. A prospective matched cohort study. Thromb Haemost. 1996;75(2):254–7.
78. Dahlman TC. Osteoporotic fractures and the recurrence of thromboembolism during pregnancy and the puerperium in 184 women undergoing thromboprophylaxis with heparin. Am J Obstet Gynecol. 1993;168(4):1265–70.
79. Pettila V, Kaaja R, Leinonen P, Ekblad U, Kataja M, Ikkala E. Thromboprophylaxis with low-molecular-weight heparin (dalteparin) in pregnancy. Thromb Res. 1999;96(4):275–82.
80. Nelson-Piercy C, Letsky EA, de Swiet M. Low-molecular-weight heparin for obstetric thromboprophylaxis: experience of sixty-nine pregnancies in sixty-one women at high risk. Am J Obstet Gynecol. 1997;176(5):1062–8.
81. Carlin AJ, Farquharson RG, Quenby SM, Topping J, Fraser WD. Prospective observational study of bone mineral density during pregnancy: low-molecular-weight heparin versus control. Hum Reprod. 2004;19(5):1211–4.
82. Le Templier G, Rodger MA. Heparin-induced osteoporosis and pregnancy. Curr Opin Pulm Med. 2008;14(5):403–7.
83. Matziolis G, Perka C, Disch A, Zippel H. Effects of fondaparinux compared with dalteparin, enoxaparin and unfractionated heparin on human osteoblasts. Calcif Tissue Int. 2003;73(4):370–9.
84. Handschin AE, Trentz OA, Hoerstrup SP, Kock HJ, Wanner GA, Trentz O. Effect of low-molecular-weight heparin (dalteparin) and fondaparinux (Arixtra) on human osteoblasts in vitro. Br J Surg. 2005;92(2):177–83.
85. Merck Sharp & Dohme. Summary of product characteristics: Orgaran (danaparoid). The electronic medicines compendium. 1998.
86. Wilde MI, Markham A. Danaparoid—a review of its pharmacology and clinical use in the management of heparin-induced thrombocytopenia. Drugs. 1997;54(6):903–24.
87. Danhof M, Deboer A, Magnani HN, Stiekema JCJ. Pharmacokinetic considerations on Orgaran (ORG-10172) therapy. Haemostasis. 1992;22(2): 73–84.
88. Farner B, Eichler P, Kroll H, Greinacher A. A comparison of danaparoid and lepirudin in heparin-induced thrombocytopenia. Thromb Haemost. 2001;85(6):950–7.
89. Newman PM, Swanson RL, Chong BH. Heparin-induced thrombocytopenia: IgG binding to PF4-heparin complexes in the fluid phase and cross-reactivity with low-molecular-weight heparin and heparinoid. Thromb Haemost. 1998;80(2):292–7.

90. Keng TB, Chong BH. Heparin-induced thrombocytopenia and thrombosis syndrome: in vivo cross-reactivity with danaparoid and successful treatment with r-Hirudin. Br J Haematol. 2001;114(2):394–6.
91. Peeters LLH, Hobbelen PMJ, Verkeste CM, Vogel GMT, Hasenack HG, Meuleman DG, et al. Placental transfer of Org-10172, a low-molecular-weight heparinoid, in the awake late pregnant guinea-pig. Thromb Res. 1986;44(3):277–83.
92. Magnani HN. An analysis of clinical outcomes of 91 pregnancies in 83 women treated with danaparoid (Orgaran). Thromb Res. 2010;125(4):297–302.
93. Chapman ML, Martinez-Borges AR, Mertz HL. Lepirudin for treatment of acute thrombosis during pregnancy. Obstet Gynecol. 2008;112(2):432–3.
94. Furlan A, Vianello F, Clementi M, Prandoni P. Heparin- induced thrombocytopenia occurring in the first trimester of pregnancy: successful treatment with lepirudin. A case report. Haematologica. 2006;91(8 Suppl):ECR40.
95. Harenberg J, Jorg I, Bayerl C, Fiehn C. Treatment of a woman with lupus pernio, thrombosis and cutaneous intolerance to heparins using lepirudin during pregnancy. Lupus. 2005;14(5):411–2.
96. Mehta R, Golichowski A. Treatment of heparin induced thrombocytopenia and thrombosis during the first trimester of pregnancy. J Thromb Haemost. 2004;2(9):1665–6.
97. Lindhoff-Last E, Bauersachs R. Heparin-induced thrombocytopenia—alternative anticoagulation in pregnancy and lactation. Semin Thromb Hemost. 2002;28(5):439–45.
98. Markwardt F, Fink G, Kaiser B, Kloecking HP, Nowak G, Richter M, et al. Pharmacological survey of recombinant hirudin. Pharmazie. 1988;43(3):202–7.
99. Bates SM, Greer IA, Pabinger I, Sofaer S, Hirsh J. Venous thromboembolism, thrombophilia, antithrombotic therapy, and pregnancy. Chest. 2008; 133(6):844S–86.
100. Mitsubishi-Pharma-Europe. Summary of product characteristics Exembol (argatroban) 100mg/mL concentrate for solution for infusion. The electronic medicines compendium. 2014. https://www.medicines.org.uk/emc/.
101. Ekbatani A, Asaro LR, Malinow AM. Anticoagulation with argatroban in a parturient with heparin-induced thrombocytopenia. Int J Obstet Anesth. 2010;19(1):82–7.
102. Tanimura K, Ebina Y, Sonoyama A, Morita H, Miyata S, Yamada H. Argatroban therapy for heparin-induced thrombocytopenia during pregnancy in a woman with hereditary antithrombin deficiency. J Obstet Gynaecol Res. 2012;38(4):749–52.
103. Young SK, Al-Mondhiry HA, Vaida SJ, Ambrose A, Botti JJ. Successful use of argatroban during the third trimester of pregnancy: case report and review of the literature. Pharmacotherapy. 2008;28(12): 1531–6.
104. Hale TW. Medication and mother's milk 2012: a manual of lactational pharmacology. 15th ed. Amarillo: Hale Publishing; 2012.
105. Wockhardt. Summary of product characteristics: Prosulf (protamine sulphate) 10mg/ml solution for injection. The electronic medicines compendium. 2010. https://www.medicines.org.uk/emc/.
106. Hirsh J, Levine MN. Low-molecular-weight heparin. Blood. 1992;79(1):1–17.
107. Majerus PW. Arachidonate metabolism in vascular disorders. J Clin Invest. 1983;72(5):1521–5.
108. Patrono C, Baigent C, Hirsh J, Roth G. Antiplatelet drugs. Chest. 2008;133(6):199S–233.
109. Loll PJ, Picot D, Garavito RM. The structural basis of aspirin activity inferred from crystal structure of inactivated prostaglandin H-2 synthase. Nat Struct Biol. 1995;2(8):637–43.
110. Roth GJ, Majerus PW. The mechanism of the effect of aspirin on human platelets. I. Acetylation of a particulate fraction protein. J Clin Invest. 1975;56(3):624–32.
111. Burch JW, Stanford N, Majerus PW. Inhibition of platelet prostaglandin synthetase by oral aspirin. J Clin Invest. 1978;61(2):314–9.
112. Patrono C, Ciabattoni G, Patrignani P, Pugliese F, Filabozzi P, Catella F, et al. Clinical-pharmacology of platelet cyclooxygenase inhibition. Circulation. 1985;72(6):1177–84.
113. Pedersen AK, Fitzgerald GA. Dose-related kinetics of aspirin—presystemic acetylation of platelet cyclooxygenase. N Engl J Med. 1984;311(19): 1206–11.
114. Bhatt DL, Scheiman J, Abraham NS, Antman EM, Chan FKL, Furberg CD, American College of Cardiology Foundation Task Force on Clinical Expert Consensus Documents, et al. ACCF/ACG/AHA 2008 expert consensus document on reducing the gastrointestinal risks of antiplatelet therapy and NSAID use. Am J Gastroenterol. 2008;103(11): 2890–907.
115. de Abajo FJ, Garcia Rodriguez LA. Risk of upper gastrointestinal bleeding and perforation associated with low-dose aspirin as plain and enteric-coated formulations. BMC Clin Pharmacol. 2001;1:1.
116. Källén BA. Use of omeprazole during pregnancy—no hazard demonstrated in 955 infants exposed during pregnancy. Eur J Obstet Gynecol Reprod Biol. 2001;96(1):63–8.
117. Diav-Citrin O, Arnon J, Shechtman S, Schaefer C, Tonningen MR, Clementi M, et al. The safety of proton pump inhibitors in pregnancy: a multicentre prospective controlled study. Aliment Pharmacol Ther. 2005;21(3):269–75.
118. Plante L, Ferron GM, Unruh M, Mayer PR. Excretion of pantoprazole in human breast milk. J Reprod Med. 2004;49(10):825–7.
119. Marshall JK, Thomson ABR, Armstrong D. Omeprazole for refractory gastroesophageal reflux disease during pregnancy and lactation. Can J Gastroenterol. 1998;12(3):225–7.
120. Tulppala M, Viinikka L, Ylikorkala O. Thromboxane dominance and prostacyclin deficiency in habitual abortion. Lancet. 1991;337(8746):879–81.

121. Ylikorkala O, Viinikka L. The role of prostaglandins in obstetrical disorders. Baillieres Clin Obstet Gynaecol. 1992;6(4):809–27.
122. Kaaja R, Julkunen H, Viinikka L, Ylikorkala O. Production of prostacyclin and thromboxane in lupus pregnancies—effect of small dose of aspirin. Obstet Gynecol. 1993;81(3):327–31.
123. Corby DG. Aspirin in pregnancy—maternal and fetal effects. Pediatrics. 1978;62(5):930–7.
124. Slone D, Siskind V, Heinonen OP, Monson RR, Kaufman DW, Shapiro S. Aspirin and congenital-malformations. Lancet. 1976;1(7974):1373–5.
125. Kozer E, Nikfar S, Costei A, Boskovic R, Nulman I, Koren G. Aspirin consumption during the first trimester of pregnancy and congenital anomalies: a meta-analysis. Am J Obstet Gynecol. 2002;187(6):1623–30.
126. Norgard B, Puho E, Czeizel AE, Skriver MV, Sorensen HT. Aspirin use during early pregnancy and the risk of congenital abnormalities: a population-based case-control study. Am J Obstet Gynecol. 2005;192(3):922–3.
127. CLASP Collaborative Group. Low dose aspirin in pregnancy and early childhood development: follow up of the collaborative low dose aspirin study in pregnancy. CLASP collaborative group. Br J Obstet Gynaecol. 1995;102(11):861–8.
128. Palmisano P, Cassady G. Salicylate exposure in the perinate. JAMA. 1969;209(4):556–8.
129. Levy G, Garretts LK. Kinetics of salicylate elimination by newborn-infants of mothers who ingested aspirin before delivery. Pediatrics. 1974;53(2):201–10.
130. Noschel H, Bonow A, Moller R, Estel C, Muller B. Placental passage of sodium salicylate. Zentralbl Gynakol. 1972;94(13):437–42.
131. Benigni A, Gregorini G, Frusca T, Chiabrando C, Ballerini S, Valcamonico A, et al. Effect of low-dose aspirin on fetal and maternal generation of thromboxane by platelets in women at risk for pregnancy-induced hypertension. N Engl J Med. 1989;321(6):357–62.
132. Viinikka L, Hartikainensorri AL, Lumme R, Hiilesmaa V, Ylikorkala O. Low-dose aspirin in hypertensive pregnant-women—effect on pregnancy outcome and prostacyclin thromboxane balance in mother and newborn. Br J Obstet Gynaecol. 1993;100(9):809–15.
133. Sibai BM, Caritis SN, Thom E, Shaw K, McNellis D. Low dose aspirin in nulliparous women—safety of continuous epidural block and correlation between bleeding time and maternal-neonatal bleeding complications. Am J Obstet Gynecol. 1995;172(5):1553–7.
134. Horlocker TT, Wedel DJ, Rowlingson JC, Enneking FK, Kopp SL, Benzon HT, et al. Regional anesthesia in the patient receiving antithrombotic or thrombolytic therapy: American Society of Regional Anesthesia and Pain Medicine Evidence-Based Guidelines (Third Edition). Reg Anesth Pain Med. 2010;35(1):64–101.
135. Gogarten W, Vandermeulen E, Van Aken H, Kozek S, Llau JV, Samama CM. Regional anaesthesia and antithrombotic agents: recommendations of the European Society of Anaesthesiology. Eur J Anaesthesiol. 2010;27(12):999–1015.
136. Lewis RB, Schulman JD. Influence of acetylsalicylic acid, an inhibitor of prostaglandin synthesis, on duration of human gestation and labor. Lancet. 1973;2(7839):1159–61.
137. Joint Formulary Committee. British National Formulary (BNF). 66th ed. London/Chicago: Pharmaceutical Press; 2013.
138. Kauffman RE, Banner W, Berlin CM, Blumer JL, Gorman RL, Lambert GH, et al. The transfer of drugs and other chemicals into human milk. Pediatrics. 1994;93(1):137–50.
139. Sweetman SC, editor. Martindale: the complete drug reference. 37th ed. London: Pharmaceutical Press; 2011.
140. Sanofi-Aventis. Summary of product characteristics: Plavix (clopidogrel) 75mg film-coated tablets. The electronic medicines Compendium. 2015. https://www.medicines.org.uk/emc/.
141. De Santis M, De Luca C, Mappa I, Cesari E, Mazza A, Quattrocchi T, et al. Clopidogrel treatment during pregnancy: a case report and a review of literature. Intern Med. 2011;50(16):1769–73.
142. Klinzing P, Markert UR, Liesaus K, Peiker G. Case report: successful pregnancy and delivery after myocardial infarction and essential thrombocythemia treated with clopidrogel. Clin Exp Obstet Gynecol. 2001;28(4):215–6.
143. Santiago-Díaz P, Arrebola-Moreno AL, Ramírez-Hernández JA, Melgares-Moreno R. Platelet antiaggregants in pregnancy. Rev Esp Cardiol. 2009;62(10):1197–8 [Article in English, Spanish].
144. Al-Aqeedi RF, Al-Nabti AD. Drug-eluting stent implantation for acute myocardial infarction during pregnancy with use of glycoprotein IIb/IIIa inhibitor, aspirin and clopidogrel. J Invasive Cardiol. 2008;20(5):E146–9.
145. Shah P, Dzavik V, Cusimano RJ, Sermer M, Okun N, Ross J. Spontaneous dissection of the left main coronary artery. Can J Cardiol. 2004;20(8):815–8.
146. Boehringer-Ingelheim. Summary of product characteristics Persantin (dipyridamol) 100mg tablets. The electronic medicines compendium. 2015.
147. Eikelboom JW, Hirsh J, Spencer FA, Baglin TP, Weitz JI. Antiplatelet drugs: Antithrombotic Therapy and Prevention of Thrombosis, 9th ed: American College of Chest Physicians Evidence-Based Clinical Practice Guidelines. Chest. 2012;141(2 Suppl):e89S–119.
148. Hall JG, Pauli RM, Wilson KM. Maternal and fetal sequelae of anticoagulation during pregnancy. Am J Med. 1980;68(1):122–40.
149. Chan WS, Anand S, Ginsberg JS. Anticoagulation of pregnant women with mechanical heart valves—a systematic review of the literature. Arch Intern Med. 2000;160(2):191–6.

150. Schaefer C, Hannemann D, Meister R, Elefant E, Paulus W, Vial T, et al. Vitamin K antagonists and pregnancy outcome—a multi-centre prospective study. Thromb Haemost. 2006;95(6):949–57.
151. Vitale N, De Feo M, De Santo LS, Pollice A, Tedesco N, Cotrufo M. Dose-dependent fetal complications of warfarin in pregnant women with mechanical heart valves. J Am Coll Cardiol. 1999;33(6): 1637–41.
152. Chong MB, Harvey D, Deswiet M. Follow-up-study of children whose mothers were treated with Warfarin during pregnancy. Br J Obstet Gynaecol. 1984;91(11):1070–3.
153. Wesseling J, Van Driel D, Heymans HSA, Rosendaal FR, Geven-Boere LM, Smrkovsky M, et al. Coumarins during pregnancy: long-term effects on growth and development of school-age children. Thromb Haemost. 2001;85(4):609–13.
154. Orme ML, Lewis PJ, Swiet MD, Serlin MJ, Sibeon R, Baty JD, et al. May mothers given warfarin breast feed their infants. Br Med J. 1977;1(6076):1564–5.
155. McKenna R, Cole ER, Vasan U. Is warfarin sodium contraindicated in the lactating mother. J Pediatr. 1983;103(2):325–7.
156. Clark SL, Porter TF, West FG. Coumarin derivatives and breast-feeding. Obstet Gynecol. 2000;95(6): 938–40.
157. Boehringer-Ingelheim. Summary of product characteristics Pradaxa 75mg, 110mg and 150mg hard capsules The electronic medicines compendium. 2013.
158. Eikelboom JW, Connolly SJ, Brueckmann M, Granger CB, Kappetein AP, Mack MJ, et al. RE-ALIGN Investigators. Dabigatran versus warfarin in patients with mechanical heart valves. N Engl J Med. 2013;369(13):1206–14.
159. Eriksson BI, Quinla DJ, Weitz JI. Comparative pharmacodynamics and pharmacokinetics of oral direct thrombin and factor Xa inhibitors in development. Clin Pharmacokinet. 2009;48(1):1–22.
160. Di Nisio M, Middeldorp S, Büller HR. Direct thrombin inhibitors. N Engl J Med. 2005;353(10): 1028–40.
161. Baetz BE, Spinler SA. Dabigatran etexilate: an oral direct thrombin inhibitor for prophylaxis and treatment of thromboembolic diseases. Pharmacotherapy. 2008;28(11):1354–73.
162. Eisert WG, Hauel N, Stangier J, Wienen W, Clemens A, van Ryn J. Dabigatran. An oral novel potent reversible nonpeptide inhibitor of thrombin. Arterioscler Thromb Vasc Biol. 2010;30(10):1885–9.
163. Perzborn E, Strassburger J, Wilmen A, Pohlmann J, Roehrig S, Schlemmer KH, et al. In vitro and in vivo studies of the novel antithrombotic agent BAY 59-7939—an oral, direct Factor Xa inhibitor. J Thromb Haemost. 2005;3(3):514–21.
164. Wong PC, Pinto DJP, Zhang D. Preclinical discovery of apixaban, a direct and orally bioavailable factor Xa inhibitor. J Thromb Thrombolysis. 2011;31(4):478–92.
165. Bayer. Summary of product characteristics Xarelto 10mg and 20mg film coated tablets. The electronic medicines compendium. 2013.
166. Bristol-Myers Squibb-Pfizer. Summary of product characteristics Eliquis (apixaban) 5mg film-coated tablets. The electronic medicines compendium. 2013.

3 Systemic Thromboembolism in Pregnancy: Heritable and Acquired Thrombophilias

Trevor Baglin

Abstract

Normal pregnancy is a hypercoagulable state. The predisposition to thrombosis may be exacerbated in women with heritable or acquired predisposition to thrombosis, known as thrombophilia. For a variety of reasons, the precise contribution of these thrombophilias to pregnancy morbidity is uncertain. However, there is evidence of an association between heritable thrombophilia and pregnancy morbidity including early and late pregnancy loss, preeclampsia, and intrauterine growth restriction. There also appears to be a weak association with placental abruption. Management of pregnant women with a thrombophilia relies on an accurate assessment of individual risk based on her personal and family history.

Keywords

Thrombophilia • Thromboembolism • Pregnancy • Hypercoagulable • Pregnancy morbidity • Pregnancy loss • Preeclampsia • Intra-uterine growth restriction

3.1 Introduction

Pregnancy results in an acquired hypercoagulable state due to pregnancy-associated changes in the hemostatic system (see Chap. 1). At delivery the placental bed spiral arteries, which lack a muscular layer, must quickly thrombose to limit and stop maternal hemorrhage. While contraction of the uterus is essential for prevention of major blood loss, it is likely that the evolutionary development of the hemostatic response to pregnancy (reviewed in Chap. 1) has provided a material survival advantage to both mother and fetus. However, the progressive hypercoagulability increases the risk of venous thrombosis during pregnancy (and the postpartum period) and in some women may contribute to pregnancy complications.

Venous thrombosis (deep vein thrombosis and pulmonary embolus, also referred to collectively as venous thromboembolism), pregnancy loss,

T. Baglin, MA, MB ChB, PhD, FRCP, FRCPath
Department of Haematology, Addenbrooke's Hospital, Cambridge University Hospitals NHS Foundation Trust, Cambridge CB2 0QQ, UK
e-mail: trevor.baglin@addenbrookes.nhs.uk

H. Cohen, P. O'Brien (eds.), *Disorders of Thrombosis and Hemostasis in Pregnancy: A Guide to Management*, DOI 10.1007/978-3-319-15120-5_3,

preeclampsia, and intrauterine growth restriction are common pregnancy complications. These risks may be amplified in women with a heritable or acquired predisposition to thrombosis, so-called thrombophilia. Testing for heritable thrombophilias in women with previous pregnancy morbidity is now common in clinical practice. Consequently, hematologists and obstetricians are frequently asked for advice on intervention with antithrombotic therapy for subsequent pregnancies in women found to have laboratory evidence of heritable thrombophilia. However, the material contribution of heritable thrombophilia to pregnancy morbidity and hence the value of testing and using the results to inform clinical management decisions are still uncertain.

- The association between a diagnosis of heritable thrombophilia and pregnancy morbidity is weak as (1) the laboratory tests are imprecise, (2) the tests performed do not comprehensively assess the genetic framework of thrombophilia, and (3) both laboratory abnormalities and pregnancy morbidity are common and so it is inevitable that abnormalities are frequently found in women who are investigated.
- If there is a true association, then causation might be expected to be related to a common underlying pathology in which the likelihood of venous thrombosis and pregnancy morbidity is increased. However, while limited, studies reported so far do not support a common underlying pathology, at least for venous thromboembolism and pregnancy loss. Furthermore, based on biological plausibility, there is reason to believe that there may be different mechanistic pathology.
- Finally, if there is a causative link between an underlying predisposition to thrombosis and pregnancy morbidity, then testing for a limited number of thrombophilias using imprecise laboratory methodology may have little theoretical or practical clinical utility as the test results do not discriminate between women with and without an underlying predisposition to pregnancy morbidity.

The management of pregnancy-associated venous thromboembolism is detailed in Chap. 5 with specific treatment in relation to heritable thrombophilia addressed in Sect. 3.4.1 below. The association of pregnancy morbidity and late pregnancy complications with hereditary and acquired thrombophilias is reviewed in detail in Chap. 4. In this chapter, generic aspects of thrombophilia are considered, and a summary is presented of:

- The spectrum of established heritable thrombophilias associated with an increased risk of venous thrombosis
- The limitations of laboratory measurement and the implications for establishing a causal relationship and developing testing strategies that might have clinical utility
- An overview of heritable thrombophilia as it relates to pregnancy-associated venous thrombosis
- An overview of heritable thrombophilia as it relates to pregnancy morbidity

Acquired conditions that predispose to venous thrombosis, which therefore increase the risk of pregnancy-associated venous thrombosis, are included for the sake of completeness alongside the definite and possible heritable thrombophilias listed in Table 3.1.

3.2 Heritable Thrombophilias Associated with an Increased Risk of Venous Thrombosis

The heritable thrombophilias shown to be associated with at least a twofold increased risk of venous thrombosis are deficiencies of the natural anticoagulants antithrombin, protein C, and protein S, due to mutations in the corresponding genes *SERPIN1*, *PROC*, and *PROS*, and the two common mutations in genes encoding pro-coagulant factor: *F5*G1691A (FVR506Q, factor V Leiden) and *F2*G20210A (commonly referred to as the prothrombin gene mutation) (Table 3.1). The causal association between these heritable thrombophilias and venous thrombosis has been confirmed by comparing the prevalence of defects in patients with venous thrombosis and controls. The expression of heritable thrombophilia as a disease (venous thrombosis) is dependent on a strong gene-environ-

Table 3.1 Heritable and acquired conditions that predispose to venous thrombosis and hence which increase the risk of pregnancy-associated venous thrombosis

Heritable thrombophilia	Possible heritable component	Acquired risk factors for venous thrombosis
Antithrombin deficiency	High factor VIII/VWF	Increasing age (over 35 in pregnancy)
Protein C deficiency	High factor IX	Pregnancy
Protein S deficiency	High factor XI	COC/HRT
*F5*G1691A (factor V Leiden)	High fibrinogen	Obesity
*F2*G20210A (Sickle and thalassaemia disorders)	Factor XIII (qualitative) High homocysteine Hypofibrinolysis	Smoking Immobility Dehydration (hyperemesis) Hospitalization Antiphospholipid syndrome (APS) Heart failure Inflammatory disease Chronic respiratory disease Nephrotic syndrome Cancer Myeloproliferative disorders (PV, ET, PMF) Paroxysmal nocturnal hemoglobinuria (PNH)

VWF Von Willebrand Factor, *COC* combined oral contraceptive, estrogen containing, *HRT* hormone replacement therapy, *PV* polycythemia vera, *ET* essential thrombocythemia, *PMF* primary myelofibrosis

ment interaction and, in this respect, there is a strong interaction with pregnancy [1].

Numerous acquired medical conditions and environmental factors increase the risk of venous thrombosis (Table 3.1). Risk factors for venous thrombosis generally interact synergistically. This means that risk factors are not additive, rather that they multiply. For example, if two risk factors A and B each increase the risk of venous thrombosis threefold, then the combination of factors increases the risk nine times (3×3), not six times (3+3). Pregnancy is an independent risk factor for venous thrombosis, so the presence of additional heritable and acquired thrombophilias and environmental factors act synergistically to increase the risk of venous thrombosis in pregnancy. The baseline risk of venous thrombosis in women of reproductive age is low at approximately 1 per 10,000. Consequently, the relative increased risk of venous thrombosis associated with pregnancy translates into an absolute risk of only 1 per 1,000 live births overall. However, in an individual woman, a relative increase in risk due to multiple interacting factors may translate into a high absolute risk. This is the basis for assessing the risk of venous thrombosis and offering thromboprophylaxis in high-risk pregnancies (see Chap. 5).

3.2.1 Antithrombin Deficiency

Antithrombin is a protease inhibitor. Based on kinetic rates of inhibition, its primary targets are thrombin and factor Xa, and hence antithrombin both regulates generation of thrombin and inhibits thrombin that has been generated. Inhibition of target proteases is increased approximately 1,000-fold by glycosaminoglycan activation of antithrombin, which is the mechanism by which heparin acts as a pharmacological anticoagulant. The activation process involves an induced conformational change in the structure of antithrombin which enables formation of an irreversible covalent complex with the target protease [2]. The complex undergoes a further dramatic conformational change involving both the inhibitor and the inhibited protein which alters the properties of each, resulting in rapid clearance from the circulation.

Two laboratory (intermediate) phenotypes of heritable antithrombin deficiency are recognized. Type I is characterized by a quantitative reduction of antithrombin with a parallel reduction in function (measured as inhibitory activity against factor Xa or thrombin) and the level of protein in the plasma (measured immunologically as the antigenic level). Type 2 deficiency is due to the production of a qualitatively abnormal antithrombin protein characterized by disturbance of the complex inhibitory mechanism of protease inhibition as a result of a mutation in the *SERPINC1* gene. The functional activity is discrepantly low compared to the antigenic level. Type 2 deficiency is subclassified according to the nature of the functional deficit:

- Type 2 reactive site (RS) in which mutations alter the sequence of the mobile reactive center loop, thus reducing the ability to inhibit thrombin or factor Xa either in the presence or absence of heparin in a laboratory assay
- Type 2 heparin binding site (HBS) in which mutations affect the ability of antithrombin to bind and be activated by glycosaminoglycans, resulting in reduced ability to inhibit thrombin or factor Xa only in the presence of heparin in a laboratory assay
- Type 2 pleiotropic (PE) in which a single mutation produces multiple effects on the structure-function relationship of the molecule which is often associated with low plasma levels due to effects on either secretion or stability

Approximately 100 point mutations (missense, nonsense, or insertions or deletions causing frameshifts) and several whole or partial gene deletions have been identified as causes of type 1 deficiency. Numerous point mutations causing qualitative type 2 deficiency have been identified. Homozygous type 1 deficiency and type 2RS mutations are incompatible with life. Type 2 HBS and some PE mutations are associated with a lower risk of thrombosis; homozygosity, and compound heterozygosity, involving these mutations is compatible with life.

Functional activity assays typically use a chromogenic substrate and factor Xa as the target protease. The total amount of antithrombin protein can be measured immunologically with antibodies, for example, by enzyme-linked immunosorbent assay (ELISA). As antithrombin antigen levels may be normal or near normal in type 2 deficiency, immunological assays may fail to identify patients with these variants and so a functional assay should be used as the initial assay.

Although there is little reported variation in the plasma concentration of antithrombin both during healthy pregnancy and following delivery (as stated in Chap. 1), antithrombin levels may be slightly reduced in pregnancy and are reduced in women taking estrogen preparations, as well as in other situations. Consequently, the clinical significance of a low antithrombin level must be interpreted by an experienced clinician who is aware of all the relevant factors that may have influenced the test result in a specific patient.

3.2.2 Protein C Deficiency

Protein C is the zymogen precursor of activated protein C (APC). Protein C is activated to APC by thrombin bound to thrombomodulin on the endothelial surface. APC inactivates the activated cofactors (VIIIa and Va) and so inhibits thrombin generation. Factors VIII and V are activated by small amounts of thrombin during initiation of coagulation to nonenzymatic cofactors required for assembly of macromolecular complexes that are required for the full thrombin explosion. The enzymatic components of these complexes are factors IXa and Xa, and so inactivation of VIIIa and Va by APC leads to disassembly of the enzymatic complexes, thus attenuating thrombin generation.

Protein C deficiency is classified into type 1 and 2 defects on the basis of functional and antigenic assays. The relative risk of thrombosis in relation to type 1 and the various type 2 defects has not been characterized. Most heritable protein C deficiency is due to type 1 abnormalities. The majority of type 1 defects are due to point mutations. Multiple type 2 defects due to mutations in the *PROC* gene have been reported affecting the catalytic active site, the phospholipid-binding Gla domain, the propeptide cleavage activation site, and the sites of interaction with substrates or cofactors. In this case, there is discordance between the functional and antigenic levels.

The laboratory diagnosis of protein C deficiency is based on a functional assay. As protein C antigen levels may be normal or near normal in type 2 deficiency, immunological assays may fail to identify patients with these variants, so a functional assay should be used as the initial assay. Most commercially available functional assays use a snake venom to activate protein C and a chromogenic substrate to quantify APC activity. A chromogenic assay will detect type 1 and most type 2 defects. The diagnosis of type 1 protein C deficiency is problematic because of the wide overlap in protein C activity between heterozygous carriers and unaffected individuals. The diagnosis of type 2 defects is problematic because a chromogenic assay will only detect defects affecting the enzymatic site.

Protein C levels are not affected by pregnancy or estrogen exposure. Acquired low levels of protein C occur during anticoagulant therapy with oral vitamin K antagonists, vitamin K deficiency, disseminated intravascular coagulation (DIC), and liver disease. Consequently, the clinical significance of a low protein C level must be interpreted by an experienced clinician who is aware of all the relevant factors that may have influenced the test result in a specific patient.

3.2.3 Protein S Deficiency

Protein S is a vitamin K-dependent glycoprotein produced in the liver, endothelial cells, and megakaryocytes. Protein S is a nonenzymatic cofactor for APC-mediated inactivation of factors VIIIa and Va and additionally is involved with tissue factor pathway inhibitor-dependent natural anticoagulation. Approximately 60 % of protein S circulates bound to C4b-binding protein and is inactive. The remaining 40 %, designated free protein S, is uncomplexed and is the active form. Free protein S increases the affinity of activated protein C for negatively charged phospholipid surfaces on platelets or the endothelium and increases complex formation of APC with the activated forms of factors VIII and V (VIIIa & Va). However, the degree of C4b binding has not yet been shown to be a determinant of thrombosis risk. In addition to APC cofactor activity, protein S has an independent anticoagulant activity as a cofactor for TFPI (tissue factor pathway inhibitor).

Protein S is usually quantified immunologically rather than measured functionally. Nowadays, monoclonal antibodies that detect only free protein are used to quantify free protein S. Functional protein S assays are imprecise and are not used in the majority of coagulation laboratories.

Protein S levels are significantly lower in females, so much so that different normal reference ranges are required for males and females. There is a significant risk of a false-positive diagnosis of protein S deficiency in women. Protein S levels are reduced by estrogens and fall progressively during normal pregnancy. Acquired low levels of protein S occur during anticoagulant therapy with oral vitamin K antagonists, vitamin K deficiency, DIC, and liver disease.

Protein S defects are divided into three types:

- In type I deficiency, both total and free protein S levels are low (and functional activity, if measured, is found to be low).
- Type II defects are characterized by reduced activity in the presence of normal total and free levels of protein S. Type II deficiency is difficult to diagnose because functional protein S assays are imprecise.
- In type III deficiency, the total protein S level is normal but the free protein S level is low. Some type III deficiency is thought to be a phenotypic variation of type 1 resulting from the same genetic mutations. However, it is now apparent that many patients with an apparent type III phenotype do not have heritable protein S deficiency. This may be related to an increase in C4b levels.

This complicated classification reflects the complexity of the biology of protein S but has no mechanistic reference to disturbance of natural anticoagulant activity. Given these limitations and the imprecision of laboratory methodology, the diagnosis of heritable protein S deficiency is less precise and the clinical implication of a low protein S level in an individual is more uncertain than it is for antithrombin or protein C.

3.2.4 *F5*G1691A (FVR506Q, Factor V Leiden)

Factor V is a cofactor required for thrombin generation. Factor V has no cofactor activity until cleaved by thrombin or factor Xa. Activated factor V (Va) is inactivated by APC (see Sect. 3.2.2 above). Resistance to activated protein C (APC resistance) is a laboratory phenomenon in which there is a suboptimal anticoagulant response to addition of APC to a patient's plasma. In 95 % of cases of familial APC resistance, this is due to the same point mutation in the gene for FV, a guanine to adenine transition at nucleotide position 1691 in exon 10 (*F5*G1691A), resulting in a mutant protein FVR506Q. The mutation is known as the factor V Leiden mutation and the mutant factor Va has normal procoagulant activity, but substitution of glutamine for arginine at position 506 (which is an APC cleavage site) results in slower inactivation by APC. Nowadays, the mutation is frequently detected by direct DNA analysis (rather than by a clotting assay) to detect the presence of the mutant protein.

The mutation is present in around 4 % of the Caucasian population and around 15 % of unselected consecutive Caucasian patients with a first venous thrombosis. The prevalence is highest in Northern Europeans. The mutation is infrequent in other populations. The high prevalence and founder effect suggest positive selection, and this may relate to a favorable effect on embryo implantation and hence reproduction [3] rather than a lower risk of fatal hemorrhage in females during childbirth, as originally thought.

Acquired APC resistance is common, in part often due to increased FVIII levels, and is observed in pregnancy and in association with estrogen exposure.

3.2.5 *F2*G20210A

A single nucleotide change of guanine to adenine at position 20210 in the 3′ untranslated region of the prothrombin gene is a mild risk factor for venous thrombosis. The prevalence of the *F2*G20210A mutation is around 2 % in Caucasians with a higher prevalence in Southern compared to Northern Europeans. The mutation increases the plasma level of prothrombin by around 30 %, but the mechanism responsible for this has not been identified. No specific clotting test for the presence of the mutation has been described, and diagnosis depends on detection of the genetic mutation by DNA analysis.

3.2.6 Other Candidate Heritable Thrombophilias

A number of other anticoagulant proteins have been investigated as potential factors causing thrombophilia, but a relationship between venous thrombosis and low protein levels or associated gene mutations has not been established.

Increased levels of factors VIII, IX, and XI are associated with an increased risk of venous thrombosis, but a heritable basis for high levels associated with venous thrombosis is not established. There is equivocal evidence for a causal relationship between fibrinogen levels and venous thrombosis. Polymorphisms in the prothrombin gene have been described that may further increase the risk of venous thrombosis associated with the *F2*G20210A mutation, but the effect is mild. It was previously thought that deficiency of factor XII was a risk factor for venous thromboembolism, but subsequent investigation strongly indicates that this is unlikely. A protective effect against venous thrombosis has been reported for a polymorphism in the factor XIII gene (FXIIIV341L).

A causal relationship between levels of specific individual proteins involved in regulating fibrinolysis and venous thrombosis has not been established. However, in a case–control study using a global measure of fibrinolytic potential, there was an approximately doubled risk of venous thrombosis in patients with clot lysis times above the 90th percentile of controls [4]. Further analysis of a larger study confirmed this finding and demonstrated that hypofibrinolysis in combination with established acquired and genetic risk factors, such as *F5*G1691A, had a synergistic effect on venous thrombosis risk [5].

The genetic basis for hypofibrinolysis in these patients was not investigated.

Hyperhomocysteinemia may be caused by genetic abnormalities but only the severe inherited abnormalities of homocysteine metabolism (homozygous cystathionine beta-synthase deficiency and homozygous deficiency of methylenetetrahydrofolate reductase) result in congenital homocystinuria associated with an increased risk of both arterial and venous thrombosis, as well as premature atherosclerosis and mental retardation, epilepsy, and skeletal and eye problems. Fifty percent of patients present with venous or arterial thrombosis before the age of 30 years. The thermolabile variant of methylenetetrahydrofolate reductase (MTHFR), due to a common genetic polymorphism (C677T), is not a risk factor for venous thrombosis [6, 7].

3.2.7 Antiphospholipid Syndrome (APS)

The antiphospholipid syndrome (APS) is the most common acquired form of thrombophilia. APS is diagnosed when a patient with arterial or venous thrombosis (or pregnancy morbidity in women) is found to have antiphospholipid antibodies (anticardiolipin, aCL; and/or lupus anticoagulant, LA; and/or anti-beta-2-glycoprotein I, aß$_2$-GPI). The updated international consensus (revised Sapporo) classification criteria for definite antiphospholipid syndrome [8] require the presence of a LA and/or IgG or IgM aCL present in medium or high titer (i.e., >40 GPL or MPL or > the 99th percentile) and/or aß$_2$GPI (IgG and/or IgM) >99th percentile. These aPL should be persistent, defined as being present on two or more consecutive occasions at least 12 weeks apart. The international consensus criteria were originally designed for scientific clinical studies, and there remains a need for firm diagnostic criteria for routine clinical use which may differ from these. APS has conventionally been divided into primary and secondary forms, the latter being associated with systemic lupus erythematosus (SLE) or a related rheumatological condition. However, this distinction was abandoned in the revised Sapporo classification [8] on the basis that it is unknown whether APS and SLE are two diseases coinciding in an individual, underlying SLE offers a setting for the development of APS, or APS and SLE represent two elements of the same process.

Laboratory test results are subject to considerable pre-analytical variation. In addition, transiently abnormal results may be found in normal healthy individuals. For these reasons, for a patient to be considered to have antiphospholipid activity (aCL, LA, or aß2-GPI), test results must be positive on two separate occasions. The probability of misdiagnosing APS has been reduced by stricter criteria for antibody titers (>40 GPL or MPL for aCL or >90th percentile for aCL or aß2-GPI) and demonstration of persistence of antibodies (present on at least 2 consecutive occasions at least 12 weeks apart) [9]. Positivity in all 3 assays (aCL, LA, aß2-GPI) is associated most strongly with thrombosis and pregnancy complications. Recent evidence suggests that the antibodies most strongly associated with thrombosis and pregnancy morbidity are against domain I of β2-GPI; these antibodies are responsible for lupus anticoagulant activity specifically associated with clinical events and are responsible for positive aCL results. While the criteria for diagnosis of APS are unlikely to change again soon, it is possible that the laboratory identification of clinically relevant antibodies to domain I β2-GPI will eventually simplify the diagnosis and improve the clinical utility of laboratory tests.

3.3 Limitations of Laboratory Measurement and the Implications for Establishing a Causal Relationship and Developing Testing Strategies with Clinical Utility

The laboratory diagnosis of heritable thrombophilias is difficult as the tests are subject to considerable pre-analytical variables. Low levels of antithrombin, protein C, and protein S occur in a variety of circumstances and test results, and the clinical implications of both positive and negative results, are frequently misinterpreted. If testing is performed during pregnancy, results must be interpreted with reference to the effect of the pregnancy.

Functional assays should be used for which accuracy and imprecision are acceptable. However, no single method will detect all defects. Even in families with characterized defects, a phenotypic assay may fail to accurately discriminate affected and nonaffected individuals. True heritable deficiencies may not be detected and false positive diagnoses are common.

Low levels of antithrombin, protein C, or protein S may relate to age, sex, acquired illness, or drug therapy, so interpretation requires knowledge of the patient's condition at the time of blood sampling. Low levels of antithrombin, protein C, or protein S suspected to be the result of heritable mutations should be confirmed on one or more separate samples. Demonstrating a low level in other family members supports a diagnosis of heritable deficiency, and characterization of the genetic mutation can be confirmatory.

As well as specific limitations relating to individual factors, there are a number of common generic issues which limit accuracy and precision of laboratory diagnosis and consequently contribute to limiting the clinical utility of thrombophilia testing. These can be summarized as follows:

- The laboratory diagnosis of heritable thrombophilias is difficult as the tests are subject to numerous biological and pre-analytical variables.
- The fact that venous thrombosis has a multiple genetic basis with incomplete penetrance and a strong gene-environment interaction makes counseling in relation to thrombophilia testing uncertain.
- In families with known heritable thrombophilias, the risk of venous thrombosis can be increased in unaffected members as well as affected, so a negative thrombophilia result does not exclude an increased risk of venous thrombosis.
- Even in families with characterized defects, a phenotypic assay may fail to accurately discriminate affected and nonaffected individuals.
- True heritable deficiencies may not be detected and false positive diagnoses are common.
- Low levels of antithrombin, protein C, and protein S occur in a variety of circumstances, and test results and the clinical implications of both positive and negative results are frequently misinterpreted.
- Testing for heritable thrombophilias in selected patients, such as those with a strong family history of unprovoked recurrent thrombosis, may influence decisions regarding duration of anticoagulation. Unfortunately, in this regard, identifying patients for testing is not straightforward as criteria for defining thrombosis-prone families have not been validated and the association between family history of thrombosis and detection of inherited thrombophilia is weak.

In order to limit inaccuracy and imprecision, the British Society for Haematology has published clinical guidelines for testing for heritable thrombophilia [10] which include the following generic recommendations:

- Testing at the time of acute venous thrombosis is not indicated as the utility and implications of testing need to be considered and the patient needs to be counseled before testing. As treatment of acute venous thrombosis is not influenced by test results, testing can be performed later.
- The prothrombin time (PT) should be measured to detect the effect of oral vitamin K antagonists which will cause a reduction in protein C and S levels.
- Functional assays should be used to determine antithrombin and protein C levels.
- Chromogenic assays of protein C activity are less subject to interference than clotting assays and are therefore preferable.
- Immunoreactive assays of free protein S antigen are preferable to functional assays. If a protein S activity assay is used in the initial screen, low results should be further investigated with an immunoreactive assay of free protein S.

- Repeat testing for identification of deficiency of antithrombin, protein C, and protein S is indicated, and a low level should be confirmed on one or more separate samples. Deficiency should not be diagnosed on the basis of a single abnormal result.

In addition to factors that limit the accuracy and precision of laboratory testing, there is potentially a fundamental flaw in attempting to quantify the degree of thrombophilia in an individual patient by using a dichotomous testing strategy in which a limited number of factors are designated normal or abnormal. The "thrombophilic condition" is dependent on a large complex genetic framework subject to strong environmental influence [1, 11, 12].

3.4 Overview of Heritable Thrombophilia as It Relates to Pregnancy-Associated Venous Thrombosis

3.4.1 Treatment of Pregnancy-Associated Venous Thrombosis

There are limited data in relation to treatment specifically of pregnancy-associated venous thrombosis in women with heritable thrombophilia. However, there is no evidence that issues that have been clarified in nonpregnant patients are different in pregnant women:

- There is no evidence that heritable thrombophilia should influence the initial intensity of anticoagulation with heparin.
- When warfarin is introduced following delivery, there is no evidence that heritable thrombophilia should influence the intensity of anticoagulation.
- Warfarin-induced skin necrosis is extremely rare, even in patients with protein C or S deficiency, such that most individuals with protein C or S deficiency do not develop skin necrosis.
- There is no evidence that recurrent venous thrombosis while on anticoagulant treatment is more likely in patients with heritable thrombophilia.

In nonpregnant patients with antithrombin deficiency, heparin resistance is infrequent and recurrence or extension of thrombosis while on treatment is no more frequent than that observed in individuals without antithrombin deficiency. However, there are anecdotes of pregnant women with heritable antithrombin deficiency who have low anti-Xa levels despite therapeutic doses of low-molecular-weight heparin. It is advisable for pregnant women with venous thrombosis and antithrombin deficiency to be referred urgently to a hematologist with appropriate expertise for supervision of treatment.

The most important clinical factor predicting likelihood of recurrent venous thrombosis is whether or not a first episode of venous thrombosis was unprovoked or provoked. Pregnancy is a relatively strong provocation for venous thrombosis and the risk of spontaneous recurrent venous thrombosis after pregnancy-associated venous thrombosis in women with heritable thrombophilia is low, and long-term anticoagulation is not indicated. Long-term prospective cohort outcome studies have shown that finding a heritable thrombophilia does not reliably predict recurrence in unselected patients even after an episode of unprovoked venous thrombosis. However, studies were not powered to exclude an increased risk of recurrence specifically in relation to rare thrombophilias, such as antithrombin or protein C deficiency. Therefore, it remains uncertain if mutations affecting the *SERPINC1*, *PROC*, and *PROS* genes causing deficiency of the corresponding protein might predict a sufficiently high risk of thrombosis to justify long-term (life-long) anticoagulation after a single episode of venous thrombosis. Following an episode of pregnancy-associated venous thrombosis, women with heritable thrombophilia should be referred to a thrombophilia specialist for consideration of future management, including duration of anticoagulation and need for thromboprophylaxis in subsequent pregnancies.

3.4.2 Prevention of Pregnancy-Associated Venous Thrombosis

Pregnancy is associated with a five to tenfold increased risk of venous thrombosis compared to nonpregnant women of comparable age and has an absolute risk of 1 per 1,000 deliveries. There is an increased relative risk of pregnancy-associated venous thrombosis in women with thrombophilia (Table 3.2), but this translates into a low absolute risk. For example, the relative risks of 34 and 8 associated with homozygosity and heterozygosity for the factor V Leiden mutation, respectively equate to absolute risks of 3.4 and 0.8 %, based on an overall absolute risk of 0.1 % (1 per 1,000 deliveries). Based on the calculated odds ratios in Table 3.2, absolute risks of pregnancy-associated venous thrombosis would only be expected to exceed 1 % for homozygosity for the factor V Leiden mutation. However, where a statistically significant increase in risk is demonstrated, the possibility of rates greater than 1 % cannot be excluded (based on the upper 95 % confidence intervals) for deficiencies of antithrombin, protein C, and protein S; heterozygosity for the *F5*G1691A (factor V Leiden); and homozygous and heterozygous *F2*G20210A mutations. Homozygosity for the thermolabile variant of MTHFR (C677T) is not associated with an increased risk of pregnancy-associated venous thrombosis (Table 3.2).

The risk of thrombosis, compared to the general age-matched female population, is increased 100-fold in pregnancy in women with a previous thrombosis. Thrombosis in pregnancy rarely occurs in women whose initial venous thrombosis was provoked, unless the provocation was use of an estrogen-containing contraceptive. In general, the absolute risk of pregnancy-associated venous thrombosis in women with heritable thrombophilia with no previous history is small, but the risk is considered greatest in women with antithrombin deficiency, those homozygous for the FVR506Q or the *F2*G20210A mutations or those who are double heterozygotes for FVR506Q and *F2*G20210A. The number of women with these defects is very small. The most appropriate management of these women is uncertain and recommendations are based on low-level evidence. Retrospective studies in women with laboratory evidence of thrombophilia and previous venous thrombosis for whom detailed information of the type of thrombophilia was available indicate that the rate of recurrence is similar in women with and without thrombophilia. However, a limitation of studies published to date is that women with high-risk thrombophilias were excluded (deficiency of antithrombin, protein C, and protein S, and combined defects).

In women with a previous history of venous thrombosis, the major factor in determining whether prophylaxis should be given is whether or not the prior venous thrombosis was provoked. If the episode was unprovoked, prophylaxis should be considered and thrombophilia testing is not required if prophylaxis is given. In women with a first provoked event, the decision to test or not should be influenced by the strength of the provocation, for example, thrombosis associated with major trauma and subsequent immobility would not be an indication for prophylaxis or testing. In women with a first-degree relative with thrombosis, the decision to test should be influenced by whether or not the event in the relative was unprovoked or provoked and the strength of the provocation. If the event in the first-degree relative was pregnancy or COC-associated, then testing and finding thrombophilia should prompt consideration of prophylaxis, particularly if the symptomatic relative was known to have the same defect, especially deficiency of antithrombin or protein C. When testing in pregnancy is performed, it is necessary to interpret the results with reference to the effect of pregnancy on the test results.

Table 3.2 Results of systematic review of thrombophilia in pregnancy

	Pregnancy-associated VTE	Recurrent pregnancy loss in first trimester	Non-recurrent second trimester loss	Late pregnancy loss	Preeclampsia	Intrauterine growth restriction
Antithrombin deficiency	(8/11)/(242/815)			(1/1)/(17/61)	(1/1)/(57/131)	
	4.7	–	–	7.6	3.9	–
	(1.3–17.0)			(0.3–196)	(0.2–97)	
Protein C deficiency	(23/32)/(232/715)			(3/234)/(18/524)	(3/3)/(60/104)	
	4.8	–	–	3.0	5.1	–
	(2.1–10.6)			(0.2–38.5)	(0.3–102)	
Protein S deficiency	(16/28)/(250/911)			(14/15)/(258/801)	(14/20)/(158/402)	
	3.2	–	–	20.1	2.8	–
	(1.5–6.9)			(3.7–109)	(0.8–10.6)	
Homozygous *F5*G1691A	(29/91)/(145/1,248)	Heterozygous and homozygous	–	(7/212)/(2/118)	(4/5)/(608/1,143)	(1/1)/(60/153)
	34.4			2.0	1.9	4.6
	(9.9–120)			(0.4–9.7)	(0.4–7.9)	(0.2–115)
Heterozygous *F5*G1691A	(96/226)/(263/1,595)	(173/287)/(1,390/2,285)	(34/58)/(98/432)	(27/382)/(124/1,121)	(161/249)/(1,790/3,673)	(25/49)/(512/1,147)
	8.3	**1.9**	**4.12**	**2.1**	**2.2**	2.7
	(5.4–12.7)	(1.01–3.6)	(1.9–8.8)	(1.1–3.9)	(1.5–3.3)	(0.6–12.1)
Homozygous *F2*G20210A	(2/2)/(40/253)	–	–	–	–	–
	26.4					
	(1.2–559)					
Heterozygous *F2*G20210A	(42/61)/(277/1,005)	(54/78)/(627/1,428)	(4/11)/(22/271)	(15/36)/(348/1,134)	(42/71)/(937/2,028)	(25/44)/(583/1,375)
	6.8	**2.7**	8.6	**2.7**	**2.5**	2.9
	(2.5–18.8)	(1.4–5.3)	(2.2–34)	(1.3–5.5)	(1.5–4.2)	(0.6–13.7)
Homozygous MTHFR (C677T)	(20/128)/(89/543)	(22/39)/(21/368)		(69/323)/(198/1,059)	(221/482)/(1,234/3,205)	(62/121)/(460/961)
	0.7	0.9	–	1.3	**1.4**	1.2
	(0.2–2.5)	(0.4–1.7)		(0.9–1.9)	(1.1–1.8)	(0.8–1.8)

(continued)

Table 3.2 (continued)

	Pregnancy-associated VTE	Recurrent pregnancy loss in first trimester	Non-recurrent second trimester loss	Late pregnancy loss	Preeclampsia	Intrauterine growth restriction
Hyperhomocysteinemia	(33/37)/(128/235)	(12/16)/(47/113)		(2/7)/(16/55)	(37/41)/(257/364)	
	6.2	4.3	–	1.0	**3.5**	–
	(1.4–28.4)	(1.3–13.9)		(0.2–5.6)	(1.2–10.1)	
Lupus anticoagulant	(59/107)/(581/1,728)		(9/17)/(13/178)	(15/242)/(124/730)	(63/89)/(426/981)	
	3.0	–	14.3	2.4	1.5	–
	(1.03–8.6)		(4.7–43)	(0.8–7.0)	(0.8–4.6)	
Anticardiolipin antibodies	(127/149)/(869/1,956)	(116/120)/(551/647)		(52/242)/(124/730)	(130/217)/(803/2,428)	(7/60)/(15/800)
	3.4	**5.0**	–	**3.3**	**2.7**	**6.9**
	(1.3–8.7)	(1.8–14.0)		(1.6–6.7)	(1.7–4.5)	(2.7–17.7)

Data from Robertson et al. [13]

Each box indicates in brackets number of women in total (women with thrombophilia/women with event)/(women with no thrombophilia/women with event), odds ratios calculated on the random effects model (not the fixed effect model) to provide a more conservative result, indicated to 1 decimal place with 95 % confidence intervals in brackets.

Statistically significant results are indicated in bold if n >20 for thrombophilia group

In summary:

- Women should be assessed for risk of pregnancy-associated venous thrombosis primarily in relation to clinical risk factors; this assessment should be performed when first seen in pregnancy and again if circumstances change during pregnancy, for example, the woman develops preeclampsia or is admitted to hospital.
- Most women with a previous unprovoked venous thrombosis or pregnancy or COC-related thrombosis will qualify for thromboprophylaxis on the basis of clinical risk alone, so testing for heritable thrombophilia may not be contributory.
- Women with a previous event due to a major provoking factor, for example, surgery or major trauma, would not usually require prophylaxis or testing.
- Women with a previous event due to a minor provoking factor, for example, travel, should be tested and considered for prophylaxis if a thrombophilia is found.
- In asymptomatic women with a family history of venous thrombosis, testing is not required if the clinical risks alone are sufficient to result in thromboprophylaxis during pregnancy.
- Asymptomatic women with a family history of venous thrombosis should be tested if an event in a first-degree relative was unprovoked or provoked by pregnancy, COC exposure, or a minor risk factor. The result will be more informative if the first-degree relative has a known thrombophilia, so the interpretation of the result in the asymptomatic woman is with reference to the defect in the symptomatic affected relative.

3.5 Overview of Heritable Thrombophilia as It Relates to Pregnancy Morbidity

There is evidence of an association between heritable thrombophilia and pregnancy morbidity including early and late pregnancy loss, preeclampsia, and intrauterine growth restriction. There also appears to be a weak association with placental abruption [13]. A simple hypothesis is that thrombophilia may increase the risk of placental insufficiency due to placental vascular thrombosis. If thrombophilia results in pathology which mechanistically results from thrombosis, it might be expected that women with a predisposition to venous thrombosis would have a higher incidence of pregnancy morbidity thought to be due to placental vascular thrombosis. However, in a case–control study, pregnancy loss was no more frequent in women with a history of venous thrombosis than in controls, although pregnancy-induced hypertension and preeclampsia were more common. The stillbirth rate was not significantly higher [14]. The placental vasculature is not formed until 10–12 weeks of gestation so a thrombotic pathology does not explain why the majority of women with thrombophilia have early pregnancy loss before 12 weeks. An alternative "non-thrombotic" hypothesis is that trophoblast apoptosis is the underlying mechanism. In vitro studies have demonstrated that antiphospholipid antibodies inhibit trophoblast differentiation and placentation [15, 16]. Experimental studies in mice with genetic disruption of the protein C pathway indicate that the fetal loss that occurs before 10 weeks is similarly due to inhibition of trophoblast growth by coagulation proteases [17].

Meta-analysis indicates an increased prevalence of thrombophilias in case–control studies comparing women with pregnancy complications to those without. However, the point estimates of odds ratios calculated from case–control studies are low, indicating that any causal association is weak. Importantly, the predictive value of a positive thrombophilia test result for recurrence of a particular pregnancy complication has not yet been determined. Randomized trials demonstrating that the presence of a thrombophilia should modify management of subsequent pregnancies have yet to be reported. Nevertheless, many clinicians have instituted a policy of offering anticoagulant drugs to women with a history of pregnancy morbidity, particularly recurrent miscarriage or stillbirth, on the basis of finding laboratory evidence of a thrombophilic defect. Thromboprophylactic dose of low-molecular-weight heparin (LMWH) is usually the preferred option and, while the risk of treatment is low, it is not zero. Allergic skin reactions occur in 1–2 % [18] although heparin-induced thrombocytopenia with thrombosis that often manifests with skin necrosis at injection sites rarely if ever occurs in pregnancy. Regional analgesia is considered to be contraindicated if within 12 h of subcutaneous prophylactic dose heparin [19]. There seems to be little if any risk of osteoporosis with the use of low-dose LMWH for the duration of a pregnancy. A review of almost 3,000 women prescribed low-dose LMWH in pregnancy revealed a very low incidence of complications including bleeding [18].

Systematic reviews of the results of studies reported up to 2005 investigating the association between heritable thrombophilia and pregnancy loss have been published [13, 20–22]. The summary of results of the most recent is shown in Table 3.2.

3.5.1 Pregnancy Loss

The largest study of pregnancy loss and thrombophilia investigated an association with the factor V Leiden mutation in over 1,000 consecutive Caucasian women [23]. No association was demonstrated with congenital APC resistance (due to the factor V Leiden mutation), but acquired APC resistance was more common in women with a history of miscarriage. Acquired APC resistance reflects the physiological hypercoagulable state of pregnancy, and there may be an association between pregnancy loss and other pregnancy morbidity; however, in this study, the women were tested in the non-pregnant state. A retrospective analysis of 64 women homozygous for the factor V Leiden mutation compared pregnancy outcomes to those in 54 age-matched control women [24]. The stillbirth rate in the affected women was 3.3 % compared to 1.7 % in the controls and rates of miscarriage were 12 and 10 % respectively, results that were not significantly different. While the statistically insignificant results may have resulted from the low power of the study, a major difference in outcome between heterozygous and homozygous women is unlikely, a finding suggested also by systematic review (Table 3.2). The only prospective controlled study investigating the association between heritable thrombophilia and pregnancy loss showed no increased risk in 48 affected women compared to 60 controls [25].

The systematic review published by Robertson and colleagues [13] showed that recurrent first trimester pregnancy loss in association with anticardiolipin antibodies was higher than for any heritable thrombophilia, and second trimester pregnancy loss was strongly associated with lupus anticoagulant activity (Table 3.2). Late pregnancy loss appeared to be most strongly associated with protein S deficiency, but the number of women with protein S deficiency was only 15 and, as indicated in Sect. 3.3, the diagnosis of heritable protein S deficiency is often inaccurate.

Individual studies have produced conflicting findings on the association between MTHFR homozygosity and recurrent pregnancy loss: some found an association [26, 27] but others did not [28–30], and a meta-analysis suggested that there is no association (Table 3.2). Adequate folic acid supplementation silences the phenotypic expression of this polymorphism.

3.5.2 Preeclampsia and Intrauterine Growth Restriction

The association between heritable thrombophilia and preeclampsia and intrauterine growth restriction appears to be similar to other pregnancy morbidity, but fewer data are available. Anticardiolipin antibodies appear to be relatively strongly associated with growth restriction (Table 3.2).

A meta-analysis suggested that MTHFR homozygosity was associated with an increased risk only for preeclampsia (Table 3.2). However, this polymorphism may be associated with an increased risk of other pregnancy complications, including placental abruption or infarction [31], preeclampsia [32, 33] and pregnancy-induced hypertension [34]. As mentioned above, adequate folic acid supplementation silences the phenotypic expression of this polymorphism.

3.5.3 Recommendations

Randomized controlled trials, with a no treatment or a placebo arm, in women with a history of pregnancy complications are in progress. The British Society for Haematology has recommended that results from these trials should be awaited before recommending that anticoagulant drugs are given to pregnant women based on testing for heritable thrombophilia, but the issue remains contentious [10]. Provisional studies suggest a benefit of intervention in women with thrombophilia but the benefit, if true, may not be restricted to women with thrombophilia. In small studies, live birth rates of around 70 % were reported compared to live birth rates of around 30 % in previous pregnancies. However, these studies involved small cohorts and there were no control groups. If hypercoagulability, and a related mechanism such as protease-induced trophoblastic apoptosis, is a material contributory factor in many cases of pregnancy morbidity, then administration of low-dose LMWH may be beneficial regardless of whether or not there is laboratory evidence of thrombophilia. If there is an increased relative risk in women with a laboratory "marker," then a beneficial effect will be more readily demonstrated in women with thrombophilia, even though the magnitude of benefit may be the same in women with the same underlying pathology but no identifiable thrombophilia "marker." Therefore, until the results of trials in women at high risk of pregnancy complications and the results of trials specifically in women with thrombophilia are known, many experts suggest that decisions to use low-dose heparin for prevention of pregnancy morbidity should not be made in relation to the results of thrombophilia tests.

In all future studies, criteria for both diagnosis of heritable thrombophilia and pregnancy morbidity must be clearly defined a priori [35]. Many studies to date have not defined criteria for the diagnosis of thrombophilia, they have often relied on results of single laboratory measurements in individuals, and they have not used strict criteria for pregnancy morbidity, for example, the use of ultrasound for accurate clinical assessment.

3.6 Purpura Fulminans in the Newborn

Purpura fulminans is a rare syndrome characterized by progressive hemorrhagic skin necrosis that occurs in neonates with congenital severe protein C or S deficiency at birth or in the first few days of life (an alternative form of the condition occurs in association with infection in children and adults, and this condition is typically associated with acquired severe protein S deficiency). If a neonate develops purpura fulminans, levels of protein C and S should be measured urgently. Levels are normally low at birth, but the condition is associated with undetectable levels. Measurement of levels in the parents may help to interpret the neonate's results. Neonatal purpura fulminans due to deficiency of protein C or S requires urgent replacement therapy with factor concentrate or fresh frozen plasma when concentrate is not immediately available.

In cases of pregnancy where one partner is known to have protein C deficiency, some experts would consider testing the other partner to determine if there is the possibility of the child having severe protein C deficiency at birth, with a view to antenatal detection of a homozygous infant. However, this approach is extremely problematic and counseling and interpretation of test results must be undertaken by an expert. Given the unreliability of phenotypic diagnosis, genetic analysis is mandatory if antenatal diagnosis is going to be considered with a view to termination. Some experts would consider this approach only if there was a previously affected infant.

References

1. Rosendaal FR. Venous thrombosis: a multicausal disease. Lancet. 1999;353:1167–73.
2. Langdown J, Johnson DJ, Baglin TP, Huntington JA. Allosteric activation of antithrombin critically depends upon hinge region extension. J Biol Chem. 2004;279:47288–97.
3. Gopel W, Ludwig M, Junge AK, Kohlmann T, Diedrich K, Moller J. Selection pressure for the factor-V-Leiden mutation and embryo implantation. Lancet. 2001;358:1238–9.

4. Lisman T, de Groot PG, Meijers JC, Rosendaal FR. Reduced plasma fibrinolytic potential is a risk factor for venous thrombosis. Blood. 2005;105: 1102–5.
5. Meltzer ME, Lisman T, Doggen CJ, de Groot PG, Rosendaal FR. Synergistic effects of hypofibrinolysis and genetic and acquired risk factors on the risk of a first venous thrombosis. PLoS Med. 2008;5:e97.
6. Bezemer ID, Doggen CJ, Vos HL, Rosendaal FR. No association between the common MTHFR 677C->T polymorphism and venous thrombosis: results from the MEGA study. Arch Intern Med. 2007;167: 497–501.
7. Brown K, Luddington R, Baglin T. Effect of the MTHFRC677T variant on risk of venous thromboembolism: interaction with factor V Leiden and prothrombin (F2G20210A) mutations. Br J Haematol. 1998;103:42–4.
8. Miyakis S, Lockshin MD, Atsumi T, Branch DW, Brey RL, Cervera R, Derksen RHWM, de Groot PG, Koike T, Meroni PL, Reber G, Shoenfeld Y, Tincani A, Vlachoyiannopoulos PG, Krilis SA. International consensus statement on an update of the classification criteria for definite antiphospholipid syndrome (APS). J Thromb Haemost. 2006;4:295–306.
9. Pengo V, Tripodi A, Reber G, Rand JH, Ortel TL, Galli M, De Groot PG. Update of the guidelines for lupus anticoagulant detection. J Thromb Haemost. 2009;7:1737–40.
10. Baglin T, Gray E, Greaves M, Hunt B, Keeling D, Machin S, Mackie I, Makris M, Nokes T, Perry D, Tait RC, Walker I, Watson H. Clinical guidelines for testing for heritable thrombophilia Br J Haematol. 2010;149:209–20
11. Baglin T. Unravelling the thrombophilia paradox: from hypercoagulability to the prothrombotic state. J Thromb Haemost. 2010;8:228–33.
12. Rosendaal FR, Bovill EG. Heritability of clotting factors and the revival of the prothrombotic state. Lancet. 2002;359:638–9.
13. Robertson L, Wu O, Langhorne P, Twaddle S, Clark P, Lowe GD, Walker ID, Greaves M, Brenkel I, Regan L, Greer IA. Thrombophilia in pregnancy: a systematic review. Br J Haematol. 2006;132:171–96.
14. Pabinger I, Grafenhofer H, Kaider A, Ilic A, Eichinger S, Quehenberger P, Husslein P, Mannhalter C, Lechner K. Preeclampsia and fetal loss in women with a history of venous thromboembolism. Arterioscler Thromb Vasc Biol. 2001;21:874–9.
15. Bose P, Black S, Kadyrov M, Weissenborn U, Neulen J, Regan L, Huppertz B. Heparin and aspirin attenuate placental apoptosis in vitro: implications for early pregnancy failure. Am J Obstet Gynecol. 2005;192: 23–30.
16. Sebire NJ, Regan L, Rai R. Biology and pathology of the placenta in relation to antiphospholipid antibody-associated pregnancy failure. Lupus. 2002;11:641–3.
17. Isermann B, Sood R, Pawlinski R, Zogg M, Kalloway S, Degen JL, Mackman N, Weiler H. The thrombomodulin-protein C system is essential for the maintenance of pregnancy. Nat Med. 2003;9:331–7.
18. Greer IA, Nelson-Piercy C. Low-molecular-weight heparins for thromboprophylaxis and treatment of venous thromboembolism in pregnancy: a systematic review of safety and efficacy. Blood. 2005;106: 401–7.
19. Royal College of Obstetricians & Gynaecologists. Greentop guideline no. 37. Thrombosis and embolism during pregnancy and the puerperium, reducing the risk. London; 2009. https://www.rcog.org.uk/guidelines.
20. Howley HE, Walker M, Rodger MA. A systematic review of the association between factor V Leiden or prothrombin gene variant and intrauterine growth restriction. Am J Obstet Gynecol. 2005;192:694–708. 2002;99:614–9.
21. Kovalevsky G, Gracia CR, Berlin JA, Sammel MD, Barnhart KT. Evaluation of the association between hereditary thrombophilias and recurrent pregnancy loss: a meta-analysis. Arch Intern Med. 2004;164: 558–63.
22. Rey E, Kahn SR, David M, Shrier I. Thrombophilic disorders and fetal loss: a meta-analysis. Lancet. 2003;361:901–8.
23. Rai R, Shlebak A, Cohen H, Backos M, Holmes Z, Marriott K, Regan L. Factor V Leiden and acquired activated protein C resistance among 1000 women with recurrent miscarriage. Hum Reprod. 2001;16:961–5.
24. Pabinger I, Nemes L, Rintelen C, Koder S, Lechler E, Loreth RM, Kyrle PA, Scharrer I, Sas G, Lechner K, Mannhalter C, Ehrenforth S. Pregnancy-associated risk for venous thromboembolism and pregnancy outcome in women homozygous for factor V Leiden. Hematol J. 2000;1:37–41.
25. Vossen CY, Preston FE, Conard J, Fontcuberta J, Makris M, van der Meer FJ, Pabinger I, Palareti G, Scharrer I, Souto JC, Svensson P, Walker ID, Rosendaal FR. Hereditary thrombophilia and fetal loss: a prospective follow-up study. J Thromb Haemost. 2004;2:592–6.
26. Nelen WL, Blom HJ, Steegers EA, den Heijer M, Eskes TK. Hyperhomocysteinemia and recurrent early pregnancy loss: a meta-analysis. Fertil Steril. 2000;74:1196–9.
27. Unfried G, Griesmacher A, Weismuller W, Nagele F, Huber JC, Tempfer CB. The C677T polymorphism of the methylenetetrahydrofolate reductase gene and idiopathic recurrent miscarriage. Obstet Gynecol. 2002;99:614–9.
28. Foka ZJ, Lambropoulos AF, Saravelos H, Karas GB, Karavida A, Agorastos T, Zournatzi V, Makris PE, Bontis J, Kotsis A. Factor V Leiden and prothrombin G20210A mutations, but not methylenetetrahydrofolate reductase C677T, are associated with recurrent miscarriages. Hum Reprod. 2000;15:458–62.

29. Holmes ZR, Regan L, Chilcott I, Cohen H. The C677T MTHFR gene mutation is not predictive of risk for recurrent fetal loss. Br J Haematol. 1999; 105:98–101.
30. Makino A, Nakanishi T, Sugiura-Ogasawara M, Ozaki Y, Suzumori N, Suzumori K. No association of C677T methylenetetrahydrofolate reductase and an endothelial nitric oxide synthase polymorphism with recurrent pregnancy loss. Am J Reprod Immunol. 2004;52:60–6.
31. Van der Molen EF, Arends GE, Nelen WL, Van der Put NJ, Heil SG, Eskes TK, Blom HJ. A common mutation in the 5,10-methylenetetrahydrofolate reductase gene as a new risk factor for placental vasculopathy. Am J Obstet Gynecol. 2000;182:1258–63.
32. Lachmeijer AM, Arngrimsson R, Bastiaans EJ, Pals G, ten Kate LP, de Vries JI, Kostense PJ, Aarnoudse JG, Dekker GA. Mutations in the gene for methylenetetrahydrofolate reductase, homocysteine levels, and vitamin status in women with a history of preeclampsia. Am J Obstet Gynecol. 2001;184:394–402.
33. Murakami S, Matsubara N, Saitoh M, Miyakaw S, Shoji M, Kubo T. The relation between plasma homocysteine concentration and methylenetetrahydrofolate reductase gene polymorphism in pregnant women. J Obstet Gynaecol Res. 2001;27:349–52.
34. Kosmas IP, Tatsioni A, Ioannidis JP. Association of C677T polymorphism in the methylenetetrahydrofolate reductase gene with hypertension in pregnancy and pre-eclampsia: a meta-analysis. J Hypertens. 2004;22:1655–62.
35. Middeldorp S. Thrombophilia and pregnancy complications: cause or association? J Thromb Haemost. 2007;5 Suppl 1:276–82.

Systemic Thromboembolism in Pregnancy: Thromboprophylaxis

4

Charlotte J. Frise, Peter K. MacCallum, Lucy H. Mackillop, and Catherine Nelson-Piercy

Abstract

Venous thromboembolism is a significant cause of maternal death in the UK, despite being a preventable condition for which clear risk factors have been identified. The introduction of routine antenatal and postnatal thromboprophylaxis for women identified by risk assessment tools has been linked to a steady reduction in the number of deaths. This chapter discusses the risk factors for the development of thromboembolism as well as the options for prophylactic intervention, and the specific clinical situations which can alter the treatment advice.

Keywords

Thromboembolism • Thromboprophylaxis • Pregnancy • Risk factors • Low-molecular-weight heparin • Puerperium • Risk assessment

4.1 Introduction

Venous thromboembolism (VTE) is a preventable condition, yet pulmonary embolus remains a leading direct cause of maternal death in the UK [1]. In recent years, attention has been drawn to the assessment of every person admitted to hospital to attempt to risk stratify individuals

C.J. Frise, BM BCh, MA, MRCP (✉)
Acute General Medicine, John Radcliffe Hospital, Oxford University Hospitals NHS Trust, Headley Way, Headington, Oxford OX3 9DU, UK
e-mail: charlotte.frise@ouh.nhs.uk

P.K. MacCallum, MB ChB, MD, FRCP, FRCPath
Wolfson Institute of Preventive Medicine, Barts Health NHS Trust, Barts and The London School of Medicine and Dentistry, Charterhouse Square, London EC1M 6BQ, UK
e-mail: p.k.maccallum@qmul.ac.uk

L.H. Mackillop, BM BCh, MA, FRCP
Nuffield Department of Obstetrics and Gynaecology, Women's Center, John Radcliffe Hospital, Oxford University Hospitals NHS Trust, Headley Way, Headington, Oxford OX3 9DU, UK
e-mail: lucy.mackillop@ouh.nhs.uk

C. Nelson-Piercy, MBBS, MA, FRCP, FRCOG
Women's Health Academic Centre, Guy's & St Thomas' Foundation Trust and Imperial College Healthcare Trust, St Thomas' Hospital, Westminster Bridge Road, London SE1 7EH, UK
e-mail: catherine.nelson-piercy@gstt.nhs.uk

H. Cohen, P. O'Brien (eds.), *Disorders of Thrombosis and Hemostasis in Pregnancy: A Guide to Management*, DOI 10.1007/978-3-319-15120-5_4, © Springer-Verlag London 2015

and institute appropriate preventive measures to reduce the rate of venous thromboembolic events [2]. Pregnancy is a prothrombotic state, meaning that women are at increased risk of venous thromboembolic disease from the first trimester, and in particular in the puerperium.

Regular assessment of a pregnant woman, repeated every time there is a change in her clinical condition (whether inpatient or outpatient), is the cornerstone of successful prevention of VTE. Low-molecular-weight heparins (LMWHs) are the most commonly used agents for thromboprophylaxis as they are safe, effective, and well tolerated in pregnancy and the postnatal period.

This chapter aims to summarize the risk factors for venous thromboembolic disease in pregnancy and the rationale for different treatment approaches depending on the risk factors present in each individual. It is based on the VTE prophylaxis guidelines of the Royal College of Obstetricians and Gynaecologists (RCOG) [2a]. The reader should also refer to the RCOG 2015 VTE prophylaxis guidelines published after this book had gone to Press [2b].

4.2 Assessment of Thromboembolic Risk

Physiological changes in the hemostatic system produce a hypercoagulable state and make pregnancy an independent risk factor for VTE. VTE is still a rare event, however, in pregnant women without other risk factors. Therefore, a search for other risk factors and stratification of those risks is critical to enable decisions about thromboprophylaxis. Known risk factors may be characterized as preexisting, those directly relating to the pregnancy, and transient risk factors that might be present for part of the pregnancy only.

The assessment and reassessment of thrombotic risk are of utmost importance. Assessment of risk should take place at the initial consultation whether that is in primary or secondary care, if clinical parameters change, on any admission to hospital and immediately postnatally. Risk factors for VTE, which are shown in Table 4.1, must be reviewed and documented. The latest evidence for risk factor assessment is presented below.

4.2.1 Thrombophilia: Heritable

A heritable thrombophilia is found in 20–50 % of women with pregnancy-related VTE [3]. However, different thrombophilias have different levels of risk. In a retrospective study of 72,000 pregnancies in which women with VTE were investigated for a thrombophilic tendency and the background prevalence of these defects was known, the risk of VTE in pregnancy was estimated to be 1:2.8 in type I antithrombin deficiency (with reduced activity and antigen), 1:42 for type II antithrombin deficiency (with reduced activity and normal antigen level), 1:113 for protein C deficiency, and 1:437 for factor V Leiden [4].

4.2.1.1 Factor V Leiden and Prothrombin G20210A

The most common heritable thrombophilic tendencies in the UK are factor V Leiden and prothrombin F2G20210A, present in around 4 and 2 % of the population, respectively. Case– control studies show that individuals heterozygous for these genes are at roughly fivefold increased risk of VTE in both the general population and pregnancy [5–7]. However, the absolute risk appears to be small (<1 %). Cohort studies undertaken in the general population and a further study in women heterozygous for factor V Leiden recorded three episodes of VTE in 752 pregnancies [8–11]. Therefore, the benefit of thromboprophylaxis at this level of risk would be limited.

The absolute risk may be higher, however, in women with a family history of VTE and a thrombophilic genotype. In a meta-analysis [8, 12], 2 % of factor V Leiden carriers had a pregnancy-related VTE. In the cohort studies where the cases were selected because of family screening, that is, two or more first-degree relatives with VTE but exclusion of the proband from analysis, 3 % of factor V Leiden carriers had a pregnancy-related VTE compared to 0.6 % in family members who were not carriers. This absolute risk is similar in magnitude to that seen in retrospective analyses in women with pregnancy-related thrombosis and with the F2G20210A prothrombin gene variant, selected because of a family history of VTE, and to those

Table 4.1 Risk factors for VTE

Preexisting	
Previous VTE	Single Estrogen or pregnancy related Thrombophilia related Unprovoked Related to temporary risk factor Recurrent events
Thrombophilia	Heritable Antithrombin deficiency Protein C deficiency Protein S deficiency Factor V Leiden Prothrombin gene G20210A Acquired Antiphospholipid syndrome – persistent lupus anticoagulant or persistent moderate/high-titre anticardiolipin or anti-β2-glycoprotein 1 antibodies
Medical comorbidities including	SLE Nephrotic syndrome Heart disease Sickle cell disease Cancer Inflammatory conditions, e.g. inflammatory bowel disease
Others	Age >35 years Obesity BMI >30 kg/m^2 either prior to pregnancy or in early pregnancy Parity ≥3 Smoking Varicose veins: gross, symptomatic, above knee, or with phlebitis or skin changes Paraplegia Family history of VTE
Obstetric	
Antenatal	Multiple pregnancy, assisted reproduction therapy (ART) Preeclampsia
Delivery	Cesarean section Prolonged labor, midcavity rotational operative delivery
Postnatal	Postpartum hemorrhage (>1 L) Blood transfusion
New onset/transient	
Early pregnancy	Hyperemesis gravidarum Ovarian hyperstimulation syndrome
Any time in pregnancy	Surgical procedure, e.g. ERPC, appendicectomy, postpartum sterilization Admission or immobility, e.g. symphysis pubis dysfunction Dehydration Systemic infection, e.g. pneumonia, pyelonephritis, wound infection Travel of duration >4 h

Adapted from RCOG guideline no. 37a [2]

observed in a retrospective family study in carriers of factor V Leiden and F2G20210A [13–15]. A review of heterozygous factor V Leiden carriers with at least one symptomatic first-degree relative estimated the incidence of the first episode of VTE occurring in association with pregnancy at 2.1 %. The risk *during* pregnancy, however, was only 0.4 % compared to 1.7 % in the postpartum period. Very similar incidences were estimated for the prothrombin variant – 0.5 % in pregnancy and 1.9 % postpartum [16].

The risk of pregnancy-related VTE also appears to increase with compound (combined defects) or homozygous states. In previously asymptomatic women, the risk is higher in compound heterozygotes for factor V Leiden and F2G20210A, with an absolute risk of approximately 4 %, although a retrospective family cohort study did not confirm this increased risk [14, 17, 18]. A systematic review suggests that women who are homozygous for factor V Leiden or F2G20210A are also at much higher risk of pregnancy-related VTE, and absolute risks of 9–16 % have been reported for homozygous factor V Leiden [11, 19].

4.2.1.2 Antithrombin, Protein C, and Protein S Deficiencies

Outside pregnancy, the risk of the first VTE appears to be higher in individuals with deficiencies of antithrombin, protein C, or protein S compared to V Leiden and the F2G20210A [20]. Asymptomatic women with protein C or protein S deficiency probably have a moderately increased risk of VTE associated with pregnancy, again with most events occurring postpartum. The risk associated with antithrombin deficiency appears to vary according to the subtype but may be associated with a very high absolute risk of 15–50 % [21].

In a more recent retrospective cohort study of women from families with hereditary antithrombin, protein C, or protein S deficiency, 12 pregnancy-related VTE episodes were objectively diagnosed in 162 pregnancies (7 %), two-thirds of which occurred in the postpartum period [22]. In a recent review, in women with a deficiency of antithrombin, protein C, or protein S and at least one symptomatic first-degree relative, the incidence of the first episode of VTE occurring in association with pregnancy was estimated at 4.1 % (1.7–8.3 %). Again, the incidence appeared to be higher during the postpartum period than during pregnancy, 3 and 1.2 %, respectively [16].

4.2.1.3 MTHFR

Homozygosity for a thermolabile variant of the gene for methylenetetrahydrofolate reductase (C677T MTHFR) is sometimes included in thrombophilia testing, but there is no evidence of an association with a clinically relevant increase in the risk of VTE in pregnancy [19].

4.2.2 Thrombophilia: Antiphospholipid Syndrome

Antiphospholipid syndrome (APS) is defined as the presence of persistently positive antiphospholipid antibodies (aPL) – lupus anticoagulant (LA) and/or anticardiolipin (aCL) and/or anti-β2-glycoprotein 1 (β2 GP1) antibodies of medium or high titre on two consecutive occasions at least 12 weeks apart ("persistently positive") in association with a history of arterial or venous thrombosis or adverse pregnancy outcome. An adverse pregnancy outcome is defined as either a fetal death after 10 weeks' gestation, a preterm birth at less than 34 weeks' gestation due to severe pre-eclampsia or intrauterine growth restriction, or the occurrence of three or more unexplained miscarriages before 10 weeks' gestation [23].

Antiphospholipid antibodies, in particular persistent LA or moderate/high-titre aCL antibodies or a β2 GP1 antibodies, are associated with an increased risk of recurrent thrombosis, and it is common for such women to be on long-term warfarin after a first event [24–26].

Optimal management for the prevention of recurrent thrombosis in pregnancy is unclear. There is a lack of randomized trials and very few prospective studies of women with APS and prior thrombosis. In one study, 98 of 565 women tested were found to have positive aPL and were divided into low, high, or very high risk based on their clinical history, that is, asymptomatic, three or more pregnancy losses, or prior venous or arterial thrombosis, respectively [27]. Women who were low risk received 2 weeks of postpartum LMWH and antenatal LMWH if there were additional risk factors. Women in the latter two groups received prophylactic or high-prophylactic-dose LMWH (dalteparin 50–100 and 100–200 IU/kg/day, respectively) from enrollment until 6 weeks postpartum (or until oral anticoagulation was recommenced). They also received low-dose aspirin from weeks 12 to 36. There were no VTE events in the low- or high-risk groups, but there were two events in the 28 patients in the very-high-risk group, suggesting a significant risk of thrombosis. In a further series of 33 women with primary APS, women who had no previous history of thrombosis and no other risk factors were given 3–5 days of thromboprophylaxis postpartum only, and there were no thrombotic events in this subgroup [28].

4.2.3 Previous Venous Thromboembolism

Women with previous VTE have an increased risk of recurrence in pregnancy and postpartum, with reported recurrence rates of 1.4–11.1 %, and this risk appears to be constant over the whole duration of pregnancy [29, 30]. A retrospective comparison of the recurrence rate of VTE during pregnancy and the nonpregnant period revealed recurrence rates of 10.9 % during and 3.7 % outside pregnancy, giving a relative risk during pregnancy of 3.5 (95 % CI 1.6–7.8) [31].

In order to aid risk assessment, women with previous VTE can be stratified into those with recurrent or single previous VTE. The latter group may be further subdivided into those with:

- A temporary risk factor associated with the VTE, for example, major trauma or surgery
- Estrogen-provoked, that is, pregnancy or estrogen-containing contraception
- Unprovoked
- Thrombophilia, either heritable or acquired or associated with a family history of VTE

4.2.3.1 Recurrent VTE

Individuals with recurrent VTE are at increased risk of further recurrence [32]. Many will therefore be on long-term therapeutic dose warfarin. Although data are lacking, these women would be expected to have a high risk of recurrence in pregnancy.

4.2.3.2 Temporary Risk Factor-Associated VTE

Outside pregnancy, there is a low risk of recurrence of VTE which resulted from a transient major risk factor. This is also likely to be the case in pregnancy, as both a prospective and a retrospective study suggested that the risk of antenatal recurrence is very low if the prior VTE was provoked by a transient major risk factor that is no longer present [33, 34]. Examples of this include a DVT post surgery or trauma or in an intravenous drug user who is no longer injecting.

4.2.3.3 Single Previous Estrogen Related

Although prior estrogen-provoked VTE was not found to be a risk factor for VTE in subsequent pregnancy in the study by Brill-Edwards and colleagues [33], other retrospective studies suggest the contrary [30, 31, 34]. For example, in women whose previous VTE was associated with the use of estrogen-containing contraception, the recurrence rate was 9.5 % in subsequent pregnancies where thromboprophylaxis was withheld [34]. The risk was very similar (9.8, 95 % CI 4.2–20.9 %) if the prior VTE had occurred during a previous pregnancy. In another study comparing pregnant women whose prior episode was provoked by estrogen-containing contraception and those women without a history of contraceptive use at the time of VTE, the recurrence rates were 10 and 2.7 %, respectively [30].

A retrospective study using Californian hospital discharge data analyzed recurrence rates in women with a previous single pregnancy-related VTE and in women with a previous unprovoked thromboembolic event [35]. The overall recurrence rates over the following 6–60 months were lower in the group with pregnancy-related VTE initially (5.8 % compared to 10.4 %), but the rate of recurrence in subsequent pregnancies was higher (4.5 % compared to 2.7 %). Of the recurrent events in the women who had previously had a pregnancy-related VTE, 35 % occurred in a subsequent pregnancy, compared to 8.7 % in the group with previous unprovoked VTE. Furthermore, 71 % of the recurrences were antenatal in the former group compared to 54 % in the latter. This adds further support to the stratification of women with previous estrogen-related VTE as being at high risk of VTE in subsequent pregnancy and the puerperium.

4.2.3.4 Single Previous Unprovoked

In non-pregnant populations, unprovoked VTE has been shown to be associated with an increased risk of recurrence compared to those provoked by a temporary risk factor that is no longer present [32]. A prospective study of 125 pregnant women with a single prior episode of VTE showed that 5.9 % of women with VTE that was unprovoked or associated with a thrombophilia had a recurrence, in contrast to women with a previous VTE that was associated with a temporary risk factor and no thrombophilia, in whom no recurrences were seen [33]. In this study, estrogen-provoked VTE was included as a temporary risk factor. A retrospective study of 155 pregnancies in 88 women with a previous VTE compared the recurrence rate in women with a previous unprovoked VTE who were not given thromboprophylaxis to that in women where the prior VTE was associated with a transient risk factor. The recurrence rate was 4.2 % in the former group and none in the latter [34].

In contrast, Pabinger and colleagues [31] found that the presence or absence of a temporary risk factor did not affect the risk of recurrence in a subsequent pregnancy, although again estrogen-provoked VTE was included as a temporary risk factor, which may have influenced the results.

4.2.3.5 Thrombophilia Related

Outside pregnancy, the most common heritable thrombophilias do not substantially increase the risk of recurrence after a single event. This was shown in a systematic review of prospective studies [36] where being a heterozygote carrier of factor V Leiden increased the relative risk of recurrence with an OR of 1.39 (95 % CI 1.15–1.67). Data regarding the effect of heritable thrombophilia on the risk of recurrent VTE in pregnancy are extremely sparse.

4.2.4 Obesity

Obesity is common in the non-pregnant population, and a body mass index (BMI) above 30 kg/m^2 was seen in 19 % of women aged 25–34 and 25 % of women aged 35–44 years [37]. Any increase in weight above a normal BMI appears to be associated with an increased risk of VTE in pregnancy. Being overweight (BMI 25–30 kg/m^2) is very common in pregnancy, with a prevalence of approximately 50 %, and this is a risk factor for pregnancy-related VTE. The risk of VTE appears to increase further with increasing obesity, although the data are limited [38]. In one study, obesity was more strongly associated with pulmonary embolism than with deep vein thrombosis, with odds ratios of 14.9 (95 % CI 3.0–74.8) and 4.4 (95 % CI 1.6–11.9), respectively [39].

Obesity has been identified as a particular concern in two reports from the UK's Centre for Maternal and Child Enquiries (CMACE). For the triennium 2003–2005, there were 33 deaths from pulmonary embolus [40]. In the 21 cases where BMI was recorded, 12 women were obese, that is, BMI >30 kg/m^2. In the report from 2006 to 2008, 30 % of mothers who died from direct causes and for whom the BMI was known were obese, as were 24 % of women who died from indirect causes (27 % overall) [1].

4.2.5 Age

Age greater than 35 years increases the risk of antenatal and postnatal VTE, with an odds ratio of 1.3 (95 % CI 1.0–1.7) compared to that of women aged 20–34 years [41]. Simpson and colleagues [42] also showed that postnatal events were significantly associated with maternal age greater than 35 years (OR 1.4, 95 % CI 1.0–2.0).

4.2.6 First-Trimester Events

The risk of VTE may increase further in the first trimester due to other complications such as hyperemesis gravidarum (OR 2.5, 95 % CI 2.0–3.2) or ovarian hyperstimulation (OR 4.3, 95 % CI 2.0–9.4) [29, 43]. Women with ovarian hyper-stimulation are at particular risk of internal jugular vein VTE [44]. There is also an increased risk of VTE associated with surgery during pregnancy, including termination of pregnancy and ectopic pregnancy. Postsurgical thromboprophylaxis is therefore advised if indicated in these circumstances, as it is after delivery.

4.2.7 Mode of Delivery

Compared with vaginal birth, Cesarean section increases the risk of postpartum VTE. In a Canadian retrospective population-based cohort study of 46,766 women who underwent a planned Cesarean section for breech presentation and 2,292,420 women who planned to deliver vaginally, an increased risk of postpartum VTE with Cesarean section was demonstrated, with an odds ratio of 2.2 (95 % CI 1.5–3.2) [45].

Compared to elective Cesarean section, emergency Cesarean further increases the risk of VTE. A Swedish study included both elective and emergency Cesarean sections and showed a relative risk of VTE of 6.7 compared to vaginal delivery [46]. A Scottish study also compared emergency with elective Cesarean section and showed that the risk of VTE was doubled following emergency [47].

RCOG guidelines were published in 1995 that recommended thromboprophylaxis after emergency Cesarean section [48]. The CEMACE reports for the subsequent four triennia show that during this period (1997–2008), there were 26 deaths from VTE following Cesarean section compared to 27 following vaginal delivery [1]. As the latter make up 70–80 % of all deliveries, this suggests that Cesarean section remains a risk factor for fatal PE despite the published guidelines on thromboprophylaxis.

4.2.8 Immobility

Immobility is known to be a risk factor for the development of VTE in non-pregnant patients, but the information available for pregnant patients is limited. One case–control study looked at antepartum immobilization, defined as strict bed rest for 1 week or more prior to delivery, in patients with a BMI of greater than 25 kg/m^2. The results showed a multiplicative effect on the risk of antepartum and postpartum VTE with odds ratios of 62.3 and 40.1, respectively [43].

The UK's National Institute for Health and Care Excellence (NICE) guideline on antenatal care [49] and the UK's RCOG Scientific Advisory Committee Opinion Paper on air travel in pregnancy [50] state that long-haul air travel increases the risk of VTE, but the current RCOG guideline considers all long-distance travel longer than 4 h duration, and not just by air, to be a risk factor for VTE in pregnancy [2].

4.2.9 Hospital Admission

In non-pregnant medical and surgical patients, hospitalization is now recognized as a major risk factor for VTE, and it is believed that at least 25,000 deaths per year in England resulting from PE complicating hospital admission may be preventable. An independent expert working group set up by the UK Chief Medical Officer recommended that it be mandatory for all patients to be risk assessed for VTE on admission to hospital, and this report has been accepted by the Department of Health [51]. NICE guidelines on prevention of VTE in patients admitted to hospital recommend consideration of VTE prophylaxis with LMWH for women who are pregnant or have given birth within 6 weeks who are admitted to hospital and have one or more risk factors [52].

4.3 Thromboprophylaxis

4.3.1 Efficacy

Thromboprophylaxis has been shown to reduce the incidence of VTE in pregnancy. In a study of 284 pregnancies in women with a prior event, there were no recurrent events in the 87 in which thromboprophylaxis was administered compared with eight in the 197 pregnancies where it was not [30]. In a prospective cohort study in families with antithrombin, protein C, or protein S deficiency or factor V Leiden, two VTEs occurred in 28 pregnancies (7 %) in women who did not receive thromboprophylaxis, whereas there were no episodes in 43 women who did receive thromboprophylaxis [53]. Another study compared the incidence of postpartum VTE before and after the introduction of thromboprophylaxis across Scottish maternity hospitals in 1995. There were approximately 1.55 million maternities between 1980 and 2005, and there was a significant reduction in the incidence of VTE between 1996 and 2004 compared to 1980–1995 [54].

4.3.2 Pharmacological Agents

4.3.2.1 Low-Molecular-Weight Heparins (LMWHs)

LMWHs have been shown to be as effective as, and safer than, unfractionated heparin (UFH) when used to prevent VTE in pregnancy [55, 56]. UFH can cause heparin-induced thrombocytopenia (HIT), but the risk of this is much lower when LMWHs are used. Current guidelines support monitoring the platelet count in patients on LMWH only when there has been previous exposure to UFH. Prolonged use of UFH during pregnancy can result in osteoporosis and fractures, but this risk is very low with LMWH [57]. In a systematic review of prophylactic and treatment dose LMWH use in 2,777 pregnancies, there were no cases of HIT; the incidence of osteoporotic fractures was 0.04 % and of allergic skin reactions was 1.8 % [55]. Significant bleeding was seen in 1.98 % and was usually related primarily to obstetric causes.

Table 4.2 gives suggested prophylactic and therapeutic subcutaneous doses of LMWH in pregnancy and postpartum. Doses of LMWH are based on booking weight rather than BMI or weight later in pregnancy (although some authorities calculate the dose according to current weight). Data from the UK Obstetric Surveillance Study (UKOSS) show that overweight and obese women develop VTE while on prophylactic LMWH at doses appropriate for those of lower weight [58]. There is no consensus on the appropriate prophylactic dosing of obese women, so some units may prescribe the usual prophylactic dose twice daily for women over 90 kg.

It may be appropriate to use higher doses of LMWH as prophylaxis in women who are usually on long-term oral anticoagulation because of previous recurrent VTE or thrombophilia. Anti-Xa level monitoring may also be helpful in guiding therapy in women at very high risk because of antithrombin deficiency, but this should be done in association with an expert in hemostasis.

4.3.2.2 Unfractionated Heparin

UFH has a shorter half-life than LMWH, and there is more complete reversal of its activity by protamine sulfate. UFH has several disadvantages compared to LMWH. In addition to the association with HIT and osteoporosis, when used for thromboprophylaxis, more frequent administration is required due to its shorter half-life [59].

Table 4.2 Suggested doses for antenatal and postnatal LMWH thromboprophylaxis

Weight	Enoxaparin	Dalteparin	Tinzaparin
<50 kg	20 mg daily	2,500 units daily	3,500 units daily
50–90 kg	40 mg daily	5,000 units daily	4,500 units daily
91–130 kg	60 mg daily[a]	7,500 units daily[a]	7,000 units daily[a]
131–170 kg	80 mg daily[a]	10,000 units daily[a]	9,000 units daily[a]
>170 kg	0.6 mg/kg/day[a]	75 u/kg/day[a]	75 u/kg/day[a]
50–90 kg, high prophylactic	40 mg twice daily	5,000 units twice daily	4,500 units twice daily
Treatment dose (antenatal)	1 mg/kg/twice daily	100 u/kg/twice daily	175 u/kg/day
Treatment dose (postnatal)	1.5 mg/kg/day	200 u/kg/day	175 u/kg/day

[a]Can be given in two divided doses

In some women, for example those at very high risk of thrombosis or increased risk of hemorrhage, UFH may be preferred around the time of delivery so that use of regional anesthesia or analgesia is not prevented. For example, if no LMWH has been given for 24 h but the woman has not yet delivered and there is concern about delaying further doses of LMWH, a prophylactic dose of 5,000 units subcutaneously of UFH could be used and repeated every 12 h until LMWH can be safely resumed after delivery. The required interval between a prophylactic dose of UFH and regional analgesia or anesthesia is less than with LMWH (4 and 12 h, respectively), and there is less concern regarding neuraxial hematoma with UFH [60].

4.3.2.3 Danaparoid

Danaparoid, a heparinoid with a half-life of approximately 24 h, is used mostly in patients intolerant of heparin. A recent review of the use of prophylactic and treatment doses of danaparoid in pregnant women with (current or a history of) HIT or skin allergy to heparin (32 and 19 cases, respectively) showed four maternal bleeding events, two of which were fatal due to placental problems (previa and abruption) [61]. In three lactating women with measurable plasma levels, no anti-Xa activity was detected in the cord blood of five infants tested, and no anti-Xa activity was found in breast milk. There were no adverse fetal outcomes attributed to danaparoid. Use of this agent should be managed in conjunction with a consultant hematologist with expertise in this area.

4.3.2.4 Fondaparinux

Fondaparinux is a synthetic indirect factor Xa inhibitor, licensed in the UK for the prevention and treatment of VTE outside pregnancy, and is similar in efficacy to LMWH [62]. No placental transfer of fondaparinux was found in a human cotyledon model [63], but anti-Xa activity of approximately 10 % of that in maternal plasma was found in the umbilical cord plasma in newborns of five mothers being treated with fondaparinux [64]. There is limited experience of its use in pregnancy, where it may be useful in women with a history of HIT. Although no adverse effects were observed in the newborns, it is premature to conclude that it is safe, and its use should be reserved for women intolerant of heparin compounds. The regular prophylactic dose is 2.5 mg subcutaneously daily, and it does not seem necessary to alter this dose in pregnancy [65].

It is unknown whether fondaparinux is excreted in breast milk and, although oral absorption seems unlikely, its use in the postpartum setting is not currently advised.

4.3.2.5 Low Dose Aspirin

There are no controlled trials on the use of aspirin for thromboprophylaxis in pregnancy, so conclusions about its efficacy have been extrapolated from other trials in the non-pregnant population. A meta-analysis of trials of short-term antiplatelet therapy in surgical and medical patients showed a significant reduction in both DVT and PE with antiplatelet prophylaxis [66]. Another meta-analysis, focusing on patients at high risk for occlusive vascular events, found a statistically significant 25 % reduction in the odds of pulmonary embolism associated with antiplatelet therapy [67]. Another trial, much criticized, suggested that, compared to placebo, low dose aspirin reduces by 36 % the risk of VTE after orthopedic surgery, even in some patients taking concomitant heparin therapy [68]. The Women's Health Study, however, found aspirin to be no better than placebo for long-term primary prevention of VTE in older women in a secondary end-point analysis [69]. The American College of Chest Physicians' guidelines recommend against the use of aspirin for VTE prophylaxis in any patient group [70, 71].

No adverse fetal outcomes were reported in the meta-analyses of large randomized controlled trials of low dose aspirin in pregnancy for the prevention of preeclampsia [72]. Use of low dose aspirin is appropriate for women with APS to improve fetal outcome [73] and as conjunctive therapy when LMWH is used in pregnant women with mechanical heart valves.

4.3.2.6 Warfarin

Warfarin use in pregnancy is restricted to a few situations where heparin is considered unsuitable, that is, in some patients with mechanical heart valves. It is therefore generally not used for thromboprophylaxis antenatally.

Warfarin can be safely used following delivery and in breastfeeding mothers, although it requires close monitoring and visits to an anticoagulant clinic and, compared with LMWH, carries an increased risk of postpartum hemorrhage and perineal hematoma. It is appropriate for those on maintenance warfarin outside pregnancy to restart postnatally, but this should be delayed for at least 5–7 days after delivery to minimize the risk of hemorrhage during the period of overlap of LMWH and warfarin. It is not appropriate for those women who require short-term postpartum prophylaxis, for example, 7 days.

Table 4.3 Risk factors for bleeding

Active antenatal or postpartum bleeding
Increased risk of major hemorrhage (e.g. placenta previa)
Bleeding diathesis, for example, von Willebrand's disease, some types of hemophilia, acquired coagulopathy
Thrombocytopenia (platelet count <75 × 10⁹ per liter)
Acute stroke in the last 4 weeks (ischemic or hemorrhagic)
Uncontrolled hypertension (BP >200 mmHg systolic or >120 mmHg diastolic)
Severe liver disease (prothrombin time above normal range or known varices)
Severe renal disease (creatinine clearance <30 ml/min)

4.3.2.7 Dextran

Dextran should be avoided antenatally and intrapartum, primarily because of the risk of anaphylactoid reaction, which has been associated with uterine hypertonus, fetal distress, fetal neurological abnormalities, and death [74, 75]. As there are now many alternatives, dextran is of little value in modern obstetric practice.

4.3.2.8 Oral Thrombin and Xa Inhibitors

Dabigatran and rivaroxaban are licensed for the prevention of VTE after major orthopedic surgery and the latter is now licensed for treatment of acute DVT. They are not licensed for use in pregnancy where there is no experience in their use and thus should be avoided.

4.3.3 Contraindications to Pharmacological Thromboprophylaxis

LMWH should be avoided, discontinued, or postponed in women who are at risk of bleeding, after careful consideration of the balance of risks of bleeding and thrombosis. Nonpregnancy-related risk factors for bleeding in pregnancy are extrapolated from data obtained from non-pregnant populations.

Women with major antepartum hemorrhage, progressive wound hematoma, suspected intra-abdominal bleeding, and postpartum hemorrhage are at high risk of further hemorrhage and may be more appropriately managed with UFH or antiembolism stockings. If a woman develops a hemorrhagic problem while on LMWH, the treatment should be stopped and expert hematological advice sought. Excessive blood loss and blood transfusion are also risk factors for VTE, so thromboprophylaxis should be begun or reinstituted as soon as the immediate risk of hemorrhage is reduced, again emphasizing the need for repeated review of the individual patient [43, 76].

Renal impairment is not an absolute contraindication to LMWH use, but a dose reduction is required in severe renal impairment (because of the risk of accumulation of LMWH and the association of platelet dysfunction with uremia). The dose reduction depends on the specific LMWH. For example, the dose of enoxaparin and dalteparin should be reduced in patients with creatinine clearance less than 30 mL/min, but the dose of tinzaparin should be reduced if the creatinine clearance is less than 20 mL/min. Table 4.3 summarises risk factors for bleeding.

4.3.4 Graduated Compression Stockings

Previous British Committee for Standards in Haematology (BCSH) guidelines advised that all women with a history of VTE should be encouraged to wear graduated compression stockings (GCSs) throughout their pregnancy and for 6–12 weeks after delivery [77]. This guidance was based on evidence extrapolated from studies using GCS in hospitalized, non-pregnant populations as there are no trials specifically looking at pregnant women. Small studies have shown that GCSs significantly improve venous emptying in pregnant women and increase the blood flow while decreasing the lumen diameter of the superficial femoral and common femoral veins in late pregnancy and early postpartum [78, 79].

The advantages and limitations of GCS and other mechanical methods of VTE prevention in the nonpregnancy setting were reviewed by the ACCP [71]. The conclusion was that such methods should be used primarily in patients at high risk of bleeding and thus unable to receive pharmacological thromboprophylaxis and as an adjunct to anticoagulant thromboprophylaxis where this had been shown to improve efficacy, for example, in surgical patients. Attention should be given to their proper application. In hospitalized medical patients, their recommended use was limited to those who had a contraindication to anticoagulant thromboprophylaxis.

In the 2008 ACCP guidelines on thromboprophylaxis in pregnancy [70], the use of GCS was recommended for women considered to be at high risk of VTE after Cesarean section, and antenatally and postpartum for all women with a previous DVT. However, this latter indication was not included in the 2012 ACCP guidelines [80]. In patients with a symptomatic DVT, a tighter-fitted GCS should be worn during the day, that is, with an ankle pressure gradient of 30–40 mmHg. This should be worn for 2 years to reduce the risk of post-thrombotic syndrome and longer if there are post-thrombotic sequelae [32]. This recommendation should apply in pregnancy where possible.

GCSs of an appropriate size are therefore suggested in pregnancy for those who are hospitalized in whom LMWH is contraindicated, those who are at particularly high risk of VTE (previous VTE or more than three risk factors) and hospitalized post-Cesarean section, outpatients with prior VTE, and women traveling for more than 4 h.

There are few data regarding the most efficacious length of GCS to use in pregnancy. Calf vein DVTs are more common in the nonpregnant population in comparison to pregnant populations in whom most DVTs are iliofemoral. Reviews outside pregnancy suggest equivalent efficacy of knee- and thigh-length GCS but better compliance with the former [81, 82]. Studies in pregnancy have assessed only thigh-length stockings [79]. Hydrostatic pressures on standing tend to counteract venous compression from GCS, so GCS may be of less benefit in the ambulant population compared with those confined to bed [83, 84]. On balance, therefore, properly applied thigh-length GCSs are advocated for pregnant women, but knee-length GCS should be considered if thigh-length GCSs are ill-fitting or compliance is poor.

4.3.5 Monitoring

Anti-Xa levels can be used to monitor the effect of LMWH. Anti-Xa levels are only an indication of the concentration of LMWH present, and levels provide little or no evidence on the efficacy in relation to prevention of thrombosis. Experience indicates that monitoring of anti-Xa levels is not required when LMWH is used for thromboprophylaxis, provided that the woman has normal renal function [85]. In women at extremes of body weight, it may be reasonable to check anti-Xa levels. Due to the relatively short half-life of LMWH, it is important to check with the local laboratory as to when to check the levels. Many laboratories have a reference range for 4 h post dose, whereas some use a trough level.

4.3.6 Timing

Many studies have shown that the VTE risk in the first trimester is significant. A meta-analysis shows that most VTEs occur antenatally with an equal distribution throughout gestation [86]. CMACE found that two-thirds of antenatal fatal pulmonary VTE in 2003–2005 occurred in the first trimester [40] and half in the 2006–2008 report [1]. Women at high risk of VTE either because of a previous event, thrombophilia, or multiple risk factors should therefore be offered pre-pregnancy counseling to ensure that treatment is started as soon as pregnancy is confirmed. It is advisable that an assessment of risk factors should occur at first contact with a healthcare professional and be repeated at every hospital admission or intercurrent illness. The

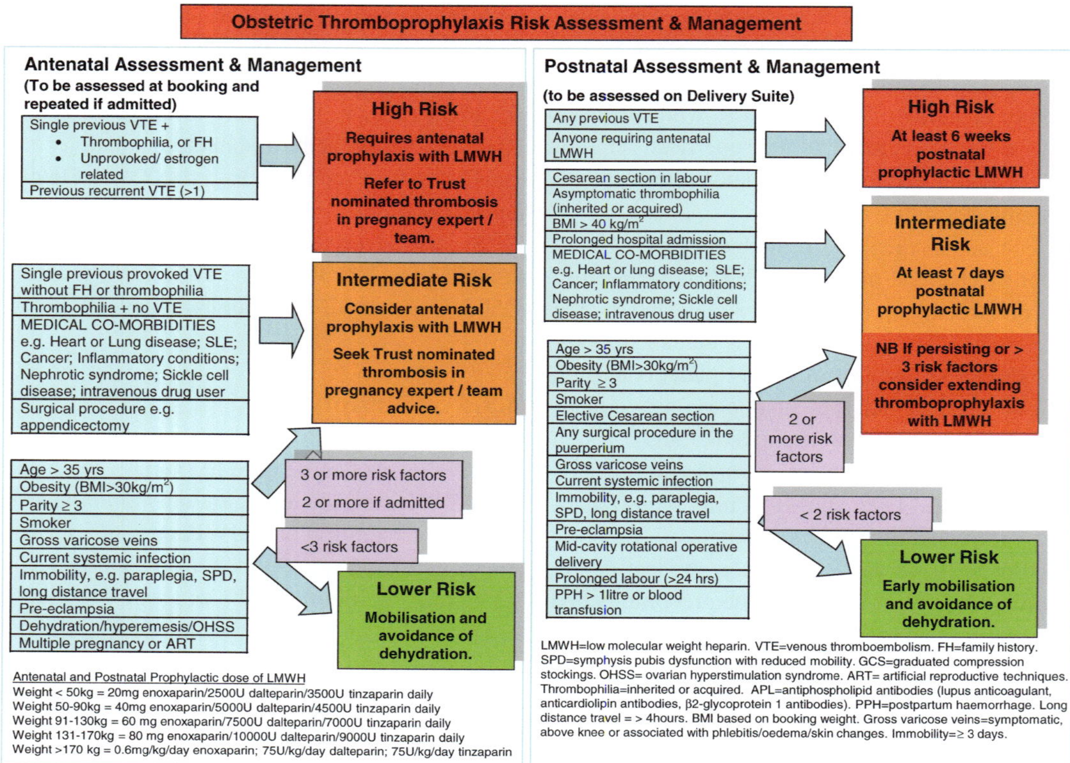

Fig. 4.1 An example of a risk assessment tool

period of greatest risk per day is postpartum [70, 76]. Therefore, many women who did not meet the threshold for significant risk antenatally should be reconsidered for thromboprophylaxis postnatally. Any woman taking antenatal thromboprophylaxis should continue it postnatally unless contraindications have developed, and all women with prior VTE should receive postpartum prophylaxis. Given this increased risk postnatally, further assessment of the risk of VTE is required following delivery, taking into consideration mode of delivery, bleeding risk, and any complications or comorbidities that may have developed.

4.3.7 Duration

As detailed in Chap. 1, the prothrombotic changes associated with pregnancy can take several weeks to normalize. A study of thromboelastography (TEG) data from 71 women after normal delivery showed that all parameters remain abnormal at 1 week postpartum but normalize over the subsequent 3 weeks [87], although pro-thrombotic coagulation factor and naturally occurring anticoagulant abnormalities may persist for longer (see Chap. 1). The clinical data from several observational studies, however, show that the risk persists for up to 6 weeks postpartum, although to a lesser degree in weeks 5 and 6 [6, 10, 48, 76, 88].

In view of this persistent increased risk, it is advisable for high-risk women, that is, those on antenatal thromboprophylaxis, to continue for 6 weeks postpartum. There has been much debate as to the optimal duration of thromboprophylaxis in women at intermediate risk of VTE (Fig. 4.1 and Table 4.4). There is little evidence to support recommendations regarding duration of thromboprophylaxis in such women, and research in this area is needed. In view of the

Table 4.4 Stratification of VTE risk by type of thrombophilia and history

Very high risk	*Treatment recommendation*
Previous VTE on long-term warfarin Antithrombin deficiency Antiphospholipid syndrome + previous VTE	Antenatal high-dose LMWH and at least 6 weeks' postnatal LMWH or warfarin
High risk	***Treatment recommendation***
Previous recurrent or unprovoked VTE Previous estrogen-related VTE Previous VTE + thrombophilia Previous VTE + family history of VTE Asymptomatic thrombophilia – combined defects, homozygous FVL	Antenatal and 6 weeks' postnatal LMWH
Intermediate risk	***Treatment recommendation***
Single previous VTE associated with transient risk factor, no family history, or thrombophilia Asymptomatic thrombophilia (other than those above)	7 days postnatal prophylactic LMWH 6 weeks if other risk factors present

data regarding postpartum prothrombotic changes, a minimum of 7 days' thromboprophylaxis is suggested. In addition, women with ongoing additional risk factors should be considered potentially high risk, and it may be necessary to extend the 7-day period of prophylaxis for up to 6 weeks, for example, if hospital discharge is delayed due to sepsis.

4.4 Management in Specific Situations

The management of pregnant women with respect to their risk of VTE starts with accurate assessment of risk factors at their first presentation in pregnancy or ideally before, together with regular reassessment throughout the pregnancy and puerperium. Management also requires accurate and sensitive counseling of women and their families so that they understand the risks of VTE, the signs and symptoms of VTE, and the requirement for thromboprophylaxis. Women should be taught how to give the subcutaneous injections and require support from primary and secondary care to facilitate continued compliance. They should be counseled about delivery and management of their LMWH and require sensitive discussion around how this might influence their birth plan. Women receiving thromboprophylaxis require referral to an obstetric anesthetist, preferably antenatally, for discussion of pain management during labor.

The decision about the threshold for thromboprophylaxis in a woman with risk factors is discussed under each risk factor below. This is summarized in Fig. 4.1, an algorithm to aid thromboprophylaxis decision making, based on that in the recent RCOG guidelines [2].

4.4.1 Thrombophilia

Current evidence supports antenatal thromboprophylaxis and postnatal thromboprophylaxis for 6 weeks in women with an identified thrombophilia and previous VTE. For very-high-risk individuals (those with a compound thrombophilia or antithrombin deficiency or previous recurrent VTE on long-term anticoagulation), discussion with a clinician with expertise in hemostasis and pregnancy is imperative to determine the appropriate level of anticoagulation for pregnancy, as high prophylactic (twice daily) dose or therapeutic anticoagulation may be indicated.

Management of asymptomatic women (without prior VTE) with a known heritable thrombophilia is not straightforward because there are limited reliable data on the benefits of thromboprophylaxis in this setting. It is desirable to discuss the options as fully as possible with the woman, ideally in conjunction with a clinician with expertise in this area. It is important that laboratory thrombophilia results are not viewed in isolation but considered along with the family history and other risk factors before a conclusion is reached about the risk of VTE, and therefore the benefit of thromboprophylaxis, in the individual. In the family history, factors considered should include the number of affected relatives, the age at which thrombosis developed, and the presence or absence of additional risk factors in the affected relatives [77].

Since the risk of VTE is lower in asymptomatic women, antenatal thromboprophylaxis is usually necessary only in those with antithrombin deficiency or with combined or homozygous defects [77, 89, 90]. However, since asymptomatic thrombophilia is a risk factor, if combined with other risk factors such as increased age, obesity, or immobility, it may be justified to use antenatal thromboprophylaxis. Similarly, for asymptomatic women with thrombophilia without either a personal or family history of VTE, 6 weeks of postpartum thromboprophylaxis may be unnecessary. Again, decisions regarding whether to recommend postnatal thromboprophylaxis should be based on a risk assessment for that individual immediately after delivery.

The validity of this approach was reported in a prospective study in which women classified as low risk were managed by clinical surveillance alone unless there were additional risk factors [27]. This group included those with heritable thrombophilia (excluding antithrombin deficiency) and no prior VTE. Of the 225 women in this group, 70 % had either a heritable laboratory-detected thrombophilia or a positive family history in a first-degree relative, and none developed a pregnancy-related episode of VTE. However, in practice, 85 % of the women in this group received antenatal thromboprophylaxis because of additional risk factors, and the median time of treatment initiation was at 24 weeks' gestation (range 4–41 weeks). The duration of postpartum thromboprophylaxis the women received was intended to be 2 weeks, but other studies suggest that the risk of VTE remains elevated for up to 6 weeks postpartum, and therefore, if thromboprophylaxis is given antenatally for a persisting risk factor, it should be continued postpartum for 6 weeks [10, 76].

4.4.1.1 Antithrombin Deficiency

Women with antithrombin deficiency, particularly type 1, have a very high risk of first and recurrent thrombosis and probably require higher doses of LMWH in pregnancy. They are likely to be on long-term anticoagulation with warfarin, and therefore an intermediate or treatment dose of LMWH may be indicated throughout pregnancy and continued postpartum for a minimum of 6 weeks or until converted back to long-term warfarin. Heparins may not be as effective in antithrombin deficiency as their mode of action is antithrombin dependent, and it is reasonable to monitor anti-Xa levels in this setting, aiming for a level 4 h post injection of 0.35–0.5 u/mL [77]. Such women should be managed in collaboration with a hematologist with expertise in thrombosis in pregnancy.

4.4.1.2 Antiphospholipid Syndrome

On the basis of the perceived high risk of recurrent thrombosis, it is recommended in the most recent ACCP guidelines that pregnant women with APS and previous VTE should receive antenatal thromboprophylaxis with LMWH [70]. It is suggested that women on warfarin convert to LMWH before the sixth week of pregnancy and that those not on warfarin commence LMWH in the first trimester as soon as possible after diagnosis of the pregnancy. For women with a single previous VTE event, a high prophylactic (i.e. twice daily) dose of LMWH is often used [28]. For women with a history of recurrent VTE, particularly where this has entailed an increase in the usual target INR from 2.0 to 3.0, a high prophylactic, that is, 75 % of treatment dose, or full treatment dose can be used. Low dose aspirin is recommended for all women with APS [73]. A survey by the European Antiphospholipid Forum of clinicians who regularly manage patients with APS concluded that in women with APS associated with a previous VTE event, the majority would advise therapeutic dose LMWH during pregnancy, aiming for a 4-h anti-Xa level of 0.5–1.0 (Boffa MC, 2009, personal communication). The presence of antiphospholipid antibodies alone, even if persistent, without previous APS-classifiable pregnancy loss or thrombosis, does not equate to APS, and such women do not generally require antenatal LMWH [91].

After delivery, women on antenatal LMWH should continue at the same dose until reestablished on long-term oral anticoagulation or for a minimum of 6 weeks if not on long-term therapy. In women with APS featuring recurrent miscarriage or fetal loss without thrombosis, the risk of postpartum VTE is unclear, but data from randomized trials suggest the risk is likely to be low. Antenatal antithrombotic therapy administered to improve pregnancy outcome in these trials was typically stopped between 34 weeks and delivery, and no maternal VTE events were reported [92, 93]. However, many clinicians advocate postpartum thromboprophylaxis for 6 weeks in a similar way to those with asymptomatic inherited thrombophilia [70]. In women with persistent lupus anti-coagulant or high-titre antiphospholipid antibodies but without APS, that is, no prior thrombosis, recurrent miscarriage, or fetal loss, the risk of VTE is small. It is, however, reasonable to administer LMWH postnatally at a prophylactic dose for 7 days, even in the absence of additional risk factors.

4.4.2 Previous VTE

It is recommended that women with previous VTE are stratified into intermediate-risk, high-risk, and very high risk groups (Table 4.3) [70].

Women in the high and very high risk groups will therefore benefit from referral for pre-pregnancy counseling to construct a prospective management plan for thromboprophylaxis in pregnancy. Those who become pregnant before receiving such counseling require early referral for specialist management by an expert in hemostasis and pregnancy.

Women with recurrent VTE or a previous unprovoked or estrogen-related VTE or a previous VTE along with a family history of VTE are at higher risk than the normal population and should be offered thromboprophylaxis both antenatally and for 6 weeks postpartum. All women with a previous history of confirmed VTE should have postpartum prophylaxis.

Women on warfarin for recurrent VTE should be counseled about the risks to the fetus and advised to stop warfarin and change to LMWH as soon as pregnancy is confirmed, ideally within 2 weeks of the missed period, i.e., before 6 weeks' gestation. Women with recurrent VTE but not on warfarin should be advised to start LMWH as soon as they have a positive pregnancy test. For some women in this category, higher doses of LMWH may be appropriate. Advice should be sought from a clinician with expertise in hemostasis and pregnancy.

Where objective documentation is not available, the previous diagnosis of VTE can be assumed in cases where the woman gives a good history and received prolonged (>6 weeks) therapeutic anticoagulation. Any woman with objective documentation of previous VTE should have a careful history documented and undergo testing for both heritable and acquired thrombophilias if appropriate, preferably before pregnancy (see below).

4.4.2.1 Thrombophilia Testing

Testing for an underlying heritable thrombophilia is indicated only in certain circumstances in pregnancy and should be performed only when the outcome of the test will influence subsequent management. Pregnancy can also affect circulating coagulation factors; for example, protein S levels are reduced by pregnancy, deficiency cannot be diagnosed in pregnancy. If testing is planned, counseling is required to ensure that the woman and her family are aware of the potential implications of a positive diagnosis.

In women with a previous VTE, if this was unprovoked or estrogen related, then thrombophilia testing is not required as thromboprophylaxis is already indicated.

Testing is therefore useful in two main settings. In women with a previous VTE related to a minor temporary risk factor, if a thrombophilia is detected, then they would be offered antenatal prophylaxis. If antiphospholipid antibodies or antithrombin deficiency is detected, then the dose of LMWH would be increased during pregnancy.

4.4.3 Obesity

All women with class 3 obesity (BMI >40 kg/m^2) should be considered for thromboprophylaxis for 7 days after delivery (whether vaginal or Cesarean section), even if young and no other risk factors are present. The weight-related doses for different types of LMWH are provided in Table 4.2.

4.4.4 Mode of Delivery

The increased risk of VTE following Cesarean section, particularly as an emergency procedure, supports the routine prescription of postpartum prophylactic LMWH in all women undergoing an emergency Cesarean section and any woman with additional risk factors that undergoes elective Cesarean section. The duration of this should be at least 7 days, but extension of this period is recommended if additional risk factors are present or persisting, as the numbers of VTE after elective and emergency Cesarean sections are similar in weeks 1, 2, and 3 post delivery [43].

4.4.5 Thromboprophylaxis at Delivery

Pregnancy-associated prothrombotic changes are maximal soon after delivery. However, continuing thromboprophylaxis during labor to cover this time risks significant bleeding at the time of delivery and conflicts with techniques for administering regional anesthesia. The main concern with respect to regional anesthetic techniques is the potential for increasing the risk of epidural hematoma formation, either at the time of epidural or spinal injection or at removal of the epidural catheter. There is also an increased risk of wound hematoma following Cesarean section with both UFH and LMWH of around 2 % [55]. Women on LMWH should therefore be advised to discontinue it at the onset of labor or in the event of any vaginal bleeding and restart only after medical review and reassessment of risks of VTE and bleeding.

Regional techniques are not advised until at least 12 h after the previous prophylactic dose of LMWH or 24 h after a therapeutic dose (i.e. given on a 12-hourly basis). If an epidural has been sited, the catheter should not be removed within 12 h of the most recent prophylactic LMWH injection. A further 4 h should pass before the next dose of prophylactic LMWH is given. Prophylactic LMWH can be safely given 4 h after spinal anesthesia [60].

If women have been receiving antenatal prophylactic LMWH and an elective Cesarean section is planned, the normal dose can be given on the day prior to delivery. On the day of delivery, any morning dose can be omitted and the operation performed that morning. The same prophylactic dose of LMWH should be given 4 h postoperatively or 4 h post epidural catheter removal. For example, if the woman normally takes her dose of LMWH at 6 p.m., she can take this the evening prior to delivery and then have the elective Cesarean section the following morning. If the epidural catheter is removed before 2 p.m., the next prophylactic dose of LMWH can be given as normal at 6 p.m.

If regional techniques cannot be used for a patient presenting in spontaneous labor as a result of insufficient time since the last dose, alternative analgesia such as opiate-based intravenous patient-controlled analgesia should be offered. This restriction of anesthetic options means that planned induction of labor can be an attractive option for patients on high-prophylactic-dose or treatment dose LMWH therapy so that treatment can be planned around delivery. For example, a multiparous woman could take the morning dose on the day prior to induction and then omit the evening dose. An elective epidural could then be sited the following day (24 h after the last dose) prior to induction. Alternatively, the dose could be reduced to the standard prophylactic dose on the day prior to induction of labor and continued at this dose during labor if appropriate, if plans had been made to use alternative methods of analgesia. This group of women would therefore benefit from antenatal anesthetic review.

4.5 Case Studies

Case Study 1

A 30 year old woman in her first pregnancy booked at 12 weeks' gestation. At the age of 22 she had an above knee deep vein thrombosis whilst taking the combined oral contraceptive pill. She takes no regular medication and has no other risk factors for VTE.

What advice do you give her?

She needs to take a prophylactic dose of LMWH, starting as soon as possible, to be continued until 6 weeks postpartum. She should also be advised that in future pregnancies, she should start the prophylaxis earlier, i.e. as soon as she has a positive pregnancy test.

Case Study 2

A 38 year old woman is pregnant following in vitro fertilization. She has a body mass index of 32 kg/m^2.

What advice do you give her?

She has three risk factors for the development of venous thromboembolism, so current guidelines would suggest commencing thromboprophylaxis with LMWH, in the absence of any contraindications.

Case Study 3

A 28 year old woman has a postpartum hemorrhage following a spontaneous vaginal delivery at term. Her booking weight was 100 kg.

What advice do you give her?

Current guidelines advise at least 7 days of LMWH prophylaxis following delivery in any woman with two or more risk factors for the development of VTE. The dose prescribed depends on her booking weight, and a higher dose would therefore be advised for this woman (see weight specific doses) [2].

Case Study 4

A 32 year old woman undergoes an elective cesarean section for breech presentation. She has no other risk factors for venous thromboembolism.

What advice do you give her?

She has one risk factor for the development of VTE so should be advised to stay mobile and well hydrated, but she does not warrant prophylactic LMWH unless other risk factors develop.

Case Study 5

A 30 year old woman is readmitted 2 weeks after an emergency cesarean section with a wound infection requiring intravenous antibiotics.

What advice do you give her?

This woman requires prophylactic LMWH for the duration of her in-patient stay.

Key Learning Points

- Assessment of risk factors for VTE is required at booking and postpartum and should be reassessed at every hospital admission or development of intercurrent illness.
- The increased risk of VTE is present from early pregnancy. Therefore, if thromboprophylaxis is indicated antenatally, it should be instituted at the earliest opportunity.
- Low-molecular-weight heparin is the agent of choice for thromboprophylaxis in pregnancy, and the dose depends on maternal weight and any risk factors present.
- Anti-embolism stockings can be useful if pharmacological thromboprophylaxis is contraindicated, and these should be thigh length and properly fitted.
- All women with a previous history of confirmed VTE should be offered thromboprophylaxis for 6 weeks postpartum.

References

1. Centre for Maternal and Child Enquiries (CMACE). Saving mothers' lives: reviewing maternal deaths to make motherhood safer: 2006–08. The eighth report on confidential enquiries into maternal deaths in the United Kingdom. BJOG. 2011;118 Suppl 1:1–203.

2a. Royal College of Obstetricians and Gynaecologists. Reducing the risk of thrombosis and embolism during pregnancy and the puerperium, Green-top guideline no. 37a. London: RCOG; 2009. https://www.rcog.org.uk/guidelines.
2b. Royal College of Obstetricians and Gynaecologists. Reducing the risk of venous thromboembolism during pregnancy and the puerperium, Green-top guideline no 37a. London RCOG; 2015. https://www.rcog.org.uk/guidelines.
3. Lim W, Eikelboom JW, Ginsberg JS. Inherited thrombophilia and pregnancy associated venous thromboembolism. BMJ. 2007;334:1318–21.
4. McColl MD, Ramsay JE, Tait RC, Walker ID, McCall F, Conkie JA, Carty MJ, Greer IA. Risk factors for pregnancy associated venous thromboembolism. Thromb Haemost. 1997;78(4):1183–8.
5. Gerhardt A, Scharf RE, Beckman MW, et al. Prothrombin and factor V mutations in women with thrombosis during pregnancy and the puerperium. N Engl J Med. 2000;342:374–80.
6. Pomp ER, Lenselink AM, Rosendaal FR, Doggen CJ. Pregnancy, the postpartum period and prothrombotic defects: risk of venous thrombosis in the MEGA study. J Thromb Haemost. 2008;6(4):632–7.
7. Rosendaal FR, Koster T, Vandenbroucke JP, Reitsma PH. High risk of thrombosis in patients homozygous for factor V Leiden (activated protein C resistance). Blood. 1995;85(5):1504–8.
8. Biron-Andreani C, Schved J-F, Daures J-P. Factor V Leiden mutation and pregnancy-related venous thromboembolism. Thromb Haemost. 2006;96:14–8.
9. Dizon-Townson D, Miller C, Sibai B, Spong CY, Thom E, Wendel G Jr, Wenstrom K, Samuels P, Cotroneo MA, Moawad A, Sorokin Y, Meis P, Miodovnik M, O'Sullivan MJ, Conway D, Wapner RJ, Gabbe SG, for the National Institute of Child Health and Human Development Maternal-Fetal Medicine Units Network. The relationship of the factor V Leiden mutation and pregnancy outcomes for mother and fetus. Obstet Gynecol. 2005;106(3):517–24.
10. Heit JA, Kobbervig CE, James AH, Petterson TM, Bailey KR, Melton 3rd LJ. Trends in the incidence of venous thromboembolism during pregnancy or postpartum: a 30-year population-based study. Ann Intern Med. 2005;143:697–706.
11. Lindqvist PG, Svensson PJ, Marsal K, Grennert L, Luterkort M, Dahlback B. Activated protein C resistance (FV:Q506) and pregnancy. Thromb Haemost. 1999;81(4):532–7.
12. Bezemer ID, van der Meer FJ, Eikenboom JC, Rosendaal FR, Doggen CJ. The value of family history as a risk indicator for venous thrombosis. Arch Intern Med. 2009;169(6):610–5.
13. Bank I, Libourel EJ, Middeldorp S, van Pampus ECM, Koopman MMW, Hamulyak K, Prins MH, van der Meer J, Buller HR. Prothrombin 20210A mutation: a mild risk factor for venous thromboembolism but not for arterial thrombotic disease and pregnancy-related complications in a family study. Arch Intern Med. 2004;164(17):1932–7.
14. Martinelli I, Battaglioli T, De Stefano V, Tormene D, Valdre L, Grandone E, Tosetto A, Mannucci PM, on behalf of the GIT (Gruppos Italiano Trombofilia). The risk of first venous thromboembolism during pregnancy and puerperium in double heterozygotes for factor V Leiden and prothrombin G20210A. J Thromb Haemost. 2008;6:494–8.
15. Samama MM, Rached RA, Horellou M-H, Aquilanti S, Mathieux VG, Plu-Bureau G, Elalamy I, Conard J. Pregnancy-associated venous thromboembolism (VTE) in combined heterozygous factor V Leiden (FVL) and prothrombin (FII) 20210 A mutation and in heterozygous FII single gene mutation alone. Br J Haematol. 2003;123:327–34.
16. Middeldorp S, van Hylckama Vlieg A. Does thrombophilia testing help in the clinical management of patients? Br J Haematol. 2008;143:321–35.
17. Danilenko-Dixon DR, Heit JA, Silverstein MD, Yawn BP, Petterson TM, Lohse CM, Melton 3rd LJ. Risk factors for deep vein thrombosis and pulmonary embolism during pregnancy or post partum: a population-based, case–control study. Am J Obstet Gynecol. 2001;184(2):104–10.
18. Martinelli I, Legnani C, Bucciarelli P, Grandone E, De Stefano V, Mannucci PM. Risk of pregnancy-related venous thrombosis in carriers of severe inherited thrombophilia. Thromb Haemost. 2001;86:800–3.
19. Robertson L, Wu O, Langhorne P, Twaddle S, Clark P, Lowe GDO, Walker ID, Greaves M, Brenkel I, Regan L, Greer IA. The thrombosis: risk and economic assessment of thrombophilia screening (TREATS) study. Br J Haematol. 2005;132(2):171–96.
20. Lijfering WM, Brouwer JLP, Veeger NJGM, Coppens M, Middeldorp S, Hamulyak K, Prins M, Buller HR, van der Meer J. Selective testing for thrombophilia in patients with first venous thrombosis: results from a retrospective family cohort study on absolute thrombotic risk for currently known thrombophilic defects in 2479 relatives. Blood. 2009;113(21):5314–22.
21. Conard J, Horellou MH, van Dreden P, Le Compte T, Samama M. Thrombosis in pregnancy and congenital deficiencies in AT III, protein C or protein S: study of 78 women. Thromb Haemost. 1990;63:319–20.
22. Folkeringa N, Brouwer JLP, Korteweg FJ, Veeger JGM, Erwich JJHM, van der Meer J. High risk of pregnancy-related venous thromboembolism in women with multiple thrombophilic defects. Br J Haematol. 2007;138:110–6.
23. Miyakis S, Lockshin MD, Atsumi T, Branch DW, Brey RL, Cervera R, Derksen RHWM, De Groot PG, Koike T, Meroni PL, Reber G, Shoenfeld Y, Tincani A, Vlachoyannopoulos PG, Krilis SA. International consensus statement on an update of the classification criteria for definite antiphospholipid syndrome. J Thromb Haemost. 2006;4:295–306.
24. Crowther MA, Ginsberg JS, Julian J, Denburg J, Hirsh J, Douketis J, Laskin C, Fortin P, Anderson D, Kearon C, Clarke A, Geerts W, Forgie M, Green D, Costantini L, Yacura W, Wilson S, Gent M, Kovacs MJ. A com-

parison of two intensities of warfarin for the prevention of recurrent thrombosis in patients with the antiphospholipid antibody syndrome. N Engl J Med. 2003;349:1133–8.
25. Finazzi G, Marchioli R, Brancaccio V, Schinco P, Wisloff F, Musial J, Baudo F, Berrettini M, Testa S, D'Angelo A, Tognoni G, Barbui T. A randomized clinical trial of high-intensity warfarin vs. conventional antithrombotic therapy for the prevention of recurrent thrombosis in patients with the antiphospholipid syndrome (WAPS). J Thromb Haemost. 2005;3:848–53.
26. Galli M, Luciani D, Bertolini G, Barbui T. Anti-beta 2-glycoprotein I, antiprothrombin antibodies, and the risk of thrombosis in the antiphospholipid syndrome. Blood. 2003;102(8):2717–23.
27. Bauersachs RM, Dudenhausen J, Faridi A, Fischer T, Fung S, Geisen U, et al. Risk stratification and heparin prophylaxis to prevent venous thromboembolism in pregnant women. Thromb Haemost. 2007;98(6):1237–45.
28. Stone S, Hunt BJ, Khamashta MA, Bewley SJ, Nelson-Piercy C. Primary antiphospholipid syndrome in pregnancy: an analysis of outcome in a cohort of 33 women treated with a rigorous protocol. J Thromb Haemost. 2005;3(2):243–5.
29. James AH, Jamison MG, Brancazio LR, Myers ER. Venous thromboembolism during pregnancy and the postpartum period: incidence, risk factors, and mortality. Am J Obstet Gynecol. 2006;194(5):1311–5.
30. Pabinger I, Grafenhofer H, Kaider A, Kyrle PA, Quehenberger P, Mannhalter C, Lechner K. Risk of pregnancy-associated recurrent venous thromboembolism in women with a history of venous thrombosis. J Thromb Haemost. 2005;3(5):949–54.
31. Pabinger I, Grafenhofer H, Kyrle PA, Quehenberger P, Mannhalter C, Lechner K, Kaider A. Temporary increase in the risk for recurrence during pregnancy in women with a history of venous thromboembolism. Blood. 2002;100:1060–2.
32. Kearon C, Kahn SR, Agnelli G, Goldhaber S, Raskob GE, Comerota AJ. Antithrombotic therapy for venous thromboembolic disease: American College of Chest Physicians Evidence-Based Clinical Practice Guidelines (8th Edition). Chest. 2008;133: 454–545.
33. Brill-Edwards P, Ginsberg JS, for the Recurrence of Clot in this Pregnancy (ROCIT) Study Group. Safety of withholding antepartum heparin in women with a previous episode of venous thromboembolism. N Engl J Med. 2000;343:1439–44.
34. De Stefano V, Martinelli I, Rossi E, Battaglioli T, Za T, Mannuccio Mannucci P, Leone G. The risk of recurrent venous thromboembolism in pregnancy and puerperium without antithrombotic prophylaxis. Br J Haematol. 2006;135(3):386–91.
35. White RH, Chan WS, Zhou H, Ginsberg JS. Recurrent venous thromboembolism after pregnancy-associated versus unprovoked thromboembolism. Thromb Haemost. 2008;100(2):246–52.
36. Marchiori A, Mosena L, Prins MH, Prandoni P. The risk of recurrent venous thromboembolism among heterozygous carriers of factor V Leiden or pro-thrombin G20210A mutation. A systematic review of prospective studies. Haematologica. 2007;92: 1107–14.
37. Health Survey for England – 2008 trend tables. Department of Health, http://www.ic.nhs.uk/statistics-and-data-collections/health-and-lifestyles-related-surveys/health-survey-for-england. Accessed 26 Jan 2010.
38. Robinson HE, O'Connell CM, Joseph KS, McLeod NL. Maternal outcomes in pregnancies complicated by obesity. Obstet Gynecol. 2005;106(6): 1357–64.
39. Larsen TB, Sorensen HT, et al. Maternal smoking, obesity, and risk of venous thromboembolism during pregnancy and the puerperium: a population-based nested case–control study. Thromb Res. 2007;120(4):505–9.
40. Confidential Enquiry into Maternal and Child Health (CEMACH). Saving mothers' lives: reviewing maternal deaths to make motherhood safer, 2003–05. In: Lewis G, editor. The seventh report of the confidential enquiries into maternal deaths in the United Kingdom. London: CEMACH; 2007.
41. Lindqvist P, Dahlbäck B, Marŝál K. Thrombotic risk during pregnancy: a population study. Obstet Gynecol. 1999;94:595–9.
42. Simpson EL, Lawrenson RA, Nightingale AL, Farmer RDT. Venous thromboembolism in pregnancy and the puerperium: incidence and additional risk factors from a London perinatal database. BJOG. 2001;108:56–60.
43. Jacobsen AF, Skjeldestad FE, Sandset PM. Ante- and postnatal risk factors of venous thrombosis: a hospital-based case – control study. J Thromb Haemost. 2008;6(6):905–12.
44. Arya R, Shehata HA, Patel RK, Sahu S, Rajasingam D, Harrington K, Nelson-Piercy C, Parsons J. Internal jugular vein thrombosis following assisted conception therapy. Br J Haematol. 2001;115:153–6.
45. Liu S, Liston RM, Joseph KS, Heaman M, Sauve R, Kramer MS, et al. Maternal mortality and severe morbidity associated with low-risk planned cesarean delivery versus planned vaginal delivery at term. CMAJ. 2007;176(4):455–60.
46. Ros HS, Lichtenstein P, Bellocco R, Petersson G, Cnattingius S. Pulmonary embolism and stroke in relation to pregnancy: how can high-risk women be identified? Am J Obstet Gynecol. 2002;186(2):198–203.
47. Macklon NS, Greer IA. Venous thromboembolic disease in obstetrics and gynaecology: the Scottish experience. Scott Med J. 1996;41(3):83–6.
48. Royal College of Obstetricians and Gynaecologists. Report of the RCOG Working Party on prophylaxis against thromboembolism in gynaecology and obstetrics. London: RCOG Press; 1995. https://www.rcog.org.uk/guidelines.
49. National Institute for Health and Care Excellence. Clinical guideline no. 62. Antenatal care. Routine care for the healthy pregnant woman. London: NICE: https://www.nice.org.uk/ March 2008.

50. Royal College of Obstetricians and Gynaecologists. Air travel and pregnancy, Scientific advisory committee opinion paper, vol. 1. London: RCOG Press; 2008. https://www.rcog.org.uk/guidelines.
51. Department of Health. Report of the independent expert working group on the prevention of venous thromboembolism in hospitalised patients. http://www.dh.gov.uk/dr_consum_dh/groups/dh_digitalas-sets/documents/digitalasset/dh_073953.pdf. Accessed Jan 2010.
52. National Institute for Health and Clinical Excellence. Clinical guideline no. 92. Venous thromboembolism: reducing the risk of venous thromboembolism (deep vein thrombosis and pulmonary embolism) in patients admitted to hospital. London: NICE: https://www.nice.org.uk/ Jan 2010.
53. Vossen CY, Conard J, Fontcuberta J, Makris M, van der Meer FJM, Pabinger I, Palareti G, Preston FE, Scharrer I, Souto JC, Svensson P, Walker ID, Rosendaal FR. Risk of a first venous thrombotic event in carriers of a familial thrombophilic defect. The European Prospective Cohort on Thrombophilia (EPCOT). J Thromb Haemost. 2005;3:459–64.
54. Greer IA. Reduction in incidence of postpartum VTE following the introduction of thromboprophylaxis. Abstract presented at the International Society of Obstetric Medicine, Washington, 2008.
55. Greer IA, Nelson-Piercy C. Low-molecular-weight heparins for thromboprophylaxis and treatment of venous thromboembolism in pregnancy: a systematic review of safety and efficacy. Blood. 2005;106:401–7.
56. Sanson BJ, Lensing AWA, Prins MH, et al. Safety of low-molecular-weight heparin in pregnancy: a systematic review. Thromb Haemost. 1999;81:668–72.
57. Pettila V, Leinonen P, Markkola A, Hiilesmaa V, Kaaja R. Postpartum bone mineral density in women treated for thromboprophylaxis with unfractionated heparin or LMW heparin. Thromb Haemost. 2002;87:182–6.
58. Knight M, on behalf of UKOSS. Antenatal pulmonary embolism: risk factors, management and outcomes. BJOG. 2008;115(4):453–61.
59. Verstraete M. Pharmacotherapeutic aspects of unfractionated and low-molecular-weight heparins. Drugs. 1990;40(4):498–530.
60. Horlocker TT, et al. Regional anesthesia in the anticoagulated patient: defining the risks (the second ASRA Consensus Conference on Neuraxial Anesthesia and Anticoagulation). Reg Anesth Pain Med. 2003;28:172–97.
61. Lindhoff-Last E, Kreutzenbeck H-J, Magnani HN. Treatment of 51 pregnancies with danaparoid because of heparin intolerance. Thromb Haemost. 2005;93:63–9.
62. Mazzolai L, Hohlfeld P, Spertini F, Hayoz D, Schapira M, Duchosal MA. Fondaparinux is a safe alternative in case of heparin intolerance during pregnancy. Blood. 2006;108:1569–70.
63. Lagrange F, Vergnes C, Brun JL, Paolucci F, Nadal T, Leng JJ, Saux MC, Banwarth B. Absence of placental transfer of pentasaccharide (fondaparinux, Arixtra®) in the dually perfused human cotyledon in vitro. Thromb Haemost. 2002;87:831–5.
64. Dempfle CH. Minor transplacental passage of fondaparinux in vivo. N Engl J Med. 2004;350:1914–5.
65. Gerhardt A, Zotz RB, Stockschlaeder M, Scharf RE. Fondaparinux is an effective alternative anticoagulant in pregnant women with high risk of venous thromboembolism and intolerance to low-molecular-weight heparins and heparinoids. Thromb Haemost. 2007;97:496–7.
66. Antiplatelet Trialists' Collaboration. Collaborative overview of randomised trials of antiplatelet therapy – III: reduction in venous thrombosis and pulmonary embolism by antiplatelet prophylaxis among surgical and medical patients. BMJ. 1994;308:235–46.
67. Antithrombotic Trialists' Collaboration. Collaborative meta-analysis of randomised trials of antiplatelet therapy for prevention of death, myocardial infarction, and stroke in high risk patients. BMJ. 2002;324: 71–86.
68. Pulmonary Embolism Prevention (PEP) Trial Collaborative Group. Prevention of pulmonary embolism and deep venous thrombosis with low dose aspirin: pulmonary embolism prevention (PEP) trial. Lancet. 2000;355:1295–302.
69. Glynn RJ, Ridker PM, Goldhaber SZ, Buring JE. Effect of low-dose aspirin on the occurrence of venous thromboembolism: a randomized trial. Ann Intern Med. 2007;147(8):525–33.
70. Bates SM, Greer IA, Pabinger I, Sofaer S, Hirsh J. Venous thromboembolism, thrombophilia, antithrombotic therapy, and pregnancy: American College of Chest Physicians Evidence-Based Clinical Practice Guidelines (8th Edition). Chest. 2008;133(6 Suppl):844S–86.
71. Geerts WH, Bergqvist D, et al. Prevention of venous thromboembolism. American College of Chest Physicians Evidence-Based Clinical Practice Guidelines (8th Edition). Chest. 2008;133:381–453.
72. Duley L, Henderson-Smart DJ, Meher S, King JF. Antiplatelet agents for preventing pre-eclampsia and its complications. Cochrane Database Syst Rev. 2007;(2):CD004659. doi:10.1002/14651858.CD004659.pub2.
73. Robertson B, Greaves M. Antiphospholipid syndrome: an evolving story. Blood Rev. 2006;20(4):201–12.
74. Barbier P, Jongville AP, Autre TE, Coureau C. Fetal risks with dextran during delivery. Drug Saf. 1992;7:71–3.
75. Berg EM, Fasting S, Sellevold OF. Serious complications with dextran-70 despite hapten prophylaxis. Is it best avoided prior to delivery? Anaesthesia. 1991;46:1033–5.
76. Jacobsen AF, Skjeldestad FE, Sandet PM. Incidence and risk patterns of venous thromboembolism in pregnancy and puerperium – a register-based case–control study. Am J Obstet Gynecol. 2008;198:223–34.
77. Walker ID, Greaves M, Preston FE, British Society for Haematology Guideline. Investigation and man-

agement of heritable thrombophilia. Br J Haematol. 2001;114:512–28.
78. Buchtemann AS, Steins A, Volkert B, Hahn M, Klyscz T, Junger M. The effect of compression therapy on venous haemodynamics in pregnant women. Br J Obstet Gynaecol. 1999;106:563–9.
79. Jamieson R, Calderwood CJ, Greer IA. The effect of graduated compression stockings on blood velocity in the deep venous system of the lower limb in the postnatal period. BJOG. 2007;114:1292–4.
80. Bates SM, Greer IA, Middeldorp S, Veenstra DL, Prabulos A-M, Vandvik PO. VTE, thrombophilia, antithrombotic therapy, and pregnancy. Antithrombotic Therapy and prevention of Thrombosis, 9th ed: American College of Chest Physicians Evidence-Based Clinical Practice Guidelines. Chest. 2012;141(2 Suppl):e691S–736.
81. Brady D, Raingruber B, Peterson J, Varnau W, Denman J, Resuello R, De Contreaus R, Mahnke J. The use of knee-length versus thigh-length compression stockings and sequential compression devices. Crit Care Nurs Q. 2007;30(3):255–62.
82. Phillips S, Gallagher M, Buchan H. Use graduated compression stockings postoperatively to prevent deep vein thrombosis. BMJ. 2008;336:943–4.
83. Lord RA, Hamilton D. Graduated compression stockings (20–30 mmHg) do not compress leg veins in the standing position. ANZ J Surg. 2004;74:581–5.
84. Partsch B, Partsch H. Calf compression pressure required to achieve venous closure from supine to standing positions. J Vasc Surg. 2005;42:734–8.
85. Baglin T, Barrowcliffe TW, Cohen A, Greaves M, for the British Committee for Standards in Haematology. Guidelines on the use and monitoring of heparin. Br J Haematol. 2006;133:19–34.
86. Ray JG, Chan WA. Deep vein thrombosis during pregnancy and the puerperium: a meta-analysis of the period of risk and the leg of presentation. Obstet Gynecol Surv. 1999;54(4):265–71.
87. Maybury H, Waugh JJ, Gornall AS, Pavord S. There is a return to non-pregnant coagulation parameters after four not six weeks postpartum following spontaneous vaginal delivery. Obstet Med. 2008; 1:92–4.
88. Ros HS, Lichtenstein P, Bellocco R, Petersson G, Cnattingius S. Increased risks of circulatory diseases in late pregnancy and puerperium. Epidemiology. 2001;12(4):456–60.
89. Gerhardt A, Scharf RE, Zotz RB. Effect of hemostatic risk factors on the individual probability of thrombosis during pregnancy and the puerperium. Thromb Haemost. 2003;90:77–85.
90. McColl MD, Ellison J, Reid F, et al. Prothrombin 20210GA, MTHFR C677T mutations in women with venous thromboembolism associated with pregnancy. Br J Obstet Gynaecol. 2000;107:565–9.
91. Stone S, Langford K, Nelson-Piercy C, Khamashta M, Bewley S, Hunt BJ. Antiphospholipid antibodies do not a syndrome make. Lupus. 2002;11:130–3.
92. Laskin CA, Spitzer CA, Clark C, et al. Low-molecular-weight heparin and aspirin for recurrent pregnancy loss: results from the randomized, controlled Hep ASA trial. J Rheumatol. 2009;36:279–87.
93. Rai R, Cohen H, Dave M, Regan L. Randomised controlled trial of aspirin and aspirin plus heparin in pregnant women with recurrent miscarriage associated with phospholipid antibodies (or antiphospholipid antibodies). BMJ. 1997;314:253–7.

Systemic Thromboembolism in Pregnancy: Venous Thromboembolism

5

Asma Khalil, Louise Bowles, Patrick O'Brien, and Hannah Cohen

Abstract

Venous thromboembolism (VTE), which includes deep venous thrombosis, pulmonary embolism and cerebral vein and venous sinus thrombosis, remains a leading cause of maternal morbidity and mortality, despite improvements in prevention in recent years. Low-molecular-weight heparin (LMWH) is the mainstay of treatment of pregnancy-associated VTE. The primary aim in peripartum management is to balance the risk of major postpartum hemorrhage versus the risk of extension or recurrence of VTE when anticoagulation is interrupted. In general, being on a treatment dose of anticoagulation is often an indication for timing of delivery, but would not be an indication for elective Cesarean section; induction of labor is usually preferable unless there is an obstetric indication for Cesarean section. Therapeutic anticoagulation should be continued for the duration of the pregnancy and for at least 6 weeks postnatally, and until at least 3 months of anticoagulation has been given in total.

Keywords

Pregnancy • Venous thromboembolism • Deep venous thrombosis • Pulmonary embolism • Lung imaging • Low-molecular-weight heparin

A. Khalil, MB BCh, MD, MRCOG, MSc, DFSRH (✉)
Department of Obstetrics and Gynaecology,
St. George's Hospital,
St. George's Healthcare NHS Trust,
Blackshaw Road, Tooting, London SW17 OQT, UK
e-mail: asmakhalil79@googlemail.com

L. Bowles, MBBS, BSc, MRCP, FRCPath
Department of Clinical Haematology,
The Royal London Hospital,
Whitechapel, London E1 1BB, UK
e-mail: Louise.Bowles@bartshealth.nhs.uk

P. O'Brien, MB BCh, FRCOG, FICOG, FFSRH
Institute for Women's Health, University College
London Hospitals NHS Foundation Trust,
250 Euston Road, London NW1 2PG, UK
e-mail: patobrien64@yahoo.co.uk

H. Cohen, MB ChB, MD, FCRP, FRCPath
Department of Haematology, University College
London Hospitals NHS Foundation Trust,
250 Euston Road, London NW1 2PG, UK
e-mail: hannah.cohen@uclh.nhs.uk

H. Cohen, P. O'Brien (eds.), *Disorders of Thrombosis and Hemostasis in Pregnancy: A Guide to Management*, DOI 10.1007/978-3-319-15120-5_5, © Springer-Verlag London 2015

5.1 Introduction

Venous thromboembolism (VTE) remains a leading cause of maternal mortality and morbidity worldwide, although the United Kingdom Centre for Maternal and Child Enquiries (CMACE) reported a significant fall in maternal death due to VTE [1, 2]. Physiological changes during pregnancy alter the balance in the hemostatic system in favor of thrombosis. The increased risk of VTE begins in early pregnancy and lasts throughout pregnancy and the puerperium. The elevated risk of VTE has been shown to persist until at least 12 weeks after delivery, although the absolute increase in risk beyond 6 weeks is low.

Pregnancy increases the risk of VTE five- to ten-fold compared with the non-pregnant state, with VTE occurring in around 1 per 1,000 deliveries [3–8]. While available data suggest that Cesarean section is associated with an increased risk of fatal and non-fatal VTE, in the four triennia between 1997 and 2008, half of all deaths followed vaginal delivery [1].

5.2 Epidemiology

The incidence of VTE in non-pregnant women of childbearing age is around 1 in 10,000 [9–13] compared with an incidence in pregnancy between 0.6 and 1.3 episodes per 1,000 births [3–8]. The hypercoagulability of pregnancy confers benefit on the pregnant woman in that it helps to reduce the risk of death from hemorrhage after delivery of the baby and placenta. However, the price paid is an increased risk of VTE throughout pregnancy and the puerperium. VTE can occur in any of the three trimesters, but the puerperium is the time of greatest risk [14]. This is consistent with the physiological hypercoagulability providing the greatest protection against the risk of hemorrhage around the time of birth and immediately afterwards.

In the UK, CMACE reported that there were 18 deaths due to VTE in the triennium 2006–2008 [1]. This was notably fewer than the 41 deaths in the 2003–2005 report and by far the lowest since the UK-wide enquiry began in 1985. The fall in deaths from pulmonary embolism (PE), from 33 to 16, was mainly the result of a reduction in antenatal deaths and deaths following vaginal delivery, though deaths following Cesarean section also fell slightly. This CMACE report noted that "this is the first full triennium following publication of the 2004 RCOG guideline 'Thromboprophylaxis during pregnancy, labor and after normal vaginal delivery' and it seems likely that the unprecedented fall in deaths is the result of better recognition of at-risk women and more widespread thromboprophylaxis."

In that 2006–2008 CMACE report, 16 of the 18 deaths were due to PE; the remaining 2 were as a result of cerebral vein thrombosis. The United Kingdom Obstetric Surveillance System (UKOSS) reported that the incidence of antenatal PE in the UK was 13.1 per 100,000 maternities (95 % confidence intervals 10.6, 16) [15, 16], with a case fatality rate of 3.5 %. In the previous two Confidential Enquires into Maternal Deaths reports (2000–2002 and 2003–2005) [2, 17], there were 25 and 33 deaths, respectively, caused by PE, representing mortality rates of 1.56 and 1.2 per 100,000, respectively. These rates are similar to those published for the United States by the Centers for Disease Control and Prevention that monitors pregnancy mortality via the Pregnancy Mortality Surveillance System. They reported rates of deaths due to PE in pregnancy of 1.8 and 2.3 per 100,000 live births for the periods 1987–1990 and 1991–1999, respectively [18, 19]. Table 5.1 shows the numbers of direct deaths from VTE and rates per 100,000 maternities in the United Kingdom in the period 1985–2008.

The incidence of deep vein thrombosis (DVT) in pregnancy and the puerperium is approximately 1 in 1000 pregnancies [20]. VTE can occur at any stage of pregnancy but the puerperium is the time of highest risk, with estimates of relative risk of approximately 20-fold [21]. In pregnancy, DVT occurs more commonly in the left leg (up to 90 %) in contrast to 55 % in the non-pregnant state. This observation may be explained by compression of the left common iliac vein by the gravid uterus, at the point where it is crossed by the overlying right common iliac artery (May-Thurner syndrome). However, this hypothesis would not seem to apply not seem to apply to DVT observed in early pregnancy. A systematic review of 6 studies, which included 124 patients, selected because they provided objective diagnostic and anatomic

Table 5.1 Direct deaths from thrombosis and thromboembolism and rates per 100,000 maternities (United Kingdom, 1985–2008)

	Pulmonary embolism				Cerebral vein thrombosis				Thrombosis and thromboembolism			
	Number	Rate	95 % CI		Number	Rate	95 % CI		Number	Rate	95 % CI	
1985–1987	30	1.32	0.83	1.89	2	0.09	0.02	0.32	32	1.41	1.00	1.99
1988–1990	24	1.02	0.68	1.51	9	0.38	0.20	0.72	33	1.40	1.00	1.96
1991–1993	30	1.30	0.91	1.85	5	0.22	0.09	0.51	35	1.51	1.09	2.10
1994–1996	46	2.09	1.57	2.79	2	0.09	0.02	0.33	48	2.18	1.65	2.90
1997–1999	31	1.46	1.03	2.07	4	0.19	0.07	0.48	35	1.65	1.19	2.29
2000–2002	25	1.25	0.85	1.85	5	0.25	0.11	0.59	30	1.50	1.05	2.14
2003–2005	33	1.56	1.11	2.19	8	0.38	0.19	0.75	41	1.94	1.43	2.63
2006–2008	16	0.70	0.43	1.14	2	0.09	0.02	0.35	18	0.79	0.49	1.25

Confidential Enquiry into Maternal and Child Health [1]

Table 5.2 Risk factors for venous thromboembolism in pregnancy and the puerperium

Pre-existing	New onset or transient
Age over 35 years	Surgical procedure in pregnancy or puerperium, e.g. evacuation of retained products of conception, postpartum sterilization, emergency CS, elective CS with other risk factors
Obesity (Weight >100 kg or BMI >30 kg/m^2) either pre-pregnancy or in early pregnancy	Hyperemesis
Parity ≥3	Dehydration
Smoker	Ovarian hyperstimulation syndrome
Gross varicose veins with phlebitis	Multiple pregnancy or assisted conception
Paraplegia	Severe infection, e.g. pyelonephritis
One or more significant medical co- morbidities, e.g. heart disease; metabolic, endocrine or respiratory pathologies; inflammatory conditions (e.g. inflammatory bowel disease)	Immobility (e.g. SPD, significantly reduced mobility for 3 or more days; long distance travel >4 h during pregnancy and up to 6 weeks post- partum)
Known thrombophilias and other thrombotic conditions, e.g. hemoglobinopathies, myeloproliferative disease (essential thrombocythemia, polycythemia vera), nephrotic syndrome	Preeclampsia Excessive blood loss Prolonged labor (>24 h) Mid-cavity instrumental delivery Immobility after delivery Critical care admission PPH >1 L or blood transfusion

CS Cesarean section, *SPD* symphysis pubis dysfunction

information for unselected or consecutive symptomatic pregnant patients with DVT, identified that proximal DVT restricted to the femoral or iliac veins occurred in over 60 % of cases [22].

The risk factors for VTE in pregnancy are shown in Table 5.2. The prevalence of many of these risk factors is increasing. For example, levels of obesity in the general and pregnant populations are rising in the UK and elsewhere. The average age of pregnancy is rising constantly and, related to this, there are more pregnant women with coexisting medical morbidities such as heart, lung, or bowel disease. Because of the increasing availability of assisted reproduction technologies, multiple pregnancy is also on the rise. It is to be hoped that more widespread recognition and assessment of these risk factors will lead to more consistent use of thromboprophylactic measures (see Chap. 4).

Most women who die from PE will have identifiable risk factors. In the CMACE report of 2006–2008 [1], 16 of the 18 women who died from PE in the UK had recognized risk factors; and in the UKOSS report of 143 antenatal PE, including 5 fatal events, 70 % had identifiable risk factors [16].

Compared with VTE, arterial thrombosis is far less common in pregnancy, possibly reflecting the lower incidence of atherosclerotic plaques in women of this age. The incidence of stroke in pregnancy is reported as 0.04–0.34 per 1,000 births [23–26] and myocardial infarction 0.1 per 1,000 births [27]. However, a proportion of stroke will be hemorrhagic, and myocardial infarction may be due to coronary artery dissection (the risk of which is increased in pregnancy). Some of the risk factors for VTE also increase the risk of arterial thrombosis; these include older age, obesity and smoking. The risk of arterial thrombosis is also increased in association with hemoglobinopathies, antiphospholipid syndrome and other acquired disorders including myeloproliferative neoplasms and paroxysmal nocturnal hemoglobinuria, and with drugs that can cause arterial spasm such as ergometrine, cocaine and marijuana.

5.3 Pathophysiology of Venous Thromboembolism

The pathophysiology of VTE has classically been described in terms of Virchow's triad of venous stasis, hypercoagulability, and vascular damage. All three of these components are affected during pregnancy. Because of the vasodilator effect of progesterone, relaxin, and other pregnancy-related hormones, and because of the physical obstruction of the gravid uterus, there is increased venous stasis in the pelvic and lower limb veins. Doppler studies of venous blood flow in the lower limbs in pregnancy show that venous flow velocity is reduced by 50 % by the end of the second trimester and reaches a nadir at 36 weeks' gestation [28]. After delivery, flow velocity takes 6 weeks to return to normal. Pregnancy is a hypercoagulable state (as detailed in Chap. 1); hemostatic changes in coagulation factors, the fibrinolytic system, and natural anticoagulants prepare the body for the challenges of implantation, placentation, and delivery. A number of coagulation factor levels increase, including fibrinogen and factor VIII as well as von Willebrand factor, whilst other coagulation factor levels remain unchanged or decrease. The rise in factor VIII leads to a shortened activated partial thromboplastin time (APTT) in late pregnancy. These increased coagulation factors are not balanced by increases in the naturally occurring anticoagulants. Both free and total protein S decrease during pregnancy. Although protein C levels remain normal or show a slight increase, there is an increase in activated protein C resistance (APCR), largely due to the increase in factor VIII and decrease in protein S levels. Antithrombin generally remains unchanged. Thrombin generation increases during pregnancy and, although global fibrinolytic activity is reduced, plasma D-dimer (a marker of activation of fibrinolysis secondary to coagulation activation) increases [29–33]. Finally, delivery, whether vaginal (normal or instrumental) or abdominal (Cesarean section), inevitably causes a degree of injury to pelvic vessels.

5.4 Diagnosis of Venous Thromboembolism

The clinical diagnosis of acute VTE is often difficult, particularly in pregnancy when edema of the lower limbs is common, as is dyspnea (which occurs in up to 70 % of all pregnant women). The accuracy of clinical diagnosis of VTE is very low (approximately 8 % for DVT and 5 % for PE) [21, 34, 35]. It is important, therefore, to maintain a high index of suspicion in women presenting with some or all of the typical symptoms or signs of DVT (leg pain and swelling, usually

Table 5.3 Symptoms and signs of venous thromboembolism in pregnancy

Deep vein thrombosis
Painful warm leg
Swelling
Erythema
Tenderness
Lower abdominal pain
Pulmonary embolism
Pleuritic chest pain
Dyspnea
Tachypnea
Cough
Hemoptysis
Tachycardia
Raised jugular venous pressure
Focal chest signs
Collapse
Shock
Cerebral vein thrombosis
Headache
Vomiting
Photophobia
Seizures
Impaired consciousness
Focal neurological signs

unilateral lower abdominal pain) or PE (dyspnea, chest pain, hemoptysis, low grade pyrexia, collapse) or CVT (headache, clouding of consciousness or confusion, or other neurological symptoms). Any woman with suggestive symptoms and signs should undergo objective testing to confirm or rule out the diagnosis. Until the diagnosis is excluded, the woman should be started on a treatment dose of low-molecular-weight heparin (LMWH), unless there is a strong contraindication to anticoagulation. The symptoms and signs of VTE are summarized in Table 5.2, and differential diagnoses in Table 5.3.

5.4.1 Diagnosis of Deep Venous Thrombosis

When there is a clinical suspicion of DVT, the woman should undergo a venous duplex or compression ultrasound scan of the whole lower limb as soon as possible. If the scan confirms the presence of a DVT, anticoagulation therapy should be continued. If the scan is negative and clinical suspicion is low, anticoagulation should be stopped. However, if the scan is negative but the clinical suspicion remains high, prophylactic or therapeutic dose LMWH should be considered for the remainder of the pregnancy and for 6 weeks postpartum, depending on the level of clinical suspicion.

Magnetic resonance imaging (MRI) should be considered to diagnose iliac DVT, where the diagnosis may be suggested by back pain and swelling of the entire lower limb. Torkzad et al. found that approximately 10 % of pregnant women with proximal DVT examined at an average gestational age of 29 weeks had iliac vein thrombosis detected on MRI that was missed on ultrasound [36]. Based on a review of published literature on the biologic effects and safety of MRI in the obstetric patient, the Society of Obstetricians and Gynecologists of Canada concluded that fetal MR imaging is safe at 3.0 T (the unit used to denote the field strength of the magnet used for MRI – the majority of systems operate at 1.5 T) or less during the second and third trimesters, and inadvertent exposure to MRI during the first trimester has not been associated with any long-term sequelae [37]. The European Society of Uroradiology Contrast Medium Safety Committee (ESUR CMSC) recommendations on the use of gadolinium contrast media in pregnant and lactating women state: (a) pregnant women: the highest risk gadolinium contrast media are contraindicated in pregnant women. The intermediate and lowest risk gadolinium contrast media may be given to pregnant women in the lowest dose required to provide essential diagnostic information; (b) lactating women: lactating women who receive the highest risk gadolinium contrast media should stop breast-feeding for 24 h and discard the expressed milk. Lactating women who receive the intermediate and lowest risk agents should discuss with their doctor whether to discontinue breast-feeding for 24 h [38, 39].

5.4.2 Diagnosis of Pulmonary Embolism

Where there is clinical suspicion of acute PE, a chest X-ray should be performed. Although the

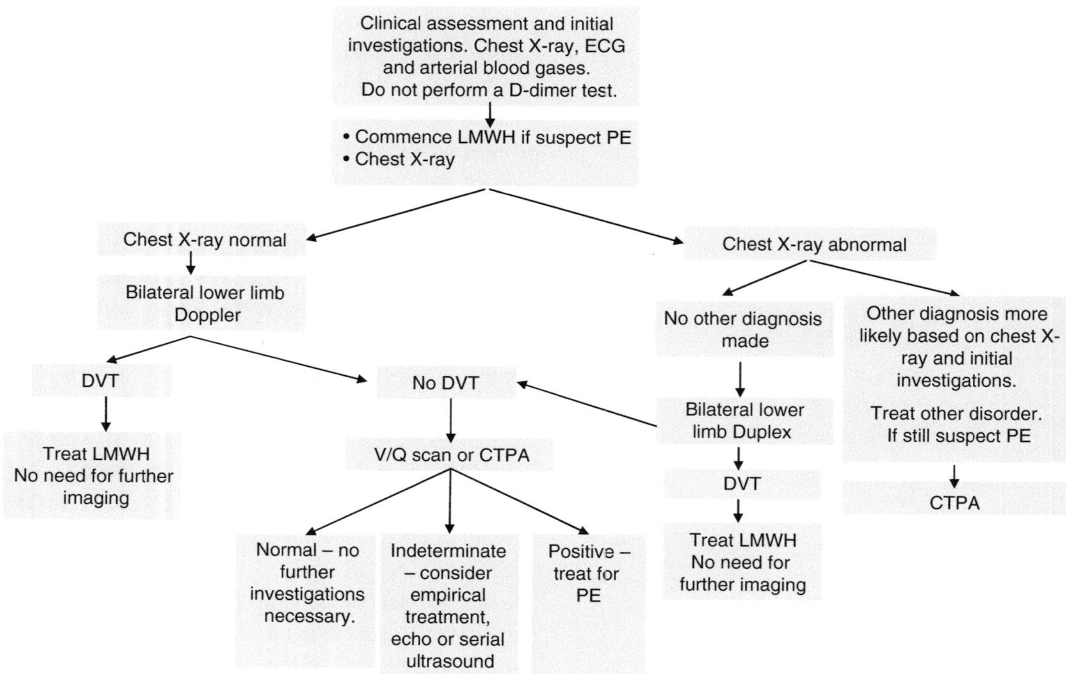

Fig. 5.1 Diagnostic algorithm for suspected pulmonary embolism in hemodynamically stable women (i.e. without shock, hypotension, signs of pulmonary hypertension) during pregnancy and the puerperium. 1) Investigations should be completed within 24 h of admission with suspected PE, 2) Chest X-ray signs include small effusion, prominent pulmonary vasculature, regional oligemia, and 3) Depending on clinical scenario, consider intervention: temporary IVC filter/thrombolysis/thrombectomy; discuss with local experts

chest X-ray is normal in over 50 % of pregnant women in whom PE is objectively diagnosed, the chest X-ray may show features of PE which include atelectasis, effusion, focal opacities, regional oligemia, or pulmonary edema.

If the chest X-ray is normal or consistent with a diagnosis of PE, bilateral whole lower limb duplex or compression ultrasound scanning should be performed. If this confirms a DVT, further imaging of the chest (and therefore the extra radiation to mother and fetus) may be avoided; the rationale is that the treatment of DVT and PE would be the same, so diagnosing or excluding PE appears to be unnecessary. If the chest X-ray is normal and the lower limb imaging is negative but the clinical suspicion remains high, a computed tomography pulmonary angiogram (CTPA) or ventilation/perfusion (V/Q) lung scan should be performed.

The chest X-ray may identify an alternative diagnosis such as pneumonia, pneumothorax or lobar collapse. If the X-ray is abnormal with a high clinical suspicion of PE, CTPA should be performed. If the CTPA or V/Q is also normal but the clinical suspicion of PE remains, either prophylactic or therapeutic dose LMWH should be given for the remainder of the pregnancy, depending on the level of clinical suspicion.

The guidance summarized above is broadly in line with the Royal College of Obstetricians and Gynaecologists' (RCOG) green top guidelines [21]. Figure 5.1 shows a suggested algorithm for suspected non-high risk PE (i.e. without shock, hypotension, signs of pulmonary hypertension) in pregnancy and the puerperium.

Initial investigations should include arterial blood gases and an electrocardiogram (ECG). Oxygen saturation measured with a pulse oximeter may show resting hypoxia. Arterial blood gases (ABG) usually show a reduced PaO_2 and normal or low $PaCO_2$. The ECG may be normal except for a sinus tachycardia. Large emboli may lead to features of acute right heart strain (right axis deviation, right bundle branch block, peaked P waves in lead II); the classical S1, Q3, T3 pattern is rare. Electrocardiography is also useful in excluding other diagnoses such as acute myocardial infarction and pericardial disease.

5.4.2.1 Lung Imaging in Pregnancy and the Puerperium and Associated Radiation Risks

The dose of radiation received by the fetus from a plain chest X-ray is negligible (0.2 mGy), particularly if lead screening is used. The National Council of Radiation Protection and Measurements in the USA states that the risk (of abnormality) is considered to be negligible at 50 mGy or less when compared to other risks of pregnancy [40, 41].

The choice between CTPA and V/Q scanning for the diagnosis of PE in pregnancy is controversial. Both CTPA and V/Q scanning have been reported to have high negative predictive value, albeit in retrospective studies [42, 43]; each has its advantages and disadvantages [21]. One advantage of CTPA is that the dose of radiation to the fetus is generally lower than that associated with a V/Q scan: 0.03–0.66 versus 0.32–0.74 mGy, respectively; The wide range of values reflects heterogeneity in the protocols and equipment used as well as differences in size and age of the fetus at the time of exposure [41]. Pregnant breast tissue is particularly sensitive to radiation and every effort should be made to minimize radiation exposure during pregnancy. Some authors recommend V/Q scan as the first-line investigation in pregnancy, as it has a high negative predictive value, lower radiation dose to the pregnant breast, and because most pregnant women in the UK will not have co-morbid pulmonary pathology [44]. If the initial chest X-ray is normal, the ventilation portion of the V/Q scan may be omitted; the perfusion scan alone will often be enough to confirm or exclude PE. Iodinated contrast medium used with CTPA has the potential to affect fetal and neonatal thyroid function, although a retrospective study of 344 pregnant women who underwent a CTPA for suspected PE found normal thyroxine levels in all neonates at the time of birth [45]. Technetium-99, which is used for perfusion scans, is excreted in the urine and secreted into breast milk. The fetal radiation dose is higher and as the contrast is often concentrated in the bladder near the fetal head.

The choice of optimal lung imaging is still debated and will be decided to some extent by local availability. The RCOG recommends that "where feasible, women should be involved in the decision to undergo CTPA or V/Q scanning. Ideally, informed consent should be obtained before these tests are undertaken" [21].

5.4.2.2 Lung Imaging in Pregnant Patients: Practice and Counseling Points

All investigations should be discussed with the patient and this should be documented in her clinical records.

- It is not clear what the absolute radiation risks are for fetus or mother; but they are small compared to the risk of a missed diagnosis of PE.
- The discussion with the patient should include an explanation of the risks of undiagnosed PE.
- Treatment of VTE with LMWH, whilst relatively safe in pregnancy, carries a risk of anticoagulant-induced bleeding. This risk is acceptable when treating a proven VTE.
- The radiation dose from a chest X-ray is very small. The fetus is shielded with a lead apron.
- A Consultant Radiologist should be involved in any imaging in a pregnant patient to ensure that the scanning process is optimized, in order to improve the diagnostic yield.
- The radiation dose to the fetus is lower in a CTPA than in a V/Q scan. However, there is a greater radiation dose to the proliferating breast tissue. The current estimated lifetime risk of breast cancer is 1 in 8 [46]. Whether or not this small amount of extra radiation translates to a measurable increase in the lifetime risk of breast cancer is not yet known [47].
- The RCOG guidelines state that women with suspected PE should be advised that, compared with CTPA, V/Q scanning may carry a slightly increased risk of childhood cancer but is associated with a lower risk of maternal breast cancer; in both situations, the absolute risk is very small [21].
- The algorithm suggested uses lower limb scanning initially as evidence of VTE. If the patient has symptoms suggestive of PE but the lower limb Doppler/Duplex scan is negative, then CTPA or V/Q scanning should be

performed, as the benefit of having direct lung imaging would outweigh risks of missed PE. CTPA also has the benefit of demonstrating other lung pathology that may cause symptoms, e.g. pneumonia, pleural effusion.

- Ventilation perfusion (V/Q) scanning can be considered for women in whom CTPA is contraindicated, i.e. contrast allergy, renal failure. Technetium-99 is used in the perfusion scan and is excreted in the urine and breast milk. Compared to CTPA, there is less radiation to the maternal breast. However, the fetal radiation dose is often higher as the contrast is concentrated in the mother's bladder near the fetal head. Women undergoing a V/Q scan should be well hydrated and encouraged to empty the bladder frequently. To follow the principle of keeping exposure as low as possible, it is reasonable to express and discard breast milk for 12 h after a V/Q scan. Neonatal thyroid testing is recommended after CTPA scanning using iodinated contrast medium and V/Q scanning [38].

5.4.3 Diagnosis of Cerebral Vein and Venous Sinus Thrombosis

Neuroimaging is the most important method for diagnosing cerebral vein or venous sinus thrombosis (CVT), which requires the clear demonstration of absence of flow and intraluminal venous thrombus by CT or MRI. CT venography, MR venography, blood-sensitive MRI sequences (e.g. gradient echo T2* or susceptibility weighted imaging) are useful techniques. Formal digital subtraction angiography may occasionally be needed in uncertain cases. Isolated thrombosis of small cortical veins may be challenging to detect. All cases must be discussed with a neurologist and neuroradiologist to ensure that the most appropriate tests are performed, and are interpreted correctly.

5.4.4 D-dimer

Measurement of D-dimer is currently not recommended in the investigation of suspected acute VTE in pregnancy. This is because D-dimer levels may be raised in normal pregnancy, particularly in the third trimester and in the puerperium. They are also increased in other pregnancy-related pathologies such as preeclampsia [21]. However, Chan et al. reported that by using higher cut-off points than those used in non-pregnant patients, the specificity of D-dimer assays for the diagnosis of DVT in pregnancy can be improved without compromising sensitivity, and recommended validation in prospective management studies [48]. Murphy et al. reported in healthy pregnant women attending for routine antenatal care, that there is a continuous increase in D-dimer levels with increasing gestation, and constructed a 95th percentile cutoff [49]. Although promising, the role of D-dimer levels in the diagnosis of pregnancy-associated VTE is not established.

5.5 Management of Acute Venous Thromboembolism

The optimal management of acute VTE requires a multidisciplinary approach, including senior obstetric, hematological and anesthetic input, liaison with the hemostasis laboratory, and additional input from a respiratory physician and neurologist in the case of suspected PE or suspected CVT, respectively.

As soon as the possibility of acute VTE is suspected, treatment dose LMWH should be started and appropriate investigations arranged. When the diagnosis is objectively confirmed, the aim of anticoagulation therapy in patients with established DVT is to prevent extension and reduce the risk of recurrence; in patients with established PE, the aim is to limit extension and prevent death [9]. It is important to realize that, while there is good (level 1) evidence guiding the treatment of acute VTE in non-pregnant patients, there is by comparison remarkably little good quality evidence in pregnancy. As a result, guidelines relating to pregnant women are generally extrapolated from the non-pregnant population [50–53].

The management of acute VTE will be primarily medical, that is, the use of anticoagulants, but non-medical therapies must not be forgotten.

Reversible risk factors for VTE, for example hyperemesis, wherever possible should be corrected, to enable optimal management.

5.5.1 Pharmacological Therapies: The Options in Patients with Acute Venous Thromboembolism

The reader should refer to Chap. 2 on Anticoagulants and Antiplatelet Agents in Pregnancy. In non-pregnant patients, therapeutic options for VTE include unfractionated heparin (UFH), LMWH, and coumarins.

LMWH is now widely used for prophylaxis and treatment of maternal thromboembolism. The change in practice from the use of UFH is based largely on the results of large trials in non-pregnant patients that show that LMWHs are at least as safe and effective as UFH for the treatment of VTE [54, 55]. Accordingly, the American College of Chest Physicians' (ACCP) guidelines recommend LMWH, rather than UFH, for the prevention and treatment of VTE in pregnant patients [56]. In the UK and Ireland, over 95 % of centers use LMWH to treat acute VTE in pregnancy [57]. The only exception is massive PE with cardiovascular compromise, when thrombolysis should be considered, and in this instance initial UFH is preferable because of its rapid onset of action and short half-life (see below).

Coumarin derivatives such as warfarin cross the placenta; if taken in early pregnancy (6–12 weeks of gestation), they can cause a typical embryopathy, and later in pregnancy may cause microcephaly, probably secondary to small fetal cerebral hemorrhages. There is also a risk of major fetal/neonatal intracerebral hemorrhage if the woman (and therefore the fetus) is anticoagulated around the time of delivery. Consequently, coumarins are avoided in pregnancy although they are an option in the highest-risk women, principally those with a metallic heart valve.

Newer oral anticoagulants, such as dabigatran, rivaroxaban, apixaban and edoxaban, are
Contraindicated in pregnancy. Fondaparinux and hirudin have not yet had their safety adequately
Established in pregnancy, and both cross the placenta, with the fondaparinux level in cord blood
Documented to be approximately 1/10 of the level in the maternal plasma [58]. Low dose aspirin
Is safe in pregnancy [56] but it is not effective for the treatment for VTE.

5.5.1.1 Unfractionated Heparin

Heparin is a natural product obtained from bovine or porcine mucosa. Naturally occurring heparin is comprised of a mix of molecules with differing molecular weights (range 5,000–35,000 Da). Only a third of these molecules contain the high-affinity pentasaccharide that mediates the primary anticoagulant effect of heparin. This accelerates its inhibition of thrombin (factor IIa) and factor Xa. Because of its large molecular weight, high degree of ionization, and poor lipid solubility, UFH does not cross the placenta and is therefore safe (from the fetal point of view) to use in pregnancy [59, 60]. Neither is it secreted into breast milk, so it is also safe to use in breast-feeding women. Heparin is cleared firstly by depolymerization after binding to macrophage receptors; this phase is rapid and can quickly become saturated. Heparin is then cleared by a much slower renal mechanism. When using concentrations of UFH in the therapeutic range, most is cleared by the rapid saturable mechanism; as a result, further rises in dosage can have a nonlinear effect on the anticoagulant effect. In general, therapeutic doses of UFH have a half-life of less than 60 min [61].

The effect of UFH is generally monitored using the APTT, with a target range for the APTT ratio of 1.5–2.5 (although each laboratory should derive its own APTT ratio based on anti-Xa levels). In pregnancy, there is increased binding of UFH to plasma proteins and increased concentrations of factor VIII and fibrinogen; as a result, pregnant women require higher doses of UFH to achieve the same prolongation of APTT. As a result of the heterogeneous mix of molecules in heparin, the clearance mechanisms discussed above, and the variable binding of heparin to plasma proteins, adjusting the dose of UFH in order to keep the APTT ratio in the therapeutic range can be problematic. Specific nomograms and, if necessary, anti-factor-Xa assays should be used (with a target anti-Xa range of 0.35–0.70 units/mL).

If prolonged therapy with UFH is used, the platelet count should be monitored from days 4–14. Heparin induced thrombocytopenia (HIT) should be suspected if the platelet count falls by 50 % or more and/or the patient develops new thrombosis or skin allergy between days 4 and 14 of heparin administration [62, 63]; in this situation, urgent hematological advice should be sought.

Protamine sulfate rapidly reverses the anticoagulant effect of UFH. The dose of protamine is determined by the heparin exposure: 1 mg of protamine neutralises 80–100 IU of UFH when administered within 15 min of the heparin dose. Less is required if protamine is given after a longer period because of the short half-life of intravenous UFH. Caution should be exercised with higher doses because of a paradoxical risk of bleeding.

5.5.1.2 Low-Molecular-Weight Heparin

Low-molecular-weight heparins are produced synthetically by cleaving UFH either enzymatically (e.g. tinzaparin) or chemically (e.g. dalteparin, enoxaparin). This process yields LMWHs which have a molecular weight around 4,300–5,000 Da, around a third the molecular weight of UFH. Both LMWH and UFH bind to antithrombin, facilitating its anticoagulant effect. However, in all LMWHs the anti-Xa activity exceeds the anti-IIa activity.

Because LMWH has far less interaction with acute-phase proteins in the blood and because its clearance is primarily by the renal route, its pharmacokinetic characteristics are quite different to those of UFH and its anticoagulant activity much more predictable. This means that, particularly in non-pregnant patients, fixed weight-adjusted dosages can be used without the need for laboratory monitoring. However, in pregnancy, weight changes with gestation, the volume of distribution of the drug increases significantly and there is a rise in renal clearance. Glomerular filtration rate increases significantly in pregnancy, resulting in more rapid renal clearance of LMWH, decreasing its half-life [64–66]. Consequently, the ACCP recommends a twice-daily therapeutic dosage regimen for LMWHs in the treatment of VTE in pregnancy, in contrast to the once-daily regimens used in non-pregnant patients [56]. A study of pharmacokinetics of enoxaparin during the antenatal period in 123 women suggests that, for enoxaparin, once daily dosing may suffice [67]. However, the optimal dosing strategy can be substantiated only with published clinical outcome data on safety and efficacy. The RCOG guidelines state that "there is insufficient evidence to recommend whether the dose of LMWH should be given once daily or in two divided doses" [21].

In non-pregnant subjects, LMWH has been shown to be at least as effective as UFH [54]; in one meta-analysis, LMWH was more effective than UFH in the initial management of VTE [68]. In addition, LMWH and UFH use compare favorably to oral anticoagulation with warfarin [53, 69, 70]. Systematic reviews have shown that LMWH is safe in pregnancy and does not cross the placenta [60, 71]. LMWHs are also much less likely than UFH to cause HIT [72] or osteoporosis [60, 73–78]. In a systematic review of 2,777 pregnancies treated for acute VTE, the use of LMWH was safe and effective, being associated with a recurrence rate of VTE of just 1.15 % [60]. Similar studies in non-pregnant women using either LMWH or UFH followed by coumarins reported a VTE recurrence rate of between 5 and 8 % up to 6 months after the initial event. Interestingly, in the 2,777 pregnancies treated with LMWH, not a single case of HIT was reported. The risk of heparin-induced osteoporosis also appears to be significantly lower with LMWH compared with UFH [35, 60, 74, 76–78]. Although clearly more data are needed, the risk of this complication appears very low, in the order of 0.04 %. In spite of this apparently low incidence, it seems reasonable to encourage these women to take vitamin D supplementation if the vitamin D level is suboptimal, together with calcium if the calcium is low or low normal.

Although rare, skin reactions to LMWH are well recognized [60, 79]. These may be due to type 1 immediate hypersensitivity reaction or type 4 delayed hypersensitivity reaction. When they occur, treatment with the LMWH preparation being used should be discontinued and an alternative LMWH preparation substituted. If a skin reaction occurs, HIT should be considered, although this is most unlikely with LMWH [60, 62, 63]. If LMWH is not tolerated, options for therapeutic anticoagulation include vitamin K antagonists, UFH, or fondaparinux (although experience in pregnancy with fondaparinux is limited).

Protamine sulfate incompletely reverses (by approximately 60 %) the effect of LMWH based on data from healthy human volunteers [80], although the limited data available suggest clinical benefit. Van Veen et al. described three patients requiring emergency surgery and 14 patients that were actively bleeding whilst receiving LMWH and who received protamine at doses suggested by the ACCP guidelines [81]. Protamine prevented excessive bleeding in all the surgical patients and was effective in 8 of 12 evaluable patients with active bleeding. Anti-Xa levels after protamine sulfate administration did not correlate with the likelihood of persistent bleeding [82]. The BCSH guideline on the management of bleeding in patients on antithrombotic agents recommends the following: (a) LMWH administration within 8 h of the time of requirement for correction of anticoagulation: give protamine sulfate (1 mg per 100 anti-Xa units of LMWH); (b) if ineffective, consider further protamine sulfate 0.5 mg per 100 anti-Xa units (2C). Protamine sulfate should be given more slowly than 5 mg/min to minimize the risk of adverse reactions; (c) LMWH administration more than 8 h from the time of requirement for correction of anticoagulation: consider smaller doses of protamine (2C); and (d) consider recombinant factor VIIa (rFVIIa) if there is continued life-threatening bleeding despite protamine sulfate and the time frame suggests there is residual effect from the LMWH contributing to bleeding (2C) [83].

5.5.2 Baseline Blood Investigations Prior to Initiating Anticoagulant Therapy

Before starting anticoagulant therapy, a full blood count, liver function tests, urea and electrolytes, and coagulation screen (APTT, prothrombin time and fibrinogen/thrombin time) should be performed.

It is controversial whether thrombophilia screening should be performed, at baseline or subsequently, in a pregnant woman diagnosed with acute VTE and this is not routinely recommended [21, 84]. Against testing is the fact that the results of thrombophilia testing are unlikely to influence management. Moreover, interpretation of the results can be misleading during pregnancy; for example, protein S levels are reduced in normal pregnancy, activated protein C resistance is found in up to 40 % of women in normal pregnancy and results of tests for antiphospholipid antibodies may not be representative. Antithrombin levels are reduced in conditions such as preeclampsia and nephrotic syndrome. Protein S and protein C are reduced in liver disease and vitamin K deficiency. For these reasons, careful consideration should be given to whether to perform thrombophilia testing and the results of thrombophilia screening tests in pregnancy should be interpreted by an experienced hematologist. The presence of a severe thrombophilia such as antithrombin deficiency may influence the management of anticoagulation during pregnancy and the puerperium.

5.5.3 Management During Pregnancy

5.5.3.1 Antithrombotic Treatment

Once VTE has been confirmed, anticoagulation should be continued. LMWH can be used in pregnancy for both initial and maintenance therapy.

As mentioned above, treatment with LMWH in non-pregnant patients is usually given once daily; however, a twice-daily regimen is recommended in pregnancy (RCOG and ACCP) [21, 56]. The RCOG advises the following doses:

Table 5.4 Calculation of initial doses of drugs by early pregnancy weight

Initial dose	Early pregnancy weight (kg)			
	<50	50–69	70–89	90–109
Enoxaparin (mg bd)	40	60	80	100
Dalteparin (iu bd)	5,000	6,000	8,000	10,000
Tinzaparin	175 units/kg once daily (all weights)			

Royal College of Obstetricians and Gynaecologists [21]
bd twice daily
>110 kg: haematologist should advise on LMWH dose

enoxaparin 1 mg/kg twice daily and dalteparin 100 units/kg twice daily. Some evidence suggests that once-daily administration of tinzaparin (175 units/kg) or enoxaparin may be adequate in pregnancy [21, 67]; however, twice-daily dosing may be preferable until once daily regimens have been substantiated. Calculation of the initial dose by early pregnancy body weight is detailed in Table 5.4 [21], although the dose may also be calculated according to current body weight. Selected patients, such as those with antiphospholipid syndrome, where low dose aspirin is useful in combination with LMWH for improved obstetric outcome [56, 85], should generally be prescribed aspirin in addition to LMWH.

In pregnant women on a treatment dose of LMWH for VTE, monitoring of anti-Xa activity is controversial and guidance is not evidence-based [86]. The RCOG [21] recommends that periodic testing of anti-Xa levels is indicated in women at extremes of weight (i.e. <50 or >90 kg), women who are bleeding (or are at increased risk of bleeding), who have recurrent VTE despite treatment with normal doses of LMWH, or who have renal disease. In such women, the target range for anti-Xa levels, measured 3–5 h after injection depending on the type of LMWH, is 0.5–1.0 units/mL.

In some studies of non-pregnant patients with acute VTE, the dose of LMWH has been reduced after an initial few weeks of therapeutic anticoagulation [87]. Currently, it is uncertain whether this would be adequate in pregnant women (bearing in mind that the prothrombotic state continues) or whether a reduction in dose would increase the risk of recurrence/propagation of the thrombosis. At present, therefore, until the safety of a reduced dose regimen in pregnancy is proved, it seems safer to continue the full therapeutic dose until at least 6 weeks after delivery.

Monitoring of the platelet count is not required when using treatment doses of LMWH during pregnancy, as LMWH is far less likely to cause HIT [60, 62, 63] when compared with UFH. Even in women who develop HIT during treated with LMWH, it is invariably the prior use of UFH that has sensitized them to heparin, even though the HIT does not develop until subsequent LMWH exposure. Consequently, if a woman is being treated with UFH alone or if she has had UFH treatment prior to treatment with LMWH, the platelet count should be checked every 3 days from day 4 to day 14, assuming heparin treatment is continued during that time.

When acute VTE is diagnosed in pregnancy, it is recommended that a treatment dose of LMWH should be continued throughout the pregnancy and for at least 6 weeks postpartum and until at least 3 months of treatment has been given in total [21, 56]. These women can invariably be managed as out-patients; the patient or her partner can almost always be taught how to administer LMWH injections safely at home.

5.5.3.2 Management of the Limb in Acute DVT

The initial management of lower limb DVT involves elevation of the leg and wearing a graduated elastic compression stocking (GCS) on the affected leg (there is no need to wear a stocking on the unaffected leg). However, studies in the non-pregnant population have shown that once the patient is stable and anticoagulated, early mobilization is not associated with an increased risk of PE; it appears likely that the same applies in pregnancy. The use of GCS is discussed below in Sect. 5.9.

5.5.3.3 Inferior Vena Cava Filter

The use of a retrievable inferior vena cava (IVC) filter should be considered in a woman in whom anticoagulation is contraindicated or who has extensive DVT close to the time (within 2 weeks) of delivery, as full anticoagulation peripartum significantly increases the risk of hemorrhage, and the thrombotic risk is high [88]. An IVC filter could also be considered in a woman with a DVT who has recurrent PE despite apparently adequate anticoagulation. However, it is preferable when possible to delay delivery and institute full anticoagulation rather than using an IVC filter; anticoagulation will then need to be managed around the time of delivery (see below). The use of an IVC filter is not without risk [89]. The IVC can be perforated during insertion. If inserted close to the time of delivery, there is a risk of filter migration due to the change in IVC pressure following delivery. On occasion, the filter may be difficult or impossible to retrieve due to filter tilt; in these situations long-term anticoagulation should be considered.

Consideration of the use of long-term anticoagulation in patients with a permanent IVC filter follows from reports that thrombus may form within the filter and propagate, reducing filter patency and lower extremity venous return, promoting stasis and increasing the risk of DVT distal to the filter [90]. In addition, impaired IVC venous return may lead to substantial collateral venous return that bypasses the IVC filter and results in PE recurrence [91]. Hajduk et al. reported on patients who had VTE, followed by treatment with permanent IVC filter placement, and were anticoagulated long-term as soon as safety allowed. Annual physical examinations and ultrasound surveillance of the lower extremity deep veins and of the IVC filter site were undertaken. Clot detected at the filter site was treated with graded intensities of anticoagulation, depending on the clot burden. Symptomatic DVT occurred in 24 of 121 patients (20 %; 95 % CI, 14–28 %); symptomatic pulmonary embolism (one fatal) was diagnosed in 6 patients (5 %; 95 % CI, 2–10 %). There were 45 episodes of filter clot in 36 patients (30 %; 95 % CI, 22–38 %). The rate of major bleeding (6.6 %) was similar to that of a concurrent persistently anticoagulated cohort without IVC filters (5.8 %). The authors concluded that if therapeutic anticoagulation can be safely begun in patients with IVC filters inserted after VTE, further management with clinical surveillance, including ultrasound examination of the IVC filter and graded degrees of anticoagulation therapy if filter clot is detected, has a favorable prognosis. The authors suggested that this approach appears valid for patients with current IVC filter and can serve as a comparison standard in subsequent clinical trials to optimize clinical management of these patients [92].

The timing and mechanism of filter tilt remains uncertain. Potential contributory factors include change in the anatomic configuration with lateral displacement of the IVC filter as a result of the gravid uterus as well as forceful uterine contractions during labor, which modify the shape and diameter of the IVC [93]. The British Society of Interventional Radiology (BSIR) IVC Filter Registry, based on analysis of 1,434 IVC filter placements and 400 attempted retrievals performed at 68 UK centers, reports that filter placement is usually a low-risk procedure, with a low major complication rate (<0.5 %). Operator inexperience (<25 procedures) was significantly associated with complications ($p<0.001$). Successful retrieval, technically successful in 83 % of those cases where retrieval was attempted, was significantly less likely for implants left in situ for >9 weeks versus those left for a shorter period. New lower limb DVT and/or IVC thrombosis was reported in 88 patients following filter placement; there was no significant difference in incidence between filter types.

5.5.3.4 Specific Situations in Pregnant Women with VTE

Very rarely, DVT can lead to venous gangrene. Management in the non-pregnant patient includes elevation of the leg, anticoagulation, and possible surgical embolectomy or thrombolytic therapy. Thrombolytic therapy may increase the risk of placental abruption and, if used immediately post-partum, may increase the risk of postpartum hemorrhage. In pregnancy and peripartum, therefore, it is reserved for women with life-threatening PE.

Patients with CVT must have input from a vascular neurologist or stroke physician. Principles of treatment are hydration, anticonvulsant therapy and therapeutic anticoagulation.

5.6 Acute Massive PE in Pregnancy

The differential diagnosis of acute maternal collapse in pregnancy includes PE, amniotic fluid embolus, myocardial infarct, and hemorrhage

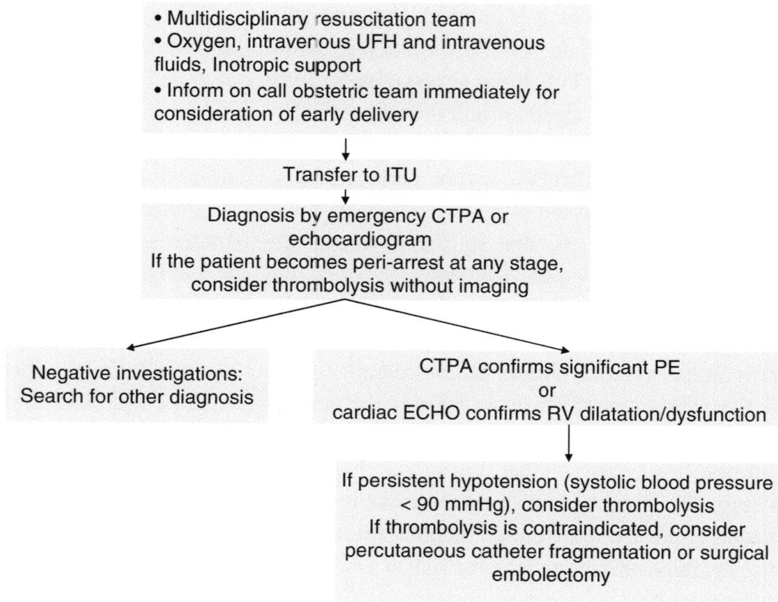

Fig. 5.2 Management of women with clinically suspected massive pulmonary embolism. *IV* intravenous, *SBP* systolic blood pressure

(concealed or revealed), among others. The immediate management is supportive, usually by a multidisciplinary team including intensivists, an obstetrician and obstetric anesthetist, a hematologist experienced in antithrombotic treatment during pregnancy; and, in addition, a respiratory physician and access to an interventional vascular radiologist and cardiothoracic surgeon.

When PE is a possibility, an echocardiogram (ECHO; bedside, if moving the patient is unfeasible) or CTPA should be arranged as a matter of urgency. Women with massive PE associated with hemodynamic compromise (low BP, tachycardia) should be managed on ITU and considered for thrombolysis, which can be lifesaving both during pregnancy and postpartum. The decision for thrombolysis should be made in conjunction with the multidisciplinary team. A suggested algorithm for the management of women with clinically suspected massive PE is illustrated in Fig. 5.2. When the diagnosis of massive acute PE is established, intravenous UFH is generally preferred because of its rapid onset of action and short half-life. Efficacy of the UFH is monitored by the APTT ratio, aiming for a range of 1.5–2.5 compared with the arithmetic mean of the normal range [21, 94], although each laboratory should define its own therapeutic range. The APTT ratio should be checked

Table 5.5 Infusion rates of unfractionated heparin (UFH) according to activated partial thromboplastin time (APTT)

APTT ratio	Dose (units/kg/h)	Additional action	Next APTT (h)
<1.2	4	Re-bolus 80 units/kg	6
1.2–1.5	2	Re-bolus 40 units/kg	6
1.5–2.5	No change		24
2.5–3.0	−2		6
>3.0	−3	Stop infusion for 1 h	6

Royal College of Obstetricians and Gynaecologists [21]

4–6 h after the initial loading dose and 6 h after any change in dose. Once the APTT ratio is in the target range (usually 1.5–2.5), it should be rechecked at least every 24 h (more frequently if there are any issues with bleeding). A suggested algorithm for managing the infusion rate of UFH is shown in Table 5.5.

While adjustment of infusion rates of UFH on the basis of repeated APTT ratios seems reasonable in theory, in practice it is problematic. This is partly because increased factor VIII levels in late pregnancy lead to apparent heparin resistance. This can lead to higher doses of UFH than necessary being used, which can cause bleeding problems. This increased risk of bleeding is particularly important soon after delivery, when the possibility of postpartum hemorrhage is a concern. In practice, in many maternity units, by the time a blood sample is taken, dispatched to the laboratory, analyzed and the result received, several hours have usually passed. As a result, dose adjustments are delayed and the risk (of either hemorrhage or thrombosis) has persisted during that time. An alternative approach is to measure anti-Xa activity. When UFH has been used, a lower level of anti-Xa is the aim (0.35–0.70 units/mL in a woman with PE which is not life-threatening; in a woman with life-threatening PE, the target is 0.5–1.0 units/mL). However, the laboratory turnaround time to measure anti-Xa activity is usually much longer than for APTT ratio measurement, making it less useful in clinical management.

There has always been a concern about the risk of using thrombolytic agents for the management of PE in pregnancy. The concern was that it might harm the fetus or increase the risk of placental abruption. In non-pregnant patients, several randomized controlled trials have shown that, while thrombolytic therapy is better than heparin in reducing clot burden and improving hemodynamic function, there is no improvement in long-term survival. Ahearn et al. [95] reviewed the many case reports of the use of thrombolytic agents in pregnancy. They found that bleeding complications occurred in 1–6 % of women, similar to the frequency in non-pregnant women receiving thrombolytic therapy. Of 172 women treated with thrombolysis, 5 had non-fatal maternal bleeding complications (2.9 %) and 3 suffered a fetal death (1.7 %). There were no maternal deaths and no reports of intracranial bleeding. Most bleeding complications were focused around catheter and puncture sites. In a woman whose life is threatened by massive PE, but in whom thrombolytic therapy also seems too risky (e.g. a woman soon after Cesarean section), consideration should be given to urgent thrombectomy by a cardiothoracic surgeon. Another option is catheter-directed thrombolysis.

5.7 Planning for Delivery

Delivery planning should ideally take place well in advance of the due date and involve detailed discussion between the woman and her multidisciplinary team. The primary aim in peripartum management of a woman who is fully anticoagulated is to balance the risk of major postpartum hemorrhage against the risk of progressive or recurrent VTE when anticoagulation is interrupted. In general, being on treatment doses of anticoagulation is often an indication for timing of delivery, but would not be an indication for elective Cesarean section; induction of labor is usually preferable. It may be particularly desirable to plan the timing of delivery (by induction of labor) in certain situations. Examples include the need to ensure delivery in the managing hospital of a woman who lives a long distance away or a woman who is certain that she wants an epidural for pain relief in labor.

In all cases, the woman should be kept well-hydrated, wear anti-embolism stockings and stay as mobile as possible peridelivery. In addition to the management of anticoagulation described below, in patients with congenital antithrombin deficiency, the peridelivery use of antithrombin concentrate, either plasma derived or recombinant, should be considered. The use of antithrombin concentrate in this situation provides thromboprophylaxis during the period when LMWH is reduced or interrupted. This approach minimizes the risk of both bleeding and VTE. Until recently, antithrombin was available only as a pooled plasma-derived product which, despite optimal viral inactivation, still carries a potential risk of transfusion-transmitted infection. A recombinant form of human antithrombin (ATryn®) is now licensed (Pan-European and USA).

5.7.1 Spontaneous Labor

Even in fully anticoagulated women, it is reasonable to aim for spontaneous labor and normal vaginal birth. The woman should be advised that, once she thinks her labor is starting, she should discontinue LMWH injections. If it turns out to be a false alarm and the contractions stop, the LMWH can be restarted. When she is admitted in labor, a blood sample should be sent for a coagulation screen, full blood count, and blood group and save. Assuming that the woman has a vaginal delivery and no postpartum hemorrhage, a prophylactic dose of LMWH can be started within 6 h after delivery (e.g. dalteparin 5,000 units SC unless at extremes of body weight). After the first dose, assuming there is no issue with bleeding, a suggested regimen is an intermediate dose of LMWH on the first day post delivery (e.g. dalteparin 5,000 units 12 hourly, with the first dose 12 h after the first post delivery dose). Treatment dose LMWH (administered as a split dose on a 12 hourly basis) is then started on the second day post delivery. The new treatment dose should be recalculated on the basis of the woman's postpartum weight.

5.7.2 Elective Cesarean Section

If elective Cesarean section is indicated for obstetric reasons, the last dose of (therapeutic dose administered as a split dose, i.e. 12 hourly) LMWH should be given 24 h before the planned operation. In practice, this will usually be the morning of the day before the Cesarean section.

After delivery by Cesarean section, if there is no problem with controlling bleeding, the first prophylactic dose of LMWH can be given within 6 h after the procedure. However, LMWH should not be given for at least 4 h after an epidural or spinal catheter has been removed. In many units, an epidural or a combined spinal epidural (CSE) is used for elective Cesarean section and the epidural catheter is removed immediately at the end of the operation; in this case, the first dose of prophylactic dose LMWH will be given 6 h after the Cesarean section (which is also 6 h after removal of the epidural catheter). Thereafter, the LMWH dose should be escalated to therapeutic dose as detailed above.

Anticoagulated women who have a Cesarean section are at increased risk of wound hematoma (in the order of 2 %), whether they are managed with UFH or LMWH. Consequently, there should be a lower threshold for using a wound drain (either pelvic or rectus sheath), and consideration should be given to using interrupted staples or sutures for closing the skin as this will allow easier drainage of any subcutaneous hematoma. The use of a pressure dressing should also be considered.

5.7.3 Induction of Labor

Labor may be induced for obstetric indications (e.g. postdates) or for logistical reasons, for example, if the woman lives distant from the hospital yet it is desirable that she delivers in the hospital because of her anticoagulation. When admitted to hospital, a blood sample should be taken for a coagulation screen, full blood count, and blood group and save. Regional anesthesia (epidural for labor or spinal anesthesia for Cesarean section) is not considered safe until 24 h after the last *treatment* dose of LMWH, assuming split dosing on a 12-hourly basis (in contrast to 12 h after the last *prophylactic* dose). In practice, women taking therapeutic dose LMWH who go into spontaneous labor are unlikely to have the option of regional anesthesia for either labor or Cesarean section.

When induction of labor is planned, a judgment needs to be made by an experienced obstetrician as to how long it is likely to take from the commencement of the induction process until labor is established. For example, in a primigravid woman at 38 weeks' gestation, this could easily take up to 24 h. On the other hand, in a woman who has had two previous vaginal births and is now at 40 weeks' gestation, labor is likely to start within 6–8 h after the first dose of prostaglandin induction agent. This estimate will help to decide when the last treatment dose of LMWH should be given. The other factor influencing this decision is whether the woman wishes to have an epidural for pain relief in labor or not. If she does, it should be borne in mind that epidural anesthesia is not considered safe until 24 h after her last treatment dose of LMWH.

In practice, this means that when inducing labor in an unfavorable primigravid woman, the last dose of treatment LMWH could be given 12 h before the first dose of prostaglandin-inducing agent. For example, she could have her final dose of LMWH at the usual time the night before induction. The following morning, induction of labor is commenced. Consideration should be given to using misoprostol rather than the usual dinoprostone in these women. Misoprostol is a stronger prostaglandin which speeds up the induction process although carries a small increased risk of hyperstimulation.

In a multiparous woman with a favorable cervix, the last dose of treatment LMWH should be given 24 h prior to commencement of the induction process, in the expectation that labor will establish quickly once induction is commenced. In practice, this would normally mean that the woman injects her last dose of LMWH on the morning of the day prior to induction. Induction commences the following morning.

Six hours after vaginal delivery, assuming there is no issue with bleeding, a prophylactic dose of LMWH can be given and, following this, the dose of LMWH should be escalated to treatment dose as detailed above.

5.7.4 Regional Anesthesia and Low-Molecular-Weight Heparin

Regional anesthesia (epidural or spinal) is not considered safe until at least 24 h after the last therapeutic dose of LMWH (administered on a 12-hourly basis) or 12 h after the last prophylactic dose of LMWH. This is because of the risk of spinal hematoma, a potentially serious complication. The patient may have an epidural/spinal 24 h following a therapeutic dose of LMWH (administered 12 hourly) provided that the coagulation screen is normal and the platelet count $>80 \times 10^9$/L. After the birth, in general the woman should be given her first dose of prophylactic dose LMWH within 6 h after delivery and at least 4 h after the epidural catheter has been removed. Epidural catheters are usually removed soon after vaginal delivery or at the end of a Cesarean section, as the woman is being moved from the operating table; in this case, the next dose of LMWH should not be given until at least 4 h later. If the epidural catheter is retained after delivery (it may, for example, be retained for further analgesia for 24 h after Cesarean section, by which time injections of LMWH have resumed), the epidural catheter should not be removed until 12 h have passed since the last injection of LMWH. In practice, this means that once the epidural catheter is removed (12 h after the previous dose of LMWH), the next dose of LMWH (which would have been due around the same time), which should be a prophylactic dose, will need to be delayed for a further 4 h.

Subcutaneous intermittent injections of UFH (which is uncommon in current management strategies for VTE in pregnancy) should be stopped 12 h before regional anesthesia can be given; a treatment dose intravenous infusion of UFH should be stopped 6 h, and the APTT ratio checked to ensure that it has normalized before regional anesthesia.

5.8 Management After Delivery

If there is a problem with continued postpartum bleeding or the woman remains at high risk of bleeding, it is better to delay resumption of LMWH. If there is active bleeding, all anticoagulation should be stopped and expert hematological advice sought; other methods of stopping the bleeding, for example, surgical, should be pursued.

Once the immediate peripartum period has been negotiated, consideration is given to the duration of further therapeutic anticoagulation. Therapeutic anticoagulation should be continued for at least 6 weeks postnatally and for a total of at least 3 months' anticoagulation [21, 56].

There are two common options for this postpartum anticoagulation, namely LMWH or warfarin. The treatment regimen of LMWH that was used antenatally may be continued, but the dose recalculated on the basis of the woman's postpartum weight. Consideration could be given to changing to once-daily injections, preferably after 5 days postpartum (i.e. from day 6) to minimize the risk of postpartum bleeding, similar to the regimen used in non-pregnant patients. The second option is to change to warfarin anticoagulation. The choice will depend on the woman's preference and the proposed duration of further anticoagulation. When this is just a further 6 weeks, a woman who is already used to administering LMWH may prefer to continue with this regimen rather than the regular testing and hospital visits that are often necessary when warfarin is initiated.

Warfarin should not generally be commenced until at least 3 days after the birth (i.e. from day 4) because there may be an increased risk of postpartum hemorrhage if started early [21]. Warfarin should be interrupted in the event of postpartum hemorrhage and should not be restarted until the bleeding has abated. In women who suffer a postpartum hemorrhage while on warfarin, consideration should be given to reversing the effect of warfarin with prothrombin complex concentrate plus intravenous vitamin K in consultation with a hematologist.

The woman should be made aware that changing to warfarin will require frequent testing of the international normalized ratio (INR), initially daily over the first few weeks until a stable INR (target 2.5, range 2–3) is achieved. When anticoagulation is planned for only a further 6 weeks, the inconvenience generally outweighs the benefits; when longer duration anticoagulation is proposed, this effort is worth it. In practice, the process of starting warfarin is often undertaken after discharge from hospital, usually in an out-patient anticoagulation clinic. LMWH should be overlapped with warfarin for at least 5 days and until the INR is 2.0 or more on two occasions at least 24 h apart [96].

Women should be advised that heparin and warfarin are safe during breast-feeding. Few data are available on whether LMWH crosses into breast milk. However, absorption of heparins from the gastrointestinal tract is minimal, so, even if some is ingested by the baby in breast milk, systemic absorption is likely to be negligible.

When it is time for anticoagulation to be stopped (often 6 weeks postnatally, assuming that the woman has had at least 3 months of anticoagulation), any continuing risk of thrombosis should be assessed. This should include a review of personal and family history of VTE. The results of any thrombophilia screen should be reviewed, on or off anticoagulation, and repeated if necessary. Where a significant thrombotic risk persists, anticoagulation may need to be continued for a further 3 months or longer.

Risk reduction measures against thrombosis should be discussed, including thromboprophylaxis in any future pregnancy and at other times of increased risk, for example, surgery, hospitalization, period of prolonged immobilization and long-haul flights. The safety or otherwise of hormonal contraception should also be addressed.

5.9 Post-thrombotic Syndrome

Post-thrombotic syndrome (PTS) is relatively common following DVT, occurring in over 60 % of cases [97]. Symptoms and signs include persistent leg swelling and pain, chronic pigmentation, eczema and telangiectasis, persistent varicose veins, and sometimes chronic ulceration and dependent cyanosis. When used for thromboprophylaxis, anti-embolism stockings have a pressure at the ankle of less than 20 mmHg; in contrast, GCS used in women with confirmed DVT have an ankle pressure of 30–40 mmHg. Accurate fitting is important and, as pregnancy progresses, repeat fittings with larger sizes may be necessary. Brandjes et al. reported, in a randomized trial in 194 patients were randomly assigned compression stockings (n=96) or no stockings (n=98) after a first episode of DVT, that the risk of PTS can be halved by wearing class II graduated elastic compression stockings on the affected limb for a period of 2 years [21, 98]. However, more recently, Kahn et al. reported, in a placebo-controlled multicenter randomized trial of active (410) versus placebo (396) elastic compression stockings (ECS), used for 2 years to prevent PTS after a first proximal DVT in centres in Canada and the USA, that ECS did not prevent PTS after a first proximal DVT. The ECS in the placebo group were manufactured to look identical to active ECS, but lacking therapeutic compression. The authors concluded that the findings do not support routine wearing of ECS after DVT [99, 100]. A secondary analysis of the SOX trials was undertaken with the objective to determine whether ECS reduce leg pain in patients with acute DVT. There were no significant differences in pain scores between groups at any assessment point (up to 60 days post randomization), and no evidence for subgroup interaction by age, sex or anatomical extent of DVT (the mean age was 55 years and 60 % of the patients were male). Results were similar in an analysis restricted to patients who reported wearing stockings every day. The authors concluded that ECS do not reduce leg pain in patients with acute proximal DVT. The RCOG guidelines advise that following a DVT, graduated ECS should be worn on the affected leg to reduce pain and swelling. They also state that clinicians should be aware that the role of compression stockings in the prevention of PTS is unclear.

5.10 Conclusions

VTE remains a leading cause of maternal morbidity and mortality, despite improvements in prevention in recent years. The optimal management of acute VTE requires a multidisciplinary approach, including senior obstetric, hematological and anesthetic input, liaison with the hemostasis laboratory, and additional input by a respiratory physician or neurologist in the case of suspected PE or suspected CVT, respectively.

Clinicians should have a low threshold for investigating women with suspected VTE during pregnancy or the puerperium. Although promising, the role of D-dimer levels in the diagnosis of pregnancy-associated VTE is not established. MRI should be considered to diagnose iliac DVT, as approximately 10 % of pregnant women with proximal DVT may have iliac vein thrombosis detected on MRI that is missed on ultrasound.

The radiation dose to the fetus is lower in a CTPA than a V/Q scan; however, there is an increase in the radiation dose to the proliferating breast tissue. The current estimated lifetime risk of breast cancer is 1 in 8. Whether or not this small additional dose of radiation translates to a measurable increase in the lifetime risk of breast cancer is not yet known. However, the risk to the mother is significant if a PE is missed. In pregnant and postpartum women with suspected PE, the first line of investigation should be lower limb scanning. It remains important however, that if the patient has symptoms suggestive of PE and the Doppler/Duplex scan is negative, then CTPA or V/Q scanning should be performed, as the benefit of having direct lung imaging would outweigh the risks. CTPA also has the benefit of demonstrating other lung pathology that may cause symptoms, e.g. pneumonia, pleural effusion.

LMWH is the mainstay in the treatment of pregnancy-associated VTE. The primary aim in peripartum management is to balance the risk of major postpartum hemorrhage versus the risk of extension or recurrence of VTE when anticoagulation is interrupted. In general, being on treatment doses of anticoagulation is often an indication for timing of delivery, but would not be an indication for elective Cesarean section; induction of labor is usually preferable. Therapeutic anticoagulation should be continued for the duration of the pregnancy and for at least 6 weeks postnatally, and until at least 3 months of anticoagulation has been given in total.

5.11 Case Study

A 33 year old woman experienced an extensive left ileo-femoral DVT, diagnosed on Doppler ultrasound, 6 weeks postpartum after an uneventful pregnancy. She was treated initially with therapeutic dose LMWH and maintained on warfarin, target INR 2.5 (range 2.0–3.0). Three months later she had a recurrent proximal lower limb DVT in the same limb and a PE, diagnosed on CTPA, when her INR was within the therapeutic range. The target INR was raised to 3.5 (range 3.0–4.0). She had erratic anticoagulant control, and experienced several episodes of superficial thrombophlebitis (STP) and a further proximal left lower limb DVT when her INR was subtherapeutic. Following this, 'step in' split dose LMWH was administered to cover INR dips below 3.0. She was referred for specialist review. A thrombophilia screen identified that she was heterozygous for factor V Leiden, with the remainder of the screen, which included detailed testing for antiphospholipid antibodies, negative. She had a post-thrombotic left lower limb with persistent swelling and discomfort in this limb. Bilateral venous duplex examination showed no evidence of acute or chronic DVT and extensive scarring and reflux in the left lower limb.

In her second pregnancy aged 39 years, her anticoagulation was switched from warfarin to dalteparin 10,000 units twice daily SC. Her booking weight was 96 kg with height 165 cm and BMI 36 kg/m^2. The dose of dalteparin was increased to 12,500 and 10,000 units 12 hourly. Anti-Xa levels at 4 h post dose ranged between 0.50 and 0.60 IU/dL. She developed vaginal bleeding at 24 weeks' gestation. This was sufficiently severe to necessitate cessation of the LMWH. An IVC filter was inserted because of her perceived risk of recurrent DVT with subsequent PE in the absence of anticoagulation. Dalteparin was reintroduced after 48 h at an initial dose of 5,000 units, with the dose gradually escalated to 7,500 units 12 hourly over a period of 3 weeks, with this dose continued for the remainder of her pregnancy. She continued to experience intermittent vaginal bleeding, the precise source of which was not identified. At 38 weeks' gestation labour was induced, and she delivered a healthy male infant, birth weight 3.5 kg. Blood loss at delivery was normal at 300 mL. The last dose of dalteparin pre-delivery of 7,500 units was administered 12 h prior to commencement of IOL. Post-delivery, she was recommenced on dalteparin, initial dose 5,000 units, 6 h after removal of the epidural. She received dalteparin 5,000 units 12 hourly on day 1 post-delivery, increasing to 10,000 units 12 hourly from day 2 onwards. She was maintained on dalteparin until removal of the IVC filter at 6 weeks post-delivery, following which her anticoagulation was switched back to her pre-pregnancy regimen.

Key Learning Points

- VTE is a leading direct cause of maternal mortality in many developed countries, including the UK.
- Pregnancy is a prothrombotic state, associated with a five- to ten-fold increased risk of VTE compared with the non-pregnant state.
- Healthcare professionals should be aware of the risk factors for venous and arterial thromboembolism.
- Clinicians should have a low threshold for investigating women with suspected VTE in pregnancy.
- Although promising, the role of D-dimer levels in the diagnosis of pregnancy-associated VTE is not established.
- MRI should be considered to diagnose iliac DVT, as approximately 10 % of pregnant women with proximal DVT may have iliac vein thrombosis detected on MRI that is missed on ultrasound.
- If the patient has symptoms suggestive of PE but the lower limb venous Doppler/Duplex scan is negative, then CTPA or V/Q scanning should be performed, as the benefit of having direct lung imaging would outweigh risks.
- LMWH is the mainstay in the treatment of pregnancy-associated VTE.

References

1. Cantwell R, Clutton-Brock T, Cooper G, Dawson A, Drife J, Garrod D, et al. Saving Mothers' Lives: reviewing maternal deaths to make motherhood safer: 2006–08. The Eighth Report on Confidential Enquiries into Maternal Deaths in the United Kingdom. BJOG. 2011;118 Suppl 1:1–203.
2. Lewis G, editor. Mothers' lives 2003–2005. Seventh report of the confidential enquiries into maternal death. London: Royal College of Obstetricians and Gynaecologists Press; 2007.
3. Andersen BS, Steffensen FH, Sorensen HT, Nielsen GL, Olsen J. The cumulative incidence of venous thromboembolism during pregnancy and puerperium – an 11 year Danish population-based study of 63,300 pregnancies. Acta Obstet Gynecol Scand. 1998;77(2):170–3.
4. Gherman RB, Goodwin TM, Leung B, et al. Incidence, clinical characteristics, and timing of objectively diagnosed venous thromboembolism during pregnancy. Obstet Gynecol. 1999;94(5 Part 1):730–4.
5. Lindqvist P, Dahlback B, Marsal K. Thrombotic risk during pregnancy: a population study. Obstet Gynecol. 1999;94(4):595–9.
6. Macklon NS, Greer IA. Venous thromboembolic disease in obstetrics and gynaecology: the Scottish experience. Scott Med J. 1996;41(3):83–6.

7. Mcoll MD, Ramsay JE, Tait RC, et al. Risk factors for pregnancy associated venous thromboembolism. Thromb Haemost. 1997;78(4):1183–8.
8. Simpson EL, Lawrenson RA, Nightingale AL, Farmer RD. Venous thromboembolism in pregnancy and the puerperium: incidence and additional risk factors from a London perinatal database. BJOG. 2001;108(1):56–60.
9. Anderson F, Wheeler H, Goldberg R, et al. A population-based perspective of the hospital incidence and case-fatality rates of deep vein thrombosis and pulmonary embolism. The Worcester DVT study. Arch Intern Med. 1991;151(5):933–8.
10. James AH, Jamison MG, Brancazio LR, Myers ER. Venous thromboembolism during pregnancy and the postpartum period: incidence, risk factors, and the mortality. Am J Obstet Gynecol. 2006;194:1311–5.
11. Nordstrom M, Lindblad B, Bergqvist D, Kjellstrom T. A prospective study of the incidence of deep-vein thrombosis within a defined urban population. J Intern Med. 1992;232(2):155–60.
12. Samuelsson E, Hagg S. Incidence of venous thromboembolism in young Swedish women and possibly preventable cases among combined oral contraceptive users. Acta Obstet Gynecol Scand. 2004;83(7):674–81.
13. White R. The epidemiology of venous thromboembolism. Circulation. 2003;107:I-4–8.
14. Jacobsen AF, Skjeldestad FE, Sandet PM. Incidence and risk patterns of venous thromboembolism in pregnancy and puerperium – a register-based case–control study. Am J Obstet Gynecol. 2008;198: 223–34.
15. Knight M, Kurinczuk JJ, Spark P, Brocklehurst P. United Kingdom Obstetric Surveillance System (UKOSS) annual report. Oxford: National Perinatal Epidemiology Unit; 2007.
16. Knight M, on behalf of UKOSS. Antenatal pulmonary embolism: risk factors, management and outcomes. BJOG. 2008;115:453–61.
17. Lewis G, editor. Why mothers die 2000–2002. Sixth report of the confidential enquiries into maternal death. London: Royal College of Obstetricians and Gynaecologists Press; 2004.
18. Berg CJ, Atrash HK, Koonin LM, Tucker M. Pregnancy-related mortality in the United States, 1987–1990. Obstet Gynecol. 1996;88:161–7.
19. Chang J, Elam-Evans LD, Berg CJ, Herndon J, Flowers L, Seed KA, Syverson CJ. Pregnancy-related mortality surveillance – United States, 1991–1999. MMWR Surveill Summ. 2003;52(2):1–8.
20. Jacobsen AF, Skjeldestad FE, Sandset PM. Incidence and risk patterns of venous thromboembolism in pregnancy and puerperium - a register-based case-control study. Am J Obstet Gynaecol 2008;198:233.e1–7.
21. Royal College of Obstetricians and Gynaecologists. Thromboembolic disease in pregnancy and the puerperium: acute management. Green-top guideline no. 37b. London: RCOG; 2015. Available at: https://www.rcog.org.uk/guidelines.
22. Chan W-S, Spencer FA, Ginsberg JS. Anatomic distribution of deep vein thrombosis in pregnancy. CMAJ. 2010;182:657–60.
23. Kittner SJ, Stern BJ, Feeser BR, Hebel R, Nagey DA, Buchholz DW, Earley CJ, Johnson CJ, Macko RF, Sloan MA, Wityk RJ, Wozniak MA. Pregnancy and the risk of stroke. N Engl J Med. 1996;335(11):768–74.
24. Jaigobin C, Silver FL. Stroke and pregnancy. Stroke. 2000;31(12):2948–51.
25. James AH, Bushnell CD, Jamison MG, Myers ER. Incidence and risk factors for stroke in pregnancy and the puerperium. Obstet Gynecol. 2005;106(3):509–16.
26. Lanska DJ, Kryscio RJ. Risk factors for peripartum and postpartum stroke and intracranial venous thrombosis. Stroke. 2000;31(6):1274–82.
27. Walker ID. Venous and arterial thrombosis during pregnancy: epidemiology. Semin Vasc Med. 2003;3:25–32.
28. Macklon NS, Greer IA, Bowman AW. An ultrasound study of gestational and postural changes in the deep venous system of the leg in pregnancy. BJOG. 1997;104:191–7.
29. Stirling Y, Woolf L, North WR, Seghatchian MJ, Meade TW. Haemostasis in normal pregnancy. Thromb Haemost. 1984;52(2):176–82.
30. Clark P, Brennand J, Conkie JA, McCall F, Greer IA, Walker ID. Activated protein C sensitivity, protein C, protein S and coagulation in normal pregnancy. Thromb Haemost. 1998;79(6):1166–70.
31. Karlsson O, Sporrong T, Hillarp A, Jeppsson A, Hellgren M. Prospective longitudinal study of thromboelastography and standard hemostatic laboratory tests in healthy women during normal pregnancy. Anesth Analg. 2012;115(4):890–8.
32. Szecsi PB, Jørgensen M, Klajnbard A, Andersen MR, Colov NP, Stender S. Haemostatic reference intervals in pregnancy. Thromb Haemost. 2010;103(4):718–27.
33. Hellgren M. Hemostasis during normal pregnancy and puerperium. Semin Thromb Hemost. 2003;29(2): 125–30.
34. British Thoracic Society Standards of Care Committee Pulmonary Embolism Guideline Development Group. British Thoracic Society guidelines for the management of suspected acute pulmonary embolism. Thorax. 2003;58:470–84.
35. Scarsbrook AF, Evans AL, Owen AR, Gleeson FV. Diagnosis of suspected venous thromboembolic disease in pregnancy. Clin Radiol. 2006;61(1):1–12.
36. Torkzad MR, Bremme K, Hellgren M, Eriksson MJ, Hagman A, Jorgensen T, et al. Magnetic resonance imaging and ultrasonography in diagnosis of pelvic vein thrombosis during pregnancy. Thromb Res. 2010;126:107–12.
37. Patenaude Y, Pugash D, Lim K, Morin L; Diagnostic Imaging Committee, Lim K, Bly S, Butt K, Cargill Y, Davies G, Denis N, et al. Society of Obstetricians and Gynaecologists of Canada. The use of magnetic resonance imaging in the obstetric patient. J Obstet Gynaecol Can. 2014;36(4):349–63.
38. ESUR guidelines on Contrast Media version 8.0. 2012. http://www.esur.org/guidelines/.

39. Thomsen HS, Morcos SK, Almen T, et al. Nephrogenic systemic fibrosis and gadolinium based contrast media: updated ESUR Contrast Medium Safety Committee Guidelines. Eur Radiol. 2013;23:307–18.
40. Patel SJ, Reede DL, Katz DS, Subramaniam R, Amorosa JK. Imaging the pregnant patient for nonobstetric conditions: algorithms and radiation dose considerations. Radiographics. 2007;27:1705–22.
41. Leung AN, Bull TM, Jaeschke R, Lockwood CJ, Boiselle PM, Hurwitz LM, et al. ATS/STR Committee on Pulmonary Embolism in Pregnancy. An official American Thoracic Society/Society of Thoracic Radiology clinical practice guideline: evaluation of suspected pulmonary embolism in pregnancy. Am J Respir Crit Care Med. 2011;184(10):1200–8.
42. Chan WS, Ray JG, Murray S, Coady GE, Coates G, Ginsberg JS. Suspected pulmonary embolism in pregnancy: clinical presentation, results of lung scanning, and subsequent maternal and pediatric outcomes. Arch Intern Med. 2002;162:1170–5.
43. Shahir K, Goodman LR, Tali A, Thorsen KM, Hellman RS. Pulmonary embolism in pregnancy: CT pulmonary angiography versus perfusion scanning. AJR Am J Roentgenol. 2010;195:W214–20.
44. Cook JV, Kyriou J. Radiation from CT and perfusion scanning in pregnancy. Br Med J. 2005;221:350.
45. Bourjeily G, Chalhoub M, Phornphutkul C, Alleyne TC, Woodfield CA, Chen KK. Neonatal thyroid function: effect of a single exposure to iodinated contrast medium in utero. Radiology. 2010;256:744–50.
46. Lifetime risk calculated using 2010 data for females and 2008–2010 data for males by the Statistical Information Team at Cancer Research UK, 2012. http://www.cancerresearchuk.org/cancer-info/cancerstats/types/breast/incidence/uk-breast-cancer-incidence-statistics.
47. Schaefer-Prokop C, Prokop M. CTPA for the diagnosis of acute pulmonary embolism during pregnancy. Eur Radiol. 2008;18(12):2705–8.
48. Chan WS, Lee A, Spencer FA, Chunilal S, Crowther M, Wu W, Johnston M, Rodger M, Ginsberg JS. D-dimer testing in pregnant patients: towards determining the next 'level' in the diagnosis of deep vein thrombosis. J Thromb Haemost. 2010;8(5):1004–11.
49. Murphy N, Broadhurst D, Khashan A, Gilligan O, Kenny L, O'Donoghue K. Gestation-specific D-dimer reference ranges: a cross-sectional study. BJOG. 2015;122(3):395–400.
50. Che Yaakob CA, Dzarr AA, Ismail AA, Zuky Nik Lah NA, Ho JJ. Anticoagulant therapy for deep vein thrombosis (DVT) in pregnancy. Cochrane Database Syst Rev. 2010;(6):CD007801.
51. James AH. Prevention and management of venous thromboembolism in pregnancy. Am J Med. 2007; 120(10 Suppl 2):S26–34.
52. Nelson S, Greer I. Thromboembolic events in pregnancy: pharmacological prophylaxis and treatment. Expert Opin Pharmacother. 2007;8(17):2917–31.
53. The Task Force for the Diagnosis and Management of Acute Pulmonary Embolism of the European Society of Cardiology. Guidelines on the diagnosis and management of acute pulmonary embolism. Eur Heart J. 2008;29:2276–315.
54. Gould MK, Dembitzer AD, Doyle RL, Hastie TJ, Garber AM. Low-molecular-weight heparins compared with unfractionated heparin for treatment of acute deep venous thrombosis. A meta-analysis of randomized, controlled trials. Ann Intern Med. 1999;130(10):800–9. 31.
55. Quinlan DJ, McQuillan A, Eikelboom JW. Low-molecular-weight heparin compared with intravenous unfractionated heparin for treatment of pulmonary embolism: a meta-analysis of randomized, controlled trials. Ann Intern Med. 2004;140(3):175–83.
56. Bates SM, Greer IA, Middeldorp S, Veenstra DL, Prabulos A-M, Vandvik PO. VTE, thrombophilia, antithrombotic therapy, and pregnancy. Antithrombotic Therapy and prevention of Thrombosis, 9th ed: American College of Chest Physicians evidence based clinical practice guidelines. Chest. 2012; 141(2 Suppl):e691S–736.
57. Voke KM, Keidan J, Parvod S, Spencer NH, Hunt BJ. The management of antenatal venous thromboembolism in the UK and Ireland: a prospective multicentre survey. Br J Haematol. 2007;139:545–58.
58. Dempfle CEH. Minor transplacental passage of fondaparinux in vivo. N Engl J Med. 2004;350(18): 1914–5.
59. Ginsberg JS, Kowalchuk G, Hirsh J, Brill-Edwards P, Burrows R. Heparin therapy during pregnancy. Risks to the fetus and mother. Arch Intern Med. 1989;149:2233–6.
60. Greer IA, Nelson-Piercy C. Low-molecular-weight heparins for thromboprophylaxis and treatment of venous thromboembolism in pregnancy: a systematic review of safety and efficacy. Blood. 2005;106:401–7.
61. Thomson AJ, Greer IA. Advances in low-molecular-weight heparin use in pregnancy. In: Garg HG, Linhardt RJ, Hales CA, editors. Chemistry and biology of heparin and heparan sulfate. Amsterdam: Elsevier; 2005. p. 745–68.
62. Watson H, Davidson S, Keeling D. Guidelines on the diagnosis and management of heparin-induced thrombocytopenia: second edition. Br J Haematol. 2012;159:528–40.
63. Linkins LA, Dans AL, Moores LK, Bona R, Davidson BL, Schulman S, Crowther M, American College of Chest Physicians. Treatment and prevention of heparin-induced thrombocytopenia: Antithrombotic Therapy and Prevention of Thrombosis, 9th ed: American College of Chest Physicians evidence-based clinical practice guidelines. Chest. 2012;141(2 Suppl):e495S–530. doi:10.1378/chest.11-2303.
64. Baglin T, et al. British Committee for Standard in Haematology (BCSH) Guidelines on the use and monitoring of heparin. Br J Haematol. 2006;133:19–34.
65. Blomback M, Bremme K, Hellgren M, Lindberg H. A pharmacokinetic study of dalteparin (Fragmin) during late pregnancy. Blood Coagul Fibrinolysis. 1998;9:343–50.

66. Casele HL, Laifer SA, Woelkers DA, Venkataramanan R. Changes in the pharmacokinetics of the low-molecular-weight heparin enoxaparin sodium during pregnancy. Am J Obstet Gynecol. 1999;181:1113–7.
67. Patel JP, Green B, Patel RK, Marsh MS, Davies JG, Arya R. Population pharmacokinetics of enoxaparin during the antenatal period. Circulation. 2013; 128(13):1462–9.
68. Van Dongen CJ, Van Den Belt AG, Prins MH, Lensing AW. Fixed dose subcutaneous low-molecular-weight heparins versus adjusted dose unfractionated heparin for venous thromboembolism. Cochrane Database Syst Rev. 2004;(4):CD001100.
69. Hull R, Delmore T, Carter C, et al. Adjusted subcutaneous heparin versus warfarin sodium in the long-term treatment of venous thrombosis. N Engl J Med. 1982;306:189–94.
70. Van Der Heijden JF, Hutten BA, Buller HR, Prins MH. Vitamin K antagonists or low-molecular-weight heparin for the long-term treatment of symptomatic venous thromboembolism. Cochrane Database Syst Rev. 2002;(1):CD002001.
71. Forestier F, Daffos F, Capella-Pavlovsky M. Low-molecular-weight heparin (PK 10169) does not cross the placenta during the second trimester of pregnancy: study by direct fetal blood sampling under ultrasound. Thromb Res. 1984;34:557–60.
72. Warkentin TE, Levine MN, Hirsh J, et al. Heparin-induced thrombocytopenia in patients treated with low-molecular-weight heparin or unfractionated heparin. N Engl J Med. 1995;332:1330–5.
73. Barbour LA, Kick SD, Steiner JF, et al. A prospective study of heparin-induced osteoporosis in pregnancy using bone densitometry. Am J Obstet Gynecol. 1994;170:862–9.
74. Carlin AJ, Farquharson RG, Quenby SM, Topping J, Fraser WD. Prospective observational study of bone mineral density during pregnancy: low-molecular-weight heparin versus control. Hum Reprod. 2004; 19:1211–4.
75. Douketis JD, Ginsberg JS, Burrows RF, et al. The effects of long-term heparin therapy during pregnancy on bone density. A prospective matched cohort study. Thromb Haemost. 1996;75:254–7.
76. Melissari E, Parker CJ, Wilson NV, Monte G, Kanthou C, Pemberton KD, et al. Use of low-molecular-weight heparin in pregnancy. Thromb Haemost. 1992;68:652–6.
77. Monreal M. Long-term treatment of venous thromboembolism: the place of low-molecular-weight heparin. Vessels. 1997;3:18–21.
78. Pettila V, Leinonen P, Markkola A, Hiilesmaa V, Kaaja R. Postpartum bone mineral density in women treated for thromboprophylaxis with unfractionated heparin or LMW heparin. Thromb Haemost. 2002; 87:182–6.
79. Bank I, Libourel EJ, Middeldorp S, Van Der Meer J, Buller HR. High rate of skin complications due to low-molecular-weight heparins in pregnant women. J Thromb Haemost. 2003;1:859–61.
80. Holst J, Lindblad B, Bergqvist D, Garre K, Nielsen H, Hedner U, Ostergaard PB. Protamine neutralization of intravenous and subcutaneous low-molecular-weight heparin (tinzaparin, Logiparin). An experimental investigation in healthy volunteers. Blood Coagul Fibrinolysis. 1994;5(5):795–803.
81. van Veen JJ, Maclean RM, Hampton KK, Laidlaw S, Kitchen S, Toth P, Makris M. Protamine reversal of low-molecular-weight heparin: clinically effective? Blood Coagul Fibrinolysis. 2011;22(7):565–70.
82. Hirsh J, Bauer KA, Donati MB, Gould M, Samama MM, Weitz JI, American College of Chest Physicians. Parenteral anticoagulants: American College of Chest Physicians evidence-based clinical practice guidelines (8th edition). Chest. 2008;133(6 Suppl):141S–59.
83. Makris M, Van Veen JJ, Tait CR, Mumford AD, Laffan M; on behalf of the British Committee for Standards in Haematology. Guideline on the management of bleeding in patients on antithrombotic agents. Br J Haematol. 2012;160:35–46.
84. Baglin T, Gray E, Greaves M, et al. Clinical guidelines for testing for heritable thrombophilia. Br J Haematol. 2010;149:209–20.
85. Keeling D, Mackie I, Moore GW, Greer IA, Greaves M. Guidelines on the investigation and management of antiphospholipid syndrome. Br J Haematol. 2012; 157:47–58.
86. Greer I, Hunt BJ. Low-molecular-weight heparin in pregnancy: current issues. Br J Haematol. 2005; 128:593–601.
87. Lee AY, Levine MN, Baker RI, Bowden C, Kakkar AK, Prins M, et al. Randomized Comparison of Low-Molecular-Weight Heparin versus Oral Anticoagulant Therapy for the Prevention of Recurrent Venous Thromboembolism in Patients with Cancer (CLOT) Investigators. Low-molecular-weight heparin versus a coumarin for the prevention of recurrent venous thromboembolism in patients with cancer. N Engl J Med. 2003;349(2):146–53.
88. British Committee for Standards in Haematology Writing Group, Baglin TP, Brush J, Streiff M. Guidelines on use of vena cava filters. Br J Haematol. 2006;134(6):590–5.
89. McConville RM, Kennedy PT, Collins AJ, Ellis PK. Failed retrieval of an inferior vena cava filter during pregnancy because of filter tilt: report of two cases. Cardiovasc Intervent Radiol. 2009;32: 174–7.
90. Tardy B, Mismetti P, Page Y, Décousus H, Da Costa A, Zeni F, et al. Symptomatic inferior vena cava filter thrombosis: clinical study of 30 consecutive cases. Eur Respir J. 1996;9(10):2012–6.
91. Piccone Jr VA, Vidal E, Yarnoz M, Glass P, LeVeen HH. The late results of caval ligation. Surgery. 1970;68(6):980–98.
92. Hajduk B, Tomkowski WZ, Małek G, Davidson BL. Vena cava filter occlusion and venous thromboembolism risk in persistently anticoagulated patients: a prospective, observational cohort study. Chest. 2010; 137(4):877–82.

93. Uberoi R, Tapping CR, Chalmers N, Allgar V. British Society of Interventional Radiology (BSIR) Inferior Vena Cava (IVC) Filter Registry. Cardiovasc Intervent Radiol. 2013;36(6):1548–61.
94. Eikelboom JW, Hirsh J. Monitoring unfractionated heparin with the aPTT: time for a fresh look. Thromb Haemost. 2006;96(5):547–52.
95. Ahearn GS, Hadjiliadis MD, Govert JA, Tapson VF. Massive pulmonary embolism during pregnancy successfully treated with recombinant tissue plasminogen activator. Arch Intern Med. 2002;162:1221–7.
96. Keeling D, Baglin T, Tait C, Watson H, Perry D, Baglin C, Kitchen S. Guidelines on oral anticoagulation with warfarin – fourth edition. Br J Haematol. 2011;154:311–24.
97. McColl MD, Ellison J, Greer IA, Tait RC, Walker ID. Prevalence of the post thrombotic syndrome in young women with previous venous thromboembolism. Br J Haematol. 2000;108:272–4.
98. Brandjes DP, Buller HR, Heijboer H, Huisman MV, de Rijk M, Jagt H, et al. Randomised trial of effect of compression stockings in patients with symptomatic proximal–vein thrombosis. Lancet. 1997;349:759–62.
99. Kahn SR, Shapiro S, Wells PS, Rodger MA, Kovacs MJ, Anderson DR, et al. SOX trial investigators. Compression stockings to prevent post-thrombotic syndrome: a randomised placebo-controlled trial. Lancet. 2014;383(9920):880–8.
100. Kahn SR, Shapiro S, Ducruet T, Wells PS, Rodger MA, Kovacs MJ, et al. Graduated compression stockings to treat acute leg pain associated with proximal DVT. A randomised controlled trial. Thromb Haemost. 2014;112(6):1137–41.

6 Systemic Thromboembolism in Pregnancy: Cerebrovascular Disease

Deepa Jayakody Arachchillage, Patrick O'Brien, Charlie Davie, and Hannah Cohen

Abstract

Stroke is a neurological emergency and one of the most common causes of long-term disability and death. Although stroke is rare at a younger age, the normal physiologic changes associated with pregnancy, combined with some of the pathophysiological processes unique to pregnancy, predispose women to develop stroke during pregnancy and the puerperium. This chapter reviews the mechanisms and risk factors for cerebrovascular disease related to pregnancy, the presenting features, diagnosis and management of these disorders, and their implications for pregnancy and delivery.

Keywords

Pregnancy • Cerebrovascular disease • Ischemic stroke • Hemorrhagic stroke • Cerebral venous and sinus thrombosis

6.1 Introduction

Cerebrovascular disease related to pregnancy can be distilled into two major categories: thrombosis/ischemia (including arterial and venous infarction) and hemorrhage (including intracerebral and subarachnoid hemorrhage). Stroke is defined by the World Health Organization [1] as a clinical syndrome consisting of "rapidly developing clinical signs of focal (at times global) disturbance of cerebral function, lasting more than 24 h or leading to death with no apparent cause other than that of vascular origin". A transient ischemic attack (TIA) is defined as stroke symptoms and signs that resolve within 24 h. However, there are limitations to these definitions. For example, they do not include retinal symptoms (sudden onset of monocular visual loss), which should be

D.J. Arachchillage, MBBS, MRCP, FRCPath (✉)
H. Cohen, MB ChB, MD, FCRP, FRCPath
Department of Haematology, University College London Hospitals NHS Foundation Trust, 250 Euston Road, London NW1 2PG, UK
e-mail: d.arachchillage@ucl.ac.uk; hannah.cohen@uclh.nhs.uk

P. O'Brien, MB BCh, FRCOG, FICOG, FFSRH
Institute of Women's Health, University College London Hospitals NHS Foundation Trust, 250 Euston Road, London NW1 2PG, UK
e-mail: patobrien64@yahoo.co.uk

C. Davie, MB ChB, MD, FRCP
Department of Clinical Neurosciences, The Royal Free Hampstead NHS Trust, Pond Street, London NW3 2QG, UK
e-mail: c.davie@ucl.ac.uk

H. Cohen, P. O'Brien (eds.), *Disorders of Thrombosis and Hemostasis in Pregnancy: A Guide to Management*, DOI 10.1007/978-3-319-15120-5_6, © Springer-Verlag London 2015

considered as part of the definition of stroke and TIA. Stroke is a neurological emergency and one of the most common causes of profound long-term disability or death.

Although arterial stroke is rare at a younger age, during pregnancy the normal physiological changes associated with pregnancy, combined with some of the pathophysiological processes unique to pregnancy or underlying prothrombotic disorders, may predispose women to develop arterial stroke and cerebral venous and sinus thrombosis (CVT) during pregnancy. The physiological changes of pregnancy, specifically venous stasis, edema, and hypercoagulability (caused by activated protein C resistance, a reduction in levels of protein S, and increased fibrinogen), combine to make pregnancy and the postpartum period a time of increased risk for venous thromboembolism (VTE). This may manifest neurologically as CVT, which may be complicated by venous and arterial infarction; or as cryptogenic stroke or TIA in association with a patent foramen ovale (PFO) and deep venous thrombosis (DVT). Pregnancy-related hypertension is the leading cause of both hemorrhagic stroke and ischemic stroke in pregnant and postpartum women [2–4]. It has been estimated that there is a mortality rate of between 10 and 13 % following pregnancy related stroke; this is disproportionately higher in black women, in older patients and those with no prenatal care [5]. Cesarean delivery is associated with an increased risk of peripartum and postpartum stroke. This may be due in part to a higher likelihood of Cesarean delivery among women who have had a stroke during pregnancy and other pregnancy related conditions such as pre-eclampsia, which increases the risk of both stroke and Cesarean section. Several underlying disorders, including antiphospholipid syndrome, hemoglobinopathies, myeloproliferative disorders, thrombotic microangiopathies and paroxysmal nocturnal hemoglobinuria, may also predispose to pregnancy-associated stroke.

Considering all of these factors, women who develop cerebrovascular disease during pregnancy and post-partum should be managed in centralised units by a multidisciplinary team, including neurology/neurosurgery, obstetric, hematology and rehabilitation services experienced in dealing with such conditions. This chapter reviews the mechanisms and risk factors for cerebrovascular disease related to pregnancy, the presenting features, diagnosis and management of these disorders, and their implications for pregnancy and delivery.

6.2 Incidence of Stroke in Pregnancy

The reported incidence of stroke during pregnancy and the puerperium ranges from 4 to 34 per 100,000 deliveries [6–9]. In a large Swedish cohort of more than 650,000 women with more than one million deliveries over 8 years, the greatest risk of ischemic and hemorrhagic stroke was found around the time of delivery, with an increased but declining risk over the subsequent 6 weeks [10]. The 2006–2008 Confidential Enquiries into Maternal Deaths (CEMD) in the United Kingdom reported that VTE in pregnancy accounts for 0.79 (n=18) deaths per 100,000 pregnancies, with 0.09 (n=2) of these deaths from CVT [11]. However, the incidence of arterial stroke related deaths was not specified. A study on 1,687,930 California residents with a first recorded hospitalization for labor and delivery between Jan 2005, and June 2010 showed an increased incidence of ischemic stroke compared with the same period 1 year later: 119 during the first 6 weeks postpartum (7.1 per 100,000 deliveries; OR 8.5; 95 % confidence interval [CI] 4.9–14.8), falling to 15 during weeks 7–12 postpartum (0.9 per 100,000 deliveries; OR 1.7 (0.7–3.8) [12].

Data addressing the risk of recurrent stroke associated with pregnancy are very limited, however, it appears to be relatively small. The risk of recurrent stroke is increased in the postpartum period but not during pregnancy, consistent with the risk period for first stroke [13]. The risk of recurrence depends on the underlying risk factors for development of stroke, and the extent to which these factors are controlled. Case series suggest an overall rate of 1 in 143, or 0.7 % (95 % CI, 0.04–4.4 %) [13–15].

6.3 Diagnosis of Cerebrovascular Disorders in Pregnancy

Prompt recognition of symptoms and signs of stroke, and distinguishing whether the stroke is due to cerebral ischemia or haemorrhage, are key to successful management. Clinical history and physical examination are insufficiently sensitive to differentiate between ischemic and hemorrhagic stroke, so brain imaging in the form of CT or MRI should be carried out as quickly as possible after symptom onset. However, several concerns about fetal exposure to radiation arise for the clinicians. The potential harmful effect of radiation depends on the stage of gestation, the total dose of radiation absorbed and the rate at which the dose is absorbed.

MRI is safe in pregnancy so is the preferred option in pregnant women. MR contrast agents should not be routinely administered to pregnant patients, and decisions about their use should be made on a case-by-case basis, based on an assessment of the risk versus benefit for the patient, by the attending senior radiologist, neurologist and obstetrician [16].

CT scanning does expose the fetus to radiation; however, if MRI is not available, the benefits of CT scanning in this scenario greatly outweigh the risks, and should be performed. As the use of iodinated contrast material during pregnancy may pose some risk to the fetus, it should be administered only in exceptional circumstances [17]. Theoretically, there is a risk that contrast medium may be absorbed by the fetus which may result in fetal thyroid suppression [18]. If iodinated contrast is administered, neonatal thyroid function should be measured during the first week after birth. With regard to lactation, a very small amount of contrast medium enters breast milk and almost nothing is absorbed across the gut, so no special precautions or cessation of breast feeding are required [17].

It is worth noting that migraine with an accompanying aura is sufficiently common in pregnancy that it should be considered in the differential diagnosis, particularly if there is evolving neurological deficit rather than a very abrupt onset. Abrupt onset headache with nausea and photophobia may suggest either a migrainous etiology or, more importantly, a subarachnoid hemorrhage [19].

6.4 Ischemic Stroke

Ischemic stroke occurs when there is a reduction of blood flow to a specific part of the brain resulting in tissue necrosis. Arterial occlusion due to atherosclerosis, embolism, thrombus, or hypotension is the most common mechanism for development of ischemic stroke. Less frequently, it can arise from a venous event (CVT), which can result in both venous ischemia and hemorrhagic infarction [15] or via a PFO associated with a DVT [20]. Physiological changes during pregnancy such as increasing levels of procoagulant factors, venous stasis or sudden reduction of blood volume during delivery, increase the risk of CVT in pregnancy [21]; there is also a risk of thrombosis related to underlying thrombotic disorders such as antiphospholipid syndrome.

6.4.1 Risk Factors for Ischemic Stroke in Pregnancy

A number of risk factors have been implicated in the development of ischemic stroke during pregnancy and the puerperium [8, 22] (Table 6.1). Migrainous headaches have been reported to be associated with a 17-fold increased risk of stroke [9], with the risk even higher for ischemic stroke (OR 30.7, CI 95 % 17.4–34.1) [23]. An analysis of approximately 3,000 pregnancy-related discharges in the United States included a diagnosis of stroke and stroke-related death in 34.2 and 1.4 per 100,000 deliveries, respectively. Medical conditions that were reported to be strongly associated with stroke included migrainous headaches, thrombophilia, systemic lupus erythematosus, heart disease, sickle cell disease, hypertension, and thrombocytopenia. Pregnancy complications that were significant risk factors included postpartum hemorrhage, pre-eclampsia and gestational hypertension, transfusion and postpartum infection [8]. Cesarean delivery has been reported to be associated with a 3–12 fold increased risk

Table 6.1 Factors for pregnancy-related stroke

Age
Greater parity
Smoking
Cardiovascular disease including: Hypertension Patent foramen ovale Metallic heart valve
Renal disease
Migraine with aura
Heritable thrombophilia
Acquired thrombophilia: antiphospholipid syndrome
Hyperhomocystinemia
Hematological disorders Thrombotic microangiopathies Paroxysmal nocturnal hemoglobinuria Sickle cell disease and thalassemias Myeloproliferative neoplasma: Primary polycythemia and essential thrombocythemia
Pregnancy-related conditions
Gestational diabetes Delivery by Cesarean section
Pregnancy Complications Postpartum sepsis Pre-eclampsia and eclampsia Amniotic fluid embolus Choriocarcinoma

of peripartum and postpartum stroke [9]. Women with a metallic heart valve are at high risk of arterial thrombotic evens including stroke, particularly in the context of suboptimal anticoagulation (see Chap. 10). The risk of ischemic events in pregnancy and the puerperium is influenced by ethnic background and by age. African American women have a significantly higher risk than Caucasians (there is a paucity of epidemiological data in Asian women). Furthermore, women over the age of 35 years have an increased risk of pregnancy related stroke [5].

6.4.2 Management of Ischemic Stroke in Pregnancy

Women affected by ischemic stroke should be managed by a multidisciplinary team, including input from neurology, obstetric, hematology and rehabilitation services experienced in dealing with such conditions.

6.4.2.1 Treatment of Acute Ischemic Stroke in Pregnancy

Treatment of acute ischemic arterial stroke in pregnancy is controversial. No data are available from clinical trials about the use of thrombolytic therapy with recombinant tissue plasminogen activator (rtPA) in pregnancy, and the experience is limited to case reports and series, including not just ischemic stroke but various other thromboembolic conditions. Randomized clinical trial evidence from non-pregnant patients demonstrates that if rtPA is administered within 3 h of ischemic stroke onset, it significantly reduces the risk of mortality and improves outcome at 90 days post stroke compared with placebo [24]. However, there is an approximately 6 % risk of hemorrhage, and this risk increases with rtPA administration more than 3 h after onset of the stroke symptoms [24]. Thrombolytic agents can be administered intra-arterially for proximal middle cerebral artery occlusion effectively and relatively safely [25]. In addition, certain devices have been approved for mechanical thrombectomy [26]. In some cases, intra-arterial rtPA can be combined with mechanical thrombectomy. Patients tend to have an optimal outcome if whatever method is used leads to partial or complete recanalization of the occluded artery. rtPA does not cross the placenta and there has been no evidence of teratogenicity in animal studies [27]. It is listed as a category C drug and pregnancy is considered a relative contraindication for administration [28], but there are multiple case reports of successful use in pregnant women, and the risk of placental abruption appears small. The risks and benefits should be carefully considered, but it appears that thrombolytic therapy can be used both intravenously and intra-arterially in pregnancy with successful outcomes [27].

6.4.2.2 Secondary Prevention of Ischemic Stroke in Pregnancy

The American Heart/American Stroke Association (AHA/ASA) stroke secondary prevention guidelines [20] and American College of Chest Physicians guidelines (ACCP) [29] recommend antiplatelet treatment for secondary prevention of non-cardioembolic ischemic stroke or TIA. The National Institute of Health and Care

Excellence (NICE) in England recommends the following for secondary prevention of ischemic stroke [30] in patients where stroke is confirmed by imaging: aspirin 300 mg daily should be given for 2 weeks, starting immediately. Clopidogrel 75 mg daily is then given long-term if it can be tolerated and is not contraindicated. If clopidogrel is contraindicated or not tolerated, a combination of modified-release dipyridamole (200 mg twice daily) and LDA is recommended. If both clopidogrel and modified-release dipyridamole are contraindicated or not tolerated, aspirin alone should be given. Clopidogrel crosses the placenta and, although there are no reliable safety data available for its use during pregnancy, case reports and anecdotal evidence suggest that it may be safe [31, 32]. There are no safety data available for the use of dipyridamole during pregnancy, but it has been used in combination with aspirin or warfarin, during both pregnancy and breastfeeding [33]. The guidance also recommends optimal management of atrial fibrillation, diabetes and hypertension if present, and to offer a statin. In a systematic review of both human and animal studies on the teratogenic effects of statins during pregnancy, most of the available data suggested that statins are unlikely to be teratogenic [34]. However, because of the disruption of gonadal stem cell development and theoretical long-term fetal neurological damage [35], statins are classified as Category X (contraindicated) for pregnancy by the FDA and contraindicated during pregnancy and lactation in the Summary of Product Characteristics (SPC) in the UK [36]. In view of this, they should not be commenced until after pregnancy and lactation are completed.

6.5 Ischemic Stroke in Specific Situations

6.5.1 Patent Foramen Ovale

A PFO is an embryonic defect in the inter-atrial septum. PFO is common, present in up to 15–25 % of the adult population [37, 38]. The meta-analysis by Overell et al. [39] published in 2000 concluded that PFO and atrial septal aneurysm were significantly associated with an increased risk of stroke in patients below the age of 55. However, older data showed no differences in rates of recurrent stroke in those with or without PFO (2 year event rate 14.8 and 15.4 %, respectively) as well as no demonstrated effect on outcomes based on PFO size or presence of atrial septal aneurysm. Overall, the importance of PFO with or without atrial septal aneurysm for a first stroke or recurrent cryptogenic stroke remains in question [20]. The American Heart Association/American Stroke Association (AHA/ASA) guidelines on secondary prevention of stroke and TIA suggest antiplatelet therapy for patients with ischemic stroke or TIA and a PFO [20]. There are insufficient data to establish whether anticoagulation is equivalent or superior to aspirin for secondary prevention in patients with PFO, and also insufficient evidence to make a recommendation regarding PFO closure in patients with stroke and PFO [20].

6.5.2 Mechanical Heart Valves

The management of anticoagulation to prevent cardiac and systemic thromboembolism, including ischemic stroke, in patients with a mechanical heart valve is covered in Chap. 10.

6.5.3 Antiphospholipid Syndrome

Antiphospholipid syndrome (APS) is a major acquired risk factor for pregnancy-associated stroke, both arterial or venous [40]. Ischemic stroke due to arterial thrombosis is the most common neurological manifestation, accounting for over 50 % of central nervous system complications in APS which presents during pregnancy or the puerperium.

6.5.3.1 Incidence of Stroke Associated with Antiphospholipid Antibodies

Estimates vary for the true frequency of antiphospholipid antibodies (aPL) in stroke. A study by the AntiPhospholipid Syndrome Alliance For Clinical Trials and InternatiOnal

Networking (APS ACTION), based on analysis of 120 full-text papers and calculation of the median frequency for positive aPL tests for clinical outcome, has estimated the overall frequency of aPL in stroke and TIA to be 13.5 and 7 %, respectively. The authors highlighted that limitations of the literature analyzed included the fact that all three criteria aPL tests (lupus anticoagulant (LA), IgG and IgM anticardiolipin (aCL) and anti-beta 2 glycoprotein I (a-β2 GPI) antibodies) were performed in only 11 % of papers, around one-third used a low-titer aCL cut-off, aPL confirmation was performed in only one-fifth and the study design was retrospective in nearly half. They concluded that best estimates of the incidence of aPL-associated events should be confirmed with appropriately designed population studies [41].

6.5.3.2 Risk of Recurrent Stroke Associated with Antiphospholipid Syndrome

Retrospective and observational studies suggest that APS related stroke is associated with a high risk of recurrence and should be treated with long-term warfarin [42]. In a meta-analysis of 16 studies (9/16 (56 %) were retrospective cohort studies, 3/16 (19 %) were prospective cohort studies and 4/16 (25 %) were randomized controlled trials), recurrence rates in patients with definite APS and previous VTE were lower than in patients with arterial and/or recurrent events, both with and without therapy. Only 3.8 % of recurrent events occurred with an INR >3.0 [43]. Antiphospholipid antibody phenotype may also be important with regard to the risk of recurrence, with high-risk triple-positive patients (i.e. with LA, aCL and a-β2 GPI) on standard intensity anticoagulation showing a 30 % recurrence rate over a 6-year follow up period [44].

Substantive data on the risk of recurrence of APS related stroke in pregnancy are lacking. In a case series of three pregnancies in women with APS and a history of stroke, all were treated with aspirin and low molecular weight heparin (LMWH) during pregnancy and remained free of cerebrovascular events. However, one woman experienced pre-eclampsia and two developed hypertension after 32–37 weeks of an otherwise uneventful pregnancy [45]. A prospective analysis of outcome in a cohort of 33 women with APS treated with a rigorous protocol (enoxaparin 40–80 mg daily according to the levels of factor Xa activity, and LDA) included six cases of pregnant women with APS and previous cerebrovascular events. In five of these six women, LDA and LMWH were inadequate in preventing further cerebral arterial thrombotic events during pregnancy [46]. A more recent prospective analysis reported on outcomes in 23 pregnancies in 20 women, 8 with TIA and 12 with stroke prior to pregnancy. Three patients experienced recurrent cerebrovascular events, one during pregnancy and two postpartum. Two of these three cases occurred in the context of pre-eclampsia, which complicated approximately 35 % of pregnancies. The authors concluded that, particularly in the context of pre-eclampsia, anticoagulation should be given rigorously to prevent recurrent cerebrovascular events [47].

6.5.3.3 Management of Antiphospholipid Syndrome Related Stroke in Pregnancy

The optimal intensity of anticoagulation following stroke associated with APS is under debate [29, 40, 42, 48]. Adequately powered prospective clinical studies are required to determine the optimal antithrombotic approach to patients with aPL-associated stroke. The risk of bleeding with increasing anticoagulant intensity needs to be balanced against the risk of profound permanent physical disability or death, or irreversible intellectual deterioration as a result of recurrent cerebral ischemic strokes. Several experts recommend a target INR of 3.5 (range 3.0–4.0) for stroke associated with persistent aPL which meet the updated Sapporo criteria, with a similar approach in patients with PL-associated TIA [48]. However, current BCSH and ACCP guidelines recommend a target INR of 2.5 (2.0–3.0) in these patients [29, 40]. The RITAPS (Rituximab for the Anticoagulation Resistant Manifestations of Antiphospholipid Syndrome) Phase II study suggested that rituximab was safe and probably effective in controlling some non-criteria manifestations of APS, such as cognitive dysfunction [49].

There is a paucity of data on the optimal management during pregnancy and postpartum of APS-related acute stroke or its secondary prevention. The general approach comprises LMWH and LDA during pregnancy and the puerperium. A survey by the European Antiphospholipid Forum of clinicians who regularly manage patients with APS concluded that, in women with APS associated with a recent or previous stroke, the majority would advise therapeutic dose LMWH during pregnancy, aiming for a peak anti-Xa level of 1.0–1.2 (Boffa MC, 2009, personal communication).

6.5.4 Thrombotic Microangiopathies

Ten to twenty-five percent of women with thrombotic thrombocytopenic purpura (TTP) or other thrombotic microangiopathies (see Chap. 17) present during pregnancy or in the postpartum period [50–52]. TTP may present with a wide variety of neurological manifestations including stroke, TIA, fluctuating neurological symptoms, headaches, seizures and confusion. The diagnosis should be considered in pregnant women who develop thrombocytopenia and anemia. Laboratory investigations may show red cell fragmentation on the blood film indicative of microangiopathic hemolytic anemia (MAHA), and other evidence of intravascular hemolysis: reticulocytosis, elevated bilirubin and lactate dehydrogenase (LDH). It is useful to distinguish between congenital and acquired antibody-mediated TTP as this influences management. In congenital TTP, activity levels of ADAMTS 13 (a disintegrin and metalloprotease with thrombospondin type 1 motif, member 13) are under 5 % and in acquired TTP ADAMTS 13 activity under 5 % and anti-ADAMTS 13 IgG autoantibodies are diagnostic [51]. Early diagnosis is crucial as intensive treatment with plasma exchange (PEX) may be lifesaving [53]; and pregnant women presenting with thrombocytopenia, MAHA, and neurological features including stroke or TIA, should be treated with PEX until the diagnosis of TTP is excluded [47]. In acute acquired TTP with neurological pathology, which is associated with a high mortality, rituximab should be considered on admission, in conjunction with PEX and steroids [47]. Adjunctive LDA and prophylactic dose LMWH may reduce the risk of pregnancy loss and late placenta-mediated vascular pregnancy morbidity such as intrauterine fetal growth restriction.

6.5.5 Heritable Thrombophilia

Heritable thrombophilic defects that are associated with an increased risk of thrombosis include factor V Leiden, prothrombin (factor II) G20210A gene mutation, deficiency of protein C, protein S and antithrombin. However, observational studies have not demonstrated a clear association between inherited thrombophilia and ischemic stroke [54–58]. Two meta-analyses have addressed the potential relationship between prothrombotic disorders and stroke. The first found a significant association between stroke and factor V Leiden, MTHFR C677T variant and the prothrombin G20210A mutation [59]. The risk of an individual suffering from a stroke associated with this polymorphism in the general population is low. The second meta-analysis [60] could not verify a significant association between stroke and factor V Leiden, but found a slight association between stroke and the prothrombin G20210A mutation and the MTHFR C677T polymorphism. These findings were more evident in younger individuals (<55 years) including women of childbearing age. There is insufficient evidence to support specific recommendations in patients with inherited thrombophilia for primary or secondary stroke prevention. With regard to secondary prevention, it appears prudent that women are investigated for DVT and a PFO, with prophylactic anticoagulation during pregnancy and 6 weeks post-partum, or long-term depending on clinical and hematological factors [20].

6.5.6 Sickle Cell Disease

Stroke is a frequent and severe complication in adults with sickle cell disease (SCD), which confers an increased risk of ischemic stroke. Ischemic stroke often causes physical and cognitive disability, while hemorrhagic stroke has a high mortality rate. As more children with SCD survive into adulthood, the number of strokes in adults is increasing, yet stroke in this patient population remains poorly understood [61].

For adults with SCD, the risk of having a first stroke can be as high as 11 % by age 20, 15 % by age 30, and 24 % by age 45 years. An analysis of administrative data from California, USA, which included individuals of all ages with SCD, identified the greatest absolute number of ischemic and hemorrhagic strokes and the highest incidence rates of ischemic stroke in adults 35–64 years of age (740/100,000 person-years), which includes women of childbearing age. The incidence is significantly higher than for ischemic stroke (excluding TIA) seen in African–Americans overall (270/100,000 person years) [62]. Numerous clinical and genetic risk factors for stroke in SCD have been identified, with the most consistently identified clinical risk factors for ischemic stroke in adults including genotype (with the risk greatest for HbSS), increasing age, increased systolic blood pressure or hypertension, lower baseline hemoglobin during pregnancy, and concomitant thalassemic syndromes [63–65].

Currently, there are no validated methods to screen for an increased risk of stroke in adults with SCD. Transcranial Doppler ultrasound (TCD) can identify children with HbSS at increased risk of stroke, and the Stroke Prevention trial in Sickle Cell Anaemia (STOP) demonstrated the efficacy of regular transfusion to maintain hemoglobin S (Hb S) <30 %, to decrease the absolute risk of stroke over 30 months from 30 to 3 %. Women with stroke associated with SCD should have an evaluation for other, potentially modifiable, risk factors for stroke. Exchange transfusion should be undertaken for all pregnant women with SCD and prior stroke or TIA to reduce the risk of stroke during pregnancy. Women with SCD and stroke should be treated in dedicated stroke units with input from both neurologists and hematologists [20].

6.5.7 Myeloproliferative Neoplasms

Myeloproliferative neoplasms (MPD) represent a group of hematological disorders caused by stem cell-derived clonal myeloproliferation. They include polycythemia (PV), essential thrombocythemia (ET), and myelofibrosis, which can all progress to acute myeloid leukemia. Thrombosis is the main cause of morbidity and mortality. The most common MPD in women of childbearing age is ET. In MPD, thrombosis can occur in any vessel, including the cerebral vasculature [66]. There is limited evidence in the literature on the management of PV in pregnancy. If the woman has a previous history of venous and arterial thrombosis (whether pregnant or not), or severe pre-eclampsia in the index pregnancy, the current pregnancy should be considered as high risk and should be managed by a multidisciplinary team including an experienced obstetrician and hematologist. All patients should receive LDA and 6 weeks of post-partum LMWH. If the patient has had previous venous or arterial thrombosis, thromboprophylaxis is indicated during pregnancy. The British Committee for Standards in Haematology (BCSH) guidelines state that LMWH should be started once the pregnancy test is positive. They recommend dalteparin 5,000 units or enoxaparin 40 mg initially once daily; at 16–20 weeks' gestation, this should be increased to twice daily; and 3 days post-partum it can be reduced again to once daily for 6 weeks, if normal body weight, no renal impairment or previous VTE or fetal morbidity. If there is previous history of stroke or other arterial event, they recommend dalteparin 5,000 units or enoxaparin 40 mg twice daily throughout the pregnancy and, if there is evidence of recurrence, to consider increasing the LMWH dose or giving warfarin after 14 weeks' gestation [67, 68]. Furthermore, regular fetal monitoring is required with serial growth scans, as well as uterine artery Doppler scan at 20 weeks (and 24 weeks, if abnormal).

6.5.8 Paroxysmal Nocturnal Hemoglobinuria

Paroxysmal nocturnal hemoglobinuria (PNH) is a rare disease of hematopoietic stem cells caused by a somatic mutation in the X-linked phosphatidylinositol glycan complementation class A (PIGA) gene. PNH is characterized by hemolytic anemia, bone marrow failure, and thromboembolism [69]. VTE constitutes the main cause of death in PNH. Cerebrovascular complications, primarily dural cerebral venous thrombosis, account for 25 % of deaths [70, 71]. Although some hypercoagulable disorders cause both venous and arterial in situ thrombosis, cases of ischemic stroke attributed to PNH may occur [72]. The diagnosis and management of PNH is discussed in detail in Chap. 19.

6.5.9 Hyperhomocysteinemia

Homocysteine is a sulphur-containing amino acid produced during metabolism of methionine. Elevated plasma levels of homocysteine are associated with an increased risk of atherosclerosis and cardiovascular ischemic events. Several mechanisms by which elevated homocysteine impairs vascular function have been proposed, including impairment of endothelial function, production of reactive oxygen species (ROS) and consequent oxidation of low-density lipids [73]. Meta-analyses have confirmed the association between hyperhomocysteinemia and stroke [74, 75]. Several studies have analyzed the efficacy of folic acid or vitamin B supplements. Although vitamin supplements reduced homocysteine levels, this did not have any significant effect on vascular risk [76–78] and a systematic review confirmed that there is insufficient evidence to determine whether treatment affecting homocysteine levels can prevent stroke recurrence [79]. The AHA/ASA guidelines advise that, although folate supplementation reduces levels of homocysteine and may be considered for patients with ischemic stroke and hyperhomocysteinemia, there is no evidence that reducing homocysteine levels prevents stroke recurrence [20].

6.5.10 Ischemic Stroke in the Context of Pregnancy Complications

There are a few specific complications of pregnancy that may cause stroke. Pre-eclampsia/eclampsia constitutes one of the highest risk situations for a cerebral event during pregnancy and the puerperium [7, 8, 21, 80–82].

Table 6.2 Recognized risk factors for hypertensive disorders of pregnancy

Obesity
Age (>40 years)
Chronic hypertension
Personal or family history of pre-eclampsia or gestational hypertension
Nulliparity
Multiple pregnancy
Pre-existing vascular disease
Collagen vascular disease
Diabetes mellitus
Renal disease

6.5.10.1 Pre-eclampsia and Eclampsia

Pre-eclampsia, a pregnancy-specific disorder, is clinically characterized by hypertension (blood pressure ≥140/90 mmHg, or if the diastolic blood pressure rises 15–25 mmHg above pre-pregnancy values) and proteinuria (≥300 mg in a 24 h urine collection) occurring after 20 weeks of gestation in a previously normotensive woman [83]. When seizures or coma develop in the context of pre-eclampsia, then it is known as eclampsia. Pre-eclampsia and eclampsia are most common during the third trimester or during labour, but can also occur after delivery, typically within the first 48 h [84]. The incidence of eclampsia in the UK is around one in 2,000 maternities, with a case fatality rate of 2 %, one of the commonest causes of maternal death in the UK [84]. In addition to the neurological features of headaches, seizures and confusion, patients may also have sudden onset focal neurological deficit consistent with stroke. The proportion of patients with pregnancy-associated stroke that have pre-eclampsia or eclampsia is between 25 and 45 % (Table 6.2) [19, 84].

Imaging may show arterial ischemic events or intracerebral hemorrhage. Intracerebral hemorrhage seems to be a poor prognostic feature; this is probably due to the fact that its occurrence is associated with more significant pre-eclampsia (i.e. higher blood pressure and greater endothelial damage) [19].

The differential diagnosis includes CVT, which is commoner in the postpartum period. A reversible posterior leucoencephalopathy (also known as reversible cerebral vasoconstriction syndrome, Call-Fleming syndrome or peripartum angiopathy) should also be considered. This is a cerebral dysregulation syndrome affecting large and medium sized cerebral arteries. It may produce a reversible posterior leucoencephalopathy, which can be associated with hemorrhagic or ischemic stroke. The clinical picture typically occurs in women aged 20–50, is usually one of abrupt onset with severe thunderclap headaches, seizures and focal neurological deficit [85]. The imaging findings may often be suggestive since white matter changes have a posterior emphasis and are usually not as extensive as in eclampsia. Diffusion weighted MR imaging may also be helpful in differentiation. The same condition has also been called post-partum cerebral angiopathy when it develops in the puerperium. Although there is likely to be an overlap with eclampsia in terms of pathogenesis, patients do not have proteinuria and may not be hypertensive. It seems that cerebral vessel vasoconstriction is a relevant mechanism in some but not all cases [19, 85].

It has been postulated that pre-eclampsia/eclampsia associated stroke may be mediated by genetic factors that predispose to both endothelial dysfunction and to a thrombophilic state. Similarly, pre-eclampsia/eclampsia associated hemorrhage may be associated with a disturbance of cerebral auto-regulation that is in part genetically determined. A more straightforward link of course is hypertension which predisposes to ischemia and hemorrhage [86]. The endothelial damage inherent in pre-eclampsia also increases the risk of thrombosis.

Treatment is aimed at first stabilising the woman's condition (lowering the blood pressure and giving magnesium to reduce the risk of eclampsia), followed by delivery of the baby, which is the definitive management of severe pre-eclampsia (Table 6.3). Management strategies include identification of those at high risk, optimization of antenatal care, early intervention and the detection and early management of complications. In the first instance, in mild to moderate pre-eclampsia, oral anti-hypertensive agents, including labetalol, nifedipine and methyldopa, should be tried. If oral anti-hypertensive agents fail to adequately control blood pressure, intravenous anti-hypertensives should be considered. Commonly used intravenous anti-hypertensives include labetalol and hydralazine [87]. In addition to anti-hypertensive agents, close attention should be given to regular clinical examination and monitoring of other vital signs, assessment of fluid balance and neurological status. Seizures should be treated with magnesium sulphate, which should also be used prophylactically in severe pre-eclampsia. Magnesium sulphate is given as a loading dose of 4 g by intravenous injection over 5–10 min, followed by a maintenance infusion of 1 g/h maintained for 24 h after delivery or the last seizure, whichever is later. Recurrent seizures should be treated with either a further bolus of 2 g magnesium sulphate or an increase in the infusion rate to 1.5 or 2.0 g/h [87].

Table 6.3 Clinical features of severe pre-eclampsia (in addition to hypertension and proteinuria)

Symptoms of severe headache
Liver tenderness
Visual disturbance
Platelet count falling to below 100 × 109/L
Epigastric pain and/or vomiting
Abnormal liver enzymes (ALT or AST rising to above 70 IU/L)
Signs of clonus
HELLP syndrome[a]
Papilledema

[a]Hemolysis, elevated liver enzymes, low platelet count

Guidance on the management of blood pressure in pre-eclampsia, as suggested by Royal College of Obstetricians and Gynaecologists' Green Top guideline [88] and NICE clinical guideline [87], is as follows:

Antihypertensive treatment should be started in women with a systolic blood pressure over 160 mmHg or a diastolic blood pressure over 110 mmHg.

In women with other markers of potentially severe disease, treatment can be considered at lower degrees of hypertension.

Labetalol given orally or intravenously, nifedipine given orally, or hydralazine given intravenously, can be used for the acute management of severe hypertension.

In moderate hypertension, treatment may assist prolongation of the pregnancy. Clinicians should use agents with which they are familiar.

Atenolol, angiotensin converting enzyme (ACE) inhibitors, angiotensin receptor-blocking drugs and diuretics should be avoided.

Nifedipine should be given orally, not sublingually. In order to avoid rapid hypotension which could lead to a reduction in uteroplacental perfusion and fetal compromise.

6.5.10.2 Other Pregnancy Complications Associated with Stroke

Amniotic fluid embolus is a rare and usually catastrophic syndrome associated with sudden cardiovascular collapse, disseminated intravascular coagulation and neurological impairment [89]. Stroke may occur secondary to venous or arterial events with rarely, paradoxical amniotic emboli causing cardio-embolic strokes. Choriocarcinoma is a malignant tumour of gestational trophoblasts. It frequently metastasises to lung and liver but also to the brain. The metastases are frequently hemorrhagic so this condition may present during pregnancy with an intracerebral or subarachnoid hemorrhage [90]. Furthermore, trophoblasts from metastatic brain lesions may invade cerebral vessels, leading to cerebral infarction. Choriocarcinoma normally occurs in the context of a molar pregnancy but may also follow an apparently normal birth, miscarriage or ectopic pregnancy.

6.6 Cerebral Venous and Sinus Thrombosis

CVT is a type of stroke caused by thrombus formation in one or more of the dural sinuses or cerebral veins, and manifesting primarily as headache [20]. Female predominance of CVT has been attributed to hormonal factors, mainly estrogen-containing oral contraceptives and pregnancy [91]. Most pregnancy-related CVT occurs in the third trimester or the puerperium and carries a fatality rate ranging from 4 to 36 % [8, 9, 91, 92]. In the majority of patients, symptoms develop within 3 weeks after delivery. The prothrombotic state of pregnancy is exacerbated after delivery by volume depletion and trauma related to delivery. Furthermore, additional risk factors such as infection and instrumental delivery or Ceesarean section can contribute further risk [93].

Approximately 2 % of strokes occurring during pregnancy can be attributed to venous thrombosis [8]. Dehydration may be an important and preventable additional risk factor, over and above the increased risk inherent in being pregnant. There is also a higher incidence of anemia in patients with CVT related to pregnancy compared with non-obstetric related cases [92]. A link between CVT and inherited heritable thrombophilia such as antithrombin deficiency, protein C deficiency, protein S deficiency and factor V Leiden [93], and also acquired thrombophilia (mainly APS) is relatively well established [94, 95]. Women with these conditions are therefore at potentially higher risk of developing CVT during pregnancy than those without thrombophilia. Lanska et al. reported that the risk of peripartum CVT increased with increasing maternal age, increasing hospital size and Cesarean section, and presence of hypertension, infections and excessive vomiting in pregnancy [9].

6.6.1 Diagnosis of Cerebral Venous and Sinus Thrombosis in Pregnancy

Typical presenting features of CVT include headache, disturbance of consciousness, focal neurological signs and seizures [19]. Papilledema has been reported in only around 50 % of cases and in this context is not a particularly reliable sign of raised intracranial pressure. Patients may present with headache and papilledema in isolation and be erroneously diagnosed as so-called ‘benign intracranial hypertension’. A very sudden onset headache at presentation may also occur and may be mistaken for a ruptured cerebral aneurysm. Involvement of cortical veins may lead to one or more areas of venous infarction, with or without hemorrhagic transformation. The presentation in such cases is often with localization related seizures and focal neurological deficit, depending on the territories involved. Deterioration in level of consciousness suggests either multiple lesions in the cerebral hemispheres, bilateral thalami or, more worryingly, transtentorial herniation and brainstem compression. A stroke-like presentation has been described as a manifestation of cortical vein thrombosis.

CVT should be seriously considered in any woman developing neurological symptoms in the immediate post-partum period, since up to 15 % of cases can occur within 2 days after uncomplicated childbirth. Cases can occur during pregnancy though these are much less common [19]. Despite the strong association with the post-partum state, it is still advisable that such patients have a thrombophilia screen to exclude any additional pro-thrombotic tendency such as APS.

The introduction of non-invasive brain imaging has resulted in a far greater recognition of intracranial venous thrombosis. Neuroradiological features include venous infarction, with or without hemorrhage. Brain CT imaging may show venous infarcts, with or without hemorrhage, that do not conform to an arterial distribution. Hyperdensity in the sagittal sinus on an unenhanced CT scan because of occlusion from fresh thrombus—the so-called delta sign—may be a useful clue. Similarly, the 'empty delta sign' may be seen in the same location after contrast has been given due to physiological enhancement in the wall of the sinus and absence of enhancement in the lumen due to the presence of thrombus [19]. MR studies may be useful in identifying CVT either with conventional studies, or with additional MR venography. MRI may also be useful in providing information about the interval from the time the thrombus began to form, although this is normally clear from the time of onset of symptoms. Although a catheter angiogram study with particular emphasis on the venous phase may be helpful in certain circumstances, it is worth noting that many normal individuals have hypoplasia and therefore non-filling of (more commonly) the left lateral sinus and occasionally absent anterior third of the superior sagittal sinus [19].

6.6.2 Treatment of Cerebral Venous and Sinus Thrombosis in Pregnancy

The mainstay of treatment of CVT is anticoagulation. A number of studies have suggested a significant improvement in survival following anticoagulation even in the presence of intracerebral hemorrhage [96, 97]. A Cochrane review based upon the limited available evidence found that anticoagulant treatment for CVT appeared to be safe and was associated with a potentially important reduction in the risk of death or dependency which did not reach statistical significance [98].

The European Federation of Neurological Societies (EFNS) [99] and the AHA/ASA guidelines [91] on the treatment of cerebral venous and sinus thrombosis in adults, recommend therapeutic dose subcutaneous LMWH or IV heparin for the treatment of CVT in patients without contraindications to anticoagulation. However, LMWH has superseded the use of unfractionated heparin in pregnancy because of safety concerns and convenience [18]. The EFNS and AHA/ASA also make the following points:

Patients with CVT without contraindications for anticoagulation should be treated either with body weight-adjusted subcutaneous LMWH or with dose-adjusted intravenous heparin (level B recommendation).

Concomitant intracranial hemorrhage (ICH) related to CVT is not a contraindication to heparin therapy.

The optimal duration of oral anticoagulant therapy after the acute phase is unclear. Oral anticoagulation may be given for:

- 3 months if CVT was secondary to a transient risk factor
- 6–12 months in patients with idiopathic CVT and in those with "mild" thrombophilia, such as heterozygous factor V Leiden or prothrombin G20210A mutation and high plasma levels of factor VIII
- Indefinite anticoagulation should be considered in patients with recurrent episodes of CVT and in those with one episode of CVT and 'severe' thrombophilia, such as antithrombin, protein C or protein S deficiency, homozygous factor V Leiden or prothrombin

G20210A mutation, antiphospholipid antibodies and combined abnormalities (good practice point).

There is insufficient evidence to support the use of either systemic or local thrombolysis in patients with CVT. If patients deteriorate despite adequate anticoagulation and other causes of deterioration have been ruled out, thrombolysis may be a therapeutic option in selected cases, possibly in those without large ICH and threatening herniation (good practice point).

There are no controlled data about the risks and benefits of certain therapeutic measures to reduce an elevated intracranial pressure (with brain displacement) in patients with severe CVT. However, in severe cases with impending herniation, craniotomy can be used as a life-saving intervention (good practice point).

Women with pregnancy-related CVT should be treated with therapeutic dose LMWH for the remainder of the pregnancy and for at least 6 weeks post-delivery. The decision regarding duration of anticoagulation should be made on an individualized basis, with a total duration of at least 6 months. The management of therapeutic dose LMWH around the time of delivery and postpartum anticoagulation is covered in Chap. 5. CVT is not a contraindication to future pregnancies, but these women should be treated with LMWH prophylaxis during pregnancy and the postpartum period.

6.7 Hemorrhagic Stroke

6.7.1 Risk of Hemorrhagic Stroke

Intracranial hemorrhage is the rarer of the two stroke subtypes but carries a greater morbidity and mortality for both the mother and the child. ICH has been estimated to account for 2–7 % of the total cases of neurological disorders related to pregnancy. Data on the frequency, risk factors, and outcomes of ICH in pregnant women are limited. However, the disease can greatly increase both maternal and perinatal morbidity and mortality, and hence merits attention. Hemorrhagic stroke occurs as a consequence of the rupture of a blood vessel, resulting in spread of blood into brain tissue [15]. The incidence varies from region to region, with the highest reported from China and Taiwan. The four most important etiological causes of ICH include pre-eclampsia/eclampsia, aneurysmal rupture, bleeding from arteriovenous malformations (AVM) and cortical venous thrombosis leading to ICH [100]. However, hypertensive disorders account for the majority of ICH seen in pregnancy, with eclampsia/pre-eclampsia accounting for 15–44 % of ICH in various series [7, 80, 101, 102]. In a large cohort study of 423 patients, Bateman et al. [2] reported that the risk of ICH associated with pregnancy is greatest in the postpartum period. Advanced maternal age, African American ethnic origin, hypertensive diseases, coagulopathy, and tobacco use were all independent risk factors for pregnancy-related ICH. Furthermore, this study reported a 10-fold increase in the odds of ICH with pre-eclampsia, a 2.6-fold increase in risk with pre-existing hypertension, and a 2.4-fold increase in risk with gestational hypertension.

6.7.2 Risk of Recurrent Hemorrhagic Stroke

The rate of recurrence of ICH in subsequent pregnancies depends on the underlying etiology [100]. Aneurysms, once secured, and AVMs once taken care of, do not recur. However, untreated lesions are prone to re-bleeding, irrespective of whether or not the patient becomes pregnant again. They should therefore be definitively treated.

6.7.3 Diagnosis of Hemorrhagic Stroke

A small but important contributor to ICH is CVT (see Sect. 6.6. above) that, although predominantly giving rise to ischemic lesions, may also lead to parenchymal hemorrhages. Presentation is usually with headaches or seizures, with or without focal deficits. Diagnosis requires brain imaging with computerized tomography or magnetic resonance imaging, and the necessity of investigation when this diagnosis is suspected supersedes the small risk of fetal malformation.

6.7.4 Management of Hemorrhagic Stroke in Pregnancy

The management of ICH in pregnancy is based on the general principles for management of this condition in the non-pregnant state. The blood pressure needs to be strictly monitored and agents used to control hypertension in pregnancy may differ from those used in the non-pregnant state due to potential teratogenic effects. For pre-eclampsia, early but safe delivery is the definitive treatment. Aneurysms and vascular malformations need to be definitively treated to prevent re-bleeding; this can be achieved through surgical or endovascular procedures. The timing of surgery depends on neurosurgical considerations. However, the timing and mode of delivery are governed by obstetric factors. The risk of future hemorrhage depends on whether the underlying etiology can be and has been definitively treated.

6.7.4.1 Arterio-venous Malformations

In women with a previously asymptomatic AVM, the risk of a hemorrhage occurring during pregnancy is approximately 3.5 % [103]. Pregnancy does not seem to increase the risk of first cerebral hemorrhage from an AVM. A study of 979 female patients with intracranial AVM admitted to Beijing Tiantan Hospital between 1960 and 2010 found that there was no increased risk of hemorrhage during pregnancy and the puerperium [104]. On the contrary, the odds ratio for rupture of AVM during pregnancy and puerperium, compared with the control period, was 0.71 (95 % confidence interval 0.61–0.82). For this reason it would seem reasonable to defer until after delivery treatment of an underlying AVM that has not previously bled. As regards methods of delivery in such patients, it makes sense to try to avoid a very strenuous and painful labour, both of which factors could lead to large surges in blood pressure and possible hemorrhage. Either elective Cesarean section or vaginal delivery with the use of epidural anesthesia to reduce pain, together with instrumental delivery if necessary to reduce pushing, is prudent [19].

In those patients who present with an ICH during pregnancy, the decision around interventional treatment is more difficult. Endovascular procedures are one potential treatment of intracranial AVM, and have a relatively low risk of mortality and morbidity. The fluoroscopy component of endovascular procedures presents a potential risk to the fetus from excessive radiation exposure. Lead shielding is considered an important method of decreasing the risk of fetal radiation exposure during fluoroscopy, and additional precautions such as decreasing the amount of beam angling, use of a collimator, and decreasing the duration of the fluoroscopy procedure should also be used to minimize risk during pregnancy [105, 106].

6.7.4.2 Subarachnoid Hemorrhage

Subarachnoid hemorrhage (SAH) is also an important contributor to pregnancy-related strokes. Most SAH are caused by aneurysmal rupture, although AVM, illicit drug abuse (in particular cocaine), and other rarer causes also have been described [100]. There are limited data to support the assumption that pregnancy increases the risk of aneurysmal SAH. A study from the Netherlands showed that the relative risk of aneurysmal SAH during pregnancy, delivery, or the puerperium was 0.4 [95 % confidence interval (CI), 0.2–0.9] when compared with non-pregnancy-related aneurysmal SAH [107]. No cases occurred during labor and delivery. This study therefore concluded that the risk of SAH is not increased during pregnancy, labor or the puerperium, and there is no need to advise against pregnancy in women with an increased risk of SAH and no evidence to advise against vaginal delivery in such women. Although epidural anesthesia is generally regarded as safe, there have been a few reports of intracranial or subarachnoid hemorrhage occurring following dural puncture. Presumably, prolonged low CSF pressure can lead to an increase in transmural pressure across an arterial wall, thus facilitating rupture of an aneurysm or AVM. For this reason, insertion of an epidural catheter in this context should be by an experienced operator to reduce the risk of a dural tap [19].

6.7.4.3 Other Causes of CNS Bleeding

Other more rare causes of CNS bleeding include septic aneurysm, arterial dissection, cerebral AVM, dural arteriovenous fistula and vascular lesions around the spinal cord. Pituitary apoplexy, a rare endocrine emergency that can occur due to hemorrhage and/or infarction of the pituitary gland, should also be considered, particularly if physical examination reveals a field defect, reduction of visual acuity or complex ophthalmoplegia. Pituitary apoplexy is often related to an underlying pituitary adenoma, and hemorrhagic infarction of a previously asymptomatic pituitary tumour may be precipitated by pregnancy. The UK Pituitary Apoplexy Guidelines Development Group under the auspices of the Society for Endocrinology has published guidelines on the management of this disorder [108].

6.8 Conclusion

Stroke, one of the most common causes of long-term disability and death, may result in a potentially devastating outcome for both mother and baby. Prompt recognition of symptoms and signs of stroke, and distinguishing between stroke due to cerebral ischemia and that due to hemorrhage, are key to success in the management of these patients. The management of ischemic stroke or hemorrhage during pregnancy and postpartum should be in centralized units with a multidisciplinary team, including neurology/neurosurgery, obstetric, hematology and rehabilitation services experienced in dealing with such conditions. Pre-eclampsia/eclampsia constitutes one of the highest risk situations for a cerebral event during pregnancy and the puerperium. Early recognition of the mother at risk of pre-eclampsia, optimization of antenatal care with institution of LDA, control of blood pressure, early intervention and the detection and early management of complications, followed by delivery of the baby, which is the definitive management of severe pre-eclampsia, are essential for improved outcomes.

6.9 Case Study

A 30-year-old woman presented with sudden onset left-sided weakness at 34 weeks' gestation in her first pregnancy. Prior to this she was well, with no significant medical history. She was a non-smoker, weight 67 kg, with no obvious risk factors for stroke. A brain CT scan showed a middle cerebral artery territory infarction. She was commenced on low dose aspirin and an urgent thrombophilia screen, including aPL antibodies, was done. She was found to be triple positive for aPL with high positive IgG anticardiolipin and anti beta 2 glycoprotein I antibodies. She was commenced on high intensity subcutaneous dalteparin 120 units/kg 12 hourly, with peak anti-Xa levels maintained at 1.0–1.2 IU/mL. The remainder of the thrombophilia screen was normal/negative. Her neurological symptoms gradually improved and she made a full recovery 3–4 weeks later. At 38 weeks gestation, she had a planned induction of labour (IOL). The last dose of daltaparin 100 units/kg was given the evening prior to the IOL. Epidural analgesia was administered as more than 24 h had elapsed since the last dose of dalteparin. She delivered a healthy female infant, birth weight 3.2 kg. Six hours after delivery, she was given dalteparin 5,000 units, and the following day commenced on split standard therapeutic dose dalteparin 100 units/kg 12 hourly. Warfarin was commenced on day 4 postpartum and the dalteparin overlapped with the warfarin until the INR was >2.5. The puerperium was uneventful. She was subsequently maintained on long-term warfarin, target INR 3.5 (range 3.0–4.0).

Key Learning Points

- Stroke is a neurological emergency and one of the most common causes of long-term disability and death.
- Although stroke is rare at a younger age, the normal physiological changes associated with pregnancy, combined with some pathophysiological processes unique to pregnancy, predispose women to develop stroke during pregnancy and the puerperium. Pre-eclampsia/eclampsia constitutes one of the highest risk situations for a cerebral event during pregnancy and the puerperium.

- Prompt recognition of symptoms and signs of stroke, and distinguishing whether the stroke is due to cerebral ischemia or hemorrhage, are key to successful management of these patients.
- The management of women who develop cerebrovascular disease during pregnancy and post-partum should be in centralized units with a multidisciplinary team, including neurology/neurosurgery, obstetric, hematology and rehabilitation services experienced in dealing with such conditions.
- MRI is safe in pregnancy so is the preferred option in pregnant women. MR contrast agents should not be routinely administered to pregnant patients and decisions about their use should be made on a case-by-case basis, based on assessment of the risk versus the benefit for the patient, by the attending consultant radiologist, neurologist and obstetrician.
- The treatment of acute arterial stroke in pregnancy is controversial. The use of thrombolytic therapy with recombinant tissue plasminogen activator in pregnancy is limited to case reports and series. It is listed as a category C drug and pregnancy is considered a relative contraindication for administration, but there are multiple case reports of successful use in pregnant women. The risks and benefits should be carefully considered, but it appears that thrombolytic therapy can be used both intravenously and intra-arterially in pregnancy with successful outcomes.
- The mainstay of treatment for cerebral venous and sinus thrombosis in pregnancy is therapeutic anticoagulation with LMWH. A number of studies have suggested a significant improvement in survival following anticoagulation even in the presence of intracerebral hemorrhage.

References

1. Hatano S. Experience from a multicentre stroke register: a preliminary report. Bull World Health Organ. 1976;54:541–53.
2. Bateman BT, Schumacher HC, Bushnell CD, Pile-Spellman J, Simpson LL, Sacco RL, et al. Intracerebral hemorrhage in pregnancy: frequency, risk factors, and outcome. Neurology. 2006;67:424–9.
3. Scott CA, Bewley S, Rudd A, Spark P, Kurinczuk JJ, Brocklehurst P, et al. Incidence, risk factors, management, and outcomes of stroke in pregnancy. Obstet Gynecol. 2012;120:318–24.
4. Tang CH, Wu CS, Lee TH, Hung ST, Yang CY, Lee CH, et al. Preeclampsia-eclampsia and the risk of stroke among peripartum in Taiwan. Stroke. 2009;40:1162–8.
5. Chang J, Elam-Evans LD, Berg CJ, Herndon J, Flowers L, Seed KA, et al. Pregnancy-related mortality surveillance–United States, 1991–1999. MMWR Surveill Summ. 2003;52:1–8.
6. Kittner SJ, Stern BJ, Feeser BR, Hebel R, Nagey DA, Buchholz DW, et al. Pregnancy and the risk of stroke. N Engl J Med. 1996;335:768–74.
7. Jaigobin C, Silver FL. Stroke and pregnancy. Stroke. 2000;31:2948–51.
8. James AH, Bushnell CD, Jamison MG, Myers ER. Incidence and risk factors for stroke in pregnancy and the puerperium. Obstet Gynecol. 2005;106:509–16.
9. Lanska DJ, Kryscio RJ. Risk factors for peripartum and postpartum stroke and intracranial venous thrombosis. Stroke. 2000;31:1274–82.
10. Salonen Ros H, Lichtenstein P, Bellocco R, Petersson G, Cnattingius S. Increased risks of circulatory diseases in late pregnancy and puerperium. Epidemiology. 2001;12:456–60.
11. Cantwell R, Clutton-Brock T, Cooper G, Dawson A, Drife J, Garrod D, et al. Saving mothers' lives: reviewing maternal deaths to make motherhood safer: 2006–2008. The Eighth Report of the Confidential Enquiries into Maternal Deaths in the United Kingdom. BJOG. 2011;118 Suppl 1:1–203.
12. Kamel H, Navi BB, Sriram N, Hovsepian DA, Devereux RB, Elkind MS. Risk of a thrombotic event after the 6-week postpartum period. N Engl J Med. 2014;370:1307–15.
13. Lamy C, Hamon JB, Coste J, Mas JL. Ischemic stroke in young women: risk of recurrence during subsequent pregnancies. French Study Group on Stroke in Pregnancy. Neurology. 2000;55:269–74.
14. Coppage KH, Hinton AC, Moldenhauer J, Kovilam O, Barton JR, Sibai BM. Maternal and perinatal outcome in women with a history of stroke. Am J Obstet Gynecol. 2004;190:1331–4.
15. Crovetto F, Somigliana E, Peguero A, Figueras F. Stroke during pregnancy and pre-eclampsia. Curr Opin Obstet Gynecol. 2013;25:425–32.

16. Kanal E, Barkovich AJ, Bell C, Borgstede JP, Bradley Jr WG, Froelich JW, et al. ACR guidance document on MR safe practices: 2013. J Magn Reson Imaging. 2013;37:501–30.
17. Board of the Faculty of Clinical Radiology. Standards for intravascular contrast administration to adult patients. 2nd ed. London: The Royal College of Radiologists; 2011. BFCR(10).4.
18. Patel SJ, Reede DL, Katz DS, Subramaniam R, Amorosa JK. Imaging the pregnant patient for non-obstetric conditions: algorithms and radiation dose considerations. Radiographics. 2007;27:1705–22.
19. Davie CA, O'Brien P. Stroke and pregnancy. J Neurol Neurosurg Psychiatry. 2008;79:240–5.
20. Bushnell C, McCullough LD, Awad IA, Chireau MV, Fedder WN, Furie KL, et al. Guidelines for the prevention of stroke in women: a statement for healthcare professionals from the american heart association/american stroke association. Stroke. 2014;45:1545–88.
21. Treadwell SD, Thanvi B, Robinson TG. Stroke in pregnancy and the puerperium. Postgrad Med J. 2008;84:238–45.
22. Kernan WN, Ovbiagele B, Black HR, Bravata DM, Chimowitz MI, Ezekowitz MD, et al. Guidelines for the prevention of stroke in patients with stroke and transient ischemic attack: a guideline for healthcare professionals from the American Heart Association/American Stroke Association. Stroke. 2014;45:2160–236.
23. Bushnell CD, Jamison M, James AH. Migraines during pregnancy linked to stroke and vascular diseases: US population based case–control study. BMJ. 2009;338:b664.
24. Tissue plasminogen activator for acute ischemic stroke. The National Institute of Neurological Disorders and Stroke rt-PA Stroke Study Group. N Engl J Med. 1995;333:1581–7.
25. Furlan A, Higashida R, Wechsler L, Gent M, Rowley H, Kase C, et al. Intra-arterial prourokinase for acute ischemic stroke. The PROACT II study: a randomized controlled trial. Prolyse in Acute Cerebral Thromboembolism. JAMA. 1999;282:2003–11.
26. Tate J, Bushnell C. Pregnancy and stroke risk in women. Womens Health (Lond Engl). 2011;7:363–74.
27. De KJ, Gdovinova Z, Uyttenboogaart M, Vroomen PC, Luijckx GJ. Intravenous alteplase for stroke: beyond the guidelines and in particular clinical situations. Stroke. 2007;38:2612–8.
28. Electronic Medicines Compendium eMC. Datapharm Communications, London. Actilyse. Summary of product characteristics (SPC). Boehringer Ingelheim: Bracknell, West Berkshire. Last updated on 13 Oct 2013. http://www.medicines.org.uk/emc/. Accessed 31 Oct 2014.
29. Lansberg MG, O'Donnell MJ, Khatri P, et al. Antithrombotic and thrombolytic therapy for ischemic stroke: antithrombotic therapy and prevention of thrombosis, 9th ed: American College of Chest Physicians Evidence-Based Clinical Practice Guidelines. Chest 2012;141:e601S–e36S.
30. National Institute for Health and Care Excellence (NICE). Stroke and TIA Clinical knowledge summaries. 2013. http://cks.nice.org.uk/stroke-and-tia. Accessed 30 Oct 2014.
31. Cuthill JA, Young S, Greer IA, Oldroyd K. Anaesthetic considerations in a parturient with critical coronary artery disease and a drug-eluting stent presenting for caesarean section. Int J Obstet Anesth. 2005;14:167–71.
32. Klinzing P, Markert UR, Liesaus KF, Peiker G. Case report: successful pregnancy and delivery after myocardial infarction and essential thrombocythemia treated with clopidrogel. Clin Exp Obstet Gynecol. 2001;28:215–6.
33. Taguchi K. Pregnancy in patients with a prosthetic heart valve. Surg Gynecol Obstet. 1977;145:206–8.
34. Kusters DM, Hassani Lahsinoui H, van de Post JA, Wiegman A, Wijburg FA, Kastelein JJ, Hutten BA. Statin use during pregnancy: a systematic review and meta-analysis. Expert Rev Cardiovasc Ther. 2012;10:363–78.
35. Lockshin MD, Pierangeli SS. Statins for the treatment of obstetric complications in antiphospholipid syndrome? J Reprod Immunol. 2010;84:206; author reply 206–7.
36. Electronic Medicines Compendium eMC. Datapharm Communications, London. Simvastatin 10mg tablets -summary product characteristics (SPC) https://www.medicines.org.uk/emc/medicine/. Accessed 31 Oct 2014.
37. Meissner I, Khandheria BK, Heit JA, Petty GW, Sheps SG, Schwartz GL, et al. Patent foramen ovale: innocent or guilty? Evidence from a prospective population-based study. J Am Coll Cardiol. 2006;47:440–5.
38. Petty GW, Khandheria BK, Meissner I, Whisnant JP, Rocca WA, Christianson TJ, et al. Population-based study of the relationship between patent foramen ovale and cerebrovascular ischemic events. Mayo Clin Proc. 2006;81:602–8.
39. Overell JR, Bone I, Lees KR. Interatrial septal abnormalities and stroke: a meta-analysis of case–control studies. Neurology. 2000;55:1172–9.
40. Keeling D, Mackie I, Moore GW, Greer IA, Greaves M. Guidelines on the investigation and management of antiphospholipid syndrome. Br J Haematol. 2012;157:47–58.
41. Andreoli L, Chighizola CB, Banzato A, Pons-Estel GJ, de Jesus GR, Erkan D. The estimated frequency of antiphospholipid antibodies in patients with pregnancy morbidity, stroke, myocardial infarction, and deep vein thrombosis. Arthritis Care Res (Hoboken). 2013;65:1869–73.
42. Arachchillage DR, Machin SJ, Cohen H. Antithrombotic treatment for stroke associated with antiphospholipid antibodies. Expert Rev Hematol. 2014;7:169–72.

43. Ruiz-Irastorza G, Hunt BJ, Khamashta MA. A systematic review of secondary thromboprophylaxis in patients with antiphospholipid antibodies. Arthritis Rheum. 2007;57:1487–95.
44. Pengo V, Ruffatti A, Legnani C, Gresele P, Barcellona D, Erba N, et al. Clinical course of high-risk patients diagnosed with antiphospholipid syndrome. J Thromb Haemost. 2010;8:237–42.
45. Langevitz P, Livneh AF, Dulitzki MF, Pauzner RF, Many AF, Soriano DF, Pras M. Outcome of pregnancy in three patients with primary antiphospholipid syndrome after stroke. Semin Arthritis Rheum. 1998;28:26–30.
46. Stone S, Hunt BJ, Khamashta MA, Bewley SJ, Nelson-Piercy C. Primary antiphospholipid syndrome in pregnancy: an analysis of outcome in a cohort of 33 women treated with a rigorous protocol. J Thromb Haemost. 2005;3:243–5.
47. Fischer-Betz R, Specker CF, Brinks RF, Schneider M. Pregnancy outcome in patients with antiphospholipid syndrome after cerebral ischaemic events: an observational study. Lupus. 2012;21:1183–9.
48. Ruiz-Irastorza G, Cuadrado MJ, Ruiz-Arruza I, Brey R, Crowther M, Derksen R, Erkan D, Krilis S, Machin S, Pengo V, Pierangeli S, Tektonidou M, Khamashta M. Evidence-based recommendations for the prevention and long-term management of thrombosis in antiphospholipid antibody-positive patients: report of a task force at the 13th International Congress on antiphospholipid antibodies. Lupus 2011;20:206–18.
49. Erkan D, Vega J, Ramón G, Kozora E, Lockshin MD. A pilot open-label phase II trial of rituximab for non-criteria manifestations of antiphospholipid syndrome. Arthritis Rheum. 2013;65(2):464–71.
50. Ridolfi RL, Bell WR. Thrombotic thrombocytopenic purpura. Report of 25 cases and review of the literature. Medicine (Baltimore). 1981;60:413–28.
51. Scully M, Yarranton H, Liesner R, Cavenagh J, Hunt B, Benjamin S, et al. Regional UK TTP registry: correlation with laboratory ADAMTS 13 analysis and clinical features. Br J Haematol. 2008;142:819–26.
52. Vesely SK, Li X, McMinn JR, Terrell DR, George JN. Pregnancy outcomes after recovery from thrombotic thrombocytopenic purpura-hemolytic uremic syndrome. Transfusion. 2004;44:1149–58.
53. Scully M, Hunt BJ, Benjamin S, Liesner R, Rose P, Peyvandi F, et al. Guidelines on the diagnosis and management of thrombotic thrombocytopenic purpura and other thrombotic microangiopathies. Br J Haematol. 2012;158:323–35.
54. Cushman M, Rosendaal FR, Psaty BM, Cook EF, Valliere J, Kuller LH, Tracy RP. Factor V Leiden is not a risk factor for arterial vascular disease in the elderly: results from the Cardiovascular Health Study. Thromb Haemost. 1998;79:912–5.
55. Feinberg WM, Pearce LA, Hart RG, Cushman M, Cornell ES, Lip GY, Bovill EG. Markers of thrombin and platelet activity in patients with atrial fibrillation: correlation with stroke among 1531 participants in the stroke prevention in atrial fibrillation III study. Stroke. 1999;30:2547–53.
56. Juul K, Tybjaerg-Hansen A, Steffensen R, Kofoed S, Jensen G, Nordestgaard BG. Factor V Leiden: The Copenhagen City Heart Study and 2 meta-analyses. Blood. 2002;100:3–10.
57. Ridker PM, Hennekens CH, Lindpaintner K, Stampfer MJ, Eisenberg PR, Miletich JP. Mutation in the gene coding for coagulation factor V and the risk of myocardial infarction, stroke, and venous thrombosis in apparently healthy men. N Engl J Med. 1995;332:912–7.
58. Ridker PM, Hennekens CHFAU, Miletich JP. G20210A mutation in prothrombin gene and risk of myocardial infarction, stroke, and venous thrombosis in a large cohort of US men. Circulation. 1999;99:999–1004.
59. Casas JP, Hingorani AD, Bautista LE, Sharma P. Meta-analysis of genetic studies in ischemic stroke: thirty-two genes involving approximately 18,000 cases and 58,000 controls. Arch Neurol. 2004;61:1652–61.
60. Kim RJ, Becker RC. Association between factor V Leiden, prothrombin G20210A, and methylenetetrahydrofolate reductase C677T mutations and events of the arterial circulatory system: a meta-analysis of published studies. Am Heart J. 2003;146:948–57.
61. Boulet SL, Okoroh EM, Azonobi I, Grant A, Hooper CH. Sickle cell disease in pregnancy: maternal complications in a Medicaid-enrolled population. Matern Child Health J. 2013;17:200–7.
62. Kissela B, Schneider AF, Kleindorfer DF, Khoury JF, Miller RF, Alwell KF, et al. Stroke in a biracial population: the excess burden of stroke among blacks. Stroke. 2004;35:426–31.
63. Ohene-Frempong K, Weiner SJ, Sleeper LA, Miller ST, Embury S, Moohr JW, et al. Cerebrovascular accidents in sickle cell disease: rates and risk factors. Blood. 1998;91:288–94.
64. Pegelow CH, Colangelo L, Steinberg M, Wright EC, Smith J, Phillips G, Vichinsky E. Natural history of blood pressure in sickle cell disease: risks for stroke and death associated with relative hypertension in sickle cell anemia. Am J Med. 1997;102:171–7.
65. Powars DF, Wilson BF, Imbus CF, Pegelow CF, Allen J. The natural history of stroke in sickle cell disease. Am J Med. 1978;65(3):461–71.
66. Passamonti F, Rumi E, Pungolino E, Malabarba L, Bertazzoni P, Valentini M, et al. Life expectancy and prognostic factors for survival in patients with polycythemia vera and essential thrombocythemia. Am J Med. 2004;117:755–61.
67. Harrison CN, Bareford D, Butt N, Campbell P, Conneally E, Drummond M, et al. British Committee for Standards in Haematology Guideline for investigation and management of adults and children presenting with a thrombocytosis. Br J Haematol. 2010;149:352–75.

68. McMullin MF, Bareford D, Campbell P, Green AR, Harrison C, Hunt B, et al.; General Haematology Task Force of the British Committee for Standards in Haematology. Guidelines for the diagnosis, investigation and management of polycythaemia/erythrocytosis. Br J Haematol. 2005;130:174–95.
69. Hillmen P, Richards SJ. Implications of recent insights into the pathophysiology of paroxysmal nocturnal haemoglobinuria. Br J Haematol. 2000;108:470–9.
70. Hall C, Richards S, Hillmen P. Primary prophylaxis with warfarin prevents thrombosis in paroxysmal nocturnal hemoglobinuria (PNH). Blood. 2003;102: 3587–91.
71. Socié G, Mary JY, de Gramont A, Rio B, Leporrier M, Rose C, et al. Paroxysmal nocturnal haemoglobinuria: long-term follow-up and prognostic factors. French Society of Haematology. Lancet. 1996;348:573–7.
72. Tiu R, Yacoub HF, Maciejewski JF, Sila CA. Recurrent ischemic stroke in paroxysmal nocturnal hemoglobinuria: paroxysmal nocturnal hemoglobinuria or missed patent foramen ovale? J Stroke Cerebrovasc Dis. 2009;18:409–10.
73. Petras M, Tatarkova ZF, Kovalska MF, Mokra DF, Dobrota DF, Lehotsky JF, Drgova A. Hyperhomocysteinemia as a risk factor for the neuronal system disorders. J Physiol Pharmacol. 2014;65:15–23.
74. Martí-Carvajal AJ, Solà I, Lathyris D, Salanti G. Homocysteine lowering interventions for preventing cardiovascular events. Cochrane Database Syst Rev. 2009;(4):CD006612.
75. Casas JP, Bautista LE, Smeeth L, Sharma P, Hingorani AD. Homocysteine and stroke: evidence on a causal link from mendelian randomisation. Lancet. 2005;365:224–32.
76. Bønaa KH, Njølstad I, Ueland PM, Schirmer H, Tverdal A, Steigen T, et al.; NORVIT Trial Investigators. Homocysteine lowering and cardiovascular events after acute myocardial infarction. N Engl J Med. 2006;354:1578–8.
77. Lonn E, Yusuf S, Arnold MJ, Sheridan P, Pogue J, Micks M, et al.; Heart Outcomes Prevention Evaluation (HOPE) 2 Investigators. Homocysteine lowering with folic acid and B vitamins in vascular disease. N Engl J Med. 2006;354:1567–77.
78. Toole JF, Malinow MR, Chambless LE, Spence JD, Pettigrew LC, Howard VJ, et al. Lowering homocysteine in patients with ischemic stroke to prevent recurrent stroke, myocardial infarction, and death: the Vitamin Intervention for Stroke Prevention (VISP) randomized controlled trial. JAMA. 2004;291(5):565–75.
79. Martí-Carvajal AJ, Solà I, Lathyris D, Karakitsiou DE, Simancas-Racines D. Homocysteine-lowering interventions for preventing cardiovascular events. Cochrane Database Syst Rev. 2013;(4):CD006612.
80. Jeng JS, Tang SC, Yip PK. Stroke in women of reproductive age: comparison between stroke related and unrelated to pregnancy. J Neurol Sci. 2004;221:25–9.
81. Martin Jr JN, Thigpen BD, Moore RC, Rose CH, Cushman J, May W. Stroke and severe preeclampsia and eclampsia: a paradigm shift focusing on systolic blood pressure. Obstet Gynecol. 2005;105:246–54.
82. Wilson BJ, Watson MS, Prescott GJ, Sunderland S, Campbell DM, Hannaford P, et al. Hypertensive diseases of pregnancy and risk of hypertension and stroke in later life: results from cohort study. BMJ. 2003;326:845.
83. Mortimer AM, Bradley MD, Likeman M, Stoodley NG, Renowden SA. Cranial neuroimaging in pregnancy and the post-partum period. Clin Radiol. 2013;68:500–8.
84. Sawle GV, Ramsay MM. The neurology of pregnancy. J Neurol Neurosurg Psychiatry. 1998;64:711–25.
85. Katz BS, Fugate JE, Ameriso SF, Pujol-Lereis VA, Mandrekar J, Flemming KD, et al. Clinical worsening in reversible cerebral vasoconstriction syndrome. JAMA Neurol. 2014;71:68–73.
86. Easton JD. Severe preeclampsia/eclampsia: hypertensive encephalopathy of pregnancy? Cerebrovasc Dis. 1998;8:53–8.
87. National Institute for Health and Care Excellence (NICE). NICE clinical guideline 107. Hypertension in pregnancy: the management of hypertensive disorders during pregnancy. 2010. https://www.nice.org.uk/guidance/CG107. Accessed 31 Oct 2014.
88. RCOG Greentop guidelines. Severe pre-eclampsia/eclampsia, guideline. Guideline no. 10A. London: Royal College of Obstetricians and Gynaecologists. 2006. http://www.rcog.org.uk/guidelines.
89. Kumar S, Wong G, Maysky M, Shulman M, Olenchock S, Falzon-Kirby M, et al. Amniotic fluid embolism complicated by paradoxical embolism and disseminated intravascular coagulation. Am J Crit Care. 2010;19:379–82.
90. Huang CY, Chen CA, Hsieh CY, Cheng WF. Intracerebral hemorrhage as initial presentation of gestational choriocarcinoma: a case report and literature review. Int J Gynecol Cancer. 2007;17:1166–71.
91. Canhão P, Ferro JM, Lindgren AG, Bousser MG, Stam J, Barinagarrementeria F, ISCVT Investigators. Causes and predictors of death in cerebral venous thrombosis. Stroke. 2005;36:1720–5.
92. Cantu C, Barinagarrementeria F. Cerebral venous thrombosis associated with pregnancy and puerperium. Review of 67 cases. Stroke. 1993;24:1880–4.
93. Saposnik G, Barinagarrementeria F, Brown RD Jr, Bushnell CD, Cucchiara B, Cushman M, et al.; American Heart Association Stroke Council and the Council on Epidemiology and Prevention. Diagnosis and management of cerebral venous thrombosis: a statement for healthcare professionals from the American Heart Association/American Stroke Association. Stroke. 2011;42:1158–92.
94. Bousser MG, Ferro JM. Cerebral venous thrombosis: an update. Lancet Neurol. 2007;6:162–70.

95. Star M, Flaster M. Advances and controversies in the management of cerebral venous thrombosis. Neurol Clin. 2013;31:765–83.
96. Einhäupl KM, Villringer A, Meister W, Mehraein S, Garner C, Pellkofer M, et al. Heparin treatment in sinus venous thrombosis. Lancet. 1991;338:597–600.
97. Fink JN, McAuley DL. Safety of anticoagulation for cerebral venous thrombosis associated with intracerebral hematoma. Neurology. 2001;57:1138–9.
98. Coutinho J, de Bruijn SF, Deveber G, Stam J. Anticoagulation for cerebral venous sinus thrombosis. Cochrane Database Syst Rev. 2011;(8): CD002005.
99. Einhäupl K, Stam J, Bousser MG, De Bruijn SF, Ferro JM, Martinelli I, Masuhr F, European Federation of Neurological Societies. EFNS guideline on the treatment of cerebral venous and sinus thrombosis in adult patients. Eur J Neurol. 2010;17:1229–35.
100. Khan M, Wasay M. Haemorrhagic strokes in pregnancy and puerperium. Int J Stroke. 2013;8:265–72.
101. Liang CC, Chang SD, Lai SL, Hsieh CC, Chueh HY, Lee TH. Stroke complicating pregnancy and the puerperium. Eur J Neurol. 2006;13:1256–60.
102. Mas JL, Lamy C. Stroke in pregnancy and the puerperium. J Neurol. 1998;245:305–13.
103. Horton JC, Chambers WA, Lyons SL, Adams RD, Kjellberg RN. Pregnancy and the risk of hemorrhage from cerebral arteriovenous malformations. Neurosurgery. 1990;27:867–71; discussion 871–2.
104. Liu XJ, Wang S, Zhao YL, Teo M, Guo P, Zhang D, et al. Risk of cerebral arteriovenous malformation rupture during pregnancy and puerperium. Neurology. 2014;82:1798–803.
105. Agarwal N, Guerra JC, Gala NB, Agarwal P, Zouzias A, Gandhi CD, et al. Current treatment options for cerebral arteriovenous malformations in pregnancy: a review of the literature. World Neurosurg. 2014;81:83–90.
106. Shaw P, Duncan A, Vouyouka A, Ozsvath K. Radiation exposure and pregnancy. J Vasc Surg. 2011;53(1 Suppl):28S–34.
107. Tiel Groenestege AT, Rinkel GJ, van der Bom JG, Algra A, Klijn CJ. The risk of aneurysmal subarachnoid hemorrhage during pregnancy, delivery, and the puerperium in the Utrecht population: case-crossover study and standardized incidence ratio estimation. Stroke. 2009;40:1148–51.
108. Rajasekaran S, Vanderpump M, Baldeweg S, Drake W, Reddy N, Lanyon M, et al. UK guidelines for the management of pituitary apoplexy. Clin Endocrinol (Oxf). 2011;74:9–20.

Pregnancy Morbidity Associated with Thrombophilias: Recurrent Miscarriage

7

Raj Rai and Lesley Regan

Abstract

Components of the haemostatic pathways play a key role in the establishment and maintenance of pregnancy. Pregnancy itself is a hypercoaguable state. An exaggerated haemostatic response is associated with an increased risk not only for recurrent miscarriage but for adverse pregnancy outcome at all gestational stages. Antiphospholipid antibodies (aPL) are the most important treatable cause for recurrent miscarriage. Recent advances have allowed us to escape from the restrictive concept of pregnancy loss being purely related to thrombosis to now emphasising the role of these antibodies in decidualisation of the endometrium and in trophoblast biology. Concurrently emphasis is now placed on the potential for the non-anticoagulant effects of heparin to improve pregnancy in those with a thrombophilic defect.

Keywords

Recurrent miscarriage • Obstetric antiphospholipid syndrome • Heritable thrombophilias • Thromboelastography

7.1 Background

Miscarriage, the loss of a pregnancy before viability, is the commonest complication of pregnancy. The term therefore includes all pregnancy losses from the time of conception, which is shortly after ovulation, until 24 weeks of gestation [1]. Although 15 % of clinically recognized pregnancies miscarry, total reproductive losses are closer to 50 %. The vast majority of miscarriages occur early in pregnancy, before 10 weeks gestation. The incidence of late- or second-trimester pregnancy loss, between 10 and 24 weeks of gestation, is no more than 2 % [2].

R. Rai, MB ChB, MD, MRCOG (✉)
Department of Obstetrics and Gynaecology, Imperial College Healthcare NHS Trust, St Mary's Hospital, Mint Wing, Imperial College Hospitals NHS Trust, South Wharf Road, London W2 1PL, UK
e-mail: r.rai@imperial.ac.uk

L. Regan, MB ChB, MD, FRCOG
Department of Obstetrics and Gynaecology, Imperial College Healthcare NHS Trust, St Mary's Hospital, Mint Wing, South Wharf Road, London W2 1NY, UK
e-mail: l.regan@imperial.ac.uk

H. Cohen, P. O'Brien (eds.), *Disorders of Thrombosis and Hemostasis in Pregnancy: A Guide to Management*, DOI 10.1007/978-3-319-15120-5_7, © Springer-Verlag London 2015

Miscarriage may be divided into two types – sporadic and recurrent. Approximately 25 % of all couples will experience a single sporadic miscarriage. The most common cause of such miscarriages is a random fetal chromosome abnormality, the incidence of which increases with advancing maternal age. In contrast, only 1–2 % of couples will be diagnosed with recurrent miscarriages, the accepted definition of which is the loss of three or more consecutive pregnancies. Three strands of evidence suggest that recurrent miscarriage is a distinct clinical problem rather than one which occurs by chance alone: (a) the observed incidence is significantly higher than that expected by chance alone (0.3 %), (b) a woman's risk of miscarriage is directly related to the outcome of her previous pregnancies – the risk of miscarriage increasing with the number of previous miscarriages she has experienced, and (c) women with recurrent miscarriage tend to lose chromosomally normal rather than abnormal pregnancies [1].

Recurrent miscarriage is associated with significant psychological sequelae for both women and their partners and considerable economic cost for the state. Among the 6,000 new couples/year diagnosed with recurrent miscarriage in the UK, pronounced emotional responses, such as anxiety, depression, denial, anger, marital disruption, and a sense of loss and inadequacy, are common [3]. While the financial burden to the UK health service is in the region of £30 million/year, this does not include the much larger cost of treatment of depressive illness and of lost productivity.

7.1.1 Recurrent Miscarriage: A Defect in the Hemostatic Response?

In preparation for pregnancy, the uterine endometrium undergoes a process of "decidualization" in which the endometrium becomes receptive to implantation of an embryo. The processes of implantation of the embryo into the uterine decidua and subsequent formation of the placenta are key events in pregnancy. Defects in this process underlie adverse pregnancy outcome at all gestational ages. Implantation of the embryo can be divided into three stages – apposition of the embryo with the uterine decidua, adhesion of the embryo to the decidua, and finally invasion of primitive placental cells (trophoblast) through the decidua into the maternal uterine spiral arteries which lie within the myometrium (Fig. 7.1). Subsequent formation of the placenta in humans is termed "hemochorial placentation," as the placenta is in contact with the maternal blood supply. Components of both the coagulation and the fibrinolytic pathways are intimately involved in these processes.

Pregnancy itself is a prothrombotic state – characterized by an increase in the levels of procoagulant factors, a simultaneous decrease in the levels of anticoagulant proteins, and activation of fibrinolysis [4–6]. The evolutionary advantage of this is thought to counteract the inherent instability of hemochorial placentation. Over the last 20 years, the hypothesis has been developed that many cases of recurrent miscarriage are due to an

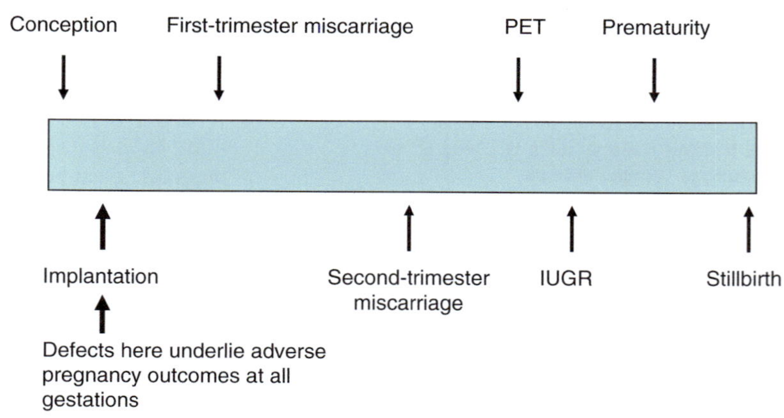

Fig. 7.1 Implantation spectrum

abnormal or exaggerated hemostatic response in pregnancy [7]. This hypothesis is supported by data reporting increased markers of thrombin generation among women with recurrent miscarriage outside of pregnancy [7, 8], an increased prevalence of coagulation defects among women with recurrent miscarriage [9–11], and histological evidence of placental thrombosis in some cases of recurrent miscarriage [12, 13].

Remarkably few studies have reported the placental histological findings among the pregnancies of women with recurrent miscarriage. Nayar and Lage [14] were the first to reported massive infarction in the first-trimester placenta from a pregnancy of a woman with antiphospholipid antibodies (aPL) and recurrent miscarriage. Our own unit reported a significantly increased prevalence of placental infarction among the pregnancies of women with recurrent miscarriage (10 %), irrespective of the presence of aPL, versus 1 % using the same criteria to assess infarction, among those with a previously uncomplicated reproductive history [12].

This chapter examines the role of thrombophilic defects – both heritable and acquired – in the pathogenesis of recurrent miscarriage.

Box 7.1: Pregnancy Morbidity Associated with Antiphospholipid Syndrome

One or more unexplained deaths of a morphologically healthy fetus at or beyond the 10th week of gestation, with healthy fetal morphology documented by ultrasound or by direct examination of the fetus

One or more premature births of a morphologically healthy newborn baby before the 34th week of gestation because of eclampsia or severe preeclampsia defined according to standard definitions or recognized features of placental failure

Three or more unexplained consecutive spontaneous abortions before the 10th week of gestation, with maternal anatomical or hormonal abnormalities and paternal and maternal chromosomal causes excluded

7.2 Antiphospholipid Syndrome

7.2.1 Introduction

Antiphospholipid syndrome (APS) is the most important treatable cause of recurrent miscarriage. Antiphospholipid antibodies are also associated with adverse pregnancy outcome at later gestational ages including preeclampsia and preterm delivery (Box 7.1). In relation to adverse pregnancy outcome, lupus anticoagulant and anticardiolipin antibodies (aCL; both IgG and IgM) together with anti-beta 2 glycoprotein I (aβ2GPI) antibodies appear to be the most important members of the family of aPL. In accordance with the revised Sapporo (Sydney) International consensus criteria [15], a diagnosis of obstetric antiphospholipid syndrome demands the presence of one of the defining criteria listed in Box 7.1 together with persistently positive tests for one or more of lupus anticoagulant, aCL and aβ2GPI.

7.2.2 Prevalence

Approximately 15 % of women with recurrent miscarriage have obstetric APS [10, 16]. In contrast, the prevalence of aPL in women with a "low-risk" obstetric history is less than 2 % [17, 18]. The largest prevalence study (500 consecutive women with recurrent miscarriage attending a specialist recurrent miscarriage clinic) reported the prevalence of persistently positive tests for lupus anticoagulant to be 9.6 %, IgG aCL 3.3 %, and IgM aCL 2.2 %. Importantly, among the miscarriage population there appears to be little crossover between lupus anticoagulant and aCL positivity and a large number of women have only transiently positive tests (66 % lupus anticoagulant and 37 % for either IgG or IgM aCL).

7.2.3 Outcome of Untreated Pregnancies

The outcome of pregnancy in untreated women with aPL and a history of recurrent miscarriage is poor. The earliest studies reported that the fetal loss rate in women with APS was in the range of 50–70 % [17, 19]. It was subsequently realized that these figures underestimated the scale of the problem because recruitment only took place after these women had presented for antenatal care (at approximately 12 weeks) by which time the majority of miscarriages have already occurred. A prospective observational study in which women with APS were identified prior to pregnancy and followed from the time of a positive pregnancy test reported the miscarriage rate to be 90 % with no pharmacological treatment [10, 16]. In contrast, the miscarriage rate among a control group of aPL-negative women with recurrent miscarriage was significantly lower – in the region of 40 %. In untreated pregnancies, women with APS are also at significant increased risk for later pregnancy complications. In a population-based analysis of 141,286 deliveries in Florida, USA, positivity for aPL increased the risk for both preeclampsia and placental insufficiency (adjusted odds ratio 2.93 [95 % CI 1.51–5.61] and 4.58 [2.0–10.5]), respectively [20].

7.2.4 Mechanisms of aPL Pregnancy Loss

Pregnancy loss associated with aPL has traditionally been attributed to thrombosis of the placental vasculature [21–23]. However, thrombosis is neither a universal nor a specific feature in antiphospholipid-associated miscarriages [23]. Advances in our understanding of early pregnancy development and phospholipid biology have highlighted alternative mechanisms of action of these antibodies in the pathogenesis of pregnancy loss.

In vitro studies demonstrate that aPL have a direct deleterious effect on implantation by affecting both the function of the uterine decidua and of the trophoblast. Antiphospholipid antibodies (a) impair signal transduction mechanisms controlling endometrial cell decidualization and impair endometrial angio-genesis [24, 25], (b) increase trophoblast apoptosis [26], and (c) decrease trophoblast fusion and impair trophoblast invasion [26, 27]. Interestingly, the effects of aPL on trophoblast function are reversed, at least in vitro, by low molecular weight heparin (LMWH) [26–28].

More recently, attention has focused on the role of complement activation in aPL related pregnancy loss. Injection of aPL into pregnant mice results in antibody and C3 deposition in the decidua, along with focal necrosis and apoptosis and neutrophil infiltration [29]. These effects are accompanied by a fourfold increase in the frequency of fetal resorption; fetal loss can be reversed by simultaneous treatment with soluble recombinant complement receptor 1-related gene/protein y (Crry), which also prevents C3 deposition and neutrophil infiltration. Finally, a causative role for complement activation was shown conclusively by injecting aPL antibodies into C3-deficient mice, which became resistant to aPL antibody-mediated fetal loss. To reevaluate the link between aPL and thrombosis, the authors showed that aPL induce thrombus formation following local vascular injury and that soluble Crry significantly decreases the size of the thrombi. Thus, complement activation is likely to be an important upstream mediator in both aPL IgG-induced vascular thrombosis and fetal loss.

7.2.5 Management of Recurrent Miscarriage Associated with aPL

The management of women with APS depends on comprehensive investigation prior to pregnancy, definition of the management plan and counseling regarding (a) the live birth rate with treatment; (b) treatment not preventing the loss of a genetically abnormal pregnancy; (c) the increased risk of later pregnancy complications such as preeclampsia and placental insufficiency necessitating preterm delivery; (d) risks of an APS-related complications in the neonate; and (e) increased risk to the mother herself during pregnancy and postpartum and the need for thromboprophylaxis.

7.2.5.1 Treatment of Obstetric Antiphospholipid Syndrome

Over the last 25 years, a variety of pharmaceutical agents have been used, either individually or in combination, in attempts to improve the pregnancy outcome of women with obstetric

APS. Low-dose aspirin (LDA) in combination with heparin remains the mainstay of treatment, as confirmed in two meta-analyses [25, 30]. This treatment combination leads to a live birth rate of over 70 % [31, 32].

Two prospective randomized controlled trials [31, 32] and one where women were alternately assigned to treatment have reported that LDA and unfractionated heparin (UFH) improve the live birth rate in women with APS when compared to aspirin alone [33]. In the trial reported by Rai et al. [34], 90 women were randomized at the time of a positive urinary pregnancy test to receive either LDA or LDA and heparin daily until the time of miscarriage or 34 weeks gestation. The live birth rate with LDA and heparin was 71 % compared to 42 % with LDA alone (OR 3.37, 95 % CI 1.40–8.10). Importantly, there was no difference in live birth rates between the two treatment groups in those pregnancies that advanced beyond 13 weeks. This implies that the beneficial effect of adjuvant heparin therapy is conferred in the first trimester of pregnancy, at a time when the intervillous circulation has not been fully established and hence cannot be due to the anticoagulant actions of heparin. It appears that the combination of LDA and heparin promotes successful embryonic implantation in the early stages of pregnancy by protecting the trophoblast from attack by aPL. Later in pregnancy, the combination therapy helps protect against subsequent thrombosis of the uteroplacental vasculature.

Treatment with LDA and heparin significantly reduces the severity of the defective endovascular trophoblastic invasion in women with APS, allowing them to achieve a live birth. However, it is important to remember that a proportion of pregnant women with aPL will remain at risk for late pregnancy complications due to the underlying uteroplacental vasculopathy. In a prospective series of 150 treated women with APS, a high risk for preterm delivery, placental abruption, fetal growth restriction, and the development of pregnancy-induced hypertension was found [35]. Once the pregnancy advances beyond the first trimester, specialist antenatal surveillance is required. Uterine artery Doppler ultrasonography at 22–24 weeks, followed by serial fetal growth and Doppler scans during the third trimester are useful tools with which to predict preeclampsia and intrauterine growth restriction in APS pregnancies [36]. Women with a circulating lupus anticoagulant or high positive IgG aCL or aβ2GPI antibodies are at particularly high risk of these complications.

Two studies have challenged the view that LDA and heparin is the treatment of choice for pregnant women with APS. Farquharson et al. [37] reported that LDA alone is as effective as LMWH, but they included women with low positive aCL, who were randomly assigned to treatment at a late stage in the first trimester, when pregnancy outcome was more likely to be successful. In addition, nearly 25 % of the study participants switched treatment groups. The more recent study by Laskin et al. [38] aimed to investigate whether treatment with LMWH plus LDA results in an increased rate of live births compared to treatment with LDA alone, but the study group was highly heterogeneous. The authors included women with two or more unexplained pregnancy losses prior to 32 weeks of gestation, accompanied by one or more of the following: positive aPL, positive antinuclear antibodies (ANA), or an inherited thrombophilic defect. A total of 88 women were recruited to the study over a 4-year period, but the RCT was then stopped prematurely when an interim analysis showed no difference in live birth rates in the two groups and a lower rate of pregnancy loss in the aspirin group than expected.

A meta-analysis of data from five trials involving 334 patients with recurrent miscarriage [39], showed that the overall live birth rates were 74.3 and 55.9 % in women who received a combination of UFH/LMWH plus LDA versus that in those treated with LDA alone. Patients who received combination treatment had significantly higher live birth rates (RR 1.301; 95 % CI 1.040, 1.629) than with aspirin alone. No significant differences in pre-eclampsia, preterm labor and birth weight were found between two groups.

The relative effectiveness of UFH versus LMWH as regards the prevention of recurrent pregnancy loss in women with APS is not established. The results of two pilot studies suggest that the combination of LMWH and LDA might be equivalent to UFH and LDA in preventing recurrent pregnancy loss [40, 41]. The American College of Chest Physicians (ACCP) recommends prophylactic or intermediate dose UFH or prophylactic dose LMWH in combination with LDA for the treatment of obstetric APS associated with a history of recurrent miscarriages [42]. The British Committee for Standards in Haematology (BCSH) guidance is that women who fulfill the International consensus criteria for obstetric APS should be screened for aPL, and in women with obstetric APS, antenatal administration of heparin combined with low dose aspirin (LDA) is recommended throughout pregnancy, in general starting as soon as pregnancy is confirmed and continuing until 6 weeks post-partum [43].

While treatment with LDA and heparin leads to a high live birth rate, some women do experience further miscarriages despite treatment. The single most important investigation to perform if a woman miscarries while taking treatment is to obtain fetal tissue for karyotype analysis. If the fetal karyotype is abnormal, pregnancy loss was not a failure of treatment and the woman can be offered treatment with LDA and heparin again in a future pregnancy. However, if the fetal karyotype was normal, one has to assume that pregnancy loss was a failure of treatment. This situation, although uncommon, has led to the use of other adjuvant therapies including intravenous immunoglobulin (IVIg). There is however considerable evidence that IVIg is of no benefit in the treatment of obstetric APS and its use is not to be recommended [44, 45]. Potential novel therapeutic agents that may be of benefit include complement inhibitors and hydroxychloroquine. With respect to the latter, it has recently been reported that hydroxychloroquine protects the anticoagulant annexin A5 shield that surrounds the trophoblast from damage induced by antiphospholipid antibodies [46]. Bramham et al. suggest that the addition of first trimester low-dose prednisolone to conventional treatment may be useful in the management of refractory aPL-related loss(es), although complications remain increased [47].

Non-criteria Obstetric Antiphospholipid Syndrome

The international consensus (revised Sapporo) criteria for obstetric APS [15] do not include low positive aCL and aβ2GPI (i.e. <99th centile) and/or certain clinical criteria such as two unexplained miscarriages, three non-consecutive miscarriages, late preeclampsia, placental abruption, late premature birth, or two or more unexplained in vitro fertilisation failures. Prospective [48] and retrospective [49–51] cohort studies of women with pregnancy morbidity, particularly recurrent pregnancy loss, suggest that elimination of aCL and/or IgM aβ2GPI, or low positive aCL or aβ2GPI from APS laboratory diagnostic criteria may result in missing the diagnosis in a sizeable number of women who could be regarded to have obstetric APS. Such studies also suggest that women with non-criteria, clinical and/or laboratory, obstetric APS ('obstetric morbidity associated with APS (OMAPS)') may benefit from standard treatment for obstetric APS with LMWH plus LDA, with good pregnancy outcomes. Thus, non-criteria manifestations of obstetric APS may be clinically relevant, and merit investigation of therapeutic approaches [52].

7.2.5.2 Neonatal Complications

Babies born to mothers with APS are at risk of the consequences of pre-term delivery. A Pan-European study reported that among 138 pregnancies, 16.3 % of babies were delivered at less than 37 weeks of gestation, 17 % were low birth weight, and, in addition, 11.3 % of neonates were small for gestational age. During the follow-up period of 6 years, 5 of the 141 babies exhibited behavioral abnormalities [53]. Almost 30 % of babies will passively acquire aPL [54]. There have been individual case reports of neonatal stroke – both hemorrhagic secondary to thrombocytopenia, and thrombotic – as well as thrombosis of the renal and axillary veins.

7.2.6 Heritable Thrombophilias

The relationship between heritable thrombophilias and recurrent first-trimester miscarriage is controversial. Indeed, many studies have been of a small size, prone to stratification and admixture bias, in which there has been poor matching of cases and controls as a result of racial heterogeneity. In addition, publication bias is evident, as judged by the discrepancy between the number of published abstracts reporting a lack of association between congenital thrombophilia and the number of peer-reviewed papers reporting an association.

A meta-analysis of pooled data from 31 retrospective studies suggested that the magnitude of the association between inherited thrombophilias and fetal loss varies according to type of fetal loss and type of thrombophilia [55]. The association between thrombophilia and late pregnancy loss has been consistently stronger than for early pregnancy loss. In this meta-analysis, factor V Leiden was associated with recurrent first-trimester fetal loss (OR 2.01, 95 % CI 1.13–3.58), recurrent fetal loss after 22 weeks (OR 7.83, 95 % CI 2.83–21.67), and nonrecurrent fetal loss after 19 weeks (OR 3.26, 95 % CI 1.82–5.83). Activated protein C resistance was associated with recurrent first-trimester fetal loss (OR 3.48, 95 % CI 1.58–7.69). The G202310A prothrombin gene mutation was associated with recurrent first-trimester fetal loss (OR 2.32, 95 % CI 1.12–4.79), recurrent fetal loss before 25 weeks (OR 2.56, 95 % CI 1.04–6.29), and late nonrecurrent fetal loss (OR 2.3, 95 % CI 1.09–4.87).

Similarly, another meta-analysis of 16 case-control studies reported that carriers of factor V Leiden or the G20210A prothrombin gene mutation have doubled the risk of experiencing recurrent miscarriage compared to women without these thrombophilic mutations [56].

Prospective data on the outcome of untreated pregnancies in women with such thrombophilias are scarce. One small study of six hereditary thrombophilias reported no adverse effects on the live birth rate of women with recurrent miscarriage [57]. In contrast, two small prospective studies reported an increased risk of miscarriage in untreated pregnancies for women with recurrent miscarriage who carry the factor V Leiden mutation compared to those with a normal factor V genotype [58, 59].

The importance of the fetal genetic thrombophilia status in governing pregnancy outcome has not been explored in large studies. Dizon-Townson et al. reported that fetal carriage of the factor V Leiden mutation is associated with a significantly increased risk of miscarriage. This area of research demands further attention [60].

While some centers advocate the use of thromboprophylactic therapy – typically LDA in combination with heparin – for those with recurrent miscarriage and hereditary thrombophilias, there is little evidence base for this. Indeed the Habenox study, a multicenter randomized study, reported no difference in live birth rates among those with an inherited thrombophilia who were treated with heparin, heparin and LDA, or LDA alone [61]. The results of this study however have to be treated with some caution as the sample population was small (26 women with thrombophilia, including 17 women with factor V Leiden and 5 with prothrombin G20210A) and the study was stopped prematurely due to slow recruitment.

The TIPPS (Thrombophilia in Pregnancy Prophylaxis Study) compared antepartum versus no antepartum dalteparin for the prevention of placenta-mediated pregnancy complications, including sever pre-eclampsia, small-for-gestational-age infants, and placental abtuption, in pregnant women with thrombophilia. The investigators postulated that antepartum dalteparin would reduce these complications in pregnant women with thrombophilia. There were 146 and 143 women randomized to the dalteparin and no dalteparin arms respectively, between 2000 and 2014; 16 % of the women randomized to dalteparin had three or more miscarriages at <10 weeks' gestation, 8 % had two or more fetal losses at 10–16 weeks gestation, and 19 % had one or more fetal losses at ≥16 weeks gestation; and 14, 10 and 23 % to the no dalteparin arm respectively. Dalteparin did not reduce the incidence of the primary composite outcome in both intention-to-treat analysis and on-treatment analysis in this trial, and was associated with an increased risk of minor bleeding [62] Limitations of this study include that the trial design permitted commencement of dalteparin up to 20 weeks gestation (approximately 27 % at <8 weeks, 27 % at 12 weeks, and 9 % at 12–20 weeks), therefore potentially excluding women with thrombophilia at higher risk of miscarriage. In addition, statistical power calculations are based on an aggregate of adverse outcomes, and thus the study may be underpowered as regards the assessment of the results in women within the individual clinical groups.

7.3 Tests of Global Haemostasis and Coagulation Activation

Conventional hemostasis tests are expensive, time-consuming, and take no account of the fact that hemostasis in vivo is a dynamic process that involves the interaction of coagulation and fibrinolytic pathways together with cellular elements such as endothelial cell surfaces. Hence, the measurement of individual coagulation factors is of limited use in establishing an individual's thrombotic risk, particularly during pregnancy. These limitations have prompted us to investigate the value of global tests of hemostasis in the investigation and treatment of women with recurrent miscarriage.

7.3.1 Thrombin-Antithrombin Complexes

We studied levels of thrombin-antithrombin (TAT) complexes, a marker of thrombin generation, in nonpregnant women with recurrent miscarriage, with and without aPL [8]. TAT concentrations were significantly raised in both aPL-positive and aPL-negative women with a history of recurrent miscarriage compared with normal controls. There was no significant difference in TAT values between aPL-positive and aPL-negative women or between women with early or late miscarriage. This study of 130 women demonstrated that even outside of pregnancy there is a cohort of women with recurrent miscarriage who have an identifiable prothrombotic state [8].

7.3.2 Activated Protein C Resistance

Activated protein C resistance (APCR) testing examines the protein C/S anticoagulant pathway together with the level of coagulation factor VIII. Resistance to activated protein C may be either genetic (usually due to factor V Leiden) or acquired. Individuals with an impaired response to activated protein C are at increased risk of thrombosis.

A large observational study including more than 1,000 consecutive nonpregnant women attending a specialist recurrent miscarriage clinic reported that acquired APC resistance is significantly more common among women with recurrent early miscarriage (80/904, 8.8 %: $p=0.02$) and those with a previous late miscarriage (18/207, 8.7 %: $p=0.04$) compared to parous controls (17/150, 3.3 %) [9]. Furthermore, those women with acquired APC resistance were significantly less likely to have had a previous live birth ($p<0.01$) compared to those with a normal APC ratio. These data suggest that acquired APC resistance contributes to the burden of recurrent pregnancy loss, the mechanism of which is likely to be thrombosis of the placental vasculature. Since a degree of APC resistance develops during normal pregnancy, it is possible that among women who are APC resistant prior to pregnancy, this effect is amplified when they become pregnant. This theory has prompted the use of thromboprophylactic treatment regimens for women with recurrent miscarriage and APC resistance (both the inherited and acquired forms) during the next pregnancy in order to improve the live birth rate and protect the mother from the risk of venous thrombosis during the pregnancy and puerperium. Although it has not been possible to conduct a randomized controlled therapeutic trial to assess the potential benefits of low-dose heparin therapy during pregnancy in these women, current clinical practice favors the use of thromboprophylaxis from early in the first trimester until 6–12 weeks postpartum.

7.4 Thromboelastography

Thromboelastography (TEG) is a rapid, reproducible near-patient test of global haemostasis which measures the rate of formation of a blood clot, its maximum strength, and fibrinolysis [63].

An important advantage of thromboelastography over conventional hemostasis testing is that it is a dynamic test, which yields information relating to the cumulative effect of the many components of coagulation including platelet function.

Our studies have shown that TEG is a useful tool with which to identify a prothrombotic state in women with a history of previously unexplained recurrent miscarriage [7]. The maximum clot amplitude (MA) was significantly greater among women with recurrent miscarriage compared with normal parous controls. Furthermore, increases in the MA were more marked in women with a history of late miscarriage compared with women with a history of only early pregnancy losses. None of the women in these studies smoked, was taking the oral contraceptive pill or had a history of thromboembolic disease.

The MA is a reflection of the absolute strength of the fibrin clot formed and hence is a dynamic test of fibrin and platelet function. Some 30 % of nonpregnant women with recurrent miscarriage have an MA that is more than two standard deviations above the mean of a control parous population, adding further weight to the hypothesis that a significant proportion of women with recurrent miscarriage are in a prothrombotic state outside of pregnancy. Furthermore, the pre-pregnancy MA was predictive of future pregnancy outcome, being significantly higher among those women with recurrent miscarriage whose next pregnancy ended in a further miscarriage as opposed to a live birth. Once pregnancy is confirmed, serial TEG testing during the first trimester can identify increases in the MA that precede the clinical evidence of impending miscarriage by several weeks [31]. Our pilot studies suggest that variable doses of aspirin can normalize the raised MA levels in early pregnancy and improve the live birth rate.

7.5 Conclusions

There is a substantial body of evidence that thrombophilic disorders are associated with adverse pregnancy outcome at all gestational ages. Antiphospholipid syndrome remains the most important treatable cause of recurrent miscarriage. Low dose aspirin together with heparin (LMWH being the most widely used) is the first-line treatment for this condition. The relationship between heritable thrombophilias and early pregnancy loss remains controversial. Large well-designed prospective studies are needed in order to clarify the relationship or lack of relationship between these defects and pregnancy outcome and the efficacy of treatment.

Tests of global hemostasis identify a subgroup of women with recurrent miscarriage who are in a prothrombotic state prior to pregnancy. Prospective data suggest that such women are at increased risk of further miscarriages in untreated pregnancies. The long-term health consequences of this hypercoagulability are increasingly recognized. A retrospective study of 130,000 women reported that a history of first-trimester spontaneous miscarriage is associated with a significant increased risk of maternal ischemic heart disease (IHD). This risk increased with the number of miscarriages such that among those with three or more miscarriages, the risk of death or hospital admission for IHD was 2.3 times greater than that among those with no previous history of miscarriage. In contrast, there was no association between therapeutic abortion and the subsequent risk of IHD [64]. Clearly, if these retrospective data are confirmed in a large prospective study, pregnancy history will become an important criterion in the risk assessment of IHD. The Nimes Obstetricians and Haematologists Antiphospholipid Syndrome (NOH-APS) observational study reported that the annual rates of deep vein thrombosis (1.46 %; range 1.15–1.82 %), pulmonary embolism (0.43 %; range 0.26–0.66 %), superficial vein thrombosis (0.44 %; range 0.28–0.68 %), and cerebrovascular events (0.32 %; range 0.18–0.53 %) were significantly higher in women with pure obstetric APS compared with aPL-negative women with obstetric morbidity, despite low dose aspirin (LDA) primary prophylaxis [65]. Thus, pregnancy history may have implications for subsequent risk of venous thromboembolism and cerebrovascular disease.

7.6 Case Studies

Case Study 1

Patient Details:

34-year-old female

Parity 0+4

Miscarriage History:

Pregnancy 1 Miscarriage at 10 weeks gestation

Pregnancy 2 Miscarriage at 8 weeks gestation

Pregnancy 3 Miscarriage at 6 weeks gestation

Pregnancy 4 Miscarriage at 10 weeks gestation. Fetal karyotype 46 XY

Medical History:

Unremarkable. No personal or family history of thrombosis

Investigations:

Lupus anticoagulant +ve on two consecutive occasions 8 weeks apart IgG and IgM anticardiolipin antibodies and anti-beta2GPI –ve

Factor V Leiden and prothrombin G20210A negative

Parental karyotypes normal – 46 XX and 46 XY

Normal uterine anatomy

Plan of Management:

Aspirin (75 mg/day) and low molecular weight heparin (enoxaparin 20 mg daily) to commence from time of positive pregnancy test

Pregnancy 5:

Miscarriage at 7 weeks gestation

Fetal karyotype Trisomy 13, i.e., not a failure of treatment

Pregnancy 6:

Treatment with aspirin (75 mg/day) + low molecular weight heparin (enox-aparin 20 mg daily)

Outcome:

Spontaneous vaginal delivery at 39 weeks gestation

Pregnancy course uncomplicated

Case Study 2

Patient Details:

39-year-old female

Miscarriage History:

Pregnancy 1: Preterm delivery by cesarean section at 30 weeks gestation – severe intra-uterine growth restriction

Pregnancy 2: Miscarriage at 12 weeks' gestation

Pregnancy 3: Intrauterine death at 16 weeks' gestation

Medical History:

Patient: history of migraine whilst taking combined oral contraceptive pill.

No personal history of systemic thromboembolism

Non-smoker

Mother: history of deep venous thrombosis post delivery.

Investigations:

Heterozygous for prothrombin G20210A; thromboelastogram: raised clot strength

Plan of Management:

Aspirin (150 mg/day) + low molecular weight heparin (Enoxaparin 40 mg SC per day) from +ve pregnancy test. Aspirin stopped at 34 weeks gestation. Enoxaparin continued until 24 h pre-cesarean section

Delivery:

Elective Cesarean section at 38 weeks – birthweight 5th centile.

Post partum thromboprophylaxis with low molecular weight heparin (Enoxaparin 40 mg per day) for 6 weeks post delivery.

Key Learning Points

- Antiphospholipid syndrome is the most important treatable cause for recurrent miscarriage. Low dose aspirin in combination with heparin leads to a significant increase in the live birth rate.
- Both in vitro and in vivo data demonstrate that the major mechanisms by which antiphospholipid antibodies cause pregnancy loss are via excessive complement-mediated inflammatory damage; an increased rate of trophoblast apoptosis; decreased trophoblast fusion, and a direct deleterious effect on endometrial receptivity. These effects are decreased by low dose heparin.
- Tests of global haemostasis suggest that women with recurrent miscarriage are in a prothrombotic state outside of

pregnancy. This may have implications for their health beyond their reproductive years.

- Apart from antiphospholipid antibodies, the relationship between individual thrombophilic defects and recurrent miscarriage is controversial.
- The use of aspirin or aspirin together with heparin in the treatment of women with recurrent miscarriage who have no demonstrable thrombophilia remains unknown.

References

1. Rai R, Regan L. Recurrent miscarriage. Lancet. 2006;368:601–11.
2. Drakeley AJ, Quenby S, Farquharson RG. Midtrimester loss – appraisal of a screening protocol. Hum Reprod. 1998;13:1975–80.
3. Craig M, Tata P, Regan L. Psychiatric morbidity among patients with recurrent miscarriage. J Psychosom Obstet Gynaecol. 2002;23:157–64.
4. Bremme KA. Haemostatic changes in pregnancy. Best Pract Res Clin Haematol. 2003;16:153–68.
5. O'Riordan MN, Higgins JR. Haemostasis in normal and abnormal pregnancy. Best Pract Res Clin Obstet Gynaecol. 2003;17:385–96.
6. Stirling Y, Woolf L, North WR, Seghatchian MJ, Meade TW. Haemostasis in normal pregnancy. Thromb Haemost. 1984;52:176–82.
7. Rai R. Is miscarriage a coagulopathy? Curr Opin Obstet Gynecol. 2003;15:265–8.
8. Vincent T, Rai R, Regan L, Cohen H. Increased thrombin generation in women with recurrent miscarriage. Lancet. 1998;352:116.
9. Rai R, Shlebak A, Cohen H, Backos M, Holmes Z, Marriott K, Regan L. Factor V Leiden and acquired activated protein C resistance among 1000 women with recurrent miscarriage. Hum Reprod. 2001;16:961–5.
10. Rai RS, Regan L, Clifford K, Pickering W, Dave M, Mackie I, et al. Antiphospholipid antibodies and beta 2-glycoprotein-I in 500 women with recurrent miscarriage: results of a comprehensive screening approach. Hum Reprod. 1995;10:2001–5.
11. Yenicesu GI, Cetin M, Ozdemir O, Cetin A, Ozen F, Yenicesu C, et al. A prospective case-control study analyzes 12 thrombophilic gene mutations in Turkish couples with recurrent pregnancy loss. Am J Reprod Immunol. 2010;63:126–36.
12. Jindal P, Regan L, Fourkala EO, Rai R, Moore G, Goldin RD, Sebire NJ. Placental pathology of recurrent spontaneous abortion: the role of histopathological examination of products of conception in routine clinical practice: a mini review. Hum Reprod. 2007;22:313–6.
13. Rai RS, Regan L, Chitolie A, Donald JG, Cohen H. Placental thrombosis and second trimester miscarriage in association with activated protein C resistance. Br J Obstet Gynaecol. 1996;103:842–4.
14. Nayar R, Lage JM. Placental changes in a first trimester missed abortion in maternal systemic lupus erythematosus with antiphospholipid syndrome; a case report and review of the literature. Hum Pathol. 1996;27:201–6.
15. Miyakis S, Lockshin MD, Atsumi T, Branch DW, Brey RL, Cervera R, et al. International consensus statement on an update of the classification criteria for definite antiphospholipid syndrome (APS). J Thromb Haemost. 2006;4:295–306.
16. Rai RS, Clifford K, Cohen H, Regan L. High prospective fetal loss rate in untreated pregnancies of women with recurrent miscarriage and antiphospholipid antibodies. Hum Reprod. 1995;10:3301–4.
17. Lockwood CJ, Romero R, Feinberg RF, Clyne LP, Coster B, Hobbins JC. The prevalence and biologic significance of lupus anticoagulant and anticardiolipin antibodies in a general obstetric population. Am J Obstet Gynecol. 1989;161:369–73.
18. Pattison NS, Chamley LW, McKay EJ, Liggins GC, Butler WS. Antiphospholipid antibodies in pregnancy: prevalence and clinical associations. Br J Obstet Gynaecol. 1993;100:909–13.
19. Perez MC, Wilson WA, Brown HL, Scopelitis E. Anticardiolipin antibodies in unselected pregnant women. Relationship to fetal outcome. J Perinatol. 1991;11:33–6.
20. Nodler J, Moolamalla SR, Ledger EM, Nuwayhid BS, Mulla ZD. Elevated antiphospholipid antibody titers and adverse pregnancy outcomes: analysis of a population-based hospital dataset. BMC Pregnancy Childbirth. 2009;9(11):11.
21. De Wolf F, Carreras LO, Moerman P, Vermylen J, Van Assche A, Renaer M. Decidual vasculopathy and extensive placental infarction in a patient with repeated thromboembolic accidents, recurrent fetal loss, and a lupus anticoagulant. Am J Obstet Gynecol. 1982;142:829–34.
22. Hanly JG, Gladman DD, Rose TH, Laskin CA, Urowitz MB. Lupus pregnancy. A prospective study of placental changes. Arthritis Rheum. 1988;31:358–66.
23. Out HJ, Kooijman CD, Bruinse HW, Derksen RH. Histopathological findings in placentae from patients with intrauterine fetal death and antiphospholipid antibodies. Eur J Obstet Gynecol Reprod Biol. 1991;41:179–86.
24. Di Simone N, Di Nicuolo F, D'Ippolito S, Castellani R, Tersigni C, Caruso A, et al. Antiphospholipid antibodies affect human endometrial angiogenesis. Biol Reprod. 2010;83:212–9.
25. Mak IY, Brosens JJ, Christian M, Hills FA, Chamley L, Regan L, White JO. Regulated expression of signal

transducer and activator of transcription, Stat5, and its enhancement of PRL expression in human endometrial stromal cells in vitro. J Clin Endocrinol Metab. 2002;87:2581–8.
26. Bose P, Black S, Kadyrov M, Weissenborn U, Neulen J, Regan L, Huppertz B. Heparin and aspirin attenuate placental apoptosis in vitro: implications for early pregnancy failure. Am J Obstet Gynecol. 2005;192:23–30.
27. Bose P, Black S, Kadyrov M, Bartz C, Shlebak A, Regan L, Huppertz B. Adverse effects of lupus anticoagulant positive blood sera on placental viability can be prevented by heparin in vitro. Am J Obstet Gynecol. 2004;191:2125–31.
28. Di Simone N, Caliandro D, Castellani R, Ferrazzani S, De CS, Caruso A. Low-molecular weight heparin restores in-vitro trophoblast invasiveness and differentiation in presence of immunoglobulin G fractions obtained from patients with antiphospholipid syndrome. Hum Reprod. 1999;14:489–95.
29. Holers VM, Girardi G, Mo L, Guthridge JM, Molina H, Pierangeli SS, et al. Complement C3 activation is required for antiphospholipid antibody-induced fetal loss. J Exp Med. 2002;195:211–20.
30. Empson M, Lassere M, Craig J, Scott J. Prevention of recurrent miscarriage for women with antiphospholipid antibody or lupus anticoagulant. Cochrane Database Syst Rev. 2005;(2):CD002859.
31. Rai R, Tuddenham E, Backos M, Jivraj S, El'Gaddal S, Choy S, et al. Thromboelastography, whole-blood haemostasis and recurrent miscarriage. Hum Reprod. 2003;18:2540–3.
32. Goel N, Tuli A, Choudhry R. The role of aspirin versus aspirin and heparin in cases of recurrent abortions with raised anticardiolipin antibodies. Med Sci Monit. 2006;12(3):CR132–6.
33. Kutteh WH. Antiphospholipid antibody-associated recurrent pregnancy loss: treatment with heparin and low-dose aspirin is superior to low-dose aspirin alone. Am J Obstet Gynecol. 1996;174:1584–9.
34. Rai R, Cohen H, Dave M, Regan L. Randomised controlled trial of aspirin and aspirin plus heparin in pregnant women with recurrent miscarriage associated with phospholipid antibodies (or antiphospholipid antibodies). BMJ. 1997;314:253–7.
35. Backos M, Rai R, Baxter N, Chilcott IT, Cohen H, Regan L. Pregnancy complications in women with recurrent miscarriage associated with antiphospholipid antibodies treated with low dose aspirin and heparin. Br J Obstet Gynaecol. 1999;106:102–7.
36. Venkat-Raman N, Backos M, Teoh TG, Lo WT, Regan L. Uterine artery Doppler in predicting pregnancy outcome in women with antiphospholipid syndrome. Obstet Gynecol. 2001;98:235–42.
37. Farquharson RG, Quenby S, Greaves M. Antiphospholipid syndrome in pregnancy: a randomized, controlled trial of treatment. Obstet Gynecol. 2002;100:408–13.
38. Laskin CA, Spitzer KA, Clark CA, Crowther MR, Ginsberg JS, Hawker GA, Kingdom JC, Barrett J, Gent M. Low molecular weight heparin and aspirin for recurrent pregnancy loss: results from the randomized, controlled HepASA Trial. J Rheumatol. 2009;36:279–87.
39. Mak A, Cheung MW, Cheak AA, Ho RC. Combination of heparin and aspirin is superior to aspirin alone in enhancing live births in patients with recurrent pregnancy loss and positive anti-phospholipid antibodies: a meta-analysis of randomized controlled trials and meta-regression. Rheumatology (Oxford). 2010;49(2):281–8.
40. Noble LS, Kutteh WH, Lashey N, Franklin RD, Herrada J. Antiphospholipid antibodies associated with recurrent pregnancy loss: prospective, multicenter, controlled pilot study comparing treatment with low-molecular-weight heparin versus unfractionated heparin. Fertil Steril. 2005;83:684–90.
41. Stephenson MD, Ballem PJ, Tsang P, Purkiss S, Ensworth S, Houlihan E, Ensom MH. Treatment of antiphospholipid antibody syndrome (APS) in pregnancy: a randomized pilot trial comparing low molecular weight heparin to unfractionated heparin. J Obstet Gynaecol Can. 2004;26:729–34.
42. Bates SM, Greer IA, Middeldorp S, Veenstra DL, Prabulos A-M, Vandvik PO. VTE, thrombophilia, antithrombotic therapy, and pregnancy: antithrombotic therapy and prevention of thrombosis, 9th ed: American College of Chest Physicians evidence-based clinical practice guidelines. Chest. 2012;141(2 Suppl):e691S–736.
43. Keeling D, Mackie I, Moore GW, Greer IA, Greaves M. Guidelines on the investigation and management of antiphospholipid syndrome. Br J Haematol. 2012;157(1):47–58.
44. Branch DW, Peaceman AM, Druzin M, Silver RK, El-Sayed Y, Silver RM, Esplin MS, Spinnato J, Harger J. A multicenter, placebo-controlled pilot study of intravenous immune globulin treatment of antiphospholipid syndrome during pregnancy. The Pregnancy Loss Study Group. Am J Obstet Gynecol. 2000;182:122–7.
45. Triolo G, Ferrante A, Ciccia F, Accardo-Palumbo A, Perino A, Castelli A, Giarratano A, Licata G. Randomized study of subcutaneous low molecular weight heparin plus aspirin versus intravenous immunoglobulin in the treatment of recurrent fetal loss associated with antiphospholipid antibodies. Arthritis Rheum. 2003;48:728–31.
46. Rand JH, Wu XX, Quinn AS, Taatjes DJ. The annexin A5-mediated pathogenic mechanism in the antiphospholipid syndrome: role in pregnancy losses and thrombosis. Lupus. 2010;19:460–9.
47. Bramham K, Thomas M, Nelson-Piercy C, Khamashta M, Hunt BJ. First-trimester low-dose prednisolone in refractory antiphospholipid antibody–related pregnancy loss. Blood. 2011;117:6948–51.

48. Alijotas-Reig J, Ferrer-Oliveras R, EUROAPS Study Group. The European Registry on Obstetric Antiphospholipid Syndrome (EUROAPS): a preliminary first year report. Lupus. 2012;21(7):766–8.
49. Cohn DM, Goddijn M, Middeldorp S, Korevaar JC, Dawood F, Farquharson RG. Recurrent miscarriage and antiphospholipid antibodies: prognosis of subsequent pregnancy. J Thromb Haemost. 2010;8(10):2208–13.
50. Gardiner C, Hills J, Machin SJ, Cohen H. Diagnosis of antiphospholipid syndrome in routine clinical practice. Lupus. 2013;22(1):18–25.
51. Mekinian A, Loire-Berson P, Nicaise-Roland P, Lachassinne E, Stirnemann J, Boffa MC, et al. Outcomes and treatment of obstetrical antiphospholipid syndrome in women with low antiphospholipidantibody levels. J Reprod Immunol. 2012;94(2):222–6.
52. Arachchillage DR, Machin SJ, Mackie IJ, Cohen H. Diagnosis and management of non-criteria obstetric antiphospholipid syndrome. Thromb Haemost. 2015;113(1):13–9.
53. Boffa MC, Lachassinne E, Boinot C, De CS, Rovere-Querini P, Avcin T, et al. European registry of babies born to mothers with antiphospholipid syndrome: a result update. Lupus. 2009;18:900–4.
54. Tincani A, Rebaioli CB, Andreoli L, Lojacono A, Motta M. Neonatal effects of maternal antiphospholipid syndrome. Curr Rheumatol Rep. 2009;11:70–6.
55. Rey E, Kahn SR, David M, Shrier I. Thrombophilic disorders and fetal loss: a meta-analysis. Lancet. 2003;361:901–8.
56. Kovalevsky G, Gracia CR, Berlin JA, Sammel MD, Barnhart KT. Evaluation of the association between hereditary thrombophilias and recurrent pregnancy loss: a meta-analysis. Arch Intern Med. 2004;164:558–63.
57. Carp H, Dolitzky M, Tur-Kaspa I, Inbal A. Hereditary thrombophilias are not associated with a decreased live birth rate in women with recurrent miscarriage. Fertil Steril. 2002;78:58–62.
58. Jivraj S, Makris M, Saravelos S, Li TC. Pregnancy outcome in women with factor V Leiden and recurrent miscarriage. BJOG. 2009;116:995–8.
59. Rai R, Backos M, Elgaddal S, Shlebak A, Regan L. Factor V Leiden and recurrent miscarriage-prospective outcome of untreated pregnancies. Hum Reprod. 2002;17:442–5.
60. Dizon-Townson DS, Meline L, Nelson LM, Varner M, Ward K. Fetal carriers of the factor V Leiden mutation are prone to miscarriage and placental infarction. Am J Obstet Gynecol. 1997;177:402–5.
61. Visser J, Ulander VM, Helmerhorst FM, Lampinen K, Morin-Papunen L, Bloemenkamp KW, Kaaja RJ. Thromboprophylaxis for recurrent miscarriage in women with or without thrombophilia. HABENOX: a randomised multicentre trial. Thromb Haemost. 2011;105:295–301.
62. Rodger MA, Hague WM, Kingdom J, Kahn SR, Karovitch A, Sermer M, et al.; for the TIPPS Investigators. Antepartum dalteparin versus no antepartum dalteparin for the prevention of pregnancy complications in pregnant women with thrombophilia (TIPPS): a multinational open-label randomised trial. Lancet. 2014;384(9955):1673–83.
63. Nair SC, Dargaud Y, Chitlur M, Srivastava A. Tests of global haemostasis and their applications in bleeding disorders. Haemophilia. 2010;16 Suppl 5:85–92.
64. Gris JC, Bouvier S, Molinari N, Galanaud JP, Cochery-Nouvellon E, Mercier E, et al. Comparative incidence of a first thrombotic event in purely obstetric antiphospholipid syndrome with pregnancy loss: the NOH-APS observational study. Blood. 2012;119(11):2624–32.
65. Smith GC, Pell JP, Walsh D. Spontaneous loss of early pregnancy and risk of ischaemic heart disease in later life: retrospective cohort study. BMJ. 2003;326(423–424326):423–4.

Pregnancy Morbidity Associated with Thrombophilias: Late Placenta-Mediated Obstetric Complications

8

Sukrutha Veerareddy, Katherine Clesham, Hannah Cohen, and Donald Peebles

Abstract

Late pregnancy complications such as severe pre-eclampsia and placental insufficiency at less than 34 weeks gestation are relatively common, as are thrombophilic risk factors, with these risk factors associated with an increased risk of venous thromboembolism during pregnancy. This chapter will focus on associations between heritable thrombophilias and antiphospholipid antibodies with late placenta-mediated complications and the management of affected women.

Keywords

Late placenta-mediated obstetric complications • Heritable thrombophilias • Antiphospholipid antibodies • Management of adverse pregnancy outcomes

S. Veerareddy, BSc, MBBS, MRCOG, PhD
Women's Health Services, Queen Elizabeth Hospital, Lewisham and Greenwich NHS Trust, Stadium Road, London SE18 4QH, UK
e-mail: Sukrutha.veerareddy@nhs.net

K. Clesham, MB ChB, MRCP, FRCPath
Department of Haematology, University College London Hospitals NHS Foundation Trust, 235 Euston Road, London NW1 2BU, UK
e-mail: katherine.Clesham@uclh.nhs.uk

H. Cohen, MB ChB, MD, FCRP, FRCPath
Department of Haematology, University College London Hospitals NHS Foundation Trust, 250 Euston Road, London NW1 2PG, UK
e-mail: hannah.cohen@uclh.nhs.uk

D. Peebles, MA, MD, FRCOG (✉)
Institute for Women's Health, University College London Hospitals NHS Foundation Trust, 2nd floor, Medical School Building, 72 Huntley St, London WC1E 6AU, UK
e-mail: d.peebles@ucl.ac.uk

8.1 Introduction

Late pregnancy complications such as severe pre-eclampsia and placental insufficiency at less than 34 weeks gestation are relatively common, probably complicating about 0.5–1 % of pregnancies. Thrombophilic risk factors are also common and observed in approximately 20 % of Caucasian populations, with these risk factors associated with an increased risk of venous thromboembolism (VTE) during pregnancy. Since pregnancy is an acquired hypercoagulable state, women with heritable or acquired thrombophilia may also present with clinical symptoms of placental vascular-mediated obstetric complications for the first time during pregnancy. This chapter will focus on associations between heritable thrombophilias and antiphospholipid antibodies (aPL) with late

H. Cohen, P. O'Brien (eds.), *Disorders of Thrombosis and Hemostasis in Pregnancy: A Guide to Management*, DOI 10.1007/978-3-319-15120-5_8, © Springer-Verlag London 2015

placental vascular-mediated obstetric complications including preeclampsia, intrauterine growth restriction (IUGR), placental abruption, and late fetal loss (fetal loss after 24 weeks' gestation is defined as stillbirth and fetal loss between 20 and 24 weeks is generally described as late fetal loss). The reader should also refer to Chap. 3.

8.2 Hemostatic Changes in Normal Pregnancy

For a detailed description, the reader should refer to Chap. 1. There is a marked increase in blood procoagulant activity, characterized by an elevation of a number of coagulation factors [4], especially at term in normal pregnancy. This is associated with an increase in prothrombin fragment F1.2 and thrombin-antithrombin complexes [5, 6], both markers of coagulation activation. There is a decrease in physiological anticoagulants manifested by a significant reduction in protein S activity and [7] by acquired activated protein C resistance (APCR) [8]. The overall fibrinolytic activity is impaired during pregnancy but rapidly returns to normal following delivery [9]. This is largely due to placenta-derived plasminogen activator inhibitor type 2 (PAI-2), which is present in substantial quantities during pregnancy [10]. D-dimer, a specific marker of fibrinolysis resulting from breakdown of cross-linked fibrin polymer by plasmin, increases as pregnancy progresses [11]. Overall, there is a five- to ten-fold increased risk of VTE throughout gestation and the postpartum period.

8.3 Antiphospholipid Syndrome (APS) and Late Placenta-Mediated Pregnancy Complications

8.3.1 Diagnosis of Obstetric Antiphospholipid Syndrome

The antiphospholipid syndrome (APS) is the most common acquired form of thrombophilia. The International consensus (revised Sapporo) criteria for diagnosis of obstetric APS is based on clinical criteria for a diagnosis of APS and persistent positive aPL: lupus anticoagulant (LA) and/or moderate or high positive aPL (IgG and/or IgM anticardiolipin (aCL) and/or anti β_2 glycoprotein I (aβ_2GPI) antibodies) that are present on two or more consecutive occasions at least 12 weeks apart [3]. Women with aPL may present with (a) recurrent miscarriage (RM), i.e. three or more unexplained consecutive spontaneous miscarriages before the 10th week of gestation, with maternal anatomic or hormonal abnormalities and paternal and maternal chromosomal causes excluded; fetal demise beyond 10 weeks of gestation; (b) one or more unexplained deaths of a morphologically normal fetus at or beyond the 10th week of gestation, with normal fetal morphology documented by ultrasound or by direct examination of the fetus; or (c) one or more premature births of a morphologically normal neonate before the 34th week of gestation (because of: (i) eclampsia or severe pre-eclampsia defined according to standard definitions; (ii) recognised features of placental insufficiency) (Table 8.1). These obstetric complications may occur alone (obstetric APS) or in combination with thrombotic manifestations. In a study of 60 pregnancies in women with APS, the most specific clinical features were reported to be thrombosis (both venous and arterial), RM, fetal loss in the second and third trimesters, and autoimmune thrombocytopenia [12].

8.3.2 Non-criteria Obstetric Antiphospholipid Syndrome

Several obstetric manifestations additional to those in the International consensus criteria have been proposed as 'obstetric morbidity associated with APS (OMAPS)'. Non-criteria laboratory manifestations include low positive aCL and aβ_2GPI (i.e. >95 centile and <99th centile). Clinical non-criteria manifestations include two unexplained miscarriages, three non-consecutive miscarriages, late pre-eclampsia, placental abruption, late premature birth, or

Table 8.1 Revised Sapporo criteria (International consensus statement) for the diagnosis of antiphospholipid syndrome

Clinical criteria (one or more)
Vascular thrombosis: One or more objectively confirmed episodes of arterial, venous or small vessel thrombosis occurring in any tissue or organ
Pregnancy morbidity:
One or more unexplained deaths of a morphologically normal fetus <10th week of gestation; or
One or more premature births of a morphologically normal neonate <34th week of gestation because of eclampsia, severe pre-eclampsia or placental insufficiency; or
Three or more unexplained consecutive miscarriages <10th week of gestation
Laboratory criteria (one or more, present on two or more occasions at least 12 weeks apart using recommended procedures)
1. Lupus anticoagulant (LA), detected according to the guidelines of the British Committee for Standards in Haematology [1] and International Society on Thrombosis and Haemostasis [2]
2. Anticardiolipin antibodies (aCL) of IgG and/or IgM isotype, moderate or high positive (>40 GPL or MPL, or >99th centile), measured by a standardized ELISA
3. Anti-$\beta_2$2-glycoprotein-1 antibodies (aβ_2GPI) of IgG and/or IgM isotype, present at a level >99th centile, measured by a standardized ELISA

Data from Miyakis et al. [3]

two or more unexplained in vitro fertilization failures [13–17].

8.3.3 Pathogenesis of Pregnancy Complications in Antiphospholipid Syndrome

Pregnancy morbidity in the form of fetal loss or premature birth is a relatively common finding in women with APS [18]. APS is associated with placental vascular thrombosis, decidual vasculopathy, intervillous fibrin deposition, and placental infarction [19–21]. These pathological changes in the placenta may result in RM, early severe pre-eclampsia, IUGR, or stillbirth. A key mechanism of fetal loss is believed to be due to binding of aPL to trophoblast cells, resulting in defective placentation [22]. Thrombotic complications within the uteroplacental circulation have also been proposed as a contributing mechanism. aPL have been shown to reduce the levels of annexin V and accelerate the coagulation of plasma on cultured trophoblasts and endothelial cells, and therefore, the reduction of annexin V levels on vascular cells may be an important mechanism of thrombosis and pregnancy loss in APS [23]. Complement activation by aPL appears to play a major role in the pathogenesis of recurrent pregnancy loss, and may also have a role in the pathogenesis of thrombosis in APS [24]. Animal experiments indicate that aPL cause decidual tissue damage by altering the classical pathway of complement activation, followed by amplification through the alternative pathway [25].

In a mouse model of APS induced by passive transfer of human aPL antibodies, it has been shown that complement activation plays a causative role in pregnancy loss and fetal growth restriction, and that blocking activation of the complement cascade can prevent pregnancy loss.

8.3.4 Antiphospholipid Antibodies and Pre-eclampsia

An association between aPL and pre-eclampsia has been suggested in two systematic reviews and meta-analyses [26, 27]. Both these systematic analyses sought to include case–control, or controlled, cross-sectional studies until 2009. The analysis by do Prado et al. [26] included 12 of 64 studies. The key finding was an association between aPL and severe, but not mild, pre-eclampsia in pregnant women without autoimmune disease. The analysis by Abou-Nasser et al. [27] included 28 studies. LA and aCL were associated with pre-eclampsia in case-control but not cohort studies. aβ2GPI were associated with pre-eclampsia in cohort but not in case–control studies. The authors of both these analyses noted significant flaws in the available data. A prospective, observational, cohort study in 142 women suggested a significant association between aCL or IgG aβ2GPI and pre-eclampsia in women who had suffered a single previous embryonic loss (adjusted OR 3.09, 1.13–8.48 and 4.61, 1.53–13.88, respectively) [28].

8.4 Heritable Thrombophilia and Placenta-Mediated Obstetric Complications

Table 8.2 lists the thrombophilic factors that may be associated with placenta-mediated obstetric complications. For details on heritable thrombophilias, the reader should refer to Chap. 3. The prevalence of factor V Leiden (FVL), the most common cause of VTE in pregnancy [29], is very low in Asian and African populations, and higher at around 4 % in Caucasians. However, APCR may be present without FVL; the reported prevalence is 3.3 % [30, 31]. The prevalence of heterozygosity for the G20210A prothrombin gene mutation is approximately 2 % in Caucasians, and increases geographically from Northern to Southern Europe [32, 33]. Protein C and S deficiencies are quite rare, and carriers have a significantly increased risk of thrombosis when the inhibitory effect on coagulation is lost. Antithrombin (AT) deficiency may be the result of many different mutations and has a prevalence of 0.07 %. It is the most thrombogenic of the inherited thrombophilias, with a reported 70–90 % lifetime risk of thromboembolism in individuals with type 1 AT deficiency. Homozygosity for the C677T methylene tetrahydrofolate reductase (MTHFR) polymorphism has an observed prevalence varying from 15.2 % in Hispanic populations to 10.2 % in Caucasians, 8.8 % in Asians, and 2.4 % in African Americans. Several alleles (C and T) have been described. Homozygosity for the T variant results in elevated homocysteine levels, which can cause vascular injury [32–35].

Associations between various thrombophilias and placenta-mediated complications are discussed below. The reader should refer to Chap. 3. Table 3.2 summarising results of a systematic review of thrombophilic defects in women with pregnancy complications [36]. A subsequent systematic review and a meta-analysis of prospective cohort studies, to estimate the association of maternal FVL or G20210A carrier status and placenta-mediated pregnancy complications, showed that women with FVL appear to be at a small absolute increased risk of late pregnancy loss; and that women with FVL and G20210A appear not to be at increased risk of pre-eclampsia or birth of small-for-gestational age (SGA) infants [37]. Of note, more recently, a prospective cohort of unselected, pregnant women (total 7343) were assessed for a composite of pregnancy loss, SGA < 10th percentile, pre-eclampsia or placental abruption. The conclusions were that carriers of FVL or G20210A are not at significantly increased risk of these pregnancy complications [38].

Table 8.2 Classification and prevalence of thrombophilia

	Thrombophilia	% of general population
Inherited	Antithrombin deficiency	0.07
	Protein C deficiency	0.3
	Protein S deficiency	0.2
	Factor V Leiden (heterozygous)	4
	Factor V Leiden (homozygous)	0.06
	G20210A prothrombin gene mutation	2
	C677T methylenetetrahydrofolate reductase (homozygous)	10
Acquired	Antiphospholipid antibodies (Lupus anticoagulant Anticardiolipin antibodies Anti-β2-glyoprotein I antibodies)	2
	Acquired APC resistance	3.3
	In the absence of factor V Leiden	

8.5 Placental Findings Associated with Heritable Thrombophilias and Pregnancy Complications

Many et al. [39] described placental findings in women who had severe obstetric complications during pregnancy and were carriers of heritable thrombophilia, and compared them to placental findings in women without thrombophilia who experienced severe obstetric complications during pregnancy. The study population comprised 68 women with singleton pregnancies who had severe pre-eclampsia, IUGR, abruptio placentae, or stillbirth. They were evaluated after delivery for the presence of mutations of FVL, C677T MTHFR homozygosity, prothrombin G20210A, and deficiencies of protein C, protein S, and AT. All were negative for aPL. Thirty-two women carried a thrombophilia and 36 women did not. All placentas were evaluated by a single pathologist who was blinded to the results of the thrombophilia assessment. There was no difference in the maternal age, parity, type of pregnancy complication, and fetoplacental weight ratio between the groups. The proportion of women with villous infarcts was significantly higher in women with thrombophilias (72 % vs. 39 %, $p<0.01$), as was the proportion of women with multiple infarcts or fibrinoid necrosis of decidual vessels.

Conversely, in a study with a very similar design that also examined the relationship between placental histology and thrombophilia in women with severe obstetric complications, no specific histological pattern could be identified when thrombophilia-positive and thrombophilia-negative groups were compared [37]. Nevertheless, a high rate of placental infarcts (50 %) and thrombosis was confirmed in women both with and without thrombophilias. Likewise, placental pathology in early-onset pre-eclampsia and IUGR was similar in women with and without thrombophilia although a high rate of placental abnormalities was found [37, 38].

Arias et al. (1998) evaluated 13 women with thrombotic lesions of the placenta [39]. All women had obstetric complications such as pre-eclampsia, preterm labor, IUGR, or stillbirth. In 10 of the 13 (77 %), an inherited thrombophilia was found; 7 were heterozygous for the FV Leiden mutation and 3 had protein S deficiency. The most prominent placental lesions were fetal stem vessel thrombosis, infarcts, hypoplasia, spiral artery thrombosis, and perivillous fibrin deposition [39].

8.6 Heritable Thrombophilia and Intrauterine Growth Restriction (IUGR)

IUGR is an important cause of perinatal morbidity and mortality. Growth-restricted infants are at increased risk of developing neuropsychological defects and suffering educational disadvantages later in childhood [40, 41]. Moreover, there is epidemiological evidence that children whose intrauterine growth was restricted have a higher risk of cardiovascular and endocrine diseases in adulthood [42]. Numerous studies have reported on associations between obstetric complications and heritable causes of thrombophilia [43–96]. Kupferminc et al. [65] reported an association between inherited thrombophilia (FVL, prothrombin G20210A, and homozygosity for C677T MTHFR) and IUGR (defined as a birth weight below the 5th percentile for gestational age).

Martinelli et al. compared 61 women with a history of IUGR, defined as birth weight below the 10th percentile, and 93 parous women with uneventful pregnancies. Among women with IUGR, 13 % had FVL compared with 2.2 % of controls (OR, 6.9; 95 % CI 1.4–33.5), and 12 % had the G20210A prothrombin mutation compared with 1.6 % of controls (OR, 5.9; 95 % CI 1.2–29.4). In a regression-analysis model, these thrombophilias were independently associated with IUGR [68]. A subsequent report from the same group [43] tested for these mutations in neonates weighing less than 2.5 kg. Neonates delivered by mothers with FVL or prothrombin G20210A mutations accounted for 30 % of newborns weighing less than 1 kg, 18.7 % of those ranging from 1.001 to 2.499 kg, and only 9.5 % of those weighing 2.5 kg or more. Overall, 27.6 % of neonates of mothers with the mutations weighed less than 2.5 kg compared with 13.9 % of neonates of mothers without mutations (OR, 2.4; 95 % CI 1.5–3.7).

However, other studies failed to confirm an association between IUGR and thrombophilic mutations. In one such study [69], the prevalence of thrombophilia in mothers of 493 newborns with IUGR (<10th percentile) and 472 controls did not differ significantly. However, one-third of the study population was not Caucasian and the degree of IUGR was mild, with mean birth weight 2.393 ± 0.606 kg and 83 % of newborns delivered at 36–40 weeks' gestation. In contrast, in the study by Kupferminc et al. (1999), the mean birth weight was 1.387 ± 0.616 kg and mean gestational week at delivery was 33 ± 4.0 [67]. Similarly, Martinelli et al. reported a mean gestational week at delivery of 35 ± 3 and a mean birth weight of 1.584 ± 0.586 kg [68]. It is therefore suggested that these studies have addressed noncomparable fetal and neonatal populations with differing clinical relevance.

8.7 Heritable Thrombophilia and Pre-eclampsia

The association of pre-eclampsia with thrombophilia is similarly controversial; a number of case-controlled studies demonstrate an association, while others fail to do so. FVL may be associated with severe pre-eclampsia and affected women may have a higher risk of serious maternal complications and adverse perinatal outcomes than those without thrombophilia [53, 74–77]. Kupferminc et al (1999) demonstrated an increased prevalence of thrombophilia (53 %) in women with severe pre-eclampsia compared with controls (18 %) [67]. The same study also highlighted that women with obstetric complications had a significantly higher incidence of combined thrombophilias. In a sample of 140 Italian women with a history of gestational hypertension, with or without significant proteinuria, a significantly higher prevalence of thrombophilias was documented regardless of the presence of proteinuria [78]. Logistic regression showed that FVL and prothrombin G20210A mutations were independently associated with occurrence of gestational hypertension. In contrast, several studies, including a large population-based study and systematic review suggest lack of an association between thrombophilia and pre-eclampsia [62].

The meta-analysis by Robertson et al (2006) suggested that heterozygosity for FVL or the prothrombin gene mutation is associated with a two-fold-increased risk of severe early-onset pre-eclampsia [36]. Rodger et al. (2010) in a systematic review and meta-analysis of ten prospective cohort studies examining associations between FVL and prothrombin G20210A and placenta-mediated pregnancy complications found no association between FVL or prothrombin G20210A and pre-eclampsia [36].

Studies of the prevalence of thrombophilia in pre-eclampsia seem to differ in selection of controls and in ethnic backgrounds. The size of these studies of pre-eclampsia is generally small, especially if the aim was to detect any possible association between the less frequent thrombophilias, such as protein C, protein S, and AT deficiencies, and obstetric complications. Studies reporting a significant association are generally smaller than those reporting a lack of association. In many of the studies, groups of different thrombophilias or obstetric complications are pooled together, which sometimes results in significant associations that do not remain significant when the relevant sub-groups are analyzed separately. The pooling of study subjects can lead to inaccuracy in determining the exact impact of a specific mutation on each of the complications.

Excessive generation of plasminogen activator inhibitor-type 1 (PAI-1) is implicated in the pathogenesis of pre-eclampsia and related conditions. The PAI-1 (−675 4G/5G) promoter polymorphism affects transcriptional activity and is a putative genetic risk factor for pre-eclampsia. A systematic review and random effects meta-analysis of genetic association studies suggested that the fibrinolytic pathway regulated by the PAI-1 gene may contribute to the pathogenesis of pre-eclampsia and related conditions. The authors concluded that the association, if confirmed in larger genetic association studies, may inform research efforts to develop novel interventions or help to prioritise therapeutic targets that merit evaluation in randomised clinical trials [56].

Overall these data suggest that, while prothrombotic genotypes might not be causative factors for pre-eclampsia, they could be linked to the severity of disease expression once the condition arises.

8.8 Thrombophilia and Placental Abruption

van der Molen et al. investigated coagulation inhibitors and abnormalities of homocysteine metabolism as risk factors for placental vasculopathy [85]. They compared non-pregnant women with a history of placental vasculopathy with non-pregnant controls. Protein C activity was noted to be significantly lower in women that had adverse pregnancy outcome. Homozygotes for the C677T MTHFR polymorphism and carriers of the FVL mutation were significantly more common in the study group. The median levels of homocysteine, APCR ratio, protein S, and AT were not different between the groups. However, homocysteine levels above 14.4 mmol/L (the 80th percentile of control values) were associated with a significant increase in the odds ratio (OR). Also, a combination of risk factors such as homocysteine levels above 14.4 mmoL and protein S deficiency resulted in a significantly increased OR for placental vasculopathy. The risk factors for placental vasculopathy that emerged in this study were APCR and decreased levels of protein C, elevated homocysteine, and the C677T MTHFR polymorphism, or a combination of these.

Wiener-Megnagi et al. studied 27 women who had placental abruption and 29 controls and found that 63 % of cases had an APCR ratio >2.5 compared with 17 % of controls (OR 8.16, p=0.001) [49]. Eight of 15 patients (53 %) tested were found to have the FVL mutation (5 heterozygous and 3 homozygous) compared with 1 heterozygote among the control subjects (3.4 %). Similarly, Kupferminc et al. [67] found a 70 % incidence of thrombophilias in women with placental abruption, of which 60 % had thrombophilic mutations and 10 % had AT deficiency or aPL. Of the 20 women who had an abruption, 3 also had mild pre-eclampsia, 7 had antepartum or postpartum hypertension, and 11 of the neonates were below the 10th percentile for gestational age. In this early study on the association between prothrombin G20210A in women with pregnancy complications, the OR for abruption with this mutation was 8.9 (95 % CI 1.8–43.6), whereas the ORs for the FVL mutation and MTHFR polymorphism were 4.9 (95 % CI 1.0–17.4) and 2 (95 % CI 0.5–8.1), respectively. In another study, the incidence of prothrombin G20210A in 27 women with placental abruption was 18.5 % compared to 3.2 % of controls (OR, 5.8; 95 % CI 1.8–18.6, p=0.01) [60]. In the study by de Vries et al. (1997), 26 % of women with placental abruption had hyperhomocysteinemia and 29 %, protein S deficiency [48].

Prochazka et al. reported that FVL carrier status was not significantly different in women with placental abruption but was associated with a positive family history of venous thrombosis [86]. However, the same group reported that 20 of 142 (14.1 %) women with placental abruption were heterozygous for FVL, compared to 10 of 196 (5.1 %) of controls (OR 3.0, 95 % CI 1.4–6.7) [87–91].

Analysis of The New Jersey-Placental Abruption Study (2002–2007) suggested that women with lower protein C levels (<5th centile) had an increased risk of abruption, with an OR of 3.2 (95 % CI 1.2–9.9) [91]. Reduction in both protein S and APCR ratio was not associated with abruption.

In the systematic review and meta-analysis of prospective cohort studies by Rodger et al. [37], five of the ten studies analysed reported on the association between FVL mutation and placental abruption. These studies included 12,308 women with a pooled FVL prevalence of 5.1 %. The absolute risk of placenta abruption in FVL positive women was 1.3 % as compared with 0.9 % for FVL negative women. The pooled OR estimate for placental abruption in women with FVL mutation (homozygous or heterozygous) was 1.85 (95 % CI 0.92–3.70). The pooled OR estimate for placental abruption in women with PGM mutation (homozygous or heterozygous) was 2.02 (95 % CI 0.81–5.02). There was moderate statistical heterogeneity across studies, suggested to be possibly attributable to the inconsistent and unclear definition of placental abruption across studies.

8.9 Heritable Thrombophilia and Late Fetal Loss

Preston et al. reported increased fetal loss in women with heritable thrombophilic defects [92]. The authors studied 1,384 women enrolled in the European Prospective Cohort on Thrombophilia (EPCOT). Of 843 women with thrombophilia, 571 had 1,524 pregnancies; of 541 control women, 395 had 1,019 pregnancies. The authors analyzed the frequency of fetal loss (<28 weeks of gestation) and stillbirth (>28 weeks of gestation) jointly and separately. The risk of fetal loss was increased in women with thrombophilia (OR, 1.35, 95 % CI 1.01–1.82). The OR was higher for stillbirth than for miscarriage (3.6; 95 % CI 1.4–9.4 vs. 1.27; 95 % CI 0.94–1.71). The highest OR for stillbirth was in women with combined defects (OR, 14.3; 95 % CI 2.4–86.0) compared with 5.2 (1.5–18.1) in AT deficiency, 2.3 (0.6–8.3) in protein C deficiency, 3.3 (1.0–11.3) in protein S deficiency, and 2.0 (0.5–7.7) with FVL. The authors concluded that women with familial thrombophilia, especially those with combined defects or AT deficiency, have an increased risk of fetal loss, particularly stillbirth.

Gris et al. performed a case–control study in 232 women with a history of one or more second- or third-trimester losses and no history of thrombosis who were matched with 464 controls and tested for thrombophilias and APS [63]. They found at least one thrombophilia in 21.1 % of the patients and in 3.9 % of the controls ($p<0.0001$), with an OR of 5.5 (95 % CI 3.4–9.0) for stillbirth in women positive for any thrombophilia. After logistic regression analysis, four adjusted risk factors for stillbirth remained: protein S deficiency, IgG aCL, IgG aβ_2GPI, and the FVL mutation.

Studies suggest that FVL heterozygotes have a higher relative risk of late pregnancy loss than early first-trimester loss. One possible explanation is that late pregnancy losses reflect thrombosis of the placental vessels, in contrast to first-trimester losses, which are more commonly attributable to other causes, in particular fetal chromosome abnormality. This hypothesis is supported by observations in the Gris et al study that the majority of placentas from women with late fetal loss were reported to show 'maternal vascular disease of the placenta' [63].

In a study of 18 pregnancies with AT deficiency [45, 46], 10 suffered an adverse outcome (55.6 %), including stillbirth (11.1 %), IUGR (33.3 %), abruption (6.7 %), and pre-eclampsia (6.7 %). A lower incidence of pregnancy complications was observed among women with antithrombotic treatment [45]. Of note, Rey et al. [94] and Robertson et al. [36] did not observe an association between AT deficiency and pregnancy loss.

Kupferminc et al. (1999) found a 50 % prevalence of thrombophilias in women with intrauterine fetal death (IUFD) occurring after 23 weeks' gestation [67]. Martinelli et al (2000) reported on 67 women with fetal loss after 20 weeks of pregnancy and 232 controls, for FVL, prothrombin gene mutation, and MTHFR polymorphism. Sixteen percent of the 67 women with fetal loss and 6 % of the controls had either the FVL or the prothrombin gene mutation. The relative risks of late fetal loss in carriers of the FVL and prothrombin gene mutations were 3.2 (95 % CI 1.0–10.9) and 3.3 (95 % CI 1.1–10.3), respectively. Placental investigation showed histological evidence of thrombosis in 76 % of placentas examined [95]. A study that investigated women with IUFD at 27 weeks' gestation or more found that, in 40 women with unexplained IUFD, the prevalence of inherited thrombophilias was 42.5 % compared with 15 % in controls (OR, 2.8; 95 % CI 1.5–5.3, $p=0.001$) [66].

8.10 Management of Adverse Pregnancy Outcome Associated with Thrombophilia

The management of the obstetric patient with thrombophilia is complex [96–98]. Many women with an underlying thrombophilia are healthy with no history of thrombotic or pregnancy complications, while many others without identifiable thrombophilia experience medical and obstetric complications. The risk of thromboembolism and adverse pregnancy outcomes seems to arise from an interplay of medical, obstetric, and family history, along with genetic and environmental factors. Furthermore, current treatment with low molecular weight heparin (LMWH) anticoagulation, at prophylactic or therapeutic dose, is not without risks, albeit small, such as the potential for bleeding and allergic reactions, and is inconvenient. Table 8.3 summarizes observational studies on prevention of poor gestational outcome in carriers of thrombophilia [12, 99–104].

8.10.1 Obstetric Antiphospholipid Syndrome

Screening for APS is recommended in women who suffer recurrent first-trimester miscarriage or who have had late fetal losses [1]. In these patients, the evidence supports a significant increase in live births following treatment with LDA plus heparin compared with LDA alone [105, 106].

Table 8.3 Observational studies on prevention of poor gestational outcome in carriers of thrombophilia

Patients, *n*	Thrombophilia	Obstetric history	Treatment	Live birth with normal outcome	Reference no.
60	APS	RFL	LMWH LDA	70 %	Lima et al. [12]
50	Inherited and acquired	RFL	Enoxaparin (LDA for APS)	46/61 (75 %)	Brenner et al. [99]
25	Factor V Leiden or factor II 20210GA	RFL pre-eclampsia IUGR	UFH or LMWH or LDA	29/31 (93 %)	Grandone et al. [100]
33	Not specified	Pregnancy complications	40 mg enoxaparin LDA	30/33 (91 %)	Kupferminc et al. [101]
276	Inherited and acquired	pre-eclampsia and/or IUGR	40 mg enoxaparin and LDA	Higher birth weight with LMWH	Riyazi et al. [102]
160	Inherited and acquired	Pregnancy complications	40 mg enoxaparin and LDA	Higher birth weight with LMWH	Gris et al. [103]
160	Inherited	Placental abruption	40 mg enoxaparin	Lower incidence of pregnancy complications	Gris et al. [104]

APS antiphospholipid syndrome, *LDA* low-dose aspirin, *RFL* recurrent fetal loss, *IUGR* intrauterine growth restriction, *LMWH* low molecular weight heparin, *UFH* unfractionated heparin

In a meta-analysis of data from five trials involving 334 patients with recurrent miscarriage [107] the overall live birth rates were 74.3 and 55.9 % in women who received a combination of unfractionated/LMWH plus low dose aspirin (LDA) versus that in those treated with LDA alone. Patients who received combination treatment had significantly higher live birth rates (RR 1.301; 95 % CI 1.040, 1.629) than with aspirin alone. No significant differences in pre-eclampsia, preterm labour and birth weight were found between two groups. Accordingly, the British Committee for Standards in Haematology (BCSH) and American College of Chest Physicians (ACCP) recommend that women with obstetric APS with a history of pregnancy loss who meet international consensus criteria, should be treated with prophylactic or intermediate dose UFH or prophylactic LMWH combined with LDA (75–100 mg/daily), in the antepartum period after pregnancy is confirmed. The BCSH and ACCP also recommend that women with aPL should be considered for post-partum thromboprophylaxis [1, 108].

The situation is less clear as regards the management of women who exhibit the remaining International consensus criteria for obstetric APS, i.e. those who suffer one or more unexplained deaths of a morphologically normal fetus at or beyond the 10th week of gestation, one or more premature births of a morphologically normal neonate before 34th week of gestation because of eclampsia, pre-eclampsia, or placental insufficiency [13]. The BCSH and ACCP guidance is that for women with APS and a history of pre-eclampsia, LDA is recommended. However, many high-risk antenatal services extrapolate the use of LMWH and LDA during pregnancy to these cases. Support for this approach comes from observations that defects in placentation are implicated not only in recurrent miscarriage, but also in late placenta-mediated obstetric complications.

The Obstetric Task Force at of the 14th International Congress on Antiphospholipid Antibodies in Rio (2013) stated that recommended treatments for all pregnancy morbidity associated with APS lack well-designed studies to confirm their efficacy [109].

8.10.2 Heritable Thrombophilia

A Cochrane review [110] revealed a paucity of studies on the efficacy and safety of aspirin and heparin in women with a history of RM without apparent causes other than those studies that address heritable thrombophilia. Therefore, the use of anticoagulants in unexplained RM is not recommended. Our knowledge of the optimal treatment during pregnancy in patients with heritable thrombophilia (except for the role of LDA in the prevention of pre-eclampsia: see below) is also limited. Previous data suggested that certain risk groups should be screened for thrombophilia, as the evidence suggested a high recurrence rate of complications in future pregnancies. These at-risk groups included women with a personal or family history of thromboembolism, recurrent first- and second-trimester loss, severe pre-eclampsia, IUGR, stillbirth, or abruptio placentae. Ideally, testing should take place between pregnancies since protein S levels fall and APCR increases during normal pregnancy [111].

A meta-analysis by Duley et al. (2001) demonstrated that the use of low-dose aspirin is associated with a 15 % reduction in the risk of pre-eclampsia (32 trials with 29,331 women, relative risk [RR] 0.85; 95 % CI 0.78–0.92) and a 14 % reduction in the risk of fetal or neonatal death (30 trials with 30,093 women, RR, 0.86; 95 % CI 0.75–0.99). This reduction in fetal and neonatal death was greatest among high-risk women (4,134 women, RR, 0.73; 95 % CI 0.56–0.96) [112]. However, the combined role of low-dose aspirin and heparin treatment in inherited thrombophilia, particularly in later pregnancy, has not been evaluated in randomized controlled trials. Many studies suggest that they may have a complementary role.

In a large retrospective cohort study performed by North et al., women with renal disease in pregnancy were allocated to a "no-treatment" control group, a LDA group, or a group that received prophylactic heparin combined with aspirin and/or dipyridamole [113]. Pre-eclampsia was less common in the heparin group compared with the no-treatment group and the aspirin group.

A study by Kupferminc et al. included women with known thrombophilia and a history of severe pre-eclampsia, abruption, IUGR, or stillbirth [101]. Women were treated with subcutaneous enoxaparin 40 mg daily and aspirin 100 mg daily from 8 to 12 weeks' gestation onward. The mean gestational age at delivery in the untreated women was 32.1 ± 5.0 weeks as compared to 37.6 ± 2.3 weeks in women treated with enoxaparin ($p<0.001$). The mean birth weight of the infants from the control group was 1.175 ± 0.59 kg compared to 2.719 ± 0.526 kg in the treated women ($p<0.001$). Pregnancy complications occurred in only 9 % of women, and neither severe pre-eclampsia nor perinatal deaths occurred in the treated women [101].

Similarly, favorable effects were suggested in a small study that evaluated treatment with LMWH combined with aspirin in pregnant women with thrombophilia and a history of early-onset pre-eclampsia and/or IUGR [102]. Pregnant women with thrombophilia were randomized to low-dose aspirin and LMWH (n = 26) or aspirin alone (n = 19). There was no difference in the overall birth weight between the groups. However, when considering the 18 patients with a single thrombophilia (i.e. excluding 8 patients with multiple thrombophilias), birth weights were significantly higher ($p=0.019$) compared to the 19 with no coagulation abnormality. In addition, two perinatal deaths occurred in the aspirin group vs. no perinatal death in the aspirin plus LMWH group. These preliminary studies suggest that LMWH may have an additional beneficial effect on the pregnancy outcome of women with a history of severe pre-eclampsia and/or IUGR and documented thrombophilia.

In the Live-Enox study, the incidence of pre-eclampsia, placental abruption, and IUGR was substantially lower with LMWH prophylaxis than in prior untreated pregnancies [10, 114]. A favorable effect on birth weight was noted in women with thrombophilia and prior fetal loss that were treated with LMWH and aspirin [103].

A pilot study investigated the effectiveness of enoxaparin in women with a previous placental abruption and inherited thrombophilia. Women were randomized to either a prophylactic daily dose of enoxaparin starting from the time of a positive pregnancy test (n = 80) or no enoxaparin (n = 80). Enoxaparin was safe, with no obvious side-effects such as thrombocytopenia or major bleeding events. Furthermore, enoxaparin reduced the occurrence of placental vascular complications [104].

Leeda et al. studied the effects of folic acid and vitamin B6 supplementation in women with hyperhomocysteinemia and a history of pre-eclampsia or IUGR [115]. A total of 207 consecutive patients with a history of pre-eclampsia or IUGR were tested for hyperhomocysteinemia. Thirty-seven were found to have raised levels and were treated with folic acid and vitamin B6, and 27 had a second methionine-loading test after vitamin supplementation. This showed that 14 patients became pregnant while receiving vitamin B6, folic acid, and aspirin; 7 of these 14 were complicated by pre-eclampsia. Birth weights were 2.867 ± 0.648 kg compared with 1.088 ± 0.57 kg in the previous pregnancies ($p<0.001$). Therefore, in women with hyperhomocysteinemia and a history of pre-eclampsia or IUGR, vitamin B6 and folic acid can correct the methionine-loading test and appear to have a favorable effect on birth weight, but not pre-eclampsia.

The findings of the FRUIT trial, (FRactionated heparin in pregnant women with a history of Utero-placental Insufficiency and Thrombophilia), a randomized controlled trial in 139 women, have been published. This study found that adding LMWH to aspirin before 12 weeks of gestation reduces recurrent hypertensive disease (HD; pre-eclampsia, hemolysis, elevated liver enzymes and low platelets [HELLP] syndrome and eclampsia) and/or small-for- gestational age (SGA) in women with previous early-onset HD and/or SGA, in the context of an inheritable thrombophilia without aPL [116].

More recently, the Thrombophilia in Pregnancy Prophylaxis Study (TIPPS) [117] reported on the effectiveness of antenatal thromboprophylaxis in woman with confirmed thrombophilia in reducing the risk of placenta-mediated pregnancy complications (i.e. pre-eclamspia, birth of a small for gestational age baby (SGA), pregnancy loss and/or placental abruption) or pregnancy associated VTE. Inclusion criteria included a past history of obstetric morbidity, family history of thrombophilia, laboratory evidence of a thrombophilia and personal history of below knee DVT/superficial thrombophlebitis and being between 4 and 20 weeks gestation. Women with aPL, Women with aPL, 8% in the dalteparin and 7% in the no dalteparin arms respectively, were also included. Women with an indication for anticoagulation were excluded. In this study 146 and 143 women respectively, were randomised between 2000 and 2012 to receive antenatal dalteparin (5,000 units daily until 20 weeks and thereafter dalteparin 5,000 units twice daily until at least 37 weeks) versus no dalteparin in a 1:1 allocation. The mean gestational age at enrolment was 12 weeks. The authors concluded that antepartum prophylactic dalteparin does not reduce the occurrence of venous thromboembolism, pregnancy loss, or placenta-mediated pregnancy complications in pregnant women with thrombophilia at high risk of these complications and is associated with an increased risk of minor bleeding. Dalteparin did not reduce the incidence of the primary composite outcome in both intention-to-treat analysis (dalteparin 25/146 [17.1 %; 95 % CI 11.4–24.2 %] vs no dalteparin 27/143 [18.9 %; 95 % CI 12.8–26.3 %]; risk difference −1.8 % [95 % CI −10.6 to 7.1 %]) and on-treatment analysis (dalteparin 28/143 [19.6 %] vs no dalteparin 24/141 [17.0 %]; risk difference +2.6 % [95 % CI −6.4 to 11.6 %]).

The occurrence of major bleeding in the TIPPS trial did not differ between the two groups. However, minor bleeding was more common in the dalteparin group (28/143 [19.6 %]) than in the no dalteparin group (13/141 [9.2 %]; risk difference 10.4 %, 95 % CI 2.3–18.4; p=0.01) [117]. Limitations of this study include that the trial design permitted commencement of dalteparin after placentation has been completed, which may lead to an underestimate of the benefit of dalteparin as treatment after placentation is complete may potentially be ineffective [118]. In addition, the statistical power calculations are based on an aggregate of adverse outcomes, and thus the study may be underpowered as regards the assessment of the results in women with individual late placenta-mediated late obstetric complications.

A meta-analysis based on six RCTs that included a total of 848 pregnant women with prior placenta-mediated pregnancy complications, suggested that LMWH may be a promising therapy for recurrent, especially severe, placenta-mediated pregnancy complications, but further research is required [119].

8.10.3 Current Approach to Management in Women with Thrombophilia

The BCSH recommends that antithrombotic therapy should not be given to pregnant women with a history of pregnancy complications based on testing for heritable thrombophilia. They state that there would only be a rational basis for recommending that antithrombotic therapy be given to pregnant women with a history of pregnancy complications based on testing for heritable thrombophilia, if randomised controlled trials with a no-treatment or placebo arm in women with a history of pregnancy complications indicate a benefit in women with pregnancy complications and heritable thrombophilia, as compared with women without thrombophilia [120]. The ACCP advises that in women with inherited thrombophilia and a history of pregnancy complications, not to use antithrombotic prophylaxis [108]. The National Collaborating Centre for Women's and Children's Health in the UK states that the evidence on the association between thrombophilias and hypertensive disorders remains unclear and is of variable quality. Their recommendation is to not routinely perform screening for thrombophilia in women who have had pre-eclampsia [121]. For women considered at risk for preeclampsia, the ACCP recommends LDA throughout pregnancy, starting from the second trimester. Unfractionated or LMWH are not recommended for thrombophilic women with a history of pre-eclampsia or other adverse pregnancy outcomes [108].

The TIPPS trial does highlight the need for further adequately powered randomized controlled trials to determine optimal management in women with late obstetric morbidity. Such studies are needed before definitive recommendations can be made about the treatment of thrombophilias associated with late placental vascular-mediated obstetric complications in pregnancy. In the presence of the uncertainties surrounding the management of these women, decisions about antithrombotic therapy should be based on an individual risk/benefit assessment.

Assessment of the maternal thrombotic risk during pregnancy should also be incorporated into the decision-making process regarding prophylaxis. In some centers, high dose folic acid and LDA are used throughout pregnancy on an empirical basis in women with late placental vascular-mediated obstetric complications. Management should ideally be within a high risk antenatal clinic setting and treatment decisions discussed with the patient and documented.

8.11 Unresolved Issues

8.11.1 Fetal Genotype

While it has been suggested that fetal thrombophilia status is important for the outcome of pregnancy [47], there are several reasons to suggest that this may not be the case. First, most thrombophilic polymorphisms are mild risk factors for gestational vascular complications and gestational thromboembolism. Secondly, thrombotic changes are noted mainly on the maternal side of the uteroplacental unit. Thirdly, LMWH, that is known to not cross the placenta, is beneficial. Thus, unless there is a severe thrombophilic defect (e.g. homozygous protein C deficiency), fetal thrombophilic status is probably not a major contributor to gestational vascular complications or thromboembolism. However, further data from studies addressing the triad of mother, father and fetus are needed to clarify this issue.

8.11.2 Women Without Thrombophilia Who Have Late Pregnancy Loss

When evaluation for the current known thrombophilias is negative, it is theoretically possible that an as yet undiscovered thrombophilia may be implicated in placental thrombotic changes found in women with gestational vascular complications. A pilot randomized controlled trial studied the effect of LMWH prophylaxis in women without thrombophilia and previous adverse pregnancy outcome. LMWH significantly reduced the incidence of severe pre-eclampsia, IUGR, abruption, and IUFD after 20 weeks [122]. Following this preliminary experience with antithrombotic therapy in these women suggesting potential benefit, further studies are required.

8.12 Conclusions and Future Perspectives

A number of issues in this field need to be addressed. Late pregnancy complications such as severe pre-eclampsia and placental insufficiency at less than 34 weeks gestation are relatively common, as are thrombophilic risk factors, with these risk factors associated with an increased risk of venous thromboembolism during pregnancy. The precise role of the known hereditary or acquired thrombophilias and whether other genetic or acquired thrombophilias will be found to play a role remain to be determined. Polymorphisms at the thrombomodulin and endothelial protein C receptor genes [123, 124] may be associated with recurrent fetal loss. It has also been suggested that circulating microparticles may play a role in unexplained fetal loss [125]. While the mechanism(s) involved in the development of vascular gestational pathologies has(ve) not been established, it is intriguing to speculate whether antithrombotic strategies or other novel strategies (the reader should refer to Chap. 9 on potential future therapeutic options for pre-eclampsia) will be of value in this setting.

The management of the obstetric patient with thrombophilia, or with an obstetric history that could be associated with thrombophilia, is controversial due to the fact that there is a paucity of evidence-based guidelines to underpin all aspects of management. The role of antithrombotic treatment should continue to be explored in prospective, appropriately designed and adequately powered multicenter clinical trials, with the aim to improve gestational outcomes in this large population of women.

8.13 Case Studies

Case Study 1

A 35-year-old woman had a normal pregnancy with a normal vaginal delivery at 41 weeks' gestation of a healthy male infant, birth weight (BW) 3,800 g. She went on to have two early miscarriages, at 7 and 8 weeks' gestation, and then a stillbirth at 29 weeks' gestation, associated with severe intrauterine growth restriction. An autopsy showed a morphologically normal fetus, weight 750 g, with extensive placental infarction. Testing for antiphospholipid antibodies showed high positive IgG anti beta 2 glycoprotein 1 (aβ_2GPI) antibodies with the remainder of the antiphospholipid antibodies (IgM aβ_2GPI antibodies, lupus anticoagulant and IgG and gM anticardiolipin antibodies) negative. She went on to have four successful pregnancies, with four live births at term. These were managed within a high risk antenatal clinic setting, and all treated with low dose aspirin 75 mg daily and subcutaneous dalteparin 5,000 units daily throughout pregnancy and for 6 weeks postpartum. A bone mineral densitometry scan done after her last delivery showed severe osteopenia and she was referred for consideration of treatment with bisphosphonate.

Case Study 2

A 35-year-old woman had severe pre-eclampsia in her first pregnancy resulting in a stillbirth at 26 weeks gestation. She then had a miscarriage at 12 weeks gestation in her next pregnancy. In her third pregnancy she was commenced on low dose aspirin (LDA) 75 mg daily at 12 weeks gestation. Enoxaparin 40 mg daily subcutaneously was added at 26 weeks gestation and she had a stillbirth at 27 weeks gestation. Autopsy showed a morphologically normal but severely growth-restricted fetus, weight 500 g. The placenta showed extensive thrombosis and infarction. A thrombophilia screen, undertaken 3 months later, showed a low free protein S level confirmed on repeat testing (while not pregnant) and no evidence of antiphospholipid antibodies. Two subsequent pregnancies, when she was aged 39 and 41 years, were managed in a high risk antenatal clinic setting and supported with LDA, which was commenced pre-conceptually, and subcutaneous dalteparin 5,000 units daily from 6 weeks' gestation. During these pregnancies, she had regular fetal scans that showed sustained growth throughout pregnancy. These pregnancies resulted in delivery at 37 and 38 weeks' gestation respectively of two healthy male infants weighing 2,440 and 2,480 g respectively. In both supported pregnancies, fetal scans showed normal progression of fetal growth, but in the latter pregnancy there was evidence of uterine artery notching from 32 weeks' gestation onwards.

Key Learning Points

- Late pregnancy complications such as pre-eclampsia and placental insufficiency at less than 34 weeks gestation are relatively common, as are thrombophilic risk factors, with these risk factors associated with an increased risk of venous thromboembolism during pregnancy.
- Although combined treatment with low dose aspirin and low-molecular-weight heparin appears to have improved perinatal outcome in some women with a poor obstetric history and inherited thrombophilias, there is a lack of clear evidence from appropriately designed and adequately powered studies.
- Except for fetal death, there are limitations in the quality of the data supporting the association of antiphospholipid antibodies (aPL) with obstetric complications included in the current APS classification criteria. Recommended treatments for all pregnancy morbidity associated with aPL lack well-designed studies to confirm their efficacy.
- Further adequately powered RCTs are needed for definitive recommendations on the treatment of individual late placenta-mediated obstetric complications associated with thrombophilias.
- In the meantime, decisions about antithrombotic therapy should be based on an individual risk/benefit assessment. Assessment of maternal thrombotic risk during pregnancy should also be incorporated into the decision-making process regarding thromboprophylaxis. Treatment decisions should be discussed with the patient and documented.

References

1. Keeling D, Mackie I, Moore GW, Greer IA, Greaves M. Guidelines on the investigation and management of antiphospholipid syndrome. Br J Haematol. 2012;157:47–58.
2. Pengo V, Tripodi A, Reber G, Rand JH, Ortel TL, Galli M, De Groot PG. Update of the guidelines for lupus anticoagulant detection. Subcommittee on Lupus Anticoagulant/Antiphospholipid Antibody of the Scientific and Standardisation Committee of the International Society on Thrombosis and Haemostasis. J Thromb Haemost. 2009;7:1737–40.
3. Miyakis S, Lockshin MD, Atsumi T, Branch DW, Brey RL, Cervera R, et al. International consensus statement on an update of the classification criteria for definite antiphospholipid syndrome (APS). J Thromb Haemost. 2006;4(2):295–306.
4. Bremme K, Ostlund E, Almqvist I, Heinonen K, Blomback M. Enhanced thrombin generation and fibrinolytic activity in normal pregnancy and the puerperium. Obstet Gynecol. 1992;80(1):132–7.
5. Bremme KA. Haemostatic changes in pregnancy. Best Pract Res Clin Haematol. 2003;16(2):153–68.
6. Hellgren M. Hemostasis during normal pregnancy and puerperium. Semin Thromb Hemost. 2003;29:125–30.
7. Comp PC, Thurnau GR, Welsh J, Esmon CT. Functional and immunologic protein S levels are decreased during pregnancy. Blood. 1986;68(4):881–5.
8. Cumming AM, Tait RC, Fildes S, Yoong A, Keeney S, Hay CR. Development of resistance to activated protein C during pregnancy. Br J Haematol. 1995;90(3):725–7.
9. Stirling Y, Woolf L, North WR, Seghatchian MJ, Meade TW. Haemostasis in normal pregnancy. Thromb Haemost. 1984;52(2):176–82.
10. Kruithof EK, Tran-Thang C, Gudinchet A, Hauert J, Nicoloso G, Genton C, et al. Fibrinolysis in pregnancy: a study of plasminogen activator inhibitors. Blood. 1987;69(2):460–6.
11. Giavarina D, Mezzena G, Dorizzi RM, Soffiati G. Reference interval of D-dimer in pregnant women. Clin Biochem. 2001;34(4):331–3.
12. Lima F, Khamashta MA, Buchanan NM, Kerslake S, Hunt BJ, Hughes GR. A study of sixty pregnancies in patients with the antiphospholipid syndrome. Clin Exp Rheumatol. 1996;14(2):131–6.
13. Arachchillage DR, Machin SJ, Mackie IJ, Cohen H. Diagnosis and management of non-criteria obstetric antiphospholipid syndrome. Thromb Haemost. 2015;113(1):13–9.

14. Ruffatti A, Olivieri S, Tonello M, Bortolati M, Bison E, Salvan E, et al. Influence of different IgG anticardiolipin antibody cut-off values on antiphospholipid syndrome classification. J Thromb Haemost. 2008;6:1693–6.
15. Gardiner C, Hills J, Machin SJ, Cohen H. Diagnosis of antiphospholipid syndrome in routine clinical practice. Lupus. 2013;22:18–25.
16. Mekinian A, Loire-Berson P, Nicaise-Roland P, Lachassinne E, Stirnemann J, Boffa MC, et al. Outcomes and treatment of obstetrical antiphospholipid syndrome in women with low antiphospholipid antibody levels. J Reprod Immunol. 2012;94:222–6.
17. Alijotas-Reig J, Ferrer-Oliveras R. The European Registry on Obstetric Antiphospholipid Syndrome (EUROAPS): a preliminary first year report. Lupus. 2012;21:766–8.
18. Out HJ, Bruinse HW, Christiaens GC, van Vliet M, De Groot PG, Nieuwenhuis HK, et al. A prospective, controlled multicenter study on the obstetric risks of pregnant women with antiphospholipid antibodies. Am J Obstet Gynecol. 1992;167(1):26–32.
19. De Wolf F, Carreras LO, Moerman P, Vermylen J, Van Assche A, Renaer M. Decidual vasculopathy and extensive placental infarction in a patient with repeated thromboembolic accidents, recurrent fetal loss, and a lupus anticoagulant. Am J Obstet Gynecol. 1982;142:829–34.
20. Hanly JG, Gladman DD, Rose TH, Laskin CA, Urowitz MB. Lupus pregnancy. A prospective study of placental changes. Arthritis Rheum. 1988;31:358–66.
21. Out HJ, Kooijman CD, Bruinse HW, Derksen RH. Histopathological findings in placentae from patients with intrauterine fetal death and antiphospholipid antibodies. Eur J Obstet Gynecol Reprod Biol. 1991;41:179–86.
22. Di SN, Luigi MP, Marco D, Fiorella DN, Silvia D, Clara DM, et al. Pregnancies complicated with antiphospholipid syndrome: the pathogenic mechanism of antiphospholipid antibodies: a review of the literature. Ann N Y Acad Sci. 2007;1108:505–14.
23. Rand JH, Wu XX, Andree HA, Lockwood CJ, Guller S, Scher J, et al. Pregnancy loss in the antiphospholipid-antibody syndrome – a possible thrombogenic mechanism. N Engl J Med. 1997;337(3):154–60.
24. Breen KA, Seed P, Parmar K, Moore GW, Stuart-Smith SE, Hunt BJ. Complement activation in patients with isolated antiphospholipid antibodies or primary antiphospholipid syndrome. Thromb Haemost. 2012;107:423–9.
25. Salmon JE, Girardi G. Antiphospholipid antibodies and pregnancy loss: a disorder of inflammation. J Reprod Immunol. 2008;77:51–6.
26. Do Prado AD, Piovesan DM, Staub HL, Horta BL. Association of anticardiolipin antibodies with preeclampsia: a systematic review and meta-analysis. Obstet Gynecol. 2010;116:1433–43.
27. Abou-Nasser K, Carrier M, Ramsay T, Rodger MA. The association between antiphospholipid antibodies with preeclampsia: a systematic review and meta-analysis. Thromb Res. 2011;128:77–85.
28. Chauleur C, Galanaud JP, Alonso S, Cochery-Nouvellon E, Balducchi JP, Marès P, et al. Observational study of pregnant women with a previous spontaneous abortion before the 10th gestation week with and without antiphospholipid antibodies. J Thromb Haemost. 2010;8(4):699–706.
29. Bloomenthal D, von Dadelszen P, Liston R, Magee L, Tsang P. The effect of factor V Leiden carriage on maternal and fetal health. CMAJ. 2002;167(1):48–54.
30. Rees DC, Cox M, Clegg JB. World distribution of factor V Leiden. Lancet. 1995;346(8983):1133–4.
31. Rai R, Shlebak A, Cohen H, Backos M, Holmes Z, Marriott K, Regan L. Factor V. Leiden and acquired activated protein C resistance among 1000 women with recurrent miscarriage. Hum Reprod. 2001;16(5):961–5.
32. Zoller B, de Garcia FP, Hillarp A, Dahlback B. Thrombophilia as a multigenic disease. Haematologica. 1999;84(1):59–70.
33. Rosendaal FR, Doggen CJ, Zivelin A, et al. Geographic distribution of the 20210 G to A prothrombin variant. Thromb Haemostas. 1998;79:706–8.
34. Conard J, Horellou MH, Van DP, Lecompte T, Samama M. Thrombosis and pregnancy in congenital deficiencies in AT III, protein C or protein S: study of 78 women. Thromb Haemost. 1990;63(2):319–20.
35. Lockwood CJ. Inherited thrombophilias in pregnant patients: detection and treatment paradigm. Obstet Gynecol. 2002;99(2):333–41.
36. Robertson L, Wu O, Langhorne P, Twaddle S, Clark P, Lowe GD, et al. Thrombophilia in pregnancy: a systematic review. Br J Haematol. 2006;132(2):171–96.
37. Rodger MA, Betancourt MT, Clark P, Lindqvist PG, Dizon-Townson D, Said J, et al. The association of factor V Leiden and prothrombin gene mutation and placenta-mediated pregnancy complications: a systematic review and meta-analysis of prospective cohort studies. PLoS Med. 2010;7(6):e1000292.
38. Rodger MA, Walker MC, Smith GN, Wells PS, Ramsay T, Langlois NJ, Carson N, Carrier M, Rennicks White R, Shachkina S, Wen SW. Is thrombophilia associated with placenta-mediated pregnancy complications? A prospective cohort study. J Thromb Haemost. 2014;12(4):469–78.
39. Many A, Schreiber L, Rosner S, Lessing JB, Eldor A, Kupferminc MJ. Pathologic features of the placenta in women with severe pregnancy complications and thrombophilia. Obstet Gynecol. 2001;98(6):1041–4.
40. Mousa HA, Alfirevic Z. Do placental lesions reflect thrombophilia state in women with adverse pregnancy outcome? Hum Reprod. 2000;15(8):1830–3.
41. Sikkema JM, Franx A, Bruinse HW, van der Wijk NG, de Valk HW, Nikkels PG. Placental pathology

in early onset pre-eclampsia and intrauterine growth restriction in women with and without thrombophilia. Placenta. 2002;23(4):337–42.

42. Arias F, Romero R, Joist H, Kraus FT. Thrombophilia: a mechanism of disease in women with adverse pregnancy outcome and thrombotic lesions in the placenta. J Matern Fetal Med. 1998;7(6):277–86.
43. Hack M, Flannery DJ, Schluchter M, Cartar L, Borawski E, Klein N. Outcomes in young adulthood for very-low-birth-weight infants. N Engl J Med. 2002;346(3):149–57.
44. Resnik R. Intrauterine growth restriction. Obstet Gynecol. 2002;99(3):490–6.
45. Barker DJ. The fetal and infant origins of adult disease. BMJ. 1990;301(6761):1111.
46. Grandone E, Margaglione M, Colaizzo D, Pavone G, Paladini D, Martinelli P, et al. Lower birth-weight in neonates of mothers carrying factor V G1691A and factor II A(20210) mutations. Haematologica. 2002;87(2):177–81.
47. von Kries R, Junker R, Oberle D, Kosch A, Nowak-Gottl U. Foetal growth restriction in children with prothrombotic risk factors. Thromb Haemost. 2001;86(4):1012–6.
48. Sabadell J, Casellas M, Alijotas-Reig J, Arellano-Rodrigo E, Cabero L. Inherited antithrombin deficiency and pregnancy: maternal and fetal outcomes. Eur J Obstet Gynecol Reprod Biol. 2010;149(1):47–51.
49. Sanson BJ, Friederich PW, Simioni P, Zanardi S, Hilsman MV, Girolami A, et al. The risk of abortion and stillbirth in antithrombin-, protein C-, and protein S-deficient women. Thromb Haemost. 1996;75(3):387–8.
50. Dizon-Townson DS, Meline L, Nelson LM, Varner M, Ward K. Fetal carriers of the factor V Leiden mutation are prone to miscarriage and placental infarction. Am J Obstet Gynecol. 1997;177(2):402–5.
51. de Vries JI, Dekker GA, Huijgens PC, Jakobs C, Blomberg BM, van Geijn HP. Hyperhomocysteinaemia and protein S deficiency in complicated pregnancies. Br J Obstet Gynaecol. 1997;104(11):1248–54.
52. Wiener-Megnagi Z, Ben-Shlomo I, Goldberg Y, Shalev E. Resistance to activated protein C and the leiden mutation: high prevalence in patients with abruptio placentae. Am J Obstet Gynecol. 1998;179(6 Pt 1):1565–7.
53. Dudding TE, Attia J. The association between adverse pregnancy outcomes and maternal factor V Leiden genotype: a meta-analysis. Thromb Haemost. 2004;91(4):700–11.
54. Kosmas IP, Tatsioni A, Ioannidis JP. Association of Leiden mutation in factor V gene with hypertension in pregnancy and pre-eclampsia: a meta-analysis. J Hypertens. 2003;21(7):1221–8.
55. Lin J, August P. Genetic thrombophilias and pre-eclampsia: a meta-analysis. Obstet Gynecol. 2005;105(1):182–92.
56. Muetze S, Leeners B, Ortlepp JR, Kuse S, Tag CG, Weiskirchen R, et al. Maternal factor V Leiden mutation is associated with HELLP syndrome in Caucasian women. Acta Obstet Gynecol Scand. 2008;87(6):635–42.
57. Kist WJ, Janssen NG, Kalk JJ, Hague WM, Dekker GA, de Vries JI. Thrombophilias and adverse pregnancy outcome – a confounded problem! Thromb Haemost. 2008;99(1):77–85.
58. Vollset SE, Refsum H, Irgens LM, Emblem BM, Tverdal A, Gjessing HK, et al. Plasma total homocysteine, pregnancy complications, and adverse pregnancy outcomes: the Hordaland Homocysteine study. Am J Clin Nutr. 2000;71(4):962–8.
59. Morgan JA, Bombell S, McGuire W. Association of plasminogen activator inhibitor-type 1 (−675 4G/5G) polymorphism with pre-eclampsia: systematic review. PLoS One. 2013;8(2):e56907. doi:10.1371/journal.pone.0056907. Epub 2013 Feb 15.
60. Kupferminc MJ, Peri H, Zwang E, Yaron Y, Wolman I, Eldor A. High prevalence of the prothrombin gene mutation in women with intrauterine growth retardation, abruptio placentae and second trimester loss. Acta Obstet Gynecol Scand. 2000;79(11):963–7.
61. Higgins JR, Kaiser T, Moses EK, North R, Brennecke SP. Prothrombin G20210A mutation: is it associated with pre-eclampsia? Gynecol Obstet Invest. 2000;50(4):254–7.
62. Morrison ER, Miedzybrodzka ZH, Campbell DM, Haites NE, Wilson BJ, Watson MS, et al. Prothrombotic genotypes are not associated with pre-eclampsia and gestational hypertension: results from a large population-based study and systematic review. Thromb Haemost. 2002;87(5):779–85.
63. Gris JC, Quere I, Monpeyroux F, Mercier E, Ripart-Neveu S, Tailland ML, et al. Case–control study of the frequency of thrombophilic disorders in couples with late foetal loss and no thrombotic antecedent–the Nimes Obstetricians and Haematologists Study5 (NOHA5). Thromb Haemost. 1999;81(6):891–9.
64. Agorastos T, Karavida A, Lambropoulos A, Constantinidis T, Tzitzimikas S, Chrisafi S, et al. Factor V Leiden and prothrombin G20210A mutations in pregnancies with adverse outcome. J Matern Fetal Neonatal Med. 2002;12(4):267–73.
65. Kupferminc MJ, Many A, Bar-Am A, Lessing JB, Ascher-Landsberg J. Mid-trimester severe intrauterine growth restriction is associated with a high prevalence of thrombophilia. BJOG. 2002;109(12):1373–6.
66. Many A, Elad R, Yaron Y, Eldor A, Lessing JB, Kupferminc MJ. Third-trimester unexplained intrauterine fetal death is associated with inherited thrombophilia. Obstet Gynecol. 2002;99(5 Pt 1):684–7.
67. Kupferminc MJ, Eldor A, Steinman N, Many A, Bar-Am A, Jaffa A, et al. Increased frequency of genetic thrombophilia in women with complications of pregnancy. N Engl J Med. 1999;340(1):9–13.

68. Martinelli P, Grandone E, Colaizzo D, Paladini D, Scianname N, Margaglione M, et al. Familial thrombophilia and the occurrence of fetal growth restriction. Haematologica. 2001;86(4):428–31.
69. Infante-Rivard C, Rivard GE, Yotov WV, Genin E, Guiguet M, Weinberg C, et al. Absence of association of thrombophilia polymorphisms with intrauterine growth restriction. N Engl J Med. 2002;347(1):19–25.
70. Howley HE, Walker M, Rodger MA. A systematic review of the association between factor V Leiden or prothrombin gene variant and intrauterine growth restriction. Am J Obstet Gynecol. 2005;192(3):694–708.
71. Clark P, Walker ID, Govan L, Wu O, Greer IA. The GOAL study: a prospective examination of the impact of factor V Leiden and ABO(H) blood groups on haemorrhagic and thrombotic pregnancy outcomes. Br J Haematol. 2008;140(2):236–40.
72. Dudding T, Heron J, Thakkinstian A, Nurk E, Golding J, Pembrey M, et al. Factor V Leiden is associated with pre-eclampsia but not with fetal growth restriction: a genetic association study and meta-analysis. J Thromb Haemost. 2008;6(11):1869–75.
73. McCowan LM, Craigie S, Taylor RS, Ward C, McLintock C, North RA. Inherited thrombophilias are not increased in "idiopathic" small-for-gestational-age pregnancies. Am J Obstet Gynecol. 2003;188(4):981–5.
74. Facchinetti F, Marozio L, Frusca T, Grandone E, Venturini P, Tiscia GL, et al. Maternal thrombophilia and the risk of recurrence of preeclampsia. Am J Obstet Gynecol. 2009;200(1):46.e1–5.
75. Grandone E, Margaglione M, Colaizzo D, Cappucci G, Paladini D, Martinelli P, et al. Factor V Leiden, C > T MTHFR polymorphism and genetic susceptibility to preeclampsia. Thromb Haemost. 1997;77(6):1052–4.
76. Mello G, Parretti E, Marozio L, Pizzi C, Lojacono A, Frusca T, et al. Thrombophilia is significantly associated with severe preeclampsia: results of a large-scale, case-controlled study. Hypertension. 2005;46(6):1270–4.
77. Kahn SR, Platt R, McNamara H, Rozen R, Chen MF, Genest Jr J, et al. Inherited thrombophilia and preeclampsia within a multicenter cohort: the Montreal Preeclampsia Study. Am J Obstet Gynecol. 2009;200(2):151–9.
78. Grandone E, Margaglione M, Colaizzo D, Cappucci G, Scianname N, Montanaro S, et al. Prothrombotic genetic risk factors and the occurrence of gestational hypertension with or without proteinuria. Thromb Haemost. 1999;81(3):349–52.
79. Murphy RP, Donoghue C, Nallen RJ, D'Mello M, Regan C, Whitehead AS, et al. Prospective evaluation of the risk conferred by factor V Leiden and thermolabile methylenetetrahydrofolate reductase polymorphisms in pregnancy. Arterioscler Thromb Vasc Biol. 2000;20(1):266–70.
80. Benedetto C, Marozio L, Salton L, Maula V, Chieppa G, Massobrio M. Factor V Leiden and factor II G20210A in preeclampsia and HELLP syndrome. Acta Obstet Gynecol Scand. 2002;81(12):1095–100.
81. Nurk E, Tell GS, Refsum H, Ueland PM, Vollset SE. Factor V Leiden, pregnancy complications and adverse outcomes: the Hordaland Homocysteine Study. QJM. 2006;99(5):289–98.
82. Alfirevic Z, Mousa HA, Martlew V, Briscoe L, Perez-Casal M, Toh CH. Postnatal screening for thrombophilia in women with severe pregnancy com-plications. Obstet Gynecol. 2001;97(5 Pt 1):753–9.
83. Lindqvist PG, Svensson PJ, Marsaal K, Grennert L, Luterkort M, Dahlback B. Activated protein C resistance (FV:Q506) and pregnancy. Thromb Haemost. 1999;81(4):532–7.
84. De Groot CJ, Bloemenkamp KW, Duvekot EJ, Helmerhorst FM, Bertina RM, Van Der Meer F, et al. Preeclampsia and genetic risk factors for thrombosis: a case–control study. Am J Obstet Gynecol. 1999;181(4):975–80.
85. van der Molen EF, Verbruggen B, Novakova I, Eskes TK, Monnens LA, Blom HJ. Hyperhomocysteinemia and other thrombotic risk factors in women with placental vasculopathy. BJOG. 2000;107(6):785–91.
86. Prochazka M, Happach C, Marsal K, Dahlback B, Lindqvist PG. Factor V Leiden in pregnancies complicated by placental abruption. BJOG. 2003;110(5):462–6.
87. Prochazka M, Lubusky M, Slavik L, Hrachovec P, Zielina P, Kudela M, et al. Frequency of selected thrombophilias in women with placental abruption. Aust N Z J Obstet Gynaecol. 2007;47(4):297–301.
88. Facco F, You W, Grobman W. Genetic thrombophilias and intrauterine growth restriction: a meta-analysis. Obstet Gynecol. 2009;113(6):1206–16.
89. Nath CA, Ananth CV, DeMarco C, Vintzileos AM. Low birthweight in relation to placental abruption and maternal thrombophilia status. Am J Obstet Gynecol. 2008;198(3):293–5.
90. Alfirevic Z, Roberts D, Martlew V. How strong is the association between maternal thrombophilia and adverse pregnancy outcome? A systematic review. Eur J Obstet Gynecol Reprod Biol. 2002;101(1):6–14.
91. Ananth CV, Nath CA, Philipp C, New Jersey Placental Abruption Study. The Normal anticoagulant system and risk of placental abruption: protein C, protein S and resistance to activated protein C. J Matern Fetal Neonatal Med. 2010;23(12):1377–83.
92. Preston FE, Rosendaal FR, Walker ID, Briet E, Berntorp E, Conard J, et al. Increased fetal loss in women with heritable thrombophilia. Lancet. 1996;348(9032):913–6.
93. Pasquier E, Bohec C, Mottier D, Jaffuel S, Mercier B, Ferec C, et al. Inherited thrombophilias and unexplained pregnancy loss: an incident case–control study. J Thromb Haemost. 2009;7(2):306–11.

94. Rey E, Kahn SR, David M, Shrier I. Thrombophilic disorders and fetal loss: a meta-analysis. Lancet. 2003;361(9361):901–8.
95. Martinelli I, Taioli E, Cetin I, Marinoni A, Gerosa S, Villa MV, et al. Mutations in coagulation factors in women with unexplained late fetal loss. N Engl J Med. 2000;343(14):1015–8.
96. Cleary-Goldman J, Bettes B, Robinson JN, Norwitz E, Schulkin J. Thrombophilia and the obstetric patient. Obstet Gynecol. 2007;110(3):669–74.
97. Rodger MA, Carrier M, Keely E, Karovitch A, Nimrod C, Walker M, et al. The management of thrombophilia during pregnancy: a Canadian survey. J Obstet Gynaecol Can. 2002;24(12):946–52.
98. Walker ID, Kujovich JL, Greer IA, Rey E, David M, Salmon JE, et al. The use of LMWH in pregnancies at risk: new evidence or perception? J Thromb Haemost. 2005;3(4):778–93.
99. Brenner B, Hoffman R, Carp H, Dulitsky M, Younis J. Efficacy and safety of two doses of enoxaparin in women with thrombophilia and recurrent pregnancy loss: the LIVE-ENOX study. J Thromb Haemost. 2005;3(2):227–9.
100. Grandone E, Brancaccio V, Colaizzo D, Sciannamé N, Pavone G, Di MG, et al. Preventing adverse obstetric outcomes in women with genetic thrombophilia. Fertil Steril. 2002;78(2):371–5.
101. Kupferminc MJ, Fait G, Many A, Lessing JB, Yair D, Bar-Am A, et al. Low-molecular-weight heparin for the prevention of obstetric complications in women with thrombophilias. Hypertens Pregnancy. 2001;20(1):35–44.
102. Riyazi N, Leeda M, de Vries JI, Huijgens PC, van Geijn HP, Dekker GA. Low-molecular-weight heparin combined with aspirin in pregnant women with thrombophilia and a history of preeclampsia or fetal growth restriction: a preliminary study. Eur J Obstet Gynecol Reprod Biol. 1998;80(1):49–54.
103. Gris JC, Mercier E, Quere I, Lavigne-Lissalde G, Cochery-Nouvellon E, Hoffet M, et al. Low-molecular-weight heparin versus low-dose aspirin in women with one fetal loss and a constitutional thrombophilic disorder. Blood. 2004;103(10):3695–9.
104. Gris JC, Chauleur C, Faillie JL, Baer G, Mares P, Fabbro-Peray P, et al. Enoxaparin for the secondary prevention of placental vascular complications in women with abruptio placentae. The pilot randomised controlled NOH-AP trial. Thromb Haemost. 2010;104(4):771–9.
105. Rai R, Cohen H, Dave M, Regan L. Randomised controlled trial of aspirin and aspirin plus heparin in pregnant women with recurrent miscarriage associated with phospholipid antibodies (or antiphospholipid antibodies). BMJ. 1997;314(7076):253–7.
106. Goel N, et al. The role of aspirin versus aspirin and heparin in cases of recurrent abortions with raised anticardiolipin antibodies. Med Sci Monit. 2006;12:CR132–6.
107. Mak A, et al. Combination of heparin and aspirin is superior to aspirin alone in enhancing live births in patients with recurrent pregnancy loss and positive anti-phospholipid antibodies: a meta-analysis of randomized controlled trials and meta-regression. Rheumatology. 2010;49:281–8.
108. Bates SM, Greer IA, Middeldorp S, Veenstra DL, Prabulos A-M, Vandvik PO. VTE, thrombophilia, antithrombotic therapy, and pregnancy: antithrombotic therapy and prevention of thrombosis, 9th ed: American College of Chest Physicians evidence-based clinical practice guidelines. Chest. 2012;141(2 Suppl):e691S–736.
109. de Jesus GR, Agmon-Levin N, Andrade CA, Andreoli L, Chighizola CB, Porter TF, Salmon J, Silver RM, Tincani A, Branch DW. 14th International Congress on Antiphospholipid Antibodies Task Force report on obstetric antiphospholipid syndrome. Autoimmun Rev. 2014;13(8):795–813.
110. Kaandorp S, Di NM, Goddijn M, Middeldorp S. Aspirin or anticoagulants for treating recurrent miscarriage in women without antiphospholipid syndrome. Cochrane Database Syst Rev. 2009;(1):CD004734.
111. De Groot CJ, Bloemenkamp KW, Duvekot EJ, Helmerhorst FM, Bertina RM, Van Der Meer F, et al. Preeclampsia and genetic risk factors for thrombosis: a case–control study. Am J Obstet Gynecol. 1999;181(4):975–80.
112. North RA, Ferrier C, Gamble G, Fairley KF, Kincaid-Smith P. Prevention of preeclampsia with heparin and antiplatelet drugs in women with renal disease. Aust N Z J Obstet Gynaecol. 1995;35(4):357–62.
113. Duley L, Henderson-Smart D, Knight M, King J. Antiplatelet drugs for prevention of pre-eclampsia and its consequences: systematic review. BMJ. 2001;322(7282):329–33.
114. Brenner B, Hoffman R, Blumenfeld Z, Weiner Z, Younis JS. Gestational outcome in thrombophilic women with recurrent pregnancy loss treated by enoxaparin. Thromb Haemost. 2000;83(5):693–7.
115. Leeda M, Riyazi N, de Vries JI, Jakobs C, van Geijn HP, Dekker GA. Effects of folic acid and vitamin B6 supplementation on women with hyperhomocysteinemia and a history of preeclampsia or fetal growth restriction. Am J Obstet Gynecol. 1998;179(1):135–9.
116. de Vries JI, van Pampus MG, Hague WM, Bezemer PD, Joosten JH, FRUIT Investigators. Low-molecular-weight heparin added to aspirin in the prevention of recurrent early-onset pre-eclampsia in women with inheritable thrombophilia: the FRUIT-RCT. J Thromb Haemost. 2012;10(1):64–72. doi:10.1111/j.1538-7836.2011.04553.x.
117. Rodger MA, Hague WM, Kingdom J, Kahn SR, Karovitch A, Sermer M, et al.; for the TIPPS Investigators. Antepartum dalteparin versus no antepartum dalteparin for the prevention of pregnancy complications in pregnant women with thrombophilia (TIPPS): a multinational open-label randomised trial. Lancet. 2014. pii: S0140-6736(14)60793-5.

doi: 10.1016/S0140-6736(14)60793-5. [Epub ahead of print].

118. Kingdom JC, Walker M, Proctor LK, Keating S, Shah PS, McLeod A, et al. Unfractionated heparin for second trimester placental insufficiency: a pilot randomized trial. J Thromb Haemost. 2011;9(8): 1483–92.

119. Rodger MA, Carrier M, Le Gal G, Martinelli I, Perna A, Rey E, de Vries JI, Gris JC, Low-Molecular-Weight Heparin for Placenta-Mediated Pregnancy Complications Study Group. Meta-analysis of low-molecular-weight heparin to prevent recurrent placenta-mediated pregnancy complications. Blood. 2014;123(6):822–8. doi:10.1182/blood-2013-01-478958. Epub 2013 Dec 19.

120. Baglin T, Gray E, Greaves M, Hunt BJ, Keeling D, Machin S, et al. Clinical guidelines for testing for heritable thrombophilia. Br J Haematol. 2010;149(2):209–20.

121. Rey E, Garneau P, David M, Gauthier R, Leduc L, Michon N, et al. Dalteparin for the prevention of recurrence of placental-mediated complications of pregnancy in women without thrombophilia: a pilot randomized controlled trial. J Thromb Haemost. 2009;7(1):58–64.

122. National Collaborating Centre for Women's and Children's Health. Hypertension in pregnancy: the management of hypertensive disorders during pregnancy. London: RCOG Press; 2010.

123. Franchi F, Biguzzi E, Cetin I, Facchetti F, Radaelli T, Bozzo M, et al. Mutations in the thrombomodulin and endothelial protein C receptor genes in women with late fetal loss. Br J Haematol. 2001;114(3):641–6.

124. Nakabayashi M, Yamamoto S, Suzuki K. Analysis of thrombomodulin gene polymorphism in women with severe early-onset preeclampsia. Semin Thromb Hemost. 1999;25(5):473–9.

125. Laude I, Rongieres-Bertrand C, Boyer-Neumann C, Wolf M, Mairovitz V, Hugel B, et al. Circulating pro-coagulant microparticles in women with unexplained pregnancy loss: a new insight. Thromb Haemost. 2001;85(1):18–21.

9 Pre-eclampsia: The Role of Hemostasis in Its Pathophysiology and Potential Future Therapeutic Options

Chris Gardiner and Manu Vatish

Abstract

Pre-eclampsia affects 2–8 % of pregnancies worldwide. It is a syndrome of new onset hypertension and proteinuria in the second half of pregnancy, typically characterized by endothelial dysfunction and systemic activation of an inflammatory response. Both maternal and fetal complications of pre-eclampsia are potentially fatal or detrimental to long-term health. This chapter considers the role of hemostasis in the pathophysiology of pre-eclampsia and potential future therapeutic options.

Keywords

Pre-eclampsia • Pathogenesis • Hemostatic changes • Laboratory testing • Management • Potential future therapeutic options

9.1 Background

Pre-eclampsia affects 2–8 % of pregnancies worldwide. No other complication of pregnancy is so common and so dangerous for mother and baby, being potentially fatal or detrimental to long-term health in both. It is a syndrome of new onset hypertension and proteinuria in the second half of pregnancy, characterized by endothelial dysfunction and systemic activation of an inflammatory response. Maternal complications include HELLP (hemolysis, elevated liver enzymes, low platelets), eclampsia, stroke, placental abruption, disseminated intravascular coagulation (DIC), pulmonary edema, liver hemorrhage, acute renal failure and death [1]. Adverse perinatal outcomes include stillbirth, fetal growth restriction (FGR) preterm delivery, fetal distress and neonatal complications.

The *clinical* diagnosis of pre-eclampsia is defined as *de novo* hypertension (at least 140/90 mmHg on two separate occasions ≥4 h apart) and new onset of proteinuria (≥300 mg/day or a spot urine/creatinine ratio of ≥30 mg/mmol) after 20 weeks of gestation [2]. Renal insufficiency, hepatocellular dysfunction, neurological symptoms, thrombocytopenia, DIC, hemolysis and FGR are also indicative. These criteria are more inclusive than the

C. Gardiner, MSc, PhD (✉)
M. Vatish, MB BChir, MA, DPhil, MRCOG
Nuffield Department of Obstetrics and Gynaecology, Level 3, Women's Centre, John Radcliffe Hospital, University of Oxford, Oxford University Hospitals NHS Foundation Trust, Oxford, Oxfordshire OX3 9DU, UK
e-mail: chris.gardiner@obs-gyn.ox.ac.uk

H. Cohen, P. O'Brien (eds.), *Disorders of Thrombosis and Hemostasis in Pregnancy: A Guide to Management*, DOI 10.1007/978-3-319-15120-5_9, © Springer-Verlag London 2015

Table 9.1 Risk factors for pre-eclampsia at antenatal booking

History	Previous pre-eclampsia
	Chronic hypertension
	Renal disease
	Type 1 or type 2 diabetes
	Multiple pregnancy
	Family history of pre-eclampsia
	Antiphospholipid syndrome
	Chronic autoimmune disease
	Increasing maternal age beyond 34 years
	First pregnancy
	Increasing time between pregnancies
Examination	Increased body mass index
	Hypertension
	Proteinuria

Adapted from Duckitt and Harrington [4]

more specific research criteria, in recognition of the multisystem nature of the presenting symptoms of pre-eclampsia. Other hypertensive disorders of pregnancy are gestational hypertension, chronic hypertension and pre-eclampsia superimposed on chronic hypertension. Pre-eclampsia may be broadly classified as mild to severe, or early to late onset. The International Society for the Study of Hypertension in Pregnancy (ISSHP) recommend a diagnosis of severe pre-eclampsia if the blood pressure exceeds 160/110 mmHg or HELLP syndrome develops, while early-onset pre-eclampsia is generally defined as that occurring before 34 weeks [3]. Although several risk factors have been identified (Table 9.1), the underlying mechanisms remain poorly understood [4].

Activation of platelets and the vascular endothelium, hemolysis and liver damage are the main pathophysiological features characteristic of the HELLP syndrome, each of which predisposes to DIC. Overt DIC, with its characteristic laboratory features (severe thrombocytopenia, fragmented red cells, markedly elevated D-dimers, prolonged prothrombin time (PT) and activated partial thromboplastin time (APTT), and reduced concentrations of fibrinogen, clotting factors and the natural anticoagulants) occurs in approximately 40 % of women with HELLP [5].

9.2 Pathogenesis

The origins of pre-eclampsia lie in the placenta, and delivery remains the only effective treatment. It is a two stage disease [6]: the first (pre-clinical) stage comprises deficient remodeling of the utero-placental circulation (8–18 weeks), dysfunctional perfusion and placental oxidative stress; the second, clinical stage (after 20 weeks) results from maternal systemic inflammation and vascular dysfunction. However, pre-eclampsia can occur in the absence of obvious placental pathology and poor placentation does not always lead to pre-eclampsia. Anti-angiogenic and pro-inflammatory factors released from the syncytiotrophoblast into the maternal circulation as a result of oxidative stress link the two stages. sFlt-1 and sEndoglin (soluble receptors for VEGF and TGFα) are two such factors that contribute to the maternal syndrome [7], but they alone cannot explain the diversity of maternal features. Indeed, a 'non-angiogenic' form of pre-eclampsia exists with normal levels of sFlt-1 and sEndoglin [8].

There is a growing body of evidence for an immune role in the early pathogenesis of pre-eclampsia; specifically a maternal maladaptation to paternal alloantigens leading to poor placentation [9]. The resultant oxidative and placental endoplasmic reticulum stress in the placenta drive the antiangiogenic and inflammatory pathways [10, 11]. The presence of agonist autoantibodies against the angiotensin II type 1 receptor (AT-1) in the plasma of women with pre-eclampsia [12, 13] has also been implicated in its pathology. AT-1 antibodies induce signalling in trophoblasts and vascular cells, induce tissue factor in vascular cells [14] and can induce the symptoms of pre-eclampsia when injected into pregnant mice [15]. The antibodies are typically undetectable 6 weeks postpartum but have also been demonstrated in patients with other hypertensive disorders [16]. Further evidence of an immunological role in pre-eclampsia comes from the activation of the complement system [17] and the localisation of the C5b-9 membrane attack complex to sites of villous trophoblast injury [18].

In addition to the release of soluble factors from the placenta, the syncytiotrophoblast releases increased amounts of placental debris directly into the maternal circulation [19, 20] which comprises syncytiotrophoblast microvesicles (STBM), microvilli, cytokeratin fragments, and soluble RNA and DNA of fetal origin [21]. These STBM may contribute to inflammation by inducing cytokine release [22, 23], endothelial dysfunction [24] and the procoagulant and [25] hypofibrinolytic states [26]. The release of STBM during labor may play a role in the development of postpartum pre-eclampsia [27].

9.3 Hemostatic Changes in Pre-eclampsia

Many consider the hemostatic changes observed in mild pre-eclampsia as an augmentation of the normal maternal physiological response. This is in contrast to severe pre-eclampsia in which the imbalance of the hemostatic system is pathological, reflecting the systemic inflammation and endothelial dysfunction characteristic of the disease. In practice, a spectrum of hemostatic changes is observed: from minor variations seen in mild pre-eclampsia to the decompensated hemostatic changes observed in HELLP syndrome, which can proceed to DIC in severe cases.

9.3.1 Platelet Activation

Excessive platelet activation and consumption are common features of pre-eclampsia [28] and may occur several weeks prior to development of maternal symptoms [29]. It has been reported that plasma β-thromboglobulin levels correlate with urinary protein and serum creatinine [30], suggesting a link between platelet activation and renal damage. Platelets from women with pre-eclampsia are more responsive to *in vitro* agonist stimulation than those from women with a normotensive pregnancy [31]. The platelets from women with pre-eclampsia also form more platelet-leucocyte aggregates [32, 33], with this contributing to the inflammatory and procoagulant processes. Increased thromboxane A2 [34] and decreased platelet nitric oxide synthase (NOS) [35] offer further evidence for platelet mediated endothelial dysfunction in pre-eclampsia. Although platelet counts in women with pre-eclampsia are highly variable, longitudinal studies have shown that the mean platelet count falls during pre-eclamptic pregnancies with a concomitant increase in platelet volume [36–38]. A falling platelet count is associated with worsening disease, and is a maternal risk in its own right. The Royal College of Obstetricians and Gynaecologists (RCOG) recommends that consultant obstetric staff should document in the woman's notes the maternal (biochemical, hematological and clinical) and fetal thresholds for elective birth before 34 weeks in women with pre-eclampsia. The levels of biochemical and hematological markers (including proteinuria) correlate poorly with maternal and fetal outcomes, such that the National Institute for Health and Clinical Excellence (NICE) in the UK felt that recommending absolute thresholds for delivery was not warranted. In general, the decision on when to expedite delivery will be made taking into account several factors, including the severity of hypertension, biochemical and hematological disturbance, proteinuria, availability of appropriate neonatal facilities, the presence of fetal growth restriction, and the gestation [39].

9.3.2 Changes in the Coagulation/Fibrinolytic Systems

The association between coagulation activation and pre-eclampsia has been recognised since the early 1950s [40]. The shift in the hemostatic balance towards a procoagulant/hyperfibrinolytic picture observed in normal pregnancy (described in Chap. 1) is exaggerated in pre-eclampsia as evidenced by perivillous fibrin deposition and placental infarcts [41–43]. Global tests of coagulation show procoagulant changes proportional to the severity of pre-eclampsia: PT and APTT may be shortened; fibrinogen and FVIIIc are elevated [44]; D-dimer and markers of in vivo thrombin generation are raised [45, 46]; and endogenous thrombin potential is increased [32, 47]. As would be expected, a decrease in the natural anticoagulants is observed over and above that of normally pregnancy, with decreases reported in antithrombin [44, 48], protein C [45] and sensitivity to protein C resistance [47, 49, 50]. A decrease in antithrombin plasma levels is indicative of deterioration of the condition [48]. It is notable that activated protein C resistance (APCR) persists long after pregnancy in women with a history of pre-eclampsia [51, 52]. However, the most striking changes are in those proteins associated with endothelial dysfunction; tissue plasminogen activator [53], PAI-1 [54], soluble thrombomodulin [55, 56], soluble endothelial APC receptor [57] and von Willebrand factor [58, 59] are all increased, while a reduction in ADAMTS13 levels appears to be linked to the degree of inflammation [60]. Decreased circulating PAI-2 reflects decreased placental function and/or intrauterine growth restriction [54, 61].

9.4 Screening

Blood pressure measurement and testing for proteinuria have been the mainstay of screening for pre-eclampsia for decades. Women considered to be at high risk of developing pre-eclampsia have more frequent blood pressure testing and may be referred for specialist care; they should be made aware of the symptoms of pre-eclampsia and the need to seek appropriate care if they experience these symptoms. This conservative management has not changed significantly for 30 years and many women considered to be at low risk still develop pre-eclampsia.

Several Doppler ultrasound screening studies, in both the first and second trimesters, have demonstrated an association between increased impedance to flow (indicated by diastolic notching in the uterine artery waveform) and subsequent development of pre-eclampsia and FGR [62]. However, a Cochrane Database systematic review of management using uterine artery Doppler showed no improvement in maternal or perinatal outcome [63].

The use of several biochemical markers, both in isolation and in combination, for the prediction of pre-eclampsia has recently been reviewed [64]. Soluble endoglin and sFlt-1 have been extensively studied and are particularly useful for predicting women at risk of early onset disease [65]. Other biomarkers include: pregnancy associated protein A (PAPP-A); placental protein-13 (PP-13); placental growth factor/sFlt-1 ratio; cystatin C; and free fetal hemoglobin; though many other markers have been studied. A recent prospective multicentre study investigated the use of low plasma PlGF concentration (<5th centile for gestation) as a negative predictive test for the development of pre-eclampsia. The negative predictive value (0.98 for pre-eclampsia within 14 days) exceeded that of other biomarkers studied to date as being useful in the management of women at risk of pre-eclampsia [66].

9.5 Laboratory Testing for Pre-eclampsia

9.5.1 Routine Coagulation Screening

There may be a tendency to over-test in pre-eclampsia. While the gravity of pre-eclampsia and HELLP cannot be overstated, it is not until the platelet count is less than 100×10^9/L that there is likely to be an associated coagulopathy. Consequently, the NICE recommendation is that coagulation studies are not required if the platelet count is above this level. In pregnant women with platelet counts of less than 100×10^9/L, a coagulation screen and fibrinogen level should be performed as initial screening tests, with D-dimer testing in the event of an abnormal clotting screen or if HELLP is suspected [67]. Lumbar epidural may be used for labor analgesia in women with pre-eclampsia if the mothers opt for it. Early epidural should be considered as it helps to diminish the hypertensive responses to pain. A platelet count of 75×10^9/L or more in the absence of coagulation abnormalities is not associated with an increased likelihood of regional anesthetic complications in the setting of pre-eclampsia [68–70].

9.5.2 Differential Diagnosis of HELLP, TTP and HUS

Thrombotic thrombocytopenic purpura (TTP) and hemolytic uremic syndrome (HUS) (see Chap. 17) are rarely encountered during pregnancy. The differential diagnosis of thrombotic microangiopathy (TMA) – HELLP and HUS or TTP - during pregnancy may be difficult as there is considerable overlap in the symptoms and laboratory findings [71, 72]. Thrombocytopenia, hemolysis with red cell fragmentation, jaundice, raised lactate dehydrogenase (LDH) and renal impairment are common to all three. The more common form of HUS, Shiga-like toxin-producing *Eschericia coli* HUS (STEC-HUS), is triggered by the infectious agent *Escherishia coli* O157:H7. Atypical HUS (aHUS) represents 5–10 % of HUS cases and is largely due to one or several genetic mutations that cause chronic, uncontrolled, and excessive activation of complement. Delivery is the only cure for HELLP and prophylactic platelet transfusion may be necessary for the severely thrombocytopenic patient. However, delivery will not ameliorate the condition of a woman with TTP and platelet transfusion is contraindicated. In the absence of timely and aggressive plasma exchange therapy, the pregnant patient with TTP will deteriorate and may die. The laboratory may help in the differential diagnosis of these conditions. A high LDH to AST ratio (>22.12) has been reported to suggest that TTP may be a more likely diagnosis than HELLP in a woman presenting in the third trimester with findings that could be compatible with either diagnosis [73]. If a TMA cannot be fully explained by a non-TTP pregnancy-related TMA, then the diagnosis of TTP must be considered and plasma exchange (PEX) should be started (2B) [71].

9.5.3 Other Tests of Hemostasis

Thromboelastography is a technique currently underutilised in obstetrics and, while it may be of limited diagnostic value in mild pre-eclampsia, it can demonstrate hemostatic defects in severe pre-eclampsia and HELLP, and could fulfil a role in the rapid assessment and subsequent treatment of coagulopathy, platelet dysfunction and hyperfibrinolysis seen in these conditions [74].

As mentioned above, during pre-eclampsia PAI-1 is markedly increased, over and above the level seen in normal pregnancy, but PAI-2 levels are lower than in normal pregnancy, most probably due to placental insufficiency. It has been suggested that the PAI-1/PAI-2 ratio may have prognostic value in determining pregnancy outcome when used in conjunction with uterine artery Doppler ultrasound [75]. TFPI activity measured during the 20th week of pregnancy has also been suggested as a predictor of pre-eclampsia later in pregnancy [76], as have soluble thrombomodulin and soluble endothelial protein C receptor [77]. While these reports are of interest, large prospective studies are necessary to ascertain whether these tests have any clinical utility.

9.5.4 Screening for Thrombophilic Risk Factors

There has been a great deal of speculation about the usefulness of thrombophilia testing to predict the likelihood of pre-eclampsia. To date, studies of thrombophilia and risk for pre-eclampsia in future pregnancy have not identified any strong risk factors. Antiphospholipid antibodies, hyprehomocysteinemia, the factor V Leiden and G20210A prothrombin gene mutations, and homozygosity of the methyltetrahydrofolate reductate (MTHFR) C667T polymorphism have all been linked with an increased incidence of pre-eclampsia. However, most studies have been underpowered and there is a paucity of data from prospective studies. It has been reported that only 13 % of cases of placental infarction are associated with a positive maternal thrombophilia test, suggesting that thrombophilia is not the major cause of infarction [78]. The Guideline Development Group of the National Collaborating Centre for Women's and Children's Health in the UK considers that the evidence on the association between thrombophilias and hypertensive disorders remains unclear and is of variable quality. Even with an association, the value of routine screening for these disorders would be unclear as there is no good evidence that treatment (thromboprophylaxis or increased folate intake) improves outcomes related to hypertensive disorders in the next pregnancy or prevents disease occurrence. Their recommendation is to not routinely perform screening for thrombophilia in women who have had pre-eclampsia [39]. The British Committee for Standards in Haematology state that therapeutic decisions should be based on clinical circumstances and not on the results of thrombophilia testing [79]. It is clear that further studies are required in this field.

9.6 Management of Pre-eclampsia and HELLP

If a diagnosis of pre-eclampsia is made, the definitive treatment is delivery. The timing of delivery is based on several factors including the gestational age of the fetus, the severity of the disease and the effects of the disease on both maternal and fetal condition.

If the diagnosis is made after 37 weeks' gestation, then delivery is expedited [80], whilst before this a balance between the risks to the mother and fetus of continuing the pregnancy and the risks to a premature fetus must be made. This is particularly relevant at gestations near the limit of viability (24 weeks). If the disease is severe, with major maternal effects (renal failure, liver failure, pulmonary edema, etc.) or the tests of fetal wellbeing (Ultrasound Doppler of the Umbilical Artery and Middle Cerebral Artery, or CTG) show evidence of compromise, then the decision to deliver is relatively straightforward. However, in situations where both the mother and fetus are relatively stable, the management often consists of 'watchful waiting', in an attempt to extend the pregnancy for the benefit of the fetus, without jeopardizing the mother's health. A diagnosis of pre-eclampsia prior to 34 weeks' gestation, without severe features, is generally managed expectantly, whilst management between 34 and 37 weeks may vary between units, since there are no randomized trials in this population group [81].

Stable patients can have hypertensive symptoms of the disease treated using a variety of drugs (alpha-methyldopa, labetalol, nifedipine, or hydralazine), but it is important to note that these drugs are treating a manifestation of the disease, and delivery is the definitive treatment [82]. Once a decision to deliver has been made, care of these patients is largely supportive, comprising of fluid restriction, strict fluid input/output control, control of hypertension and the reduction of eclamptic seizures by the use of magnesium sulphate ($MgSO_4$). $MgSO_4$ is also increasingly used between 24 and 34 weeks for fetal neuroprotection [82]. Antenatal corticosteroids are administered to improve fetal lung, bowel and brain maturity at these gestations [83]. The speed of deterioration of these patients can be rapid, and occasionally the only sign that the situation is worsening is a change in hematological parameters.

HELLP syndrome is arguably a severe subtype of pre-eclampsia, although opinion is divided [84]. It develops in up to 0.8 % of pregnancies overall and in 10–20 % of women with pre-eclampsia [85]. It is important to note that, in contrast to pre-eclampsia, there may be no hypertension or proteinuria [86]. However, similar to severe pre-eclampsia, serious hepatic manifestations are particularly common, including infarction, hemorrhage and rupture. These patients can present in more occult ways than classically pre-eclamptic patients, with vague abdominal pain or tenderness, nausea and vomiting. The diagnosis in such patients is often missed resulting in poor outcomes for the mother [87]. Classically, blood tests reveal a hemolytic anemia, platelets below $100 \times 10^9/L$, and elevated AST, ALT, LDH and bilirubin [88]. It is clear that comparison to previous results, taken earlier in pregnancy, can give insight into the diagnosis. Coagulation tests are crucial, since DIC is a common complication of HELLP [86, 89]. In contrast to pre-eclampsia, delivery in HELLP syndrome is usually expedited, although occasionally, depending on maternal condition, $MgSO_4$ and antenatal corticosteroids for fetal benefit may be given. Treatment options for hypertension and/or seizures are the same as for pre-eclampsia. These patients may have multiple blood tests requested during the course of their stay, particularly in the delivery and postpartum period, since this is the only way that disease severity can be monitored.

9.7 Prevention of Pre-eclampsia

As previously discussed, pre-eclampsia is associated with imbalance of thromboxane and prostacyclin levels. Low dose aspirin (LDA) inhibits platelet cyclooxygenase and thus production of thromboxane, while sparing vascular prostacyclin, thus correcting this imbalance [90, 91]. It is now generally accepted that LDA provides a modest reduction in the risk of pre-eclampsia and fetal/neonatal deaths [92]. Two meta-analyses have reported that LDA started at or before 16 weeks was associated with a significant reduction in the incidence of severe pre-eclampsia, perinatal death, premature delivery and FGR [93, 94]. However, the numbers were small and this remains controversial. There is evidence that the standard low dose of aspirin (75 mg daily) used in pregnancy may be subtherapeutic and that 150 mg may be more effective [95]. A major prospective randomised trial of 80 mg versus 160 mg aspirin in the first trimester is due to start recruiting (http://www.clinicaltrials.gov/ct2/show/NCT01352234?term=aspirin+for+pre-eclampsia&rank=3).

Heparin (unfractionated (UFH) or low molecular weight (LMWH)) has been used in the treatment of the obstetric antiphospholipid syndrome for many years, and it is increasingly being used for the prevention of pre-eclampsia. UFH/LMWH treatment for women at high risk of pre-eclampsia and other complications of placental insufficiency has been shown to significantly reduce the risk of perinatal mortality, preterm birth and FGR [96]. In addition to its anticoagulant effect, heparin is also known to inhibit complement activation, TNFα production and toll like receptor mediated inflammatory responses [97]. It also has an anti-apoptotic effect on first trimester villous trophoblasts [98]. Heparin has been shown to increase circulating sFlt-1 suggesting that the protective effect of heparin cannot be explained by promotion of angiogenesis [99].

Calcium supplementation in areas of low dietary calcium intake has been reported to reduce the risk of pre-eclampsia. A systematic review concluded that the limited data are consistent with low dose calcium (<1 g per day) reducing the risk of pre-eclampsia, and that confirming this in sufficiently powered randomized controlled trials would have implications for current guidelines and their global implementation [100].

9.8 Potential Future Therapeutic Options

Investigation of antithrombin replacement in pre-eclampsia is limited to case reports and a few studies. In a placebo-controlled double-blind phase III trial in 133 patients with severe pre-eclampsia (66 treated with antithrombin concentrate 3,000 IU/day and 67 with intravenous placebo), Maki et al. [101] reported a significant prolongation of pregnancy with antithrombin replacement versus placebo (mean (+/– SD) (16.8 (2.0) days versus 10.2 (1.2) days, respectively; P=0.007) and a significantly greater gestational age at delivery (34.1 (3.2) versus 33.0 (2.7) weeks, respectively; P=0.007), with a mean increase of 6.5 days. Paternoster et al. compared two different dosing regimens of antithrombin replacement in patients with severe pre-eclampsia between 24 and 33 weeks of gestation: 3,000 IU antithrombin per day for 5 days (n=10) or antithrombin replacement to maintain 80 % antithrombin activity (mean dose, 3,370 units per patient). Pregnancies in the high-dose group were prolonged by a mean of 6 days, compared with 3.5 days in the standard-dose group (P=0.03). The high-dose group also had greater birthweights (1,185 g versus 1,005 g), but this difference was not significant [102]. A prospective randomized placebo-controlled study (A Prospective Randomized Evaluation of the Safety and Efficacy of Recombinant Antithrombin in Very Preterm Pre-eclampsia (PRESERVE-1)) to study the safety and efficacy of recombinant antithrombin in very preterm pre-eclampsia has commenced [103].

Activated protein C levels are known to fall in during normal pregnancy and there is limited evidence that this is more severe in pre-eclampsia [104]. A phase II safety and efficacy trial of recombinant APC (Drotrecogin alfa) in women with either very early-onset or severe postpartum pre-eclampsia was initiated. However, Drotrecogin alfa was subsequently withdrawn from the market after a meta-analysis showed that it was ineffective in the treatment of severe sepsis and increased bleeding risk [105]. Whether a non-anticoagulant activated protein C, which retains its cytoprotective/anti-inflammatory properties [106], could be effective in the treatment of pre-eclampsia remains to be seen.

A pilot study used dextran sulphate cellulose apheresis in five women with preterm pre-eclampsia to successfully reduce levels of circulating sFlt-1 [107]. Multiple apheresis treatments were then performed in three additional women. In all three, there was a reduction in proteinuria and stabilization of blood pressure, which allowed the prolongation of pregnancy by 15–23 days with fetal growth evident. It remains to be seen whether these improvements in clinical outcome were due solely to the reduction in circulating sFlt-1 or whether other factors removed by dextran sulphate cellulose apheresis were contributory. In a similar study, heparin-mediated extracorporeal low density lipoprotein (LDL) precipitation was used to treat nine women with pre-eclampsia. Significant reductions in circulating triglycerides, LDL, Lipoprotein a, C reactive protein, TNFα, sVCAM-1, homocysteine, and lipopolysaccharide binding protein were observed post apheresis, and pregnancy was prolonged by 3–49 days [108]. It has been suggested that a similar approach could be used to remove autoantibodies against the AT1 receptor [16]. AT-1 receptor blockade with losartan attenuates vasoconstriction in an anti-AT-1 induced animal model of pre-eclampsia [109] and while losartan itself is teratogenic, the data suggest that AT-1 autoantibodies could be an important therapeutic target.

Eculizumab (Soliris; Alexion Pharmaceuticals) is a humanized recombinant, monoclonal antibody directed against human complement component C5 (humanized anti-C5 antibody) [110]. It is effective in the treatment of aHUS [111] (see Chap. 17), and approved by the European Medicines Agency and the United States Food and Drug Administration (FDA) for the treatment of aHUS. As a recombinant IgG molecule, eculizumab is expected to cross the placenta. Animal studies using a mouse analogue of the eculizumab molecule (murine anti-C5 antibody) showed increased rates of developmental abnormalities and an increased rate of dead and moribund offspring at doses 2–8 times the human dose. The manufacturer states that eculizumab should be used during pregnancy only if the potential benefit justifies the potential risk to the fetus. Limited data of the use of eculizumab in paroxysmal nocturnal hemoglobinuria (PNH; see Chap. 19) and case reports in aHUS in pregnancy are encouraging. The latter include the use of eculizumab to successfully treat one woman with aHUS in pregnancy [112]; and a woman with HELLP at 26 weeks' gestation, who was given three doses of eculizumab over 13 days, during which time her clinical condition improved and her LDH, haptoglobin, AST, and platelet count normalised – allowing her pregnancy be prolonged by 17 days with the delivery of a healthy baby [113].

The finding that hypertriglyceridemia is associated with and precedes the onset of pre-eclampsia [114] has led researchers to consider triglyceride-lowering therapies in pregnancy for the treatment and prevention of pre-eclampsia. Pravastatin, a lipid-lowering drug with pleiotropic properties, has been shown to improve vascular reactivity [115], induce PlGF and reduce proteinuria and hypertension [116], inhibit tissue factor expression [117], and restore trophoblast invasiveness angiogenic balance and placental blood flow [118] in mouse models of pre-eclampsia. A study of women exposed to statins during the first trimester of pregnancy did not detect a teratogenic effect [119] and two prospective clinical trials commenced in 2013 to examine the safety and efficacy of pravastatin for the prevention [120] and treatment of pre-eclampsia [121].

Key Learning Points

- Pre-eclampsia is a multisystem syndrome of unknown etiology peculiar to pregnancy.
- Pre-eclampsia remains the leading cause of maternal and perinatal morbidity and mortality in the developed world.
- The only definitive treatment for pre-eclampsia is delivery of the baby and the placenta.
- HELLP syndrome is a severe variant of pre-eclampsia that may be confused with TTP and HUS.
- Recent improvements in screening tests and potential novel therapies may lead to improvements in the management of pre-eclampsia.

References

1. Ghulmiyyah L, Sibai B. Maternal mortality from pre-eclampsia/eclampsia. Semin Perinatol. 2012;36(1):56–9.
2. Brown MA, Lindheimer MD, de Swiet M, Van Assche A, Moutquin JM. The classification and diagnosis of the hypertensive disorders of pregnancy: statement from the International Society for the Study of Hypertension in Pregnancy (ISSHP). Hypertens Pregnancy. 2001;20(1):IX–XIV.
3. Tranquilli AL. Introduction to ISSHP new classification of pre-eclampsia. Pregnancy Hypertens. 2013;3(2):58–9.
4. Duckitt K, Harrington D. Risk factors for pre-eclampsia at antenatal booking: systematic review of controlled studies. BMJ. 2005;330(7491):565.
5. Abildgaard U, Heimdal K. Pathogenesis of the syndrome of hemolysis, elevated liver enzymes, and low platelet count (HELLP): a review. Eur J Obstet Gynecol Reprod Biol. 2013;166(2):117–23.
6. Redman CW, Sargent IL. Latest advances in understanding pre-eclampsia. Science. 2005;308(5728):1592–4.
7. Levine RJ, Maynard SE, Qian C, Lim K-H, England LJ, Yu KF, et al. Circulating angiogenic factors and the risk of pre-eclampsia. N Engl J Med. 2004;350(7):672–83.
8. Rana S, Schnettler WT, Powe C, Wenger J, Salahuddin S, Cerdeira AS, et al. Clinical characterization and outcomes of pre-eclampsia with normal angiogenic profile. Hypertens Pregnancy. 2013;32(2):189–201.
9. Redman CW, Sargent IL. Immunology of pre-eclampsia. Am J Reprod Immunol. 2010;63(6):534–43.
10. Burton GJ, Yung HW. Endoplasmic reticulum stress in the pathogenesis of early-onset pre-eclampsia. Pregnancy Hypertens. 2011;1(1–2):72–8.
11. Cudmore M, Ahmad S, Al-Ani B, Fujisawa T, Coxall H, Chudasama K, et al. Negative regulation of soluble Flt-1 and soluble endoglin release by heme oxygenase-1. Circulation. 2007;115(13):1789–97.
12. Wallukat G, Homuth V, Fischer T, Lindschau C, Horstkamp B, Jupner A, et al. Patients with pre-eclampsia develop agonistic autoantibodies against the angiotensin AT1 receptor. J Clin Invest. 1999;103(7):945–52.
13. Herse F, Verlohren S, Wenzel K, Pape J, Muller DN, Modrow S, et al. Prevalence of agonistic autoantibodies against the angiotensin II type 1 receptor and soluble fms-like tyrosine kinase 1 in a gestational age-matched case study. Hypertension. 2009;53(2):393–8.
14. Dechend R, Homuth V, Wallukat G, Kreuzer J, Park JK, Theuer J, et al. AT(1) receptor agonistic antibodies from preeclamptic patients cause vascular cells to express tissue factor. Circulation. 2000;101(20):2382–7.
15. Zhou CC, Zhang Y, Irani RA, Zhang H, Mi T, Popek EJ, et al. Angiotensin receptor agonistic autoantibodies induce pre-eclampsia in pregnant mice. Nat Med. 2008;14(8):855–62.
16. Xia Y, Kellems RE. Angiotensin receptor agonistic autoantibodies and hypertension: pre-eclampsia and beyond. Circ Res. 2013;113(1):78–87.
17. Derzsy Z, Prohászka Z, Rigó Jr J, Füst G, Molvarec A. Activation of the complement system in normal pregnancy and pre-eclampsia. Mol Immunol. 2010;47(7–8):1500–6.
18. Rampersad R, Barton A, Sadovsky Y, Nelson DM. The C5b-9 membrane attack complex of complement activation localizes to villous trophoblast injury in vivo and modulates human trophoblast function in vitro. Placenta. 2008;29(10):855–61.
19. Knight M, Redman CW, Linton EA, Sargent IL. Shedding of syncytiotrophoblast microvilli into the maternal circulation in pre-eclamptic pregnancies. Br J Obstet Gynaecol. 1998;105(6):632–40.
20. Goswami D, Tannetta DS, Magee LA, Fuchisawa A, Redman CW, Sargent IL, et al. Excess syncytiotrophoblast microparticle shedding is a feature of early-onset pre-eclampsia, but not normotensive intrauterine growth restriction. Placenta. 2006;27(1):56–61.
21. Redman CW, Tannetta DS, Dragovic RA, Gardiner C, Southcombe JH, Collett GP, et al. Review: Does size matter? Placental debris and the pathophysiology of pre-eclampsia. Placenta. 2012;33(Suppl):S48–54.
22. Southcombe J, Tannetta D, Redman C, Sargent I. The immunomodulatory role of syncytiotrophoblast microvesicles. PLoS One. 2011;6(5):e20245.

23. Germain SJ, Sacks GP, Sooranna SR, Sargent IL, Redman CW. Systemic inflammatory priming in normal pregnancy and pre-eclampsia: the role of circulating syncytiotrophoblast microparticles. J Immunol. 2007;178(9):5949–56.
24. Smarason AK, Sargent IL, Starkey PM, Redman CW. The effect of placental syncytiotrophoblast microvillous membranes from normal and pre-eclamptic women on the growth of endothelial cells in vitro. Br J Obstet Gynaecol. 1993;100(10):943–9.
25. Gardiner C, Tannetta DS, Simms CA, Harrison P, Redman CW, Sargent IL. Syncytiotrophoblast microvesicles released from pre-eclampsia placentae exhibit increased tissue factor activity. PLoS One. 2011;6(10):e26313.
26. Guller S, Tang Z, Ma YY, Di SS, Sager R, Schneider H. Protein composition of microparticles shed from human placenta during placental perfusion: Potential role in angiogenesis and fibrinolysis in pre-eclampsia. Placenta. 2011;32(1):63–9.
27. Reddy A, Zhong XY, Rusterholz C, Hahn S, Holzgreve W, Redman CW, et al. The effect of labour and placental separation on the shedding of syncytiotrophoblast microparticles, cell-free DNA and mRNA in normal pregnancy and pre-eclampsia. Placenta. 2008;29(11):942–9.
28. Redman CW, Bonnar J, Beilin L. Early platelet consumption in pre-eclampsia. BMJ. 1978;1(6111): 467–9.
29. Janes SL, Kyle PM, Redman C, Goodall AH. Flow cytometric detection of activated platelets in pregnant women prior to the development of pre-eclampsia. Thromb Haemost. 1995;74(4):1059–63.
30. Socol ML, Weiner CP, Louis G, Rehnberg K, Rossi EC. Platelet activation in pre-eclampsia. Am J Obstet Gynecol. 1985;151(4):494–7.
31. Holthe MR, Staff AC, Berge LN, Lyberg T. Different levels of platelet activation in preeclamptic, normotensive pregnant, and nonpregnant women. Am J Obstet Gynecol. 2004;190(4):1128–34.
32. Macey MG, Bevan S, Alam S, Verghese L, Agrawal S, Beski S, et al. Platelet activation and endogenous thrombin potential in pre-eclampsia. Thromb Res. 2010;125(3):e76–81.
33. Holthe MR, Lyberg T, Staff AC, Berge LN. Leukocyte-platelet interaction in pregnancies complicated with pre-eclampsia. Platelets. 2005;16(2):91–7.
34. Wallenburg HC, Rotmans N. Enhanced reactivity of the platelet thromboxane pathway in normotensive and hypertensive pregnancies with insufficient fetal growth. Am J Obstet Gynecol. 1982;144(5):523–8.
35. Delacretaz E, de Quay N, Waeber B, Vial Y, Schulz PE, Burnier M, et al. Differential nitric oxide synthase activity in human platelets during normal pregnancy and pre-eclampsia. Clin Sci (Lond). 1995; 88(6):607–10.
36. Hutt R, Ogunniyi SO, Sullivan MH, Elder MG. Increased platelet volume and aggregation precede the onset of pre-eclampsia. Obstet Gynecol. 1994;83(1):146–9.
37. Dundar O, Yoruk P, Tutuncu L, Erikci AA, Muhcu M, Ergur AR, et al. Longitudinal study of platelet size changes in gestation and predictive power of elevated MPV in development of pre-eclampsia. Prenat Diagn. 2008;28(11):1052–6.
38. Sill PR, Lind T, Walker W. Platelet values during normal pregnancy. BJOG. 1985;92(5):480–3.
39. National Collaborating Centre for Women's and Children's Health. Hypertension in pregnancy: the management of hypertensive disorders during pregnancy. London: RCOG Press; 2010.
40. Pritchard JA, Ratnoff OD, Weisman Jr R. Hemostatic defects and increased red cell destruction in pre-eclampsia and eclampsia. Obstet Gynecol. 1954;4(2):159–64.
41. Ferrazzi E, Bulfamante G, Mezzopane R, Barbera A, Ghidini A, Pardi G. Uterine Doppler velocimetry and placental hypoxic-ischemic lesion in pregnancies with fetal intrauterine growth restriction. Placenta. 1999;20(5–6):389–94.
42. Bonnar J, McNicol GP, Douglas AS. Coagulation and fibrinolytic systems in pre-eclampsia and eclampsia. Br Med J. 1971;2(5752):12–6.
43. Kanfer A, Bruch JF, Nguyen G, He CJ, Delarue F, Flahault A, et al. Increased placental antifibrinolytic potential and fibrin deposits in pregnancy-induced hypertension and pre-eclampsia. Lab Invest. 1996;74(1):253–8.
44. Donnelly JC, Cooley SM, Walsh TA, Smith OP, Gillan J, McMahon C, et al. Circulating pro- and anticoagulant levels in normal and complicated primigravid pregnancies and their relationship to placental pathology. J Obstet Gynaecol. 2013;33(3): 264–8.
45. de Boer K, ten Cate JW, Sturk A, Borm JJ, Treffers PE. Enhanced thrombin generation in normal and hypertensive pregnancy. Am J Obstet Gynecol. 1989;160(1):95–100.
46. Pinheiro Mde B, Junqueira DR, Coelho FF, Freitas LG, Carvalho MG, Gomes KB, et al. D-dimer in pre-eclampsia: systematic review and meta-analysis. Clin Chim Acta. 2012;414:166–70.
47. VanWijk MJ, Boer K, Berckmans RJ, Meijers JC, van der Post JA, Sturk A, et al. Enhanced coagulation activation in pre-eclampsia: the role of APC resistance, microparticles and other plasma constituents. Thromb Haemost. 2002;88(3):415–20.
48. Marietta M, Simoni L, Pedrazzi P, Facchini L, D'Amico R, Facchinetti F. Antithrombin plasma levels decrease is associated with pre-eclampsia worsening. Int J Lab Hematol. 2009;31(2):227–32.
49. Clark P, Sattar N, Walker ID, Greer IA. The Glasgow Outcome, APCR and Lipid (GOAL) Pregnancy Study: significance of pregnancy associated activated protein C resistance. Thromb Haemost. 2001;85(1):30–5.
50. Paternoster DM, Stella A, Simioni P, Girolami A, Snijders D. Activated protein C resistance in normal and pre-eclamptic pregnancies. Gynecol Obstet Invest. 2002;54(3):145–9.
51. Tchaikovski SN, Thomassen MC, Costa SD, Peeters LLH, Rosing J. Role of protein S and tissue factor pathway inhibitor in the development of activated

protein C resistance early in pregnancy in women with a history of pre-eclampsia. Thromb Haemost. 2011;106(11):914–21.
52. van Pampus MG, Dekker GA, Wolf H, Huijgens PC, Koopman MM, von Blomberg BM, et al. High prevalence of hemostatic abnormalities in women with a history of severe pre-eclampsia. Am J Obstet Gynecol. 1999;180(5):1146–50.
53. Belo L, Santos-Silva A, Rumley A, Lowe G, Pereira-Leite L, Quintanilha A, et al. Elevated tissue plasminogen activator as a potential marker of endothelial dysfunction in pre-eclampsia: correlation with proteinuria. BJOG. 2002;109(11):1250–5.
54. Estelles A, Gilabert J, Grancha S, Yamamoto K, Thinnes T, Espana F, et al. Abnormal expression of type 1 plasminogen activator inhibitor and tissue factor in severe pre-eclampsia. Thromb Haemost. 1998;79(3):500–8.
55. Rousseau A, Favier R, Van DP. Elevated circulating soluble thrombomodulin activity, tissue factor activity and circulating procoagulant phospholipids: new and useful markers for pre-eclampsia? Eur J Obstet Gynecol Reprod Biol. 2009;146(1):46–9.
56. Hsu CD, Lucas RB, Johnson TR, Hong SF, Chan DW. Elevated urine thrombomodulin/creatinine ratio in severely preeclamptic pregnancies. Am J Obstet Gynecol. 1994;171(3):854–6.
57. Saposnik B, Peynaud-Debayle E, Stepanian A, Baron G, Simansour M, Mandelbrot L, et al. Elevated soluble endothelial cell protein C receptor (sEPCR) levels in women with pre-eclampsia: a marker of endothelial activation/damage? Thromb Res. 2012;129(2):152–7.
58. Hulstein JJ, van Runnard Heimel PJ, Franx A, Lenting PJ, Bruinse HW, Silence K, et al. Acute activation of the endothelium results in increased levels of active von Willebrand factor in hemolysis, elevated liver enzymes and low platelets (HELLP) syndrome. J Thromb Haemost. 2006;4(12):2569–75.
59. Nadar SK, Al Yemeni E, Blann AD, Lip GY. Thrombomodulin, von Willebrand factor and E-selectin as plasma markers of endothelial damage/dysfunction and activation in pregnancy induced hypertension. Thromb Res. 2004;113(2):123–8.
60. Stepanian A, Cohen-Moatti M, Sanglier T, Legendre P, Ameziane N, Tsatsaris V, et al. Von Willebrand factor and ADAMTS13: a candidate couple for pre-eclampsia pathophysiology. Arterioscler Thromb Vasc Biol. 2011;31(7):1703–9.
61. Astedt B, Lindoff C, Lecander I. Significance of the plasminogen activator inhibitor of placental type (PAI-2) in pregnancy. Semin Thromb Hemost. 1998;24(5):431–5.
62. Papageorghiou AT, Yu CK, Nicolaides KH. The role of uterine artery Doppler in predicting adverse pregnancy outcome. Best Pract Res Clin Obstet Gynaecol. 2004;18(3):383–96.
63. Stampalija T, Gyte GM, Alfirevic Z. Utero-placental Doppler ultrasound for improving pregnancy outcome. Cochrane Database Syst Rev. 2010;(9):CD008363.
64. Anderson UD, Olsson MG, Kristensen KH, Akerstrom B, Hansson SR. Review: Biochemical markers to predict pre-eclampsia. Placenta. 2012; 33(Suppl):S42–7.
65. Myers JE, Kenny LC, McCowan LM, Chan EH, Dekker GA, Poston L, et al. Angiogenic factors combined with clinical risk factors to predict preterm pre-eclampsia in nulliparous women: a predictive test accuracy study. BJOG. 2013;120(10):1215–23.
66. Chappell LC, Duckworth S, Seed PT, Griffin M, Myers J, Mackillop L, et al. Diagnostic accuracy of placental growth factor in women with suspected pre-eclampsia: a prospective multicenter study. Circulation. 2013;128(19):2121–31.
67. National Institute for Health and Clinical Excellence. Hypertension in pregnancy: the management of hypertensive disorders during pregnancy. London: National Institute for Health and Clinical Excellence: Guidance; 2010.
68. Sharma SK, Philip J, Whitten CW, Padakandla UB, Landers DF. Assessment of changes in coagulation in parturients with pre-eclampsia using thromboelastography. Anesthesiology. 1999;90(2):385–90.
69. Dyer RA, Piercy JL, Reed AR. The role of the anaesthetist in the management of the pre-eclamptic patient. Curr Opin Anaesthesiol. 2007;20(3):168–74.
70. Van Veen JJ, Nokes TJ, Makris M. The risk of spinal haematoma following neuraxial anaesthesia or lumbar puncture in thrombocytopenic individuals. Br J Haematol. 2010;148(1):15–25.
71. Scully M, Hunt BJ, Benjamin S, Liesner R, Rose P, Peyvandi F, Cheung B, Machin SJ. Guidelines on the diagnosis and management of thrombotic thrombocytopenic purpura and other thrombotic microangiopathies. Br J Haematol. 2012;158(3):323–35.
72. Gernsheimer T, James AH, Stasi R. How I treat thrombocytopenia in pregnancy. Blood. 2013;121(1): 38–47.
73. Keiser SD, Boyd KW, Rehberg JF, Elkins S, Owens MY, Sunesara I, Martin Jr JN. A high LDH to AST ratio helps to differentiate pregnancy-associated thrombotic thrombocytopenic purpura (TTP) from HELLP syndrome. J Matern Fetal Neonatal Med. 2012;25(7):1059–63.
74. Whitta RK, Cox DJ, Mallett SV. Thrombelastography reveals two causes of haemorrhage in HELLP syndrome. Br J Anaesth. 1995;74(4):464–8.
75. Hunt BJ, Missfelder-Lobos H, Parra-Cordero M, Fletcher O, Parmar K, Lefkou E, et al. Pregnancy outcome and fibrinolytic, endothelial and coagulation markers in women undergoing uterine artery Doppler screening at 23 weeks. J Thromb Haemost. 2009;7(6):955–61.
76. Hillman S, Chant I, Gu M, Rose P, Vatish M. Tissue pathway factor inhibitor (TFPI) activity is elevated in pregnant patients at 20 weeks gestation who subsequently develop pre-eclampsia. Thromb Haemost. 2009;101(4):778–80.
77. Boffa MC, Valsecchi L, Fausto A, Gozin D, Vigano' D'Angelo S, Safa O, et al. Predictive value of plasma

thrombomodulin in pre-eclampsia and gestational hypertension. Thromb Haemost. 1998;79(6): 1092–5.
78. Franco C, Walker M, Robertson J, Fitzgerald B, Keating S, McLeod A, et al. Placental infarction and thrombophilia. Obstet Gynecol. 2011;117(4):929–34.
79. Baglin T, Gray E, Greaves M, Hunt BJ, Keeling D, Machin S, et al. Clinical guidelines for testing for heritable thrombophilia. Br J Haematol. 2010;149(2): 209–20.
80. Magee LA, Helewa M, Moutquin JM, von Dadelszen P, Hypertension Guideline Committee; Strategic Training Initiative in Research in the Reproductive Health Sciences (STIRRHS) Scholars. Diagnosis, evaluation, and management of the hypertensive disorders of pregnancy. J Obstet Gynaecol Can. 2008;30(3 Suppl):S1–48.
81. Martin Jr JN, Thigpen BD, Moore RC, Rose CH, Cushman J, May W. Stroke and severe pre-eclampsia and eclampsia: a paradigm shift focusing on systolic blood pressure. Obstet Gynecol. 2005;105(2):246–54.
82. Magee L, Sawchuck D, Synnes A, von Dadelszen P. SOGC Clinical Practice Guideline. Magnesium sulphate for fetal neuroprotection. J Obstet Gynaecol Can. 2011;33(5):516–29.
83. Roberts D, Dalziel S. Antenatal corticosteroids for accelerating fetal lung maturation for women at risk of preterm birth. Cochrane Database Syst Rev. 2006;(3):CD004454.
84. Sibai BM, Taslimi MM, el-Nazer A, Amon E, Mabie BC, Ryan GM. Maternal-perinatal outcome associated with the syndrome of hemolysis, elevated liver enzymes, and low platelets in severe pre-eclampsia-eclampsia. Am J Obstet Gynecol. 1986;155(3):501–9.
85. Rath W, Faridi A, Dudenhausen JW. HELLP syndrome. J Perinat Med. 2000;28(4):249–60.
86. Haram K, Svendsen E, Abildgaard U. The HELLP syndrome: clinical issues and management. A Review. BMC Pregnancy Childbirth. 2009;9:8.
87. Curtin WM, Weinstein L. A review of HELLP syndrome. J Perinatol. 1999;19(2):138–43.
88. Sibai BM. Diagnosis, controversies, and management of the syndrome of hemolysis, elevated liver enzymes, and low platelet count. Obstet Gynecol. 2004;103(5 Pt 1):981–91.
89. Sibai BM, Ramadan MK, Usta I, Salama M, Mercer BM, Friedman SA. Maternal morbidity and mortality in 442 pregnancies with hemolysis, elevated liver enzymes, and low platelets (HELLP syndrome). Am J Obstet Gynecol. 1993;169(4):1000–6.
90. Schiff E, Peleg E, Goldenberg M, Rosenthal T, Ruppin E, Tamarkin M, et al. The use of aspirin to prevent pregnancy-induced hypertension and lower the ratio of thromboxane A2 to prostacyclin in relatively high risk pregnancies. N Engl J Med. 1989;321(6):351–6.
91. Benigni A, Gregorini G, Frusca T, Chiabrando C, Ballerini S, Valcamonico A, et al. Effect of low-dose aspirin on fetal and maternal generation of thromboxane by platelets in women at risk for pregnancy-induced hypertension. N Engl J Med. 1989;321(6): 357–62.
92. Duley L, Henderson-Smart DJ, Meher S, King JF. Antiplatelet agents for preventing pre-eclampsia and its complications. Cochrane Database Syst Rev. 2007;(2):CD004659.
93. Bujold E, Roberge S, Lacasse Y, Bureau M, Audibert F, Marcoux S, et al. Prevention of pre-eclampsia and intrauterine growth restriction with aspirin started in early pregnancy: a meta-analysis. Obstet Gynecol. 2010;116(2 Pt 1):402–14.
94. Roberge S, Nicolaides KH, Demers S, Villa P, Bujold E. Prevention of perinatal death and adverse perinatal outcome using low-dose aspirin: a meta-analysis. Ultrasound Obstet Gynecol. 2013;41(5): 491–9.
95. Caron N, Rivard GE, Michon N, Morin F, Pilon D, Moutquin JM, et al. Low-dose ASA response using the PFA-100 in women with high-risk pregnancy. J Obstet Gynaecol Can. 2009;31(11):1022–7.
96. Dodd JM, McLeod A, Windrim RC, Kingdom J. Antithrombotic therapy for improving maternal or infant health outcomes in women considered at risk of placental dysfunction. Cochrane Database Syst Rev. 2013;(7):CD006780.
97. Hossain N, Schatz F, Paidas MJ. Heparin and maternal fetal interface: why should it work to prevent pregnancy complications? Thromb Res. 2009;124(6): 653–5.
98. Hills FA, Abrahams VM, Gonzalez-Timon B, Francis J, Cloke B, Hinkson L, et al. Heparin prevents programmed cell death in human trophoblast. Mol Hum Reprod. 2006;12(4):237–43.
99. Rosenberg VA, Buhimschi IA, Lockwood CJ, Paidas MJ, Dulay AT, Ramma W, et al. Heparin elevates circulating soluble fms-like tyrosine kinase-1 immunoreactivity in pregnant women receiving anticoagulation therapy. Circulation. 2011;124(23):2543–53.
100. Hofmeyr GJ, Lawrie TA, Atallah AN, Duley L. Calcium supplementation during pregnancy for preventing hypertensive disorders and related problems. Cochrane Database Syst Rev. 2010;(8): CD001059
101. Maki M, Kobayashi T, Terao T, Ikenoue T, Satoh K, Nakabayashi M, et al. Antithrombin therapy for severe pre-eclampsia: results of a double-blind, randomized, placebo-controlled trial. BI51.017 Study Group. Thromb Haemost. 2000;84(4):583–90.
102. Paternoster DM, Fantinato S, Manganelli F, Milani M, Nicolini U, Girolami A. Efficacy of AT in pre-eclampsia: a case-control prospective trial. Thromb Haemost. 2004;91(2):283–9.
103. Paidas MJ, Sibai BM, Triche EW, Frieling J, Lowry S. Exploring the role of antithrombin replacement for the treatment of pre-eclampsia: a prospective randomized evaluation of the safety and efficacy of recombinant antithrombin in very preterm pre-eclampsia (PRESERVE-1). Am J Reprod Immunol. 2013;69(6):539–44.
104. von Dadelszen P, Magee LA, Lee SK, Stewart SD, Simone C, Koren G, et al. Activated protein C in normal human pregnancy and pregnancies complicated

by severe pre-eclampsia: a therapeutic opportunity? Crit Care Med. 2002;30(8):1883–92.
105. Martí-Carvajal AJ, Solà I, Gluud C, Lathyris D, Cardona AF. Human recombinant protein C for severe sepsis and septic shock in adult and paediatric patients. Cochrane Database Syst Rev. 2012;(12): CD004388.
106. Weiler H, Ruf W. Activated protein C in sepsis: the promise of nonanticoagulant activated protein C. Curr Opin Hematol. 2008;15(5):487–93.
107. Thadhani R, Kisner T, Hagmann H, Bossung V, Noack S, Schaarschmidt W, et al. Pilot study of extracorporeal removal of soluble fms-like tyrosine kinase 1 in pre-eclampsia. Circulation. 2011;124(8): 940–50.
108. Wang Y, Walli AK, Schulze A, Blessing F, Fraunberger P, Thaler C, et al. Heparin-mediated extracorporeal low density lipoprotein precipitation as a possible therapeutic approach in pre-eclampsia. Transfus Apher Sci. 2006;35(2):103–10.
109. van der Graaf AM, Wiegman MJ, Plosch T, Zeeman GG, van Buiten A, Henning RH, et al. Endothelium-dependent relaxation and angiotensin ii sensitivity in experimental pre-eclampsia. PLoS One. 2013;8(11): e79884.
110. Ecluzimab: summary of product characteristics. Alexion Pharma UK Ltd. Available at: http://www.medicines.org.uk/emc/medicine/.
111. Wong EK, Goodship TH, Kavanagh D. Complement therapy in atypical haemolytic uraemic syndrome (aHUS). Mol Immunol. 2013;56(3):199–212.
112. Ardissino G, Wally Ossola M, Baffero GM, Rigotti A, Cugno M. Eculizumab for atypical hemolytic uremic syndrome in pregnancy. Obstet Gynecol. 2013;122(2 Pt 2):487–9.
113. Burwick RM, Feinberg BB. Eculizumab for the treatment of pre-eclampsia/HELLP syndrome. Placenta. 2013;34(2):201–3.
114. Gallos ID, Sivakumar K, Kilby MD, Coomarasamy A, Thangaratinam S, Vatish M. Pre-eclampsia is associated with, and preceded by, hypertriglyceridaemia: a meta-analysis. BJOG. 2013;120(11):1321–32.
115. Costantine MM, Tamayo E, Lu F, Bytautiene E, Longo M, Hankins GD, et al. Using pravastatin to improve the vascular reactivity in a mouse model of soluble fms-like tyrosine kinase-1-induced pre-eclampsia. Obstet Gynecol. 2010;116(1):114–20.
116. Kumasawa K, Ikawa M, Kidoya H, Hasuwa H, Saito-Fujita T, Morioka Y, et al. Pravastatin induces placental growth factor (PGF) and ameliorates pre-eclampsia in a mouse model. Proc Natl Acad Sci. 2011;108(4):1451–5.
117. Girardi G. Role of tissue factor in pregnancy complications: crosstalk between coagulation and inflammation. Thromb Res. 2011;127 Suppl 3:S43–6.
118. Singh J, Ahmed A, Girardi G. Role of complement component C1q in the onset of pre-eclampsia in mice. Hypertension. 2011;58(4):716–24.
119. Winterfeld U, Allignol A, Panchaud A, Rothuizen LE, Merlob P, Cuppers-Maarschalkerweerd B, et al. Pregnancy outcome following maternal exposure to statins: a multicentre prospective study. BJOG. 2013;120(4):463–71.
120. Costantine MM, Cleary K. Pravastatin for the prevention of pre-eclampsia in high-risk pregnant women. Obstet Gynecol. 2013;121(2 Pt 1):349–53.
121. University of Birmingham. Statins to ameliorate early onset Pre-eclampsia [ISRCTN identifier: 23410175 2013; Eudra- CT2009-012968-13; online]. Available from: http://www.stamp.bham.ac.uk.

Antithrombotic Therapy for Cardiac Disorders in Pregnancy

10

Anna S. Herrey, Hannah Cohen, and Fiona Walker

Abstract

Pregnancy is a prothrombotic state and it is therefore essential that women with heart disease embarking on pregnancy have an assessment of cardiac risk as well as their risk of venous and or arterial thromboembolism. Even in the non-pregnant state many women with heart disease require thromboprophylaxis with antiplatelet agents or oral vitamin K antagonists. In this chapter we discuss how these prior treated patients are managed during pregnancy, as well as highlighting other patient groups with heart disease that should be considered for thromboprophylaxis only while pregnant.

Keywords

Pregnancy • Congenital and Acquired heart disease • Prosthetic heart valves • Antithrombotic therapy

10.1 Introduction

It is well recognized that pregnancy is a prothrombotic state due to the many changes in the coagulation cascade (discussed in detail in Chap. 1). These changes along with lower limb venous stasis and hypertension related to chronic venous insufficiency, creating a favorable environment for thrombus formation. It is therefore essential that women with heart disease embarking on pregnancy have not only an assessment of cardiac risk but are also assessed for their risk of venous and arterial thromboembolism (detailed in Chap. 3). This risk assessment must take account of not only the usual VTE risk factors during pregnancy (such as hyperemesis/dehydration, age >35 years,

A.S. Herrey, MB ChB, MD, PhD, MRCP
F. Walker, MB ChB, BM(Hons), FRCP, FESC (✉)
Department of Cardiology, The Heart Hospital, University College London Hospitals NHS Foundation Trust, 16-18 Westmoreland St, London W1G 8PH, UK
e-mail: anna.herrey@uclh.nhs.uk, fiona.walker@uclh.nhs.uk

H. Cohen, MB ChB, MD, FCRP, FRCPath
Department of Haematology, University College London Hospitals NHS Foundation Trust, 250 Euston Road, London NW1 2PG, UK
e-mail: hannah.cohen@uclh.nhs.uk

H. Cohen, P. O'Brien (eds.), *Disorders of Thrombosis and Hemostasis in Pregnancy: A Guide to Management*, DOI 10.1007/978-3-319-15120-5_10,

multiparity, pre-eclampsia, obesity, smoking, inherited or acquired thrombophilia) but also thromboembolic risks associated with the underlying cardiac malformation, for example, chamber dilatation, sluggish intracardiac blood flow, and arrhythmias.

Even in the nonpregnant state, many women with heart disease require thromboprophylaxis with antiplatelet agents or oral vitamin K antagonists. In this chapter, we will discuss how these prior treated patients are managed during pregnancy and will highlight other patient groups with heart disease that should be considered for thromboprophylaxis only when pregnant. It is, however, important to note that it is only in recent years that there have been sizable numbers of women with such complex heart disease embarking on pregnancy, so scientific data on this subject are sparse. This new and unique cohort of women will define their pregnancy outcome not only with regard to thromboembolic risk and its prevention but also as regards their underlying heart disease. This chapter is therefore based largely on our single-center experience, using scientific data if and when available.

10.2 Background

Cardiovascular disease complicates around 1–3 % of pregnancies in the developed world [1]. The improved survival of patients with complex congenital disease well into childbearing age has contributed a large number to the cohort of women with heart disease embarking on pregnancy. Another important but smaller group are women with acquired heart disease, including rheumatic heart disease (RHD) and ischemic heart disease (IHD). RHD nowadays is confined to immigrant populations, but the number of younger women with IHD has increased, due to advancing maternal age and an increase in risk factors for IHD (smoking, obesity, and diabetes) in this younger age group. Although accurate prevalence data for maternal heart disease in the UK are not available, heart disease is the single leading cause of maternal death in the UK, with the majority of deaths in those with undiagnosed acquired heart disease [2].

In the largest prospective study of pregnancy outcome in women with heart disease (CARPREG study), the outcome of 562 pregnancies was reported. Around 75 % of women had congenital heart disease and 25 % acquired heart disease. There were three deaths and four pregnancies were complicated by embolic stroke [3]. Both this study and the UK Centre for Maternal and Child Enquiries (CMACE) highlight the fact that there are risks for women with heart disease during pregnancy. A pre-pregnancy risk assessment, which allows stratification of antenatal care to an appropriate level of surveillance and specialist input, should be undertaken where possible [4, 5] (Table 10.1).

Table 10.1 Hierarchy of care for adults with Congenital Heart Disease (CHD)

Level I	*Highly complex lesions*
Exclusive care in a specialist unit	Repairs with conduits, Rastelli, Fontan, MFS, Ebstein's, pulmonary atresia, Eisenmenger syndrome, repaired TGA (arterial switch or atrial switch), CCTGA, PHT, cyanotic CHD
Level II	*Lesions of moderate complexity*
Shared care with regional adult cardiology unit	CoA (repaired/native), repaired AVSD, AS, PS/PR, TOF, VSD + AR, mechanical valves, HCM, DCM
Level III	*Simple lesions*
Care predominantly in general adult cardiology unit	Repaired PDA/VSD/TAPVD/ ASD, mild PS/PR, small VSD

Adapted from Heart Disease and Pregnancy – study group statement (http://www.rcog.org.uk/womens-health/clinical-guidance/heart-disease-and-pregnancy-study-group-statement)

TGA complete transposition of great arteries, *CCTGA* congenitally corrected transposition of great arteries, *ASD* atrial septal defect, *AVSD* atrioventricular septal defect, *AS* aortic stenosis, *PS* pulmonary stenosis, *PR* pulmonary regurgitation, *TOF* tetralogy of Fallot, *VSD* ventricular septal defect, *AR* aorta regurgitation, *PDA* patent ductus arteriosus, *MFS* Marfan syndrome, *HCM* hypertrophic cardiomyopathy, *DCM* dilated cardiomyopathy, *CoA* coarctation of the aorta, *TAPVD* total anomalous pulmonary venous drainage

10.3 Thromboprophylactic Agents Commonly Used in Heart Disease

The reader should also refer to Chap. 2.

10.3.1 Aspirin

Aspirin is the most widely used antithrombotic agent in patients with cardiovascular disease. It is given to patients with coronary artery disease and those with low a low TE risk. It crosses the placenta but at a thromboprophylactic dose (75–150 mg once daily; low dose aspirin (LDA)) is considered safe during all trimesters of pregnancy. Higher anti-inflammatory and analgesic doses are not recommended.

10.3.2 Clopidogrel

Clopidogrel is mostly used at a dose of 75 mg od in combination with aspirin (75 mg od) as part of a dual antiplatelet regimen following coronary (or other vascular) interventions. For bare metal coronary stents, dual antiplatelet therapy is given for 1 month, with aspirin lifelong thereafter, and for drug-eluting coronary stents, dual therapy (doses as above) is recommended for a minimum of 12 months with aspirin lifelong (75 mg od). Clopidogrel crosses the placenta and, although there are no reliable safety data available for its use during pregnancy, case reports and anecdotal evidence suggest that it may be safe [6, 7].

10.3.3 Dipyridamole

Dipyridamole is an antiplatelet agent often used alone or in combination with aspirin for secondary thromboprophylaxis, most commonly in patients with cerebrovascular disease. The usual dose is 200 mg twice daily. There are no safety data for its use during pregnancy, but it has been used in combination with aspirin or warfarin, during both pregnancy and breastfeeding [8].

10.3.4 Warfarin

Warfarin (or oral coumarol derivatives) is the most commonly used oral vitamin K antagonist (VKA). It is used in patients at high risk of thromboembolism, for example, patients with prosthetic valves, a previous history of VTE (pulmonary embolism (PE) or deep venous thrombosis (DVT)), atrial fibrillation, or dilated cardiomyopathy with poor systolic function. The dose is adjusted to achieve a target international normalized ratio (INR), which is determined by the indication for treatment. Warfarin crosses the placental barrier and increases the risk of spontaneous miscarriage and perinatal death [9–12]. It also causes an embryopathy [13–15] and fetal coagulopathy, which may lead to spontaneous fetal intracerebral hemorrhage [16, 17]. The risk of warfarin embryopathy (WE) is particularly high between 6 and 12 weeks of gestation. It is characterized by nasal hypoplasia and epiphyseal changes, and some evidence of lower intelligence in the long term [18, 19]. The reported incidence of WE is between 0 and 20 % [20] and appears to be greater if the warfarin dose is in excess of 5 mg per day [21]. In a systematic review of the literature published between 1966 and 1997 on anticoagulation in pregnant women with mechanical heart valves, Chan et al. found that the use of vitamin K antagonists throughout pregnancy was associated with congenital anomalies in 35 of 549 live births (6.4 %) [22]. A subsequent systematic review covering the years 2000–2009 reported a slightly lower risk (3.7 %) [23]. A multicenter observational, prospective study not included in the systematic reviews, using data collected by institutes collaborating in the European Network of Teratology Information Services (ENTIS) during individual risk counseling between 1988 and 2004, reported an increased frequency of structural defects in 666 pregnant women exposed to VKA during the first trimester compared to a non-exposed group of 1,094 women. However, there were only two cases of coumarin embryopathy among 356 live births (0.6 %; both phenprocoumon). The authors concluded that elective termination of a wanted pregnancy is not recommended if (inadvertent) exposure took place in early pregnancy, and that close follow-up by the obstetrician including level II (3D) ultrasound should be recommended in any case of VKA exposure during pregnancy [24].

10.3.5 Unfractionated Heparin

Unfractionated heparin (UFH) is an antithrombotic agent that can be given intravenously (IV) or subcutaneously (SC). At a dose of 5,000 IU SC two to three times daily, it can be used for thromboembolism prophylaxis. Therapeutic UFH may be used for patients with mechanical heart valves, pulmonary embolism, and acute coronary syndromes. Dosing is largely empirical, with different centers often using different dosing regimens. Most regimens require a bolus intravenous dose followed by a maintenance dose of 1,000–1,500 IU/h by continuous IV infusion, with a target activated partial thromboplastin time (APTT) ratio between 1.5 and 2.5 compared with the arithmetic mean of the normal range [25, 26] (or the laboratory reference range). It is well documented that achievement of a target APTT ratio within the first 24 h is difficult, because results vary considerably, even when measured every 4 h [27]. UFH does not cross the placenta and therefore has no fetal side effects. Maternal side effects include heparin-induced thrombocytopenia (HIT) in 1–3 % of patients [28–30] and osteoporosis. The latter is rare with short-term use and at low dose, however in a small prospective study to evaluate subclinical heparin-induced osteoporosis in pregnancy, a 10 % or greater decrease in bone density from baseline was reported in around 36 % of 14 women and none of the controls, with no dose-response relationship demonstrated. Furthermore, Dahlman [32] reported a symptomatic vertebral fracture rate of 2.2 % at therapeutic dose, in 4 of 184 women for whom the dosage of heparin ranged from 15,000 to 30,000 (mean 24,500) IU per 24 h, and the duration of treatment ranged from 7 to 27 (mean 17) weeks [31, 32].

10.3.6 Low Molecular Weight Heparin (LMWH)

Low molecular weight heparin (LMWH) has replaced UFH as the anticoagulant of choice for the majority of prothrombotic conditions during pregnancy [33]. Its use in patients with mechanical valves in pregnancy, however, remains contentious, with reports of high rates of thromboembolic complications in this group [34, 35]. It is administered SC and does not cross the placenta; there are therefore no adverse fetal effects. It has a better side-effect profile than UFH, with substantially less HIT <0.1 % [26, 28, 36] and osteoporosis (<0.1 %) [37, 38], has a longer half-life than UFH (3–6 h after SC injection), and has a more predictable anticoagulant effect. LMWH is eliminated by the kidneys. In the presence of renal insufficiency, the half-life is prolonged and dose adjustment is needed [39]. Prophylactic dose LMWH (LMWH-P) is generally administered once daily (the dose varies between different preparations), whereas high prophylactic (LMWH-HP) and therapeutic doses (LMWH-T) have twice daily (12 hourly) dosing regimens (see Tables 10.2 and 10.3). For the treatment and prevention of DVT and PE, routine anti-Xa monitoring is not recommended except in specific situations including at the extremes of body weight (<50 or >90 kg) or if there is renal insufficiency [26]. If used in patients with mechanical heart valves, however, anti-Xa must be measured every 1–2 weeks (peak levels at 3–5 h post-dose depending on the preparation) with regular dose adjustment to maintain anti-Xa levels between 1.0 and 1.2 IU/mL [40].

10.4 Maternal Heart Disease Associated with Increased Thromboembolic Risk

For simplicity heart disease will be categorized as acquired, inherited, or congenital. The focus will be on those conditions associated with increased thromboembolic risk, rather than an exhaustive list

Table 10.2 Indications and recommended regimens for anticoagulation and low dose aspirin in pregnancy

Cardiac lesion	Thromboprophylactic agent during pregnancy	Dose
Mitral stenosis (mild)/SR	LDA	75 mg od
Mitral stenosis (>mild)/SR	LMWH	P/HP/T
LV dilatation EF <40 %	LMWH	P/HP/T
LV dilatation EF >50 %	LDA	75 mg od
Persistent AF	LMWH	HP/T
Paroxysmal AF	LMWH	HP/T
LVNC EF >50 %	Aspirin	75 mg od
LVNC EF <40 %	LMWH	P/HP
Severe LA dilatation (> xcm^2)	LMWH	P/HP
Fontan (any)	LMWH	HP/T
Unrepaired ASD/PFO	LDA	75 mg od
Unrepaired ASD/PFO with a history of stroke	LMWH	HP/T
>Mild Ebstein's	LMWH	P/HP
ARVC RVEF <40 %	LMWH	P/HP
Prosthetic heart valves	LMWH ± LDA	HI

LMWH low molecular weight heparin, *P* prophylactic dose, *HP* high prophylactic dose, *T* therapeutic ("treatment" dose), *HI* high intensity, *LDA* low dose aspirin, *EF* ejection fraction, *SR* sinus rhythm, *AF* atrial fibrillation, *LA* left atrium, *LVNC* left ventricular non-compaction, *ASD* atrial septal defect, *PFO* persistent foramen ovale, *ARVC* Arrhythmogenic Right Ventricular Cardiomyopathy, *RVEF* right ventricular ejection fraction

Table 10.3 Weight-adjusted dosing regimens for LMWH

Weight (kg)	Enoxaparin	Dalteparin	Tinzaparin (75 U/kg od)
P dose			
<50	20 mg od	2,500 U od	3,500 U od
50–90	40 mg od	5,000 U od	4,500 U od
91–130	60 mg od	7,500 U od	7,000 U od
131–170	80 mg od	10,000 U od	9,000 U od
>170	0.6 mg/kg od	75 U/kg od	75 U/kg od
HP dose	40 mg bd	5,000 U bd	4,500 U bd
T dose	1 mg/kg bd antenatally 1.5 mg/kg od postnatally	100 U/kg bd or 200 U/kg od postnatally	175 U/kg od (ante- and postnatally)

If the creatinine clearance (Cockcroft and Gault) is <30 mL/min (<20 mL/min for tinzaparin), the LMWH dose should be reduced accordingly

Doses above as per RCOG guidelines for prevention of VTE in pregnancy [33] and the Heart Disease and Pregnancy – study group statement (http://www.rcog.org.uk/womens-health/clinical-guidance/heart-disease-and-pregnancy-study-group-statement)

of all cardiac disorders. Indications and recommended regimens for anticoagulation and low dose aspirin in pregnancy are summarized in Table 10.2.

10.4.1 Acquired Heart Disease

10.4.1.1 Valvular Heart Disease

Native Obstructive Valvular Disease

There are two main valve lesions associated with increased thromboembolic risk, both in the pregnant and nonpregnant state, namely, mitral stenosis (usually rheumatic [RHD]) and tricuspid stenosis (rare and due to RHD or abnormality of valve leaflets or its apparatus). Mitral stenosis (MS) is more common, but it is now rare in the developed world (0.02 % prevalence [41]), whereas in some parts of the developing world, the incidence is much higher (0.2–0.5 % in rural India and parts of Arabia) [42, 43]. There has been a resurgence of RHD in some areas of the UK where there are large immigrant communities, and some UK centers report that around 10–15 % of maternal heart disease is rheumatic in origin [44].

Rheumatic mitral valve disease may cause valvular stenosis (MS) or regurgitation (MR). As a consequence of these valve lesions, the left atrium dilates which leads to a high incidence of atrial arrhythmias (flutter [AFL] and/or fibrillation [AF]). Most women with more than mild mitral or tricuspid stenosis will be anticoagulated with warfarin or another VKA (target INR 2.5 (range 2.0–3.0)) even if in sinus rhythm, due to the presence of sluggish intra-atrial blood flow and the risk of atrial arrhythmia. Too often the first presentation of mitral stenosis is cerebral thromboembolism associated with new onset of AF. If there is persistent AF or a prior history of paroxysmal atrial fibrillation or flutter (PAF/PAFL), this is also an indication for anticoagulation with warfarin, irrespective of the degree of valve obstruction. If there is only mild stenosis (MVA >1.6 cm^2) and mild left atrial (LA) dilatation (<3.9 cm or 20 cm^2) and no prior history of arrhythmia, aspirin alone is used for thromboprophylaxis. During pregnancy, patients previously on warfarin are converted to LMWH-T, while those previously taking aspirin are commenced on prophylactic dose LMWH.

Other acquired obstructive valve lesions such as aortic stenosis (AS) are not associated with an increased risk of thrombus formation per se, as there is a high velocity of blood flow across the valve. Thromboembolism risk assessment in AS should, however, take into account the degree of valvar calcification/thickening and left ventricular size and function. In the presence of a heavily calcified valve or significant LV dilatation (LV end-diastolic diameter >6.2 cm or >3.8 cm/m^2) [45] and or dysfunction (EF <40 %), there may be an increased thromboembolic risk, and treatment with aspirin or LMWH should be considered during pregnancy.

Regurgitant Valve Lesions

The most common regurgitant valve lesions are mitral (MR) and aortic regurgitation (AR).

The common causes of MR are valve leaflet prolapse, myxomatous degeneration, annular dilatation, or following infective endocarditis. Irrespective of etiology, when important MR is present, it causes left atrial dilatation, and there is a risk of atrial arrhythmias, which is an indication for thromboprophylaxis (see Table 10.2).

AR frequently occurs in the context of aortic root dilatation secondary to aortopathy and connective tissue disease such as Marfan syndrome or bicuspid aortic valve (BAV), but endocarditis is also a common cause. Thromboprophylaxis is rarely indicated in those with aortopathy because the assessment of risk versus benefits of treatment must take into account the increased risk of aortic dissection in this patient group.

Ischemic Heart Disease (IHD)

The number of women with IHD in pregnancy is increasing due to advancing maternal age and increasing risk factors for IHD in younger people. It is therefore not surprising that pregnant women with acute coronary syndromes including myocardial infarction, coronary dissection, and long-term sequelae of IHD now account for the largest number of maternal cardiac deaths in the UK, a trend likely to continue [46]. Women with a prior history of IHD and prior coronary intervention are treated with dual antiplatelet therapy (aspirin and clopidogrel) for 4 weeks if a bare metal stent is deployed [47, 48] and 12 months for a drug-eluting stent [49, 50]. Aspirin 75 mg od is safe in pregnancy, but there is only anecdotal evidence for the safety of clopidogrel in pregnancy. However, when assessing the risks versus benefits of stopping clopidogrel, it must be borne in mind that stent thrombosis may be a fatal event and continuation of therapy is usually indicated.

Prosthetic Heart Valves

Prosthetic valves may be tissue/bioprosthetic (homografts/xenografts/pericardial) or mechanical (metal). Mechanical valves are highly thrombogenic and require anticoagulation with warfarin to prevent valve thrombosis [51]; bioprosthetic valves, on the other hand, do not require formal anticoagulation with warfarin.

The European Society of Cardiology (ESC) offers guidance on target INR levels for different types of metallic prostheses and patient-related factors influencing thromboembolic risk in the nonpregnant state, as follows [52]:

(a) Prostheses
Low thromboembolic risk prostheses include Carbomedics (aortic position), Medtronic Hall, St. Jude Medical and ON-X. Medium thromboembolic risk prostheses are other bileaflet valves; and high thromboembolic risk prostheses are Lillehei-Kaster, Omniscience, Starr-Edwards valves, Bjork Shiley and other tilting-disc valves.

(b) Patient-Related Factors
Mitral, tricuspid, or pulmonary valve replacement; previous history of thromboembolism; atrial fibrillation; left atrial diameter >50 mm; left atrial spontaneous echo contrast; mitral stenosis of any degree; LVEF <35 %; and hypercoagulable states such as pregnancy. If more than one patient-related risk factor is present, the INR target is increased to a higher value.

(c) Recommended INR Levels
Low-risk prosthesis and no patient risk factor: INR target 2.5 (range 2.0–3.0); ≥1 risk factor: target INR 3.0 (range 2.5–3.5)

Medium-risk prosthesis and no patient risk factor: INR target 3.5 (range 3.0–4.0); ≥1 risk factor: target INR 4.0 (range 3.0–4.0)

High-risk prosthesis and no patient risk factor: INR target 3.5 (range 3.0–4.0); >1 risk factor: target INR 4.0 (range 3.5–4.5).

The American Heart Association/American College of Cardiology (AHA/ACC) guidelines, on the other hand, recommend a target INR of 3.0, regardless of valve type and patient risk, with additional LDA if this is felt to be necessary [51].

The British Committee for Standards in Haematology (BCSH) guidelines recommend that the target INR should be raised from 2.5 to 3.0 and 3.0 to 3.5 in the low risk and medium risk groups, respectively, taking into account any additional patient risk factors for thrombosis, namely: mitral, tricuspid or pulmonary position; previous arterial thromboembolism; atrial fibrillation; left atrium diameter >50 mm; mitral stenosis of any degree; left ventricular ejection fraction <35 %; left atrial dense spontaneous echo contrast [53].

The main challenge regarding the use of anticoagulation for mechanical valves during pregnancy is that there is no ideal anticoagulant that is both safe and effective for both mother and fetus. Warfarin therapy throughout pregnancy results in the lowest observed rate of thromboembolism (3.9 %). However, VKA use is associated with fetal and neurodevelopmental problems [19, 22]. In these women, the rate of thromboembolism with UFH is high at 25 % if used throughout pregnancy and 9 % if used for the first trimester [54]. Therapeutic dose LMWH is an attractive alternative to warfarin and UFH however, in the HIP-CAT study, which compared enoxaparin with sequential UFH and warfarin in pregnant women with mechanical valves, 2/7 women receiving therapeutic dose enoxaparin 1 mg/kg 12-hourly developed fatal valve thrombosis [54]. James et al. found an overall thromboembolism rate of 22 % and a maternal mortality of 4 % [35]. Another study [34] found an overall incidence of valve thrombosis of 8.6 % (7/81) and an overall thromboembolism rate of 12.4 % (10/81). Notably, 9 of these 10 patients received a fixed dose of LMWH, and in 2 of these a low fixed dose was used. Among 51 pregnancies where anti-Xa levels were monitored, only one patient was reported to have had thromboembolism. Subsequent studies [12, 40] reported that compliance with therapeutic dose enoxaparin and aspirin is associated with a low risk of valve thrombosis: 5 thromboembolism events in 34 pregnancies treated with enoxaparin and one event in 12 pregnancies treated with LMWH (8 with dalteparin and 4 with enoxaparin) respectively, with non-compliance or subtherapeutic anti-Xa levels contributory in each case of thromboembolism. However, other authors reported fatal valve thrombosis despite therapeutic anti-Xa levels in 1 of 23 pregnancies and other adverse cardiac events in 22 % (5/23) [55]. Women must therefore be counseled of the pros and cons, regarding the choice of anticoagulant and anticoagulant regimen, in order to make an informed decision about which treatment regimen to use during pregnancy. Goland et al. reported that adjusted dose LMWH for women with mechanical heart valves is commonly associated with subtherapeutic trough levels, and suggest measurement of trough as well as peak anti-Xa levels to assure an adequate level of anticoagulation [56].

There is no consensus between cardiac societies on the optimal regimen, and current guidelines (ACCP, AHA/ACC and the ESC [28, 51, 52]) offer different advice. In practice most cardiologists consider three possible treatment regimens:

1. Warfarin throughout pregnancy, if the dose is <5 mg od, until week 36, then conversion to UFH or LMWH in preparation for delivery.
2. Stop warfarin before week 6 and convert to adjusted therapeutic dose UFH or LMWH for weeks 6–12. Then resume warfarin until week 36 when UFH or LMWH is restarted in preparation for delivery.
3. Stop warfarin before week 6 and convert to adjusted high intensity LMWH, and continue LMWH for duration of pregnancy until the time of delivery [40, 55].

If UFH or LMWH is used at any stage of pregnancy, the APTT (UFH) or anti-Xa (LMWH) must be monitored. For UFH administered by continuous intravenous infusion, the APTT ratio is measured within 4 h of starting treatment and thereafter every 6 h or after every dose adjustment, aiming for an APTT ratio which is 1.5–2.5 times that of normal controls [57] (or the laboratory reference therapeutic range). If LMWH is used, the anti-Xa is measured every 1–2 weeks. The ACCP guidelines (2012) advise that if LMWH is used, doses are adjusted to achieve 'the manufacturer's peak anti-Xa LMWH 4 h post-SC injection' (that is, approximately 1.0 IU/mL). As detailed above, therapeutic dose LMWH can be associated with thromboembolic events. We reported that high intensity adjusted LMWH, aiming for a peak level (4 h post-dose) of 1.0–1.2 IU/mL is associated with absence of thromboembolism unless levels of LMWH are subtherapeutic [40] (for suggested LMWH doses, see Table 10.3; in patients with prosthetic heart valves, considerable increases in LMWH doses may be needed during pregnancy, with a mean increase of >50 % reported by Quinn et al. [40]). LDA may be added to anticoagulation in women who are at particularly high risk of thrombosis, for example, those with atrial fibrillation.

In our practice, patients have a planned delivery at around 37–38 weeks gestation. A written delivery plan is formulated by the multidisciplinary team, which includes peripartum anticoagulation management and anesthetic options. For a vaginal delivery, patients are admitted for induction of labor (IOL), taking the last dose of LMWH (dalteparin 100 units/kg or equivalent) on the morning (or the evening in primigravidae) of the day prior to the day of IOL. In women also receiving LDA, this is stopped 1 week prior to elective delivery. The timeline for completion of delivery is 36 h and if unsuccessful a Cesarean section (CS) should be performed.

For elective CS, no LMWH should be administered for 24 h prior to admission, with the last dose half standard therapeutic dose (e.g. dalteparin 100 units/kg), allowing use of regional anaesthesia. Postdelivery, the management of LMWH is along the lines detailed in Chap. 4, aiming to start warfarin on day 4 postdelivery.

Tissue valves generally do not require anticoagulation, unless there is concomitant atrial arrhythmia, poor ventricular function, or significant chamber dilatation. Depending on thromboembolic risk assessment, LDA may also be given.

Acquired Dilated Cardiomyopathies (ADCM)

There are many causes of acquired DCM. In the younger age group, the most common causes are viral myocarditis, toxins, drugs, and pregnancy-associated cardiomyopathy that will be discussed in more detail below. Irrespective of the etiology, if there is only mild residual impairment of LV function, a subsequent pregnancy may precipitate a decline in function, and regular echo surveillance is advisable (monthly in our service). In the presence of severe LV or RV dilatation, there is blood stasis within the chamber, in addition to reduced endothelial antithrombotic properties and increased platelet adhesion [58–60]. There is no clear consensus as to whether patients with DCM and low LV ejection fraction (<40 %) should receive thromboprophylaxis in the absence of other prothrombotic risk factors, but many are treated with warfarin, especially if there is spontaneous echo contrast on transthoracic echocardiography (TTE) [61, 62]. During pregnancy, those with DCM and poor function (EF <40 %) will be given LMWH, although the majority with this degree of LV impairment will have been advised against pregnancy as they rep-resent a high-risk group with important maternal morbidity and mortality [63]. For those with DCM and an EF >40 %, LMWH or aspirin 75 mg od should be considered.

Peripartum Cardiomyopathy (PPCM)

PPCM is defined as an idiopathic cardiomyopathy presenting with heart failure secondary to LV systolic dysfunction towards the end of pregnancy or in the months following delivery where no other cause is found. Patients may present acutely in pulmonary edema or may develop progressive signs and symptoms of congestive cardiac failure. There is important morbidity and mortality from thromboembolic complications [64], and women with a new diagnosis of PPCM should be treated with LMWH during pregnancy and converted to warfarin postpartum. Around 50 % have recovery of LV function over a timeframe of approximately 6 months and during this time they remain should warfarinized [65]. If LV function recovers, warfarin can be stopped. For subsequent pregnancies, a recurrence risk of up to 50 % is quoted, especially if there is persistent LV dysfunction following the index pregnancy [66]. If there is persistent LV dysfunction with EF <50 %, pregnancy is inadvisable, but some patients will accept risk and become pregnant and they should be considered for treatment with LMWH. If LV function is normal, aspirin should be considered.

10.4.1.2 Inherited Heart Diseases

Familial Dilated Cardiomyopathy (FDCM)

In FDCM, both the right and left ventricles are dilated and dysfunctional. Approximately 25 % of DCM cases have a familial etiology. The most common inheritance pattern is autosomal dominant but an X-linked inheritance is also reported. Atrial arrhythmias and atrial dilatation are common, and warfarin anticoagulation is often needed (target INR of 2.5, range 2–3). In pregnancy warfarin is converted to LMWH.

Left Ventricular Non-compaction (LVNC)

LVNC is characterized by excessive trabeculation and recesses within the left ventricular myocardium (Fig. 10.1). The natural history of this disorder is poorly defined, but some develop progressive dilatation and LV dysfunction. If

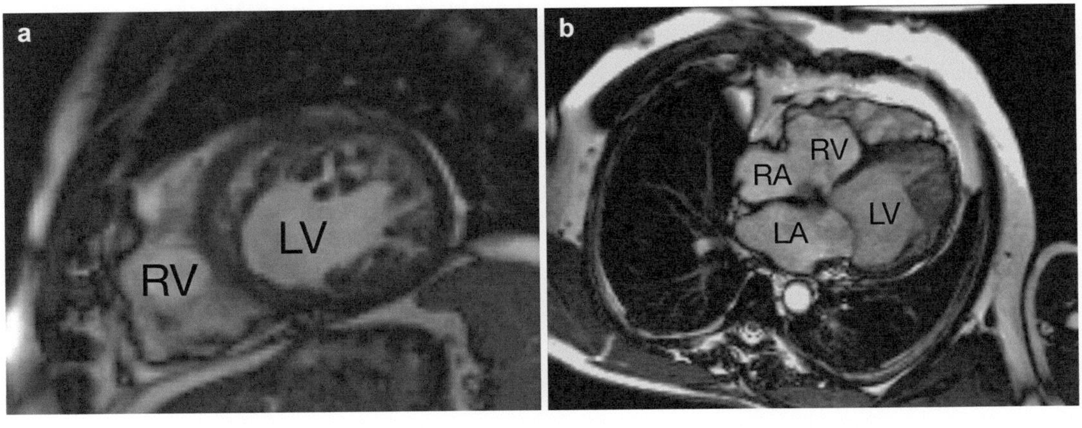

Fig. 10.1 Magnetic resonance images of left ventricular non-compaction (LVNC). (**a**) Short axis view with increased trabeculations and recesses in the anterior, lateral, and inferior wall. (**b**) Four-chamber view showing the distribution of non-compacted myocardium in both LV and RV toward the apex. *RA* right atrium, *RV* right ventricle, *LA* left atrium, *LV* left ventricle (Images courtesy Dr. Andrew Flett, University Hospital Southampton)

the LV is non-dilated, patients are given aspirin thromboprophylaxis, but in the presence of LV dysfunction and or dilatation, warfarin is used to reduce thromboembolic risk. During pregnancy, those taking warfarin are converted to LMWH, while all others are treated with aspirin.

Familial Hypertrophic Cardiomyopathy (FHCM)

FHCM is the most common form of inherited cardiomyopathy with an incidence of 1 in 500. It is inherited in a mostly autosomal dominant pattern. It is characterized by asymmetrical hypertrophy predominantly of the left ventricle and occasion-ally the right ventricle. The distribution of hypertrophy can vary, but basal septal hypertrophy is common, and this may cause left ventricular outflow tract obstruction (LVOTO). The myocardium is abnormal in structure and there is systolic and diastolic dysfunction. Diastolic (relaxation) abnormalities cause an elevation in LV filling pressure, which in turn leads to left atrial dilatation and atrial arrhythmias (30 % affected). The presence of LVH per se does not increase thromboembolic risk, but if there is a history of atrial arrhythmias, patients are anticoagulated with warfarin, which is converted to LMWH during pregnancy.

Arrhythmogenic Right Ventricular Cardiomyopathy (ARVC)

ARVC is a rare inherited cardiomyopathy characterized by right ventricular (RV) dilatation, malignant ventricular arrhythmias (ventricular tachycardia [VT] or ventricular fibrillation [VF]), and sudden cardiac death (SCD). Atrial arrhythmias are less common. Many patients have implantable defibrillators in situ for primary or secondary prevention of SCD. Over time there is progressive remodeling and dilatation of the RV, and RV dysfunction is common. In the presence of RV dilatation and paroxysmal VT/VF, patients require anticoagulation with warfarin, which is converted to LMWH during pregnancy.

10.4.2 Congenital Heart Disease

10.4.2.1 Unrepaired Atrial Septal Defect (ASD)

ASDs are the most common congenital abnormality, accounting for ~10 % of all congenital defects. Although the majority are diagnosed and repaired in infancy or childhood, some are newly detected in adulthood, especially during pregnancy. The most common defect is the ostium secundum ASD, which represents 75 % of all ASDs. Other defects including the ostium primum defect and sinus venosus defect are less common. In the presence of any type of ASD, there is a left-to-right shunt at atrial level, which causes volume overload of the right heart, leading to right atrial and right ventricular dilatation. Atrial arrhythmias are therefore common. During pregnancy, if there is no history of atrial arrhythmias, patients are given aspirin, but if there is a prior history of atrial arrhythmias, they will be anticoagulated with LMWH.

10.4.2.2 Atrioventricular Septal Defects (AVSDs)

The majority of adults with AVSD will have been diagnosed and surgically repaired in infancy or childhood. Residual problems in adulthood include left AV valve (LAVV) regurgitation and atrial arrhythmias. If arrhythmias are persistent or paroxysmal, patients are anticoagulated with warfarin and converted to LMWH during pregnancy.

10.4.2.3 Mustard or Senning Repair of Transposition of the Great Arteries (TGA)

The Mustard and Senning operations for TGA physiologically correct blood flow by complex intra-atrial baffling, whereby deoxygenated caval blood is directed across the interatrial septum (IAS), through the mitral valve into the left ventricle and via the pulmonary artery to the lungs, and oxygenated pulmonary venous blood is diverted across the IAS, through the tricuspid valve into the right ventricle (RV) and into the aorta (Fig. 10.2). Although blood flow is physiologically corrected, the anatomy remains uncorrected, and the right ventricle is the systemic/subarterial ventricle

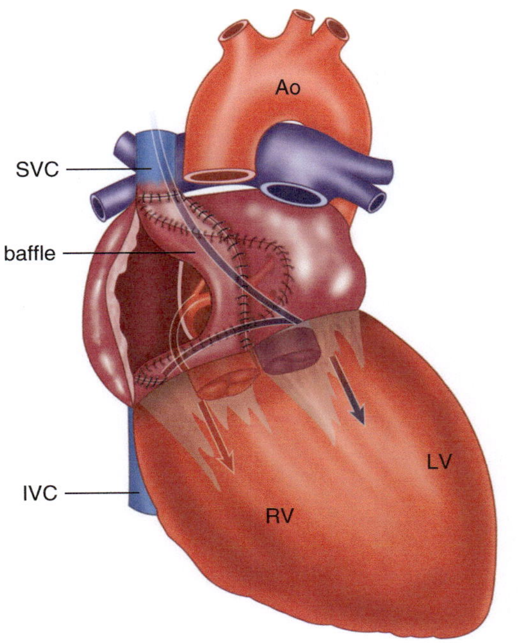

Fig. 10.2 Transposition of the great arteries (TGA), status post Mustard operation: systemic venous return is directed across to the left atrium, then subpulmonary left ventricle and the pulmonary artery. Pulmonary venous return is into the right atrium, then systemic right ventricle, then aorta. *RV* right ventricle, *LV* left ventricle, *IVC* inferior vena cava, *SVC* superior vena cava, *Ao* aorta (Image courtesy Dr. JPM Hamer, The Netherlands)

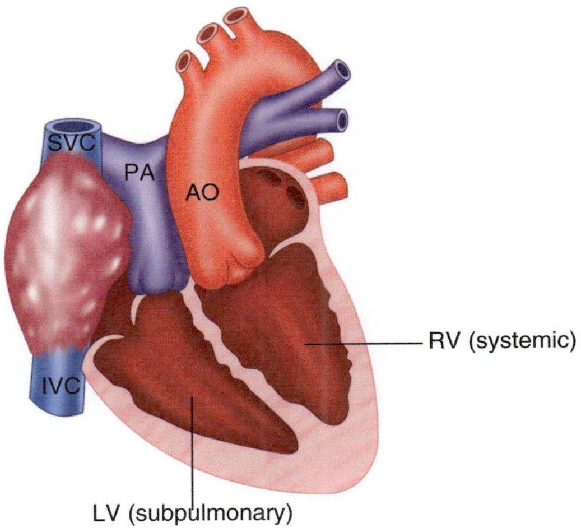

Fig. 10.3 Congenitally corrected TGA (CCTGA): systemic venous return via IVC and SVC into the right atrium, then subpulmonary left ventricle, then pulmonary artery. Pulmonary venous return via left atrium, systemic right ventricle to aorta. *TGA* transposition of the great arteries, *RV* right ventricle, *LV* left ventricle, *IVC* inferior vena cava, *SVC* superior vena cava, *Ao* aorta, *PA* pulmonary artery (Image courtesy Dr. Raquel Prieto, Hospital General Universitario Gregorio Marañon, Madrid, Spain)

(SRV). As a consequence, the RV dilates and hypertrophies and over time becomes dysfunctional. Atrial arrhythmias are also common. Patients with SRV impairment (EF <50 %) are advised that pregnancy is high risk and SRV function may deteriorate. Those with only mild impairment (EF >50 %) who embark on pregnancy are given aspirin thromboprophylaxis, unless there is a history of ARR whereby LMWH is indicated. Any patients taking warfarin prior to pregnancy will be converted to LMWH during pregnancy.

10.4.2.4 Congenitally Corrected TGA (CCTGA)

The anatomy of this rare lesion is such that the left atrium connects to a morphological RV via a tricuspid valve and the right atrium connects to the LV via a mitral valve (Fig. 10.3). There is often a VSD or pulmonary stenosis (PS), and patients with this more complex form of anatomy will often have undergone surgery in childhood to close the VSD and relieve the PS. Late complications include SRV dysfunction, atrial arrhythmias, and complete heart bock. The indication for anticoagulation is the same as for patients with the Mustard/Senning repairs.

10.4.2.5 Ebstein's Anomaly

In Ebstein's anomaly the tricuspid valve is displaced caudally toward the RV apex. This causes atrialization of the RV, reducing the functional size of the RV cavity (Fig. 10.4). The majority have a PFO or small ASD. Accessory electrophysiological pathways are common, leading to a high prevalence of ARR and supraventricular tachycardia (SVT). In its mildest form there is near-normal RV volume and function and only mild tricuspid regurgitation (TR), but with more severe TV displacement, the functional RV is small and severely restrictive, which leads to right heart failure and severe TR with cyanosis (right-to-left shunting across the PFO/ASD). The indication

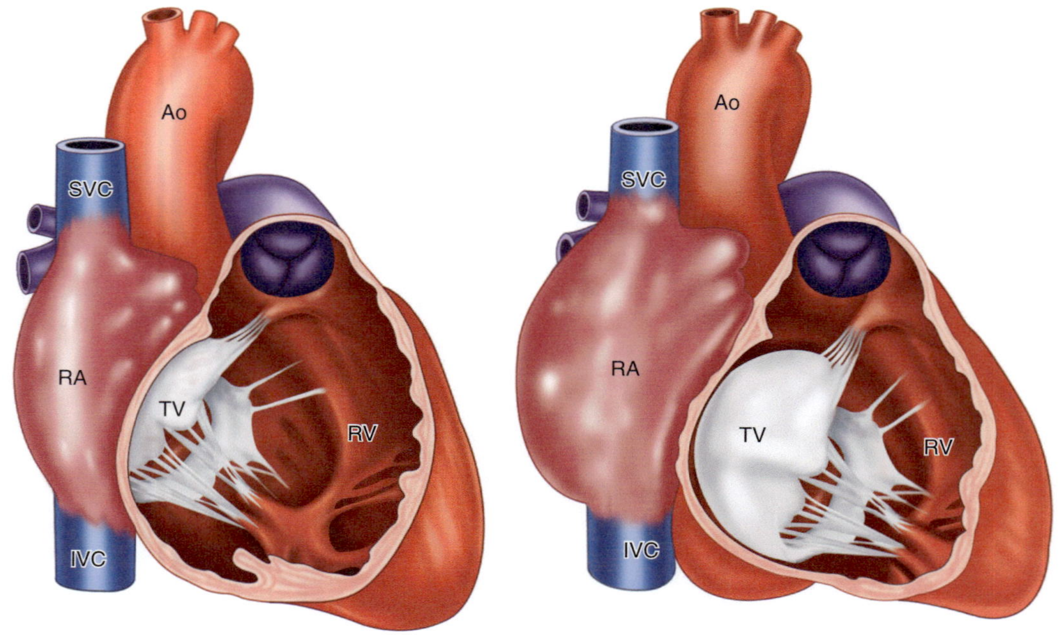

Fig. 10.4 Normal heart (*left*) versus Ebstein's anomaly (*right*): the tricuspid valve is displaced apically, resulting in a dilated right atrium and a small right ventricle. *RA* right atrium, *TV* tricuspid valve, *RV* right ventricle, *Ao* aorta, *SVC* superior vena cava, *IVC* inferior vena cava (Image courtesy Dr. JPM Hamer, The Netherlands)

for anticoagulation in this heterogeneous group of patients must be considered on an individual case-by-case basis. Those with atrial arrhythmias and severe atrialization of the RV will be anticoagulated with warfarin and converted to LMWH during pregnancy.

10.4.2.6 The Fontan Circulation

The Fontan operation is a palliative surgery for those born with complex congenital heart disease and in whom a biventricular repair is not possible. Since the original Fontan operation, there have been many modifications, but all represent a form of right heart bypass, whereby caval blood is diverted directly into the pulmonary arteries, negating the need for a subpulmonary ventricle. The total cavopulmonary connection (TCPC) is now the preferred palliation (Fig. 10.5). Although the Fontan circulation is a single ventricle circulation, unlike those born with a single ventricle, there is separation of the systemic venous and arterial circulations, and oxygen saturations are therefore normal. In the Fontan circulation, blood flow into the pulmonary artery (PA)

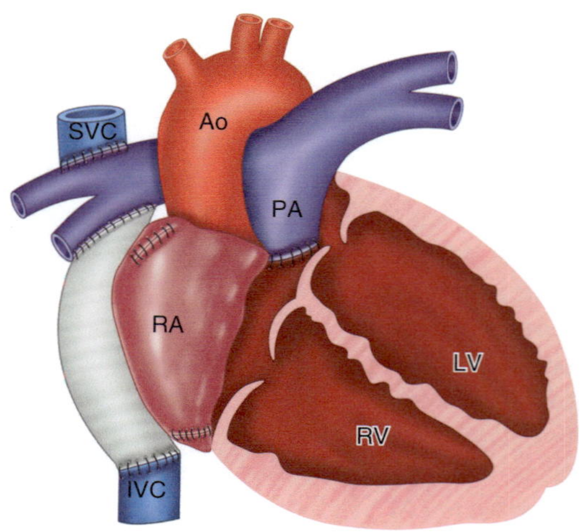

Fig. 10.5 Tricuspid atresia and status post Fontan operation (TCPC total cavopulmonary connection): the SVC is connected to the PA (bidirectional Glenn Shunt), and the IVC is connected to the PA via an extracardiac conduit. A functionally univentricular heart. *RV* right ventricle, *LV* left ventricle, *IVC* inferior vena cava, *SVC* superior vena cava, *Ao* aorta, *PA* pulmonary artery (Image courtesy Dr. Raquel Prieto, Hospital General Universitario Gregorio Marañon, Madrid, Spain)

is passive, assisted by spontaneous respiration and negative intrathoracic pressure. Blood flow is therefore sluggish, and when coupled with the coagulation abnormalities inherent to Fontan patients (increased platelet activation, impaired endothelial function, acquired protein C deficiency), there is a high risk of thromboembolic complications [67, 68] (Figs. 10.6 and 10.7). Studies have shown around 20 % incidence of asymptomatic PE in Fontan patients [69, 70]. The majority of patients with a Fontan circulation and/or severe RA dilatation are anticoagulated with warfarin, which is converted to LMWH during pregnancy. The remainder take LDA, but during pregnancy all Fontan patients should be treated with LMWH.

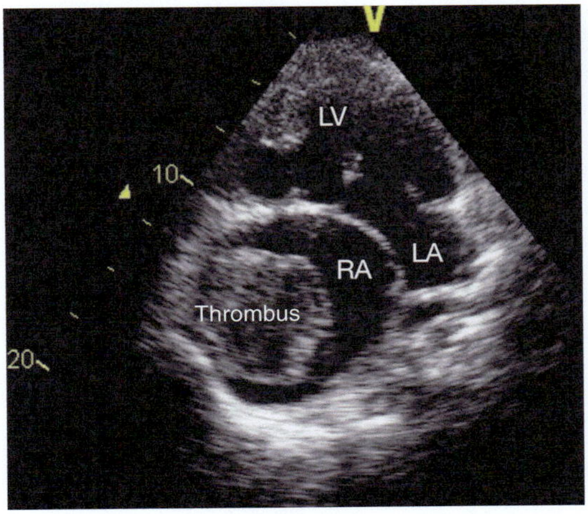

Fig. 10.6 Transthoracic echo image showing thrombus within the right atrium in a patient with APC Fontan circulation. *RA* right atrium, *LA* left atrium, *LV* left ventricle (Image courtesy Justin O'Leary, The Heart Hospital, UCLH)

10.4.2.7 Eisenmenger Syndrome (ES)

ES is a syndrome characterized by cyanosis, pulmonary hypertension, and a right-to-left shunt at atrial, ventricular, or great vessel level. The most common causes of ES are VSD, PDA, and AVSD [71]. The initial left-to-right shunt and consequent increased pulmonary blood flow cause remodeling of the pulmonary microvasculature with subsequent increase in pulmonary vascular resistance (PVR). The elevated PVR causes secondary RV hypertension and reversal of the shunt. Right-to-left shunting of deoxygenated blood causes cyano-sis and secondary polycythemia that leads to a multitude of hematological abnormalities including erythrocytosis, hyperviscosity, and iron deficiency [72]. There is both a prothrombotic (increased fibrinogen levels in the presence of reduced fibrinolytic activity) and bleeding tendency (thrombocytopenia secondary to reduced platelet production, increased activation, and increased destruction) [73, 74]. Up to a third of patients have evidence of pulmonary

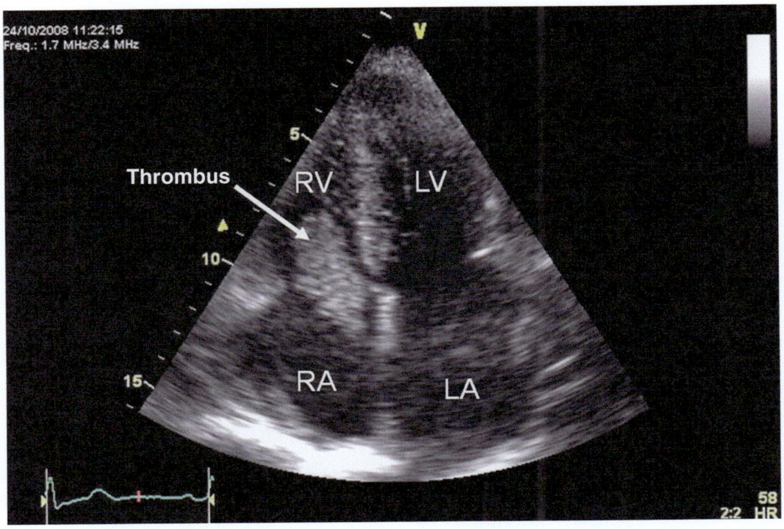

Fig. 10.7 Transthoracic echo image showing thrombus attached to internal cardiac defibrillator (ICD) lead prolapsing through the tricuspid valve into the RV in a patient with hypertrophic cardiomyopathy. *RA* right atrium, *RV* right ventricle, *LA* left atrium, *LV* left ventricle (Image courtesy Ruth Valland, The Heart Hospital, UCLH)

thromboemboli [75, 76], and around 20 % will have hemoptysis secondary to bronchial collaterals [77]. There is therefore no consensus as to whether these patients should be routinely anticoagulated, although warfarin treatment is indicated if there has been a proven thrombotic event. Pregnancy in ES is associated with a 30–50 % maternal mortality, and women are therefore advised against pregnancy [78, 79]. Fetal complications are also common, and the live-birth rate is closely associated with maternal oxygen saturation, such that if maternal resting O_2 saturation is <85 %, the chance of a live birth is approximately 12 % but if >90 % the live-birth rate is approximately 92 % [80]. If a woman with ES embarks on pregnancy, she will require anticoagulation with LMWH.

Conclusions

Thromboembolism is a major risk for women with heart disease embarking on pregnancy. While thromboembolic events are seen in 1 in 1,000 to 1 in 2,000 normal pregnancies [81, 82], the ZAHARA review of pregnancy outcomes in approximately 2,500 women with congenital heart disease concluded that thromboembolic risk in this group is 50 times higher than that in the normal pregnant population [83]. The CARPREG study also found that thromboembolic events were a major cause of morbidity and mortality within a similar pregnant population. Assessment of thromboembolic risk in any woman with heart disease embarking on pregnancy is therefore essential. Currently, however, there are no good data or guidelines specific to this patient group, with the exception of patients with mechanical valves. Clearly guidelines are needed, but until they are available, clinical practice and experience provide some insight into how to reduce thromboembolic risk in women with heart disease during pregnancy.

From our own institutional experience of managing over 500 pregnancies in women with heart disease, 90 women have received thromboprophylaxis. Their underlying cardiac lesions are shown in Fig. 10.8. There have been a total of five thromboembolic complications. Three thromboembolic events were in women prescribed thromboprophylaxis (LDA [1], LMWH [2]) and 2 were in patients on no antithrombotic therapy. There was one major thromboembolic event of mechanical valve thrombosis in a young woman with a Bjork-Shiley mitral

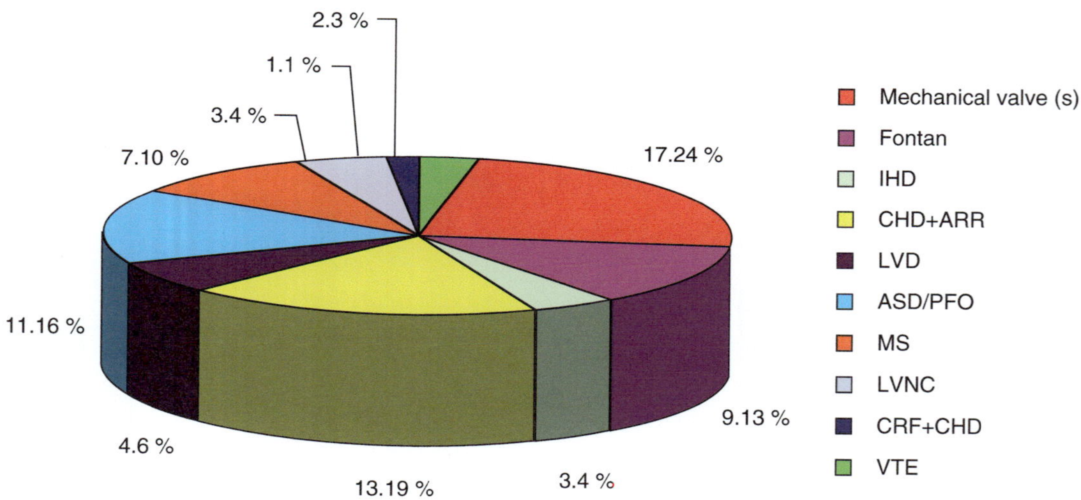

Fig. 10.8 Diagnoses of pregnant women with cardiac disorders on thromboprophylaxis at UCLH. *IHD* ischemic heart disease, *ARR* atrial arrhythmia, *LVD* left ventricular dysfunction, *ASD* atrial septal defect, *PFO* persistent foramen ovale, *MS* mitral stenosis, *LVNC* left ventricular non-compaction, *CRF* chronic renal failure, *VTE* venous thromboembolism (Chart courtesy of Ruth Valland, The Heart Hospital, UCLH)

prosthesis anticoagulated with LMWH (Case Study 1). Of the other two events on treatment, a patient with HOCM and an ICD in situ developed a large thrombus on the ICD lead at 24 weeks' gestation. She had been noncompliant with aspirin therapy and was found to be heterozygous for factor V Leiden. On further questioning she reported a family history of VTE, a sibling having had a prior PE. The other patient with a TCPC Fontan presented with a pulmonary embolism at 20 weeks' gestation. She had been noncompliant with LMWH therapy. Two thromboembolic events were in women on no VTE prophylaxis. One patient with anthracycline cardiomyopathy and near-normal LV function pre-pregnancy had a spontaneous pregnancy loss at 24 weeks' gestation and was found to have poor LV function and LV thrombus at review 2 weeks later. The second patient had moderate to severe valvular aortic stenosis and 48 h post vaginal delivery had a left-sided CVA. This clinical experience provides several learning points.

10.5 Case Studies

Case Study 1

This 25 year old patient, who had undergone mitral-valve replacement (Bjork-Shirley) at the age of 6 years for left atrio-ventricular valve regurgitation, had a valve-related thrombosis, which occurred at 26 weeks gestation. She had a past history of subclavian vein thrombosis at the age of 21. Thrombophilia testing showed that she was heterozygous for the G20210A prothrombin gene mutation. This was her second pregnancy, the first ending in an early spontaneous miscarriage 1 year previously whilst on warfarin treatment. She switched to therapeutic dose LMWH, dalteparin 5,000 IU 12 hourly (weight 50 kg) at 8 weeks gestation. Optimal anti-Xa monitoring was not possible due to geographical remoteness. By week 26, her dalteparin dose was 8,750 IU 12 hourly (peak dose during pregnancy) and she developed progressive dyspnea. Pulmonary edema secondary to mitral valve thrombosis was diagnosed. She underwent emergency CS with delivery of a female infant weighing 1,000 g followed by emergency mitral valve replacement. Importantly, anti-Xa levels at 14 and 20 weeks gestation were subtherapeutic (0.6 and 0.64 IU/mL, respectively). She made a good recovery and after a prolonged period in the neonatal intensive care unit, her daughter subsequently achieved normal growth and development [40].

Case Study 2

A 32-year-old woman contacted her anticoagulation clinic when she was 5 weeks pregnant. Her first pregnancy when aged 18 years was uncomplicated. Three months post partum she developed heart failure, and subsequently underwent mechanical mitral valve replacement a year later. Following this, she was anticoagulated with warfarin, target INR 3.5 (range 3.0–4.0) and moved to the UK. Prior to her current pregnancy, she attended a specialist cardiology clinic for preconceptual counseling, where echocardiography showed good ventricular function and normal aortic mechanical valve function, and the risks and benefits of anticoagulation with a vitamin K antagonist versus LMWH were discussed. Her warfarin was stopped and she was commenced on dalteparin at an initial dose of 5,000 units 12 hourly (weight 49 kg). She was also commenced on LDA 75 mg daily. The anti Xa 1 week later was 0.65 IU/mL, and the dalteparin dose was increased, with the maximum dose approximately 50 % above baseline by 22 weeks' gestation, to maintain peak anti-Xa levels at a target of 1.0–1.2 IU/mL. This necessitated fortnightly anti Xa testing throughout pregnancy. Her antenatal care was managed in a high risk multidisciplinary antenatal clinic. Induction of labour was planned to be undertaken at 38 weeks gestation. A peri-delivery plan was written with input from the obstetrician, cardiologist, hematologist and anesthetist, and discussed with the patient. LDA was stopped at 37 weeks gestation. The last dose of dalteparin (100 units/kg) was administered the morning 24 h before induction. She had an emergency CS for obstetric reasons following a failed induction of labour, with delivery of a healthy female infant, BW 2,800 g. The CS was performed under spinal anaesthesia, (as more than 24 h had elapsed since the last therapeutic dose of dalteparin). Post-partum she received dalteparin 5,000 units within 6 h of the CS. She developed a wound haematoma 12 h after delivery and she was taken back to theatre for evacuation under general anesthesia. Dalteparin was restarted cautiously, with an initial dose of 5,000 units 6 h post operatively, increasing to 2,500 units am and 5,000 units pm (12 h later) on day 1 post operatively (postpartum weight 53 kg). This was increased to Dalteparin 5,000 twice daily on day 2 post-delivery. She had no further bleeding and was switched to once daily dosing from day 6 post-delivery. Warfarin was restarted on day 5 and dalteparin was stopped once the INR was in the therapeutic range. She did not have any thrombotic complications [40].

Key Learning Points

- If LMWH is used for mechanical valves in pregnancy, it must be monitored meticulously every 1–2 weeks and the dose up-titrated promptly to maintain target anti-Xa levels.
- Any patient at risk of a deterioration in ventricular function during pregnancy should be considered for LMWH thromboprophylaxis.
- Inherited or acquired thrombophilias should be excluded in those with a past or family history of VTE.
- Calcified valves pose a thromboembolic risk and patients with these should be considered for thromboprophylaxis.
- Patient compliance with any treatment regimen is of paramount importance, and thromboembolic risk and its prevention needs to be highlighted and reiterated at clinic review.

Acknowledgements The authors would like to thank Ruth Brooks, cardiac specialist nurse for the maternal cardiology service at the Heart Hospital, for her input.

References

1. Arafeh JM, Baird SM. Cardiac disease in pregnancy. Crit Care Nurs Q. 2006;29:32–52.
2. Cantwell R, Clutton-Brock T, Cooper G, Dawson A, Drife J, Garrod D, Harper A, Hulbert D, Lucas S, McClure J, Millward-Sadler H, Neilson J, Nelson-Piercy C, Norman J, O'Herlihy C, Oates M, Shakespeare J, de Swiet M, Williamson C, Beale V, Knight M, Lennox C, Miller A, Parmar D, Rogers J, Springett A. Saving mothers' lives: reviewing maternal deaths to make motherhood safer: 2006–2008. The Eighth Report of the Confidential Enquiries into Maternal Deaths in the United Kingdom. BJOG. 2011;118 Suppl 1:1–203.
3. Siu SC, Sermer M, Colman JM, Alvarez AN, Mercier LA, Morton BC, Kells CM, Bergin ML, Kiess MC, Marcotte F, Taylor DA, Gordon EP, Spears JC, Tam JW, Amankwah KS, Smallhorn JF, Farine D, Sorensen S, Cardiac Disease in Pregnancy (CARPREG) Investigators. Prospective multicenter study of pregnancy outcomes in women with heart disease. Circulation. 2001;104(5):515–21.
4. Siu SC, Sermer M, Harrison DA, Grigoriadis E, Liu G, Sorensen S, Smallhorn JF, Farine D, Amankwah KS, Spears JC, Colman JM. Risk and predictors for pregnancy-related complications in women with heart disease. Circulation. 1997;96:2789–94.
5. Walker F. Antenatal care of women with cardiac disease: a cardiologists perspective. In: Steer PJ, Gatzoulis MA, Baker P, editors. Heart disease and pregnancy. London: RCOG Press; 2006.
6. Klinzing P, Markert UR, Liesaus K, Peiker G. Case report: successful pregnancy and delivery after myocardial infarction and essential thrombocythemia treated with clopidrogel. Clin Exp Obstet Gynecol. 2001;28:215–6.
7. Cuthill JA, Young S, Greer IA, Oldroyd K. Anaesthetic considerations in a parturient with critical coronary artery disease and a drug-eluting stent presenting for caesarean section. Int J Obstet Anesth. 2005;14:167–71.
8. Taguchi K. Pregnancy in patients with a prosthetic heart valve. Surg Gynecol Obstet. 1977;145:2068.
9. Nassar AH, Hobeika EM, Abd Essamad HM, Taher A, Khalil AM, Usta IM. Pregnancy outcome in women with prosthetic heart valves. Am J Obstet Gynecol. 2004;191:1009–13.
10. Blickstein D, Blickstein I. The risk of fetal loss associated with Warfarin anticoagulation. Int J Gynaecol Obstet. 2002;78:221–5.
11. Srivastava AK, Gupta AK, Singh AV, Husain T. Effect of oral anticoagulant during pregnancy with prosthetic heart valve. Asian Cardiovasc Thorac Ann. 2002;10:306–9.
12. McLintock C, McCowan LM, North RA. Maternal complications and pregnancy outcome in women with mechanical prosthetic heart valves treated with enoxaparin. BJOG. 2009;116(12):1585–92.

13. Hall JG. Embryopathy associated with oral anticoagulant therapy. Birth Defects Orig Artic Ser. 1965;12:133–40.
14. Iturbe-Alessio I, Fonseca MC, Mutchinik O, Santos MA, Zajarias A, Salazar E. Risks of anticoagulant therapy in pregnant women with artificial heart valves. N Engl J Med. 1986;315:1390–3.
15. Sadler L, McCowan L, White H, Stewart A, Bracken M, North R. Pregnancy outcomes and cardiac complications in women with mechanical, bioprosthetic and homograft valves. BJOG. 2000;107:245–53.
16. Meschengieser SS, Fondevila CG, Santarelli MT, Lazzari MA. Anticoagulation in pregnant women with mechanical heart valve prostheses. Heart. 1999;82:23–6.
17. Chen WW, Chan CS, Lee PK, Wang RY, Wong VC. Pregnancy in patients with prosthetic heart valves: an experience with 45 pregnancies. Q J Med. 1982;51:358–65.
18. Hall JAG, Paul RM, Wilson KM. Maternal and fetal sequelae of anticoagulation during pregnancy. Am J Med. 1980;68:122–40.
19. Wesseling J, Van Driel D, Heymans HSA, Rosendaal FR, Geven-Boere LM, Smrkovsky M, Touwen BCL, Van der Sauer PJJ, Veer E. Coumarins during pregnancy: long-term effects on growth and development of school-age children. Thromb Haemost. 2001;85(4): 609–13.
20. Hung L, Rahimtoola SH. Prosthetic heart valves and pregnancy. Circulation. 2003;107:1240–6.
21. Cotrufo M, De Feo M, De Santo LS, Romano G, Della Corte A, Renzulli A, Gallo C. Risk of warfarin during pregnancy with mechanical valve prostheses. Obstet Gynecol. 2002;99:35–40.
22. Chan WS, Anand S, Ginsberg JS. Anticoagulation of pregnant women with mechanical heart valves: a systematic review of the literature. Arch Intern Med. 2000;160(2):191–6.
23. Allam H. Anticoagulation of pregnant women with mechanical heart valve prosthesis: a systematic review of the literature (2000–2009). J Coagul Disord. 2010;2(1):81–8.
24. Schaefer C, Hannemann D, Meister R, Eléfant E, Paulus W, Vial T, et al. Vitamin K antagonists and pregnancy outcome. A multi-centre prospective study. Thromb Haemost. 2006;95(6):949–57.
25. Eikelboom JW, Hirsh J. Monitoring unfractionated heparin with the aPTT: time for a fresh look. Thromb Haemost. 2006;96(5):547–52.
26. Royal College of Obstetricians and Gynaecologists. Green-top guideline no.37b. Thromboembolic disease in pregnancy and the puerperium: acute management. 2015. London: RCOG; https://www.rcog.org.uk/guidelines.
27. Schaefer DC, Hufnagle J, Williams L. Rapid heparin anticoagulation: use of a weight-based nomogram. Am Fam Physician. 1996;54:2517–21.
28. Bates SM, Greer IA, Middeldorp S, Veenstra DL, Prabulos A-M, Vandvik PO. VTE, thrombophilia, antithrombotic therapy, and pregnancy: Antithrombotic Therapy and Prevention of Thrombosis, 9th ed: American College of Chest Physicians Evidence-Based Clinical Practice Guidelines. Chest. 2012;141(2):e691S–736.
29. Warkentin TE, Levine MN, Hirsh J, Horsewood P, Roberts RS, Gent M, Kelton JG. Heparin-induced thrombocytopenia in patients treated with low-molecular-weight-heparin or unfractionated heparin. N Engl J Med. 1995;332:1330–6.
30. Girolami B, Prandoni P, Stefani PM, Tanduo C, Sabbion P, Eichler P, Ramon R, Baggio G, Fabris F, Girolami A. The incidence of heparin-induced thrombocytopenia in hospitalized medical patients treated with subcutaneous unfractionated heparin: a prospective cohort study. Blood. 2003;101:2955–9.
31. Barbour LA, Kick SD, Steiner JF, LoVerde ME, Heddleston LN, Lear JL, Baron AE, Barton PL. A prospective study of heparin-induced osteoporosis in pregnancy using bone densitometry. Am J Obstet Gynecol. 1994;170:862–9.
32. Dahlman TC. Osteoporotic fractures and the recurrence of thromboembolism during pregnancy and the puerperium in 184 women undergoing thromboprophylaxis with heparin. Am J Obstet Gynecol. 1993; 168(4):1265–70.
33. Royal College of Obstetricians and Gynaecologists. Green-top guideline no. 37a. Thrombosis and embolism during pregnancy and the puerperium, reducing the risk. London: Royal College of Obstetricians and Gynaecologists; 2009. https://www.rcog.org.uk/guidelines.
34. Oran B, Lee-Parritz A, Ansell J. Low molecular weight heparin for the prophylaxis of thromboembolism in women with prosthetic mechanical heart valves during pregnancy. Thromb Haemost. 2004;92:747–51.
35. James AH, Brancazio LR, Gehrig TR, Wang A, Ortel TL. Low-molecular-weight heparin for thromboprophylaxis in pregnant women with mechanical heart valves. J Matern Fetal Neonatal Med. 2006;19:543–9.
36. Bazzan M, Donvito V. Low molecular weight heparin during pregnancy. Thromb Res. 2001;101:V175–86.
37. Sanson BJ, Lensing AW, Prins MH, Ginsberg JS, Barkagan ZS, Lavenne-Pardonge E, et al. Safety of low-molecular-weight heparin in pregnancy: a systematic review. Thromb Haemost. 1999;81(5):668–72.
38. Greer IA, Nelson-Piercy C. Low-molecular-weight heparins for thromboprophylaxis and treatment of venous thromboembolism in pregnancy: a systematic review of safety and efficacy. Blood. 2005;106:401–7.
39. Hirsh J, Bauer KA, Donati MB, Gould M, Samama MM, Weitz JI, American College of Chest Physicians. Parenteral anticoagulants: American College of Chest Physicians Evidence-Based Clinical Practice (8th Edition). Chest. 2008;133 Suppl 6:141S–59.

40. Quinn J, Von Klemperer K, Brooks R, Peebles D, Walker F, Cohen H. Use of high intensity adjusted dose low molecular weight heparin in women with mechanical heart valves during pregnancy: a single-center experience. Haematologica. 2009;94:1608–12.
41. Nkomo VT, Gardin JM, Skelton TN, Gottdiener JS, Scott CG, Enriquez-Sarano M. Burden of valvular heart diseases: a population-based study. Lancet. 2006;368(9540):1005–11.
42. Vijaykumar M, Narula J, Reddy KS. Incidence of rheumatic fever and prevalence of rheumatic heart disease in India. Int J Cardiol. 1994;43:221–8.
43. Agarwal AK. Rheumatic fever and rheumatic heart disease in Arabia. Int J Cardiol. 1994;43:221–8.
44. Personal communication with Dr. Lorna Swan, consultant cardiologist, Royal Brompton Hospital, London, and Dr. Sara Thorne, consultant cardiologist, University Hospital Birmingham, Birmingham. 2010.
45. British Society of Echocardiography guidelines for chamber quantification. www.bsecho.org.
46. Curry R, Swan L, Steer PJ. Cardiac disease in pregnancy. Curr Opin Obstet Gynecol. 2009;21:508–13.
47. Leon MB, Baim DS, Popma JJ, Gordon PC, Cutlip DE, Ho KK, et al. A clinical trial comparing three antithrombotic-drug regimens after coronary-artery stenting. Stent Anticoagulation Restenosis Study Investigators. N Engl J Med. 1998;339(23):1665–71.
48. Urban P, Macaya C, Rupprecht HJ, Kiemeneij F, Emanuelsson H, Fontanelli A, et al. Randomized evaluation of anticoagulation versus antiplatelet therapy after coronary stent implantation in high-risk patients: the multicenter aspirin and ticlopidine trial after intracoronary stenting (MATTIS). Circulation. 1998;98(20):2126–32.
49. Brener SJ, Steinhubl SR, Berger PB, Brennan DM, Topol EJ, CREDO Investigators. Prolonged dual antiplatelet therapy after percutaneous coronary intervention reduces ischemic events without affecting the need for repeat revascularization: insights from the CREDO trial. J Invasive Cardiol. 2007;19(7):287–90.
50. Galla JM, Lincoff AM. The role of clopidogrel in the management of ischemic heart disease. Curr Opin Cardiol. 2007;22:273–9.
51. Nishimura RA, Otto CM, Bonow RO, Carabello BA, Erwin 3rd JP, Guyton RA, ACC/AHA Task Force Members, et al. 2014 AHA/ACC guideline for the management of patients with valvular heart disease: a report of the American College of Cardiology/American Heart Association Task Force on Practice Guidelines. Circulation. 2014;129(23):e521–643.
52. Joint Task Force on the Management of Valvular Heart Disease of the European Society of Cardiology (ESC), European Association for Cardio-Thoracic Surgery (EACTS), Vahanian A, Alfieri O, Andreotti F, Antunes MJ, Barón-Esquivias G, Baumgartner H, Borger MA, et al. Guidelines on the management of valvular heart disease (version 2012). Eur Heart J. 2012;33(19):2451–96.
53. Keeling D, Baglin T, Tait C, Watson H, Perry D, Baglin C, British Committee for Standards in Haematology, et al. Guidelines on oral anticoagulation with warfarin – fourth edition. Br J Haematol. 2011;154(3):311–24.
54. Ginsberg JS, Chan WS, Bates SM, Kaatz S. Anticoagulation of pregnant women with mechanical heart valves. Arch Intern Med. 2003;163:694–8.
55. Yinon Y, Siu SC, Warshafsky C, Maxwell C, McLeod A, Colman JM, Sermer M, Silversides CK. Use of low molecular weight heparin in pregnant women with mechanical heart valves. Am J Cardiol. 2009;104(9):1259–63.
56. Goland S, Schwartzenberg S, Fan J, Kozak N, Khatri N, Elkayam U. Monitoring of anti-Xa in pregnant patients with mechanical prosthetic valves receiving low-molecular-weight heparin: peak or trough levels? J Cardiovasc Pharmacol Ther. 2014;19:451–6.
57. Raschke R, Gollihare B, Peirce J. The effectiveness of implementing the weight-based heparin nomogram as a practice guideline. Arch Intern Med. 1996;156:1645–9.
58. Elkayam U, Khan S, Mehboob A, Ahsan N. Impaired endothelium-mediated vasodilation in heart failure: clinical evidence and the potential for therapy. J Card Fail. 2002;8:15–20.
59. Ahnert AM, Freudenberger RS. What do we know about anticoagulation in patients with heart failure? Curr Opin Cardiol. 2008;23:228–32.
60. Chong AY, Freestone B, Patel J, Lim HS, Hughes E, Blann AD, Lip GY. Endothelial activation, dysfunction, and damage in congestive heart failure and the relation to brain natriuretic peptide and outcomes. Am J Cardiol. 2006;97:671–5.
61. Abdo AS, Kemp R, Barham J, Geraci SA. Dilated cardiomyopathy and role of antithrombotic therapy. Am J Med Sci. 2010;339(6):557–60.
62. Cleland JG, Findlay I, Jafri S, Sutton G, Falk R, Bulpitt C, Prentice C, Ford I, Trainer A, Poole-Wilson PA. The Warfarin/Aspirin Study in Heart failure (WASH): a randomized trial comparing antithrombotic strategies for patients with heart failure. Am Heart J. 2004;148:157–64.
63. Grewal J, Siu SC, Ross HJ, Mason J, Balint OH, Sermer M, Colman JM, Silversides CK. Pregnancy outcomes in women with dilated cardiomyopathy. J Am Coll Cardiol. 2009;55:45–52.
64. Sliwa K, Fett J, Elkayam U. Peripartum cardiomyopathy. Lancet. 2006;368:687–93.
65. Sutton MS, Cole P, Plappert M, Saltzman D, Goldhaber S. Effects of subsequent pregnancy on left ventricular function in peripartum cardiomyopathy. Am Heart J. 1991;121(6 Pt 1):1776–8.
66. Elkayam U, Tummala PP, Rao K, Akhter MW, Karaalp IS, Wani OR, Hameed A, Gviazda I, Shotan A. Maternal and fetal outcomes of subsequent pregnancies in women with peripartum cardiomyopathy. N Engl J Med. 2001;344(21):1567–71.

67. Kajimoto H, Nakazawa M, Murasaki K, Hagiwara N, Nakanishi T. Increased P-selectin expression on platelets and decreased plasma thrombomodulin in Fontan patients. Circ J. 2009;73:1705–10.
68. Odegard KC, McGowan Jr FX, Zurakowski D, Dinardo JA, Castro RA, del Nido PJ, Laussen PC. Procoagulant and anticoagulant factor abnormalities following the Fontan procedure: increased factor VIII may predispose to thrombosis. J Thorac Cardiovasc Surg. 2003;125:1260–7.
69. Varma C, Warr MR, Hendler AL, Paul NS, Webb GD, Therrien J. Prevalence of "silent" pulmonary emboli in adults after the Fontan operation. J Am Coll Cardiol. 2003;41:2252–8.
70. Monagle P, Cochrane A, McCrindle B, Benson L, Williams W, Andrew M. Thromboembolic complications after Fontan procedures – the role of prophylactic anticoagulation. J Thorac Cardiovasc Surg. 1998; 115:493–8.
71. Wood P. Pulmonary hypertension with special reference to the vasoconstrictive factor. Br Heart J. 1958;20:557–70.
72. Perloff JK, Rosove MH, Child JS, Wright GB. Adults with cyanotic congenital heart disease: hematologic management. Ann Intern Med. 1988;109:406–13.
73. Lill MC, Perloff JC, Child JS. Pathogenesis of thrombocytopenia in cyanotic congenital heart disease. Am J Cardiol. 2006;98(2):254–8.
74. Huber K, Beckmann R, Frank H, Kneussl M, Mlczoch J, Binder BR. Fibrinogen, t-PA, and PAI-1 plasma levels in patients with pulmonary hypertension. Am J Respir Crit Care Med. 1994;150: 929–33.
75. Diller GP, Gatzoulis MA. Pulmonary vascular disease in adults with congenital heart disease. Circulation. 2007;115:1039–50.
76. Broberg CS, Ujita M, Prasad S, Li W, Rubens M, Bax BE, Davidson SJ, Bouzas B, Gibbs JS, Burman J, Gatzoulis MA. Pulmonary arterial thrombosis in eisenmenger syndrome is associated with biventricular dysfunction and decreased pulmonary flow velocity. J Am Coll Cardiol. 2007;50:634–42.
77. Daliento L, Somerville J, Presbitero P, Menti L, Brach-Prever S, Rizzoli G, Stone S. Eisenmenger syndrome. Factors relating to deterioration and death. Eur Heart J. 1998;19:1845–55.
78. Warnes CA. Pregnancy and pulmonary hypertension. Int J Cardiol. 2004;97 Suppl 1:11–3.
79. Bédard E, Dimopoulos K, Gatzoulis MA. Has there been any progress made on pregnancy outcomes among women with pulmonary arterial hypertension? Eur Heart J. 2009;30:256–65.
80. Presbitero P, Somerville J, Stone S, Aruta E, Spiegelhalter D, Rabajoli F. Pregnancy in cyanotic congenital heart disease. Outcome of mother and fetus. Circulation. 1994;89(6):2673–6.
81. Toglia MR, Weg JG. Venous thromboembolism during pregnancy. N Engl J Med. 1996;335:108–14.
82. Greer IA. Thrombosis in pregnancy: maternal and fetal issues. Lancet. 1999;353:1258–65.
83. Drenthen W, Pieper PG, Roos-Hesselink JW, van Lottum WA, Voors AA, Mulder BJ, van Dijk AP, Vliegen HW, Yap SC, Moons P, Ebels T, van Veldhuisen DJ, ZAHARA Investigators. Outcome of pregnancy in women with congenital heart disease: a literature review. J Am Coll Cardiol. 2007;49(24):2303–11.

Inherited Bleeding Disorders in Pregnancy: von Willebrand Disease, Factor XI Deficiency, and Hemophilia A and B Carriers

11

Christine A. Lee and Rezan A. Kadir

Abstract

Obstetric management of women with von Willebrand Disease (VWD) and FXI deficiency, and carriers of hemophilia A and B, requires a multidisciplinary team approach with obstetricians, midwives, hematologists, anesthetists, and neonatologists. This chapter discusses these disorders with particular emphasis on their management during pregnancy, delivery and postpartum. Diagnostic (carrier) testing before becoming pregnant in order to allow appropriate preconception counselling and timely provision of prenatal diagnosis, especially in those who could potentially carry a severely affected baby, are also addressed.

Keywords

Carriers of haemophilia • von Willebrand disease • FXI deficiency • Pregnancy

11.1 von Willebrand Disease

11.1.1 History

In a classic paper published in 1926, Erik von Willebrand described 66 members of a bleeder family in the Aland Islands. It was noted that whereas 16 of 35 women had the trait, it was only present in 7 of 31 men, and therefore von Willebrand suggested that "the trait seemed especially to be seen among women…in the female bleeders, the diathesis becomes manifest both in a milder and graver form…Among the females five deaths have occurred." The index Hjordis, who had presented with epistaxis, later died at the onset of her fourth menstrual period, but her own mother produced 12 siblings and her deliveries were normal without heavy bleeding. However, the maternal grandmother had bled to death in childbirth. It is likely that this represented Type 1 and Type 3 von Willebrand Disease (VWD) in the mother and maternal grandmother, respectively [1] (Fig. 11.1).

C.A. Lee, MB ChB, MA, MD, DSc, FRCP, FRCPath
Department of Haemophilia,
University of London, London, UK
e-mail: profcalee@hotmail.com

R.A. Kadir, MB ChB, MRCOG FRCS(Ed), MD (✉)
Department of Obstetrics and Gynaecology,
Royal Free Hospital, Royal Free London NHS
Foundation Trust, Hampstead, London NW3 2QG, UK
e-mail: rezan.abdul-kadir@nhs.net

H. Cohen, P. O'Brien (eds.), *Disorders of Thrombosis and Hemostasis in Pregnancy: A Guide to Management*, DOI 10.1007/978-3-319-15120-5_11, © Springer-Verlag London 2015

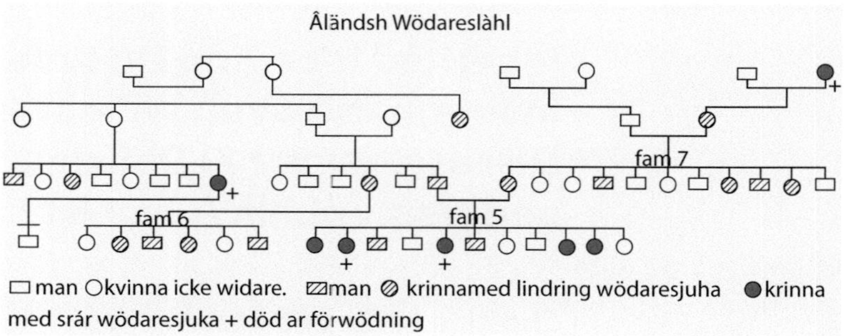

Fig. 11.1 A bleeder family from Föglö in the Aland archipelago (From von Willebrand [1])

11.1.2 Inheritance and Clinical Picture

A large epidemiological study conducted in a young normal population in Italy in 1987 showed a prevalence of VWD of 1 % or 1 in 100 [2]. In a study in which the United States Nationwide Inpatient Sample (NIS) for the years 2000–2003 was queried for pregnancy-related discharges, women with a diagnosis of VWD were compared with women without VWD; the frequency of a diagnosis of VWD among women giving birth was 0.024 % or 1 in 4,000 [3]. A study of symptomatic patients at hemostasis centers found an incidence of 0.002–0.01 % or 1 in 10,000 [4].

There are explanations for some of these discrepancies – the level of VWF in a young population tends to be lower, and it has been found that the level of VWF increases by 15 % each decade [5]. National Indicator set data are derived from discharge summaries, and there is a strong possibility of errors in coding toward underdiagnosis. Furthermore, many patients remain undiagnosed or are seen outside hemostasis centers, particularly in the USA [3]. It has also been pointed out that the wide spectrum of clinical and laboratory manifestations and the lack of strong penetrance mean that making the diagnosis can be very difficult [6].

Thus, VWD is the most common inherited bleeding disorder, and a low von Willebrand factor (VWF) may be found with a frequency of 1 % in young women [2].

11.1.3 Classification of VWD

von Willebrand disease has been classified into three main types [7].

Type 1 is a quantitative deficiency of VWF with a mild to moderate VWF level, 15–50 IU/dL, and normal VWF multimer structure. It occurs in approximately 85 % of cases.

Type 2 is a qualitative deficiency occurring in 15 % of cases and is further subdivided – type 2A, loss of high- and intermediate-weight multimers; type 2B, loss of high molecular weight multimers and often associated with thrombocytopenia; and type 2M, normal VWF multimers and poor binding to platelets. Type 2N VW involves a mutation in the VWF protein which leads to decreased binding of FVIII with resultant FVIII deficiency, and is often misdiagnosed as hemophilia A.

Type 3 is a severe quantitative deficiency with undetectable VWF protein. It is rare, occurring at a frequency of one in a million in the UK population. However, in those populations where first cousin marriage is practised, it is more common [8].

11.1.4 Prepregnancy Counseling

Type 1 and 2 von Willebrand disease is inherited as an autosomal dominant condition with variable inheritance; therefore for type 1 and 2 VWD, there is a 50 % risk of a mother transmitting VWD to her child. However, type 3 VWD is an autosomal recessive disorder, and an affected individual is either homozygote or compound heterozygote. Thus, when a child with type 3 VWD has already been born in a family, the risk of a subsequent child being affected is 25 %. This is common in first cousin marriages; the parents may request antenatal diagnosis, but this should be planned in advance to allow the causative mutation to be identified [9].

11.1.5 Antenatal Management

The physiological response to pregnancy is an increase in FVIII and VWF; thus, most women with VWD do not bleed excessively during pregnancy (Fig. 11.2) [10, 11].

Most women with type 1 VWD achieve levels in the normal nonpregnant range by the third trimester [10]. In a series of 24 pregnancies in 24 women with VWD studied retrospectively, it was found that the FVIIIC and VWF:Ag rose above baseline levels by 1.5 times in most cases. However, some women who are severely affected with type 1 VWD may fail to achieve normal VWF levels by the third trimester, and a baseline level of <15 IU/dL was predictive of a third trimester level <50 IU/dL [12].

In type 2 VWD, although FVIII and VWF:Ag levels increase, there is minimal or no increase in VWF:AC levels [12]. In type 2N VWD, the FVIII level remains low because of impaired binding by VWF. In type 2B VWD, thrombocytopenia may worsen in pregnancy because the increase in intermediate multimers induces platelet aggregation [13].

There is little or no increase of VWF in type 3 VWD [10, 14].

Regular monitoring of VWF:Ag and VWF:AC together with FVIIIC is recommended at booking, 28 and 34 weeks 'gestation, and prior to invasive procedures [9]. The platelet count should be monitored in those with type 2B VWD [13]. If the VWF:AC does not reach 50 IU/dL by the third trimester, prophylaxis with clotting factor concentrate to cover delivery should be considered [9, 15].

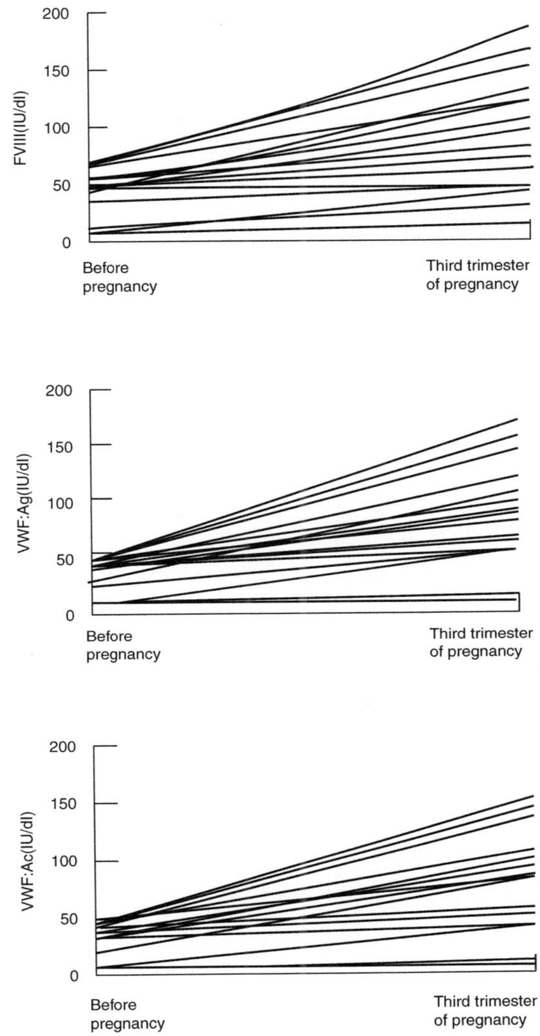

Fig. 11.2 Levels of FVIIIC, VWF:Ag, and VWF:AC during pregnancy (From Kadir et al. [10])

11.1.6 Miscarriage

The spontaneous miscarriage rate has been reported as 20 % [16]. In a review of 84 pregnancies in women with VWD during the years 1980–1996, it was found that 33 % presented with vaginal bleeding during the first trimester and there was an overall spontaneous miscarriage rate of 21 % [10]. A miscarriage rate of 21 % was reported in another study of pregnant women with VWD [17]. Thus, although women with VWD have a higher rate of bleeding during the first trimester, there is not an increased rate of miscarriage.

Spontaneous miscarriage or elective termination in women with VWD is associated with an increased risk of bleeding complications [10, 13, 17]. In one study, transfusion was required for bleeding in association with 10 % of spontaneous miscarriages or elective abortions, and intermittent bleeding occurred for 2 weeks after miscarriage in 30 % of cases [10]. Most miscarriages occur during the first trimester before the VWF: AC has increased substantially [12]. It is therefore recommended that women with VWD who present with spontaneous miscarriage or who elect for termination of pregnancy should have the VWF:AC measured and prophylactic treatment given if the VWF:AC is <50 IU/dL [9].

11.1.7 Treatment

11.1.7.1 DDAVP

The use of DDAVP in pregnancy remains controversial. A survey in the USA showed that 50 and 30 % of hematologists used intravenous and intranasal DDAVP, respectively, for postpartum hemorrhage (PPH) in type 1 VWD but 31 % considered pregnancy as a contraindication [18]. There are reports of the use of DDAVP to cover chorionic villus sampling or amniocentesis [19], to cover 52 deliveries and 20 Cesarean sections in women with a low third trimester VWF [20], and to cover mothers with VWD after cutting the cord. [21] In a systematic review of the literature including 168 pregnancies with VWD, DDAVP was shown to be effective in preventing and reducing bleeding complications associated with pregnancy and childbirth without any complications [22]. The evidence suggests that DDAVP is not contraindicated in uncomplicated pregnancy.

11.1.7.2 Clotting Factor Concentrate Containing VWF

Virally inactive plasma-derived concentrate containing VWF is the treatment of choice for those women who are unresponsive to DDAVP. If the FVIIIC and/ or VWF:AC is <50 IU/dL, a prophylactic infusion should be started at the onset of labor and a VWF:AC >50 IU/dL maintained for at least 3 days post vaginal delivery and 5 days post-Cesarean section [9]. In type 2 N VWD, recombinant FVIII has been successfully used [23]. In type 3 VWD, concentrate is always required to cover delivery because the VWF level does not increase in pregnancy [14].

11.1.8 Regional Analgesia and Anesthesia

Several case reports have described women with VWD who received epidural anaesthesia without bleeding complications [24–26]. In a series, eight women with VWD received regional anesthesia during labour and delivery without bleeding complications and only one woman received prophylactic therapy as the clotting factor levels were >50 IU/dL in the other cases [27]. Epidural anesthesia may be considered for use in the majority of women with type 1 VWD whose levels have risen to >50 IU dL. However, the decision on its use needs to be made jointly by an experienced anesthetist, obstetrician and hematologist after consideration is given to hemostatic concerns such as the degree of correction of the plasma FVIII:C and VWF levels, possible degree of residual platelet impairment, possible rate of postpartum decline of VWF and the consequent risks of bleeding/spinal hematoma. The risks of an epidural or spinal anesthetic for Cesarean section should be balanced against the risk of a general anesthetic. In all cases the epidural should be inserted by an experienced anesthetist. Epidural anesthesia is generally not recommended for use in type 2 or 3 VWD [28].

11.1.9 Postpartum Management

There is an increased risk of both primary (>500 mL blood loss in the first 24 h after delivery) and secondary (excessive bleeding from 24 h to 6 weeks postpartum) PPH in women with VWD. This is due to a fall in VWF and FVIIIC postnatally [11] (Fig. 11.3). Three series including 51 women and 92 deliveries showed a primary PPH rate of 16–29 % and a secondary PPH rate of 20–29 % [10, 12, 29]. All women with VWD should therefore be advised to have active management of the third stage of labor; this involves

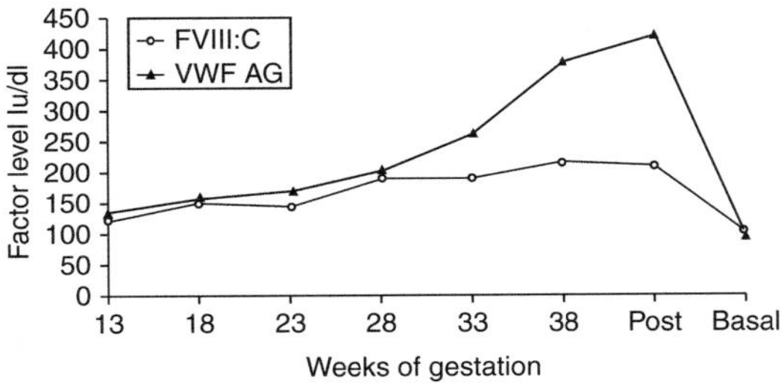

Fig. 11.3 The levels of FVIII and VWF:Ag during pregnancy and postdelivery (From Stirling et al. [11])

administration of an oxytocic drug with the birth of the baby, early cord clamping, and controlled cord traction. The VWF level should be checked postdelivery particularly in those with a low predelivery baseline. The risk of PPH is higher in types 2 and 3 VWD, and in these women, factor replacement should be given during labour and delivery to maintain VWF >50 IU/dL for at least 3 days post vaginal delivery or 5 days post-Cesarean section in addition to tranexamic acid 1 g 6 hourly until the lochia is stopped. The fall in VWF postdelivery can be very variable – there are anecdotal reports of a fall from 41 to 9 IU/dL over the course of a week [12] and a fall of 50 % within 24 h of delivery [30]. One study found that the average time of presentation of secondary PPH in women with VWD is 16 days postdelivery [31] and therefore there is a need for observation and possibly prophylaxis for several weeks postpartum. Prolonged and/or intermittent secondary PPH has also been reported in VWD [10, 12]. In a recent study, the duration of lochia was significantly longer in women with VWD compared to those with no bleeding disorders [32].

11.2 Factor XI Deficiency

11.2.1 Inheritance and Clinical Picture

The management of pregnancy and delivery for women with Factor XI (FXI) deficiency is difficult because the bleeding tendency is so unpredictable. This deficiency was first described in 1953 [33] and was termed hemophilia C. Although the inheritance was initially thought to be autosomal dominant [34], a study in 1961 showed autosomal recessive inheritance [35]. Factor XI

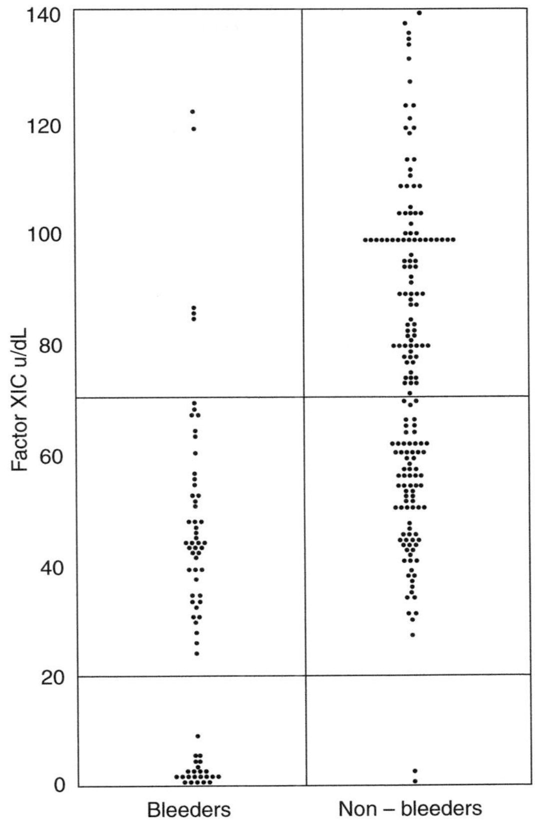

Fig. 11.4 The relationship between FXIC level and bleeding tendency. Pooled data from two UK studies [33, 34] – 249 individuals from 54 families transmitting factor XI deficiency. Of 128 heterozygotes, 45 (35 %) are bleeders. The *upper horizontal line* defines the lower limit of the normal range, and the *lower line* cut-off between severe and partial deficiency (From Bolton-Maggs [37])

deficiency was found to be very common in Jews where the frequency of the heterozygous state among Ashkenazi Jews was found to be 8 % [36].

Individuals with severe FXI deficiency, FXI below 15–20 IU/dL, are at risk of bleeding with surgery and trauma, but some individuals with this severe deficiency do not have a bleeding tendency [37]. The bleeding may be inconsistent within a particular family and is not related to the factor level, in contrast to hemophilias A and B [38, 39]. Studies of the relationship of the FXIC level and the bleeding tendency have also shown that individuals with a level between 50 and 70 IU/dL may have a bleeding tendency [37, 38] (Fig. 11.4). Thus, it is important to take a good bleeding history and to test for additional coexisting abnormalities of VWF and platelet function [40].

11.2.2 Treatment of FXI Deficiency

Comprehensive guidelines on treatment are available [41, 42].

11.2.2.1 Fresh Frozen Plasma (FFP)

FFP was the mainstay of treatment until FXI plasma-derived concentrate became available. This was used in Rosenthal's original patients [33]. FFP has been made safer with respect to possible viral transmission either by pooled solvent detergent treated plasma or single donor units treated with methylene blue [42]. However, in the UK, there remains a concern about possible transmission of abnormal prions following the large epidemic of BSE in cattle and ingestion by potential plasma donors [43].

11.2.2.2 Plasma-Derived FXI Concentrate

A plasma-derived FXI concentrate derived from German plasma is available in the UK [42]. However, there have been concerns about potential thrombogenicity [44], therefore the dose used should not raise the plasma level above 70 IU/dL, and the maximum dose should be 30 IU/dL. The use of FXI concentrate should be limited to those with severe deficiency (<20 IU/dL) or in mild deficiency (20–70 IU/dL) where there is a clear history of bleeding [42].

11.2.2.3 Tranexamic Acid

Tranexamic acid alone has been demonstrated to be sufficient to cover dental extractions in people with severe FXI deficiency [45]. It can be used in those with milder FXI deficiency (20–70 IU/dL) where bleeding is difficult to predict. However, tranexamic acid should not be used concurrently with FXI concentrate because of the potential thrombotic risk [42].

11.2.2.4 Recombinant Factor VIIa

Recombinant VIIa (rVIIa) has been used to cover surgery in FXI deficiency in order to overcome the potential risk of transfusion-transmitted infection. The dose used was 90 mcg/kg intravenously 2 h for the first 24 h, and 4 hourly for the second 24 h [46]. Low doses (30 mcg/kg) have recently been used and shown to effectively induce hemostasis in patients with FXI deficiency undergoing surgery [47]. Due to the unpredictable length of labor and short half-life of rFVIIa, its use is not practical to cover labor, but it has been used successfully to cover elective Cesarean section.

11.2.3 Genetic Counseling and Prenatal Diagnosis

Prenatal diagnosis should be offered to patients where there is a risk of severe deficiency [9]. A partner of a female with FXI deficiency should be offered screening with a FXIC assay.

There are a large number of different mutations [48, 49]. Thus, prenatal diagnosis may be difficult although Ashkenazi Jewish individuals exhibit two common mutations: type II, a stop codon in exon 5, and type III, a missense mutation in exon 9 leading to reduced expression of FXI.

11.2.4 Antenatal Management

Factor XI levels usually remain constant during pregnancy [10, 50, 51]. A study in London followed 61 pregnancies in 30 women, 2 with severe deficiency (FXI 2–8 IU/dL) and 28 with partial deficiency (FXI median 51 IU/dL, range 34–65 IU/dL). The median (range) prepregnancy and third trimester FXI levels were 55 (34–65) and 54 (37–75) IU/dL, respectively, in women with a partial deficiency, and 2 and 8 and 4 and 13 IU/dL in the two women with severe deficiency. Overall, the FXI levels did not change significantly during pregnancy ($p = 0.09$) [50]. Routine monitoring of FXI levels should ideally be carried out at booking, 28 and 34 weeks. The rate of miscarriage does not seem to be increased in these women [51], but they may be at increased risk of hemorrhage following miscarriage or termination of pregnancy, especially if there is a bleeding history [10, 51]. Therefore, consideration of prophylaxis with FXI concentrate or virally inactivated FFP should be given to those with severe FXI deficiency or a bleeding history for invasive procedures, such as CVS or amniocentesis, and termination of pregnancy. Probable "nonbleeders" can be managed expectantly, with treatment available [9].

11.2.5 Intrapartum Management

The risk of PPH can be reduced by active management of the third stage of labor and prophylactic use. FXI concentrate or solvent detergent treated fresh frozen plasma (SD-FFP) if FXI concentrate is not available [10, 52–54]. In severe deficiency (FXI<20 IU/dL), especially those with a positive bleeding history, FXI concentrate in a dose such that peak levels do not exceed 70 IU/dL (NR 70–150 IU/dL) is recommended, regardless of the mode of delivery, to be given at the onset of labour, or prior to induction of labour or Cesarean section. For women with partial deficiency and a bleeding history, or no previous hemostatic challenge, tranexamic acid 1G 6–8 hourly during labor and postdelivery for 7 days is recommended. A "wait and watch" policy is advised for those with partial deficiency and no bleeding history despite hemostatic challenge [9]. The decision to give prophylactic cover for Cesarean section in women with partial deficiency should be individualized and dependent on bleeding history and type of anesthetic or analgesia [9, 50, 55].

11.2.6 Regional Analgesia and Anesthesia

Epidural anesthesia has been carried out in FXI-deficient women without complication [10, 51, 53]. A total of 60 women with inherited bleeding disorders have been identified in the English literature describing the use of regional block during labor and delivery, and there were no reported complications [50, 55]. Epidural or spinal block should be covered with tranexamic acid or FXI concentrate depending on the mother's factor FXI level and her bleeding tendency – FFP contains a variable quantity of FXI and is not recommended [9]. Consideration can be given to the use of rFVIIa [56].

11.2.7 Postpartum Management

Women with FXI deficiency are at increased risk of postpartum hemorrhage [10, 38, 51]. A recent series documented obstetric outcome in 61 pregnancies in 30 women with FXI deficiency over 10 years (1997–2006) [51]. The rate of PPH was 11 % for both primary and secondary PPH but only 3 of the 10 PPH occurred after prophylaxis with factor XI concentrate or tranexamic acid was given – clearly prophylactic hemostatic support reduces PPH as the rate of primary PPH and secondary PPH has previously been reported as 16 and 24 %, respectively, in untreated patients (Fig. 11.5, [10, 50, 55]). Prophylactic tranexamic acid in a dose of 1G 6 hourly should be considered for 3 days post vaginal delivery partum or 5 days following Cesarean section. Since the half-life of FXI is 52 h [55], subsequent doses of FXI concentrate are rarely needed [9].

11.3 Hemophilia A and Hemophilia B

11.3.1 Inheritance

Hemophilia A and B are sex-linked recessive disorders with an incidence in male births of 1 in 5,000 and 1 in 30,000, respectively. The daughter of a male with hemophilia is an obligate carrier, and a carrier has a 50 % chance of passing the gene defect to her children – there is a 50 % chance of having an affected son and a 50 % chance of having a daughter who is a carrier (Fig. 11.6). Carriers may have a reduced clotting factor level but a wide range of values, 22–116 IU/dL, has been reported [57] because of the phenomenon of lyonization where there is random inactivation of one of the two X chromosomes [58]. Where there is extreme lyonization, the clotting factor level may be very low with an increased risk of bleeding. However, there is also

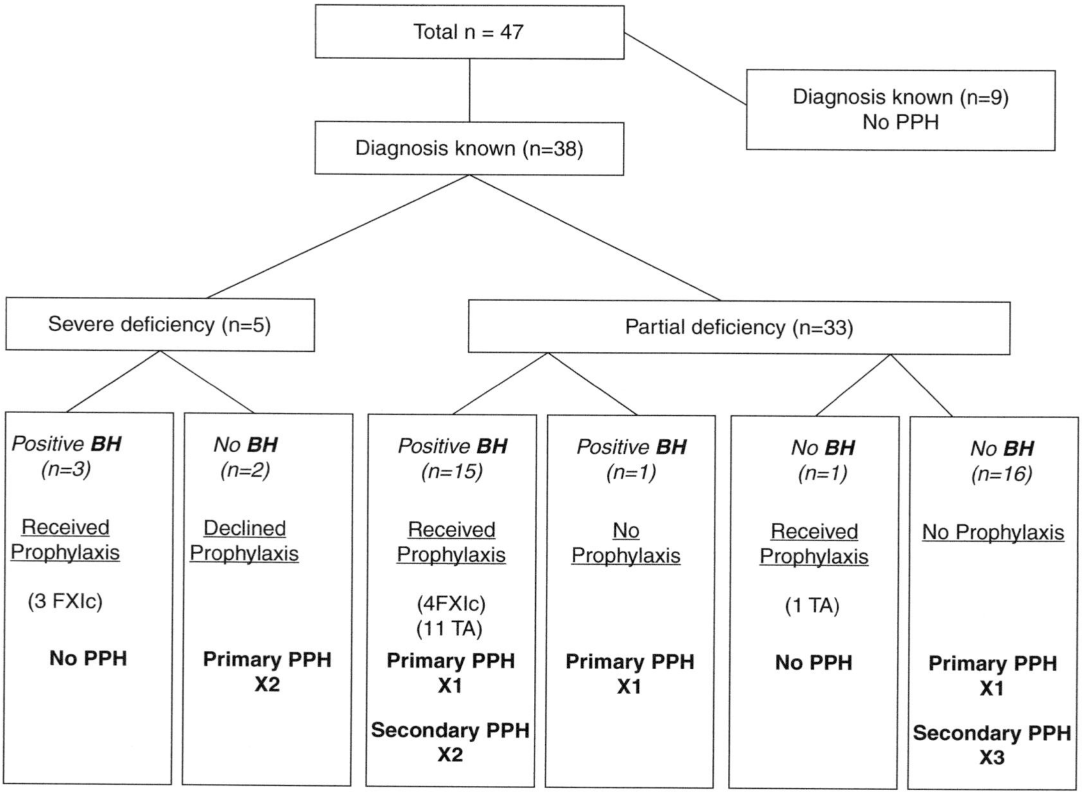

Fig. 11.5 The use of intrapartum prophylaxis and postpartum hemorrhage in women with FXI deficiency (From Chi et al. [50]). *BH* bleeding history, *TA* tranexamic acid

an increased bleeding risk at mildly reduced clotting factor levels [59]. Management of carriers of hemophilia requires a multidisciplinary approach, and ideally they should be managed in a combined clinic with both expertise and facilities to provide a management plan [60].

11.3.2 Genetic Counseling and Carrier Detection

The purpose of genetic counseling is to provide the potential carrier and her parents or partner with the information required to reach a decision about carrier testing and prenatal diagnosis and to provide support during the process [61]. Genetic counseling for hemophilia includes discussion of the medical condition – the inheritance and treatment, personal and relationship concerns related to hemophilia, and beliefs and wishes of the person discussing possible inheritance, as well as others who might be affected [61]. A framework for genetic service provision has been provided as a guideline by the UK Haemophilia Centre Doctors' Organisation (UKHCDO) [62] (Table 11.1). The first step in carrier diagnosis is the family tree – the daughter of a man with hemophilia is an obligate carrier and her sons have a 50 % chance of having hemophilia and her daughters have a 50 % chance of being a carrier (Fig. 11.6). Within a family where an index patient with hemophilia has been identified, there may be many females at risk of being carriers. However, newly diagnosed cases of hemophilia may be sporadic – one study reported this as being 50 % of newly diagnosed cases [63]. However, in a mother of a sporadic case of hemophilia, there is the possibility of mosaicism – a mixture of normal and mutation carrying cells. Carriership should be established before pregnancy and before prenatal diagnosis.

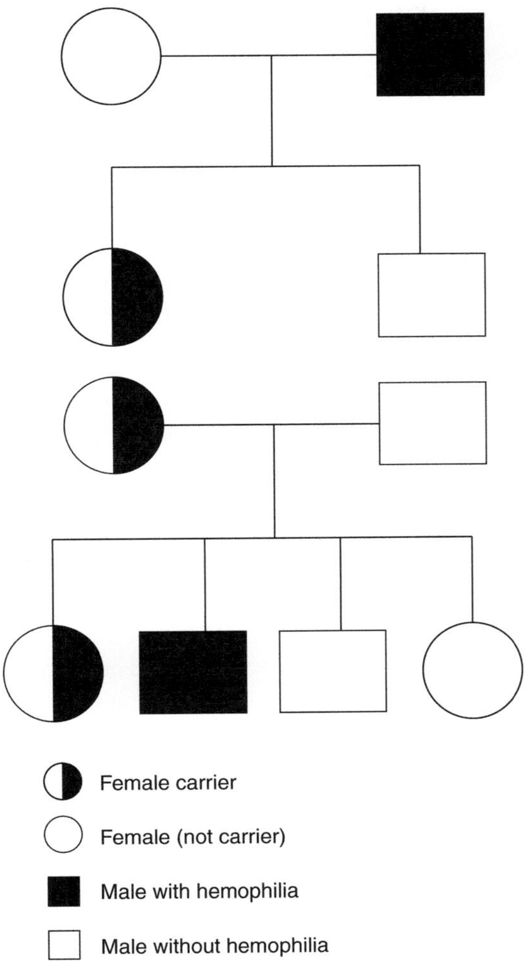

Fig. 11.6 The inheritance of hemophilia

Table 11.1 Counseling and consent for genetic testing in hemophilia

Establish that hemophilia is present in the family and determine its type and severity
Establish family pedigree (tree) to identify possible or definite (obligate) carriers
Provide a full explanation of the potential clinical effects of being a hemophilia carrier or affected male
Provide a full explanation of mode of inheritance of hemophilia
Discuss the rationale for identifying the genetic defect in patients with hemophilia
Outline the means by which carrier status is assessed
Discuss what is involved in genetic testing: sample collection, transfer/storage of data, research projects on stored material, insurance issues, and risk of error
If appropriate, advise on the techniques for prenatal testing
Provide an opportunity to ask questions
Provide an opportunity for the individual being consulted to present her understanding of the information that has been discussed
Provide patient information sheet and an opportunity for follow-up appointment

11.3.3 Testing the Carrier Status of Healthy Girls

There has been a review of the testing of healthy children for recessively inherited conditions [64]. The United Nations Convention on the Rights of the Child has declared that any action or decision affecting this group should be in their "best interests" [65]. The World Health Organization (WHO) has proposed that the reason for genetically testing children was to improve their medical care [66]. The British Medical Association (BMA) has presented a more flexible approach which suggests that the dynamics within the family should be taken into account when considering carrier testing of children [67]. A systematic review of guidelines and position papers has found that, although there were some exceptions, there was general agreement to wait until children can give informed consent for themselves [67].

In a study considering "the attitudes towards and beliefs about genetic testing in the hemophilia community," female carriers and family members thought testing was necessary for adolescent girls to determine carrier status [64].

Women who are hemophilia carriers may have a low level of FVIII or IX, and it is therefore recommended that the respective clotting factor is measured in young obligate carriers [62]. The ethical debate is redundant in this situation.

11.3.4 Genetic Diagnosis

It is now possible to perform genetic diagnosis for the specific mutation causing hemophilia in a family. In severe hemophilia A, approximately 50 % of families carry an inversion of intron 22 which is a rearrangement of the long arm of the X chromosome [68]. In this situation, it may be possible to establish carriership without knowledge of the mutation in the index member of the family. For most potential carriers, it is necessary to know the mutation in the index family member, and mutations for hemophilia A are listed on the HAMSTeRS database (http://europium.csc.mrc.ac.uk). In hemophilia B, almost all families have a unique mutation, and in the UK most of these are identified [69].

11.3.5 Reproductive Options

The options possible for families known to be at risk of transmitting an inherited bleeding disorder include:

- Conceiving naturally, having prenatal diagnosis (PND), and the option of terminating an affected fetus
- Taking the risk and consequences of having an affected child
- Not having a child
- Adoption
- Assisted conception with egg donation
- Assisted conception with preimplantation diagnosis (PGD)

The decision will be influenced by ethnic and cultural issues, the severity of hemophilia in the family, and the personal and family experience of the disorder [70].

11.3.6 Prenatal Diagnosis

The noninvasive determination of fetal sex is now often possible in the first trimester through the analysis of free fetal DNA in the maternal circulation and/or ultrasound examination of the fetal genital tubercle [71]. This means that invasive prenatal diagnostic tests can usually be avoided in female pregnancies. Chorionic villus sampling (CVS) is the most widely used method in the prenatal diagnosis of hemophilia. It is important to arrange prophylactic treatment with clotting factor concentrate if the clotting factor level is <50 IU/dL. Since invasive testing may cause feto-maternal hemorrhage, anti-D should be given to Rhesus D-negative mothers. CVS is performed between 11 and 14 weeks' gestation under ultrasound guidance to obtain a sample of placenta for genetic analysis. It is associated with a 1–2 % risk of miscarriage [72]. CVS should not be performed before 10 weeks' gestation because of the risk of fetal limb deformity [73, 74]. Amniocentesis can also be used for PND– this is usually performed between 15 and 18 weeks of gestation. Fetal cells within the amniotic fluid can be sexed by in situ hybridization (FISH), and/or DNA can be extracted for PCR-based linkage analysis or mutation detection [75]. Cordocentesis or percutaneous umbilical cord sampling can be performed to measure the FVIII or FIX – this is considered if the causative mutation in the family is unknown. There is a 1–2 % risk of fetal loss [76] and probably increased if the fetus has a bleeding tendency, so this is not commonly performed.

Preimplantation Genetic Diagnosis (PGD) uses in vitro fertilization (IVF) to create embryos. One or two cells from each fertilized embryo are tested for the specific genetic diagnosis, and unaffected embryos are identified for transfer to the uterus. In hemophilia the technique was initially used for diagnosis of fetal sex, but there are reports of specific diagnosis [77]. However, IVF is expensive, invasive and stressful, and the success rate is lower than for spontaneous conception [78].

11.3.7 Management of Pregnancy

The FVIII levels increase in carriers of hemophilia A during pregnancy, and most carriers will have a normal FVIII level (>50 IU/dL) at term. In contrast, FIX levels do not change during pregnancy [79]. Clotting factor levels should be checked at booking, 28 and 34 weeks, and prophylaxis should be given to cover invasive procedures when the level is <50 IU/dL [9].

11.3.8 Management of Delivery

For women with low factor levels, intravenous access should be established, the third stage of labor should be actively managed, and prophylactic treatment should be given to cover labor and delivery when the clotting factor level is <50 IU/dL. The optimal mode of delivery for affected infants, especially those affected by severe haemophilia, remains controversial. A planned Cesarean section is associated with least risk of intracranial bleeding in relation to delivery. Thus, delivery by a planned Cesarean section has been suggested by many authorities for affected foetuses [80]. If vaginal delivery is opted for, invasive intrapartum monitoring techniques, such as fetal scalp blood sampling and application of a fetal scalp electrode, should be avoided. The risk factors for cranial bleeding in affected newborns include prolonged labor and instrumental delivery, particularly vacuum (ventouse) extraction, which can cause cephalhematoma, or the use of high or rotational forceps. Potentially difficult instrumental delivery (high or rotational forceps) should be avoided because of the risk of intracranial bleeding in an affected baby, and there should be a low threshold for early recourse to Cesarean section. However, instrumental delivery is not completely contraindicated; there are some situations where an easy "lift-out" forceps delivery may be safer for an affected baby than a difficult Cesarean delivery of a head deeply impacted in the pelvis. It is important that a cord plasma sample is obtained to measure FVIII or FIX levels in order to make or exclude a diagnosis of hemophilia. Delivery at a tertiary referral unit is necessary only for symptomatic carriers and those carrying affected fetuses. This ensures availability of laboratory testing and treatment with factor VIII or IX concentrates if required [81].

After birth, IM injections for the baby should be avoided until the results of the cord blood factor levels are known (results should be requested urgently). The first dose of vitamin K should therefore be given orally. Circumcision should not be performed unless and until factor levels in the baby have been shown to be normal. These factor levels should be rechecked when the baby is 2–3 months old in order to establish its true status.

11.3.9 Regional Analgesia and Anesthesia

The management plan should be made in consultation with the anesthetist prior to labor. The use of regional blockade is of some concern because of the potential risk of epidural or spinal hemorrhage and hematoma. However, provided the factor VII or IX level is >50 IU/dL, regional block is not contraindicated and has been shown to be safe [55].

11.3.10 Postpartum Management

The incidence of primary and secondary PPH has been reported as 22 and 11 %, respectively [82] compared to 5–8 and 0.8 % in the general population (in whom routine prophylactic oxytocics are used). Therefore, the factor level should ideally be checked after delivery, and it should be maintained at >50 IU/dL. Tranexamic acid can be used to treat heavy lochia, if necessary [76].

11.4 Case Studies

Case Study 1

A 23-year-old Caucasian woman registered with our hemophilia center with severe type 1 VWD (VWF: Ag 5 IU/dL, VWF: Ac 4 IU/dL, FVIII 10 IU/dL at diagnosis) reported pregnant at 5 weeks' gestation in her first pregnancy. She was from a traveler family and decided against medical advice to travel to Italy with her husband during pregnancy due to her worries about infection with swine flu in the UK. She did not have regular antenatal care in Italy and had repeated episodes of mild to moderate vaginal bleeding during pregnancy that was managed with tranexamic acid (TA). At 32 weeks' gestation, she had a significant antepartum hemorrhage and required factor replacement therapy. After discharge from hospital in Italy, she returned to London and reported to our center. The scan showed normal fetal well-being and a posterior high placenta. Her factor levels were unchanged from prepregnancy, and her bleeding was minimal. We managed her with TA 1 g 6 hourly with the plan to give factor replacement if the bleeding increased.

For delivery, it was planned to continue TA and start factor replacement using Haemate P (CSL Behring UK LTD) with the first sign of labor, aiming to maintain her VWF and FVIII above 50 IU/dL for at least 2 weeks. She presented in spontaneous labor at 39 weeks of gestation and during labor was managed according to the plan. She progressed well, did not require epidural analgesia, and delivered a girl by vaginal delivery with the aid of an episiotomy.

The third stage of labor was actively managed, and she also received misoprostol 600 mcg rectally prophylactically after delivery of the placenta. Her episiotomy was sutured without any complications. She required twice daily factor replacement. On day 3 postpartum, her TA was stopped, and her factor replacement was reduced to once daily by the on-call team, due to concern about an increased risk of thrombosis, contrary to the plan of management pro-vided by the joint hemophilia/obstetric team, due to concerns of an increased risk of thrombosis.

On day 4, she had an episode of severe secondary PPH, requiring a 4-unit red cell transfusion, uterine balloon insertion, and vaginal packing. Her FVIII and VWF factor levels had dropped to 28 and 26 IU/dL, respectively. TA and twice daily factor replacement were restarted. She recovered well and was discharged home on day 7 on TA and once daily factor replacement. Her hemoglobin was 9.5 g/dL and she was given iron therapy. Three weeks after delivery, her lochia had reduced but remained moderate. Factor replacement was reduced to twice weekly until 5 weeks postdelivery. A combined oral contraceptive pill was then started and her factor replacement stopped. She continued taking TA 1 g 6 h until her lochia had completely stopped.

On review at 8 weeks, she had stopped bleeding, and her hemoglobin had risen to 10.9 g/dL. Her daughter was progressing well. Her cord blood factor level was borderline. It was advised that mild VWD could not be excluded and that repeat testing would be organized at a later stage and to inform the center if there was any concern regarding bleeding in her daughter.

Case Study 2

A 30-year-old carrier of hemophilia A was in her first pregnancy. Free fetal DNA testing at 10 weeks' gestation showed a male fetus. The mother declined CVS and was aware that there was a 50 % chance of her son being affected. Her prepregnancy FVIII level was 38 IU/dL. The pregnancy progressed without any complication, and her third trimester FVIII level normalized, rising to 140 IU/dL. She was therefore advised that there would be no need for hemostatic cover for labor and delivery, including for regional block.

She did not go into spontaneous labor by 42 weeks of gestation, so her cervix was assessed by ultrasound scan and reported to be 3.8 cm long and closed. The woman was counseled about induction of labor and the high chance of prolonged labor and operative delivery when the cervix is >3 cm long in a primip at the start of induction. She was aware that her unborn son had a 50 % chance of being affected, thus very prolonged labor and, in particular, difficult operative delivery needed to be avoided to avoid the risk of cranial bleeding. Following this counseling, the mother opted for an elective Cesarean section. This was per-formed under combined spinal/epidural block without any complications. Her estimated blood loss during delivery was 400 mL. Cord blood confirmed her son to be affected with severe hemophilia A.

Key Learning Points

- Obstetric management of women with VWD and FXI deficiency and carriers of hemophilia requires a multidisciplinary team approach with obstetricians, midwives, hematologists, anesthetists, and neonatologists.

- Women in families with such inherited bleeding disorders should undergo diagnostic (carrier) testing before becoming pregnant in order to allow appropriate preconception counseling and timely provision of prenatal diagnosis, especially in those who could potentially carry a severely affected baby.
- Women with VWD and FXI deficiency and carriers of hemophilia are at risk of postpartum hemorrhage, especially those with low factor (>50 iu/dL) levels at term. Appropriate hemostatic cover, based on the mother's factor level, her bleeding tendency, and mode of delivery, minimizes the risk, and the third stage of labor should be actively managed.
- Regional block is not contraindicated in these women provided the clotting defects have normalized during pregnancy or been corrected by replacement therapy. The decision should be made on an individual basis prior to labor after careful evaluation of the potential risks and benefits.
- Affected newborns are also at risk of bleeding during the process of birth. Cranial bleeding, including cephalhematoma and intracranial hemorrhage, is the most common and serious site. Thus, very prolonged labor and difficult instrumental delivery, in particular vacuum extraction, should be avoided, and delivery achieved by the least traumatic method with early recourse to Cesarean section.
- Umbilical cord blood should be taken at birth to measure factor levels in the baby. IM injections and surgical procedures, including circumcision, should be avoided until the levels are known to be normal.

References

1. von Willebrand EA. Hereditar pseudohenofili. Finska Lakarsallskapets Handl. 1926;67:87–112.
2. Rodeghiero F, Castaman G, Dini E. Epidemiological investigation of the prevalence of von Willebrand's disease. Blood. 1987;69:454–9.
3. James AH, Jamison MG. Bleeding events and other complications during pregnancy and childbirth in women with von Willebrand disease. J Thromb Haemost. 2007;5:1165–9.
4. Sadler JE, Mannucci PM, Berntorp E, Bochkov N, Meyer D, Peake I, Rodeghiero F, Srivastava A. Impact, diagnosis and treatment of von Willebrand disease. Thromb Haemost. 2000;84(2):160–74.
5. Kadir RA, Economides DL, Sabin CA, Pollard D, Lee CA. Variations in coagulation factors in women: effects of age, ethnicity, menstrual cycle and combined oral contraceptive. Thromb Haemost. 1999;82:1456–61.
6. Rodgiero F, Castaman G. von Willebrand Disease: epidemiology. In: Lee CA, Berntorp EE, Hoots WK, editors. Textbook of hemophilia. 2nd ed. London: Wiley-Blackwell; 2010. p. 286–93.
7. Sadler JE, Budde U, Eikenboom JC, Favaloro EJ, Hill FG, Holmberg L, Ingerslev J, Lee CA, Lillicrap D, Mannucci PM, Mazurier C, Meyer D, Nichols WL, Nishino M, Peake IR, Rodeghiero F, Schneppenheim R, Ruggeri ZM, Srivastava A, Montgomery RR, Federici AB, Working Party on von Willebrand Disease Classification. Update on the pathophysiology and classification of von Willebrand disease: a report of the Subcommittee on von Willebrand Factor. J Thromb Haemost. 2006;4(10):2103–14.
8. Lak M, Peyvandi F, Mannucci PM. Clinical manifestations and complications of childbirth and replacement therapy in 385 Iranian patients with type 3 von Willebrand disease. Br J Haematol. 2000;4:1236–9.
9. Lee CA, Chi C, Pavord SR, Bolton-Maggs PHB, Pollard D, Hinchcliffe-Wood A, Kadir RA. The obstetric and gynaecological management of women with inherited bleeding disorders – review with guidelines produced by a taskforce of UK Haemophilia Centre Doctors' Organisation. Haemophilia. 2006;12:301–36.
10. Kadir RA, Lee CA, Sabin CA, Pollard D, Economides DL. Pregnancy in women with von Willebrand's disease or factor XI deficiency. Br J Obstet Gynaecol. 1998;105:314–21.
11. Stirling Y, Woolf L, North WR, Seghatchian MJ, Meade TW. Haemostasis in normal pregnancy. Thromb Haemost. 1984;52:176–82.
12. Ramsahoye BH, Davies SV, Dasani H, Pearson JF. Obstetric management in von Willebrand's disease: a report of 24 pregnancies and a review of the literature. Haemophilia. 1995;1:140–4.

13. Rick ME, Williams SB, Sacher RA, McKeown LP. Thrombocytopenia associated with pregnancy in a patient with type IIB von Willebrand disease. Blood. 1987;69:786–9.
14. Caliezi C, Tsakiris DA, Behringer H, Kuhne T, Marbet GA. Two consecutive pregnancies and deliveries in a patient with von Willebrand's disease type 3. Haemophilia. 1998;4:845–9.
15. James AH, Kouides PA, Kadir RA, et al. von Willebrand disease and other bleeding disorders in women: consensus on diagnosis and management from an international panel. Am J Obstet Gynecol. 2009;201:12e.1–8.
16. National Institute for Health and Care Excellence. Ectopic pregnancy and miscarriage, clinical guideline CG154, London NICE. 2012. Available at: http://guidance.nice.org.uk/CG154.
17. Foster PA. The reproductive health of women with von Willebrand disease unresponsive to DDAVP: the results of an international survey. On behalf of the subcommittee on VWF of the SSC of the ISTH. Thromb Haemost. 1995;74:784–90.
18. Cohen AJ, Kessler CM, Ewenstein BM. Management of von Willebrand disease: a survey on the current clinical practice from the haemophilia centres of North America. Haemophilia. 2001;7:235–41.
19. Mannucci PM. How I, treat patients with von Willebrand disease. Blood. 2001;97:1915–9.
20. Sanchez-Luceros A, Meschengieser SS, Turdo K, et al. Evaluation of desmopressin during pregnancy in women with low plasmatic von Willebrand factor level and bleeding history. Thromb Res. 2007;120:387–90.
21. Castaman G, Tosetto A, Rodeghiero F. Pregnancy and delivery in women with von Willebrand disease and different von Willebrand factor mutations. Abstract As-Mo-029 XXII congress ISTH, Boston. 2009.
22. Trigg DE, Stergiotou I, Peitsidis P, Kadir RA. A systematic review: the use of desmopressin for treatment and prophylaxis of bleeding disorders in pregnancy. Haemophilia. 2012;18(1):25–33.
23. Dennis MW, Clough V, Toh CH. Unexpected presentation of type 2N von Willebrand disease in pregnancy. Haemophilia. 2000;6(6):696–7.
24. Caliezi C, Tsakiris DA, Behringer H, Kuhne T, Marbet GA, Jones BP, Bell EA, Maroof M. Epidural labor analgesia in a parturient with von Willebrand's disease type IIA and severe preeclampsia. Anesthesiology. 1999;90:1219–20.
25. Milaskiewicz RM, Holdcroft A, Letsky E. Epidural anaesthesia and von Willebrand's disease. Anaesthesia. 1990;45:462–4.
26. Cohen S, Daitch JS, Amar D, Goldiner PL. Epidural analgesia for labor and delivery in a patient with von Willebrand's disease. Reg Anesth. 1989;14:95–7.
27. Kadir RA, Lee CA, Sabin CA, Pollard D, Economides DL. Pregnancy in women with von Willebrand's disease or factor XI deficiency. Br J Obstet Gynaecol. 1998;105:314–32.
28. Pasi KJ, Collins PW, Keeling DM, et al. Management of von Willebrand disease: a guideline from the UK Haemophilia Centre Doctors' Organization. Haemophilia. 2004;10:218–31.
29. Greer IA, Lowe GD, Walker JJ, Forbes CC. Haemorrhagic problems in obstetrics and gynaecology in patients with congenital coagulopathies. BJOG. 1991;98:909–18.
30. Hanna W, McCarroll D, McDonald T, et al. Variant von Willebrand disease and pregnancy. Blood. 1981; 58:873–9.
31. Roque H, Funai E, Lockwood CJ. von Willebrand disease and pregnancy. J Matern Fetal Med. 2000;9:257–66.
32. Chi C, Bapir M, Lee CA, Kadir RA. Puerperal loss (lochia) in women with or without inherited bleeding disorders. Am J Obstet Gynecol. 2010;203(1):56.e1–5.
33. Rosenthal RL, Dreskin OH, Rosenthal N. New hemophilia-like disease caused by deficiency of a third plasma thromboplastin factor. Proc Soc Exp Biol Med. 1953;82:171–4.
34. Seligsohn U, Bolton-Maggs PH. Factor XI deficiency. In: Lee CA, Berntorp EE, Hoots WK, editors. Textbook of hemophilia. 2nd ed. London: Wiley-Blackwell; 2010. p. 355–61.
35. Rapaport SI, Proctor RR, Patch NJ, Yettra M. The role of inheritance of PTA deficiency: evidence for the existence of major PTA deficiency and minor PTA deficiency. Blood. 1961;18:149–65.
36. Seligsohn U. Factor XI, deficiency. Thromb Haemost. 1993;70:68–71.
37. Bolton-Maggs PHB. Factor XI, deficiency. In: Lee CA, editor. Bailliere's clinical haematology: haemophilia. London: Bailliere Tindall; 1996. p. 356–67.
38. Bolton-Maggs PH, Young Wan-Yin B, McCraw AH, Slack J, Kernoff PB. Inheritance and bleeding in factor XI deficiency. Br J Haematol. 1988;69:521–8.
39. Bolton-Maggs PH, Patterson DA, Wensley RT, Tuddenham EG. Definition of bleeding tendency in factor-XI deficient kindred's – a clinical and laboratory study. Thromb Haemost. 1995;73:194–202.
40. Bolton-Maggs PHB. The management of factor XI deficiency. Haemophilia. 1998;4:683–8.
41. Bolton-Maggs PH, Perry DJ, Chalmers EA, Parapia LA, Wilde JT, Williams MD. The rare coagulation disorders – review with guidelines for management from the UK Doctors' Organisation. Haemophilia. 2004;10:593–628.
42. Keeling D, Tait C, Makris M. Guideline on the selection and use of therapeutic products to treat haemophilia and other hereditary bleeding disorders. Haemophilia. 2008;14:671–84.
43. Peden A, Fairfoul G, Lowrie S, McCardle L, Head MW, Love S, Ward HJT, Cousens SN, Keeling D, Millar CM, Hill FGH, Ironside JW. Variant CJD infection in the spleen of an asymptomatic adult patient with haemophilia. Haemophilia. 2010;16: 296–304.

44. Bolton-Maggs PH, Colvin BT, Satchi BT, Lee CA, Lucas GS. Thrombogenic potential of factor XI concentrate. Lancet. 1994;344(8924):748–9.
45. Berliner S, Horowitz I, Martinowitz U, Brenner B, Seligsohn U. Dental surgery in patients with severe factor XI deficiency without plasma replacement. Blood Coagul Fibrinolysis. 1992;3:465–74.
46. O'Connell NM, Riddell AF, Pascoe G, Perry DJ, Lee CA. Recombinant factor VIIa to prevent surgical bleeding in factor XI deficiency. Haemophilia. 2008;14:775–81.
47. Kenet G, Lubetsky A, Luboshitz J, Ravid B, Tamarin I, Varon D, Martinowitz U. Lower doses of rFVIIa therapy are safe and effective for surgical interventions in patients with severe FXI deficiency and inhibitors. Haemophilia. 2009;15(5):1065–73. Epub 2009 May 26.
48. Seligsohn U. Factor XI, deficiency in humans. J Thromb Haemost. 2009;7 Suppl 1:84–7.
49. O'Connell NM. Factor XI, deficiency. Semin Hematol. 2004;41:76–81.
50. Chi C, Kulkarni A, Lee CA, Kadir RA. The obstetric experience of women with factor XI deficiency. Acta Obstet Gynecol Scand. 2009;88(10):1095–100.
51. Myers B, Pavord S, Kean L, Hill M, Dolan G. Pregnancy outcome in factor XI deficiency: incidence of miscarriage, antenatal and postnatal haemorrhage in 33 women with FXI deficiency. BJOG. 2007;114:643–6.
52. Collins P, Goldman E, Lilley P, Pasi KJ, Lee CA, et al. Clinical experience of factor XI deficiency: the role of fresh frozen plasma and factor XI concentrate. Haemophilia. 1995;1:227–31.
53. David AL, Paterson-Brown S, Letsky EA. Factor XI deficiency presenting in pregnancy: diagnosis and management. BJOG. 2002;109:840–3.
54. Mavromatidis G, Dinas K, Delkos D, Goutzioulis F, Vosnakis C, Hatzipantelis E. Uneventful caesarean delivery with administration of factor XI concentrate in a patient with severe factor XI deficiency. Int J Hematol. 2007;86:222–4.
55. Chi C, Lee CA, England A, Hingorani J, Paintsil J, Kadir RA. Obstetric analgesia and anaesthesia in women with inherited bleeding disorders. Thromb Haemost. 2009;101:1104–11.
56. Bolton-Maggs PH, Wensley RT, Kernoff PB, et al. Production and therapeutic use of a factor XI concentrate from plasma. Thromb Haemost. 1992;67: 314–9.
57. Rizza CR, Rhymes IL, Austen DE, Kernoff PB, Aroni SA. Detection of carriers of haemophilia: a 'blind' study. Br J Haematol. 1975;30:447–56.
58. Lyon MF. Chromatin and gene action in the mammalian X-chromosome. Am J Hum Genet. 1962;14:135–48.
59. Plug I, Mauser-Bunschoten EP, Brocker-Vriends AH, van Amstel HK, van der Bom JG, van Diemen-Homan JE, Willemse J, Rosendaal FR. Bleeding in carriers of haemophilia. Blood. 2008;111:1811–5.
60. Lee CA, Chi C, Shiltagh N, Pollard D, Griffioen A, Dunn N, Kadir RA. Review of a multidisciplinary clinic for women with inherited bleeding disorders. Haemophilia. 2009;15:359–60.
61. Miller R. Genetic counselling for haemophilia. WFH treatment monograph: No 25 World Federation of Haemophilia. 2002. www.wfh.org.
62. Ludlam CA, Pasi KJ, Bolton-Maggs P, Collins P, Cumming AM, Dolan G. A framework for genetic service provision for haemophilia and other inherited bleeding disorders. Haemophilia. 2005;11:145–63.
63. Ljund R, Petrini P, Nilsson IM. Diagnostic symptoms of severe and moderate haemophilia A and B – a survey of 140 cases. Acta Paediatr Scand. 1990;79:196–200.
64. Dunn NF, Miller R, Griffioen A, Lee CA. Carrier testing in haemophilia A and B: adult carriers and their partners experiences and their views on the testing of young females. Haemophilia. 2008;14:584–92.
65. United Nations Convention on the Rights of the Child 20. Xi. 1989: TS 44: Cm. 1976. http://www.un.org/Docs/journal/asp/ws.asp?m=A/RES/44/25.
66. World Health Organization. Proposed international guidelines on ethical issues in medical genetics and genetic services. Geneva: World Health Organization; 1998. p. 1998.
67. BMA. Consent, rights and choices in health care for children and young people. London: BMJ Books; 2001.
68. Antonarakis S, Rossiter JP, Young M, Horst J, de Moerloose P, Sommer SS, Ketterling RP, et al. Factor VIII gene inversions in severe hemophilia A: results of an international consortium study. Blood. 1995;86:2206–12.
69. Giannelli F, Green PM, Somner S. Haemophilia B (sixth edition); a database of point mutations and short editions and deletions. Nucleic Acids Res. 1996;24:103–18.
70. Kadir RA, Sabin C, Gouldman E, Pollard D, Lee C, Economides DL. Reproductive experience and attitude of carriers of haemophilia. Haemophilia. 2000;6:33–40.
71. Chi C, Hyett JA, Finning KM, Lee CA, Kadir RA. Non-invasive first trimester determination of fetal gender: a new approach for prenatal diagnosis of haemophilia. BJOG. 2006;113:239–42.
72. Mujezinovic F, Alfirevic Z. Procedure-related complications of amniocentesis and chorionic villous sampling: a systematic review. Obstet Gynecol. 2007;110:687–94.
73. Firth HV, Boyd PA, Chamberlain PF, et al. Analysis of limb reduction defects in babies exposed to chorionic villus sampling. Lancet. 1994;343:1069–71.
74. RCOG. Amniocentesis and chorionic villus sampling. Green-top guideline no. 8. London: RCOG; 2005. https://www.rcog.org.uk/guidelines.
75. Kadir RA, Lee CA. Obstetrics and gynaecology: haemophilia. In: Lee CA, Berntorp EE, Hoots WK, editors. Textbook of hemophilia. 2nd ed. London: Wiley-Blackwell; 2010. p. 355–61.

76. Buscaglia M, Ghisoni L, Bellotti M, et al. Percutaneous umbilical blood sampling: indication changes and procedure loss rate in a nine years' experience. Fetal Diagn Ther. 1996;11:106–13.
77. Michaelides K, Tuddenham EG, Turner C, Lavender B, Lavery SA. Live birth following the first mutation specific pre-implantation genetic diagnosis. Thromb Haemost. 2006;95:373–9.
78. Human Fertilization and Embryology Authority. HFEA guide to infertility and directory of clinics 2005/6. London: Human Fertilisation and Embryology Authority; 2006.
79. Chi C, Lee CA, Shiltagh N, Khan A, Pollard D, Kadir RA. Pregnancy in carriers of haemophilia. Haemophilia. 2008;14:56–64.
80. James AH, Hoots K. The optimal mode of delivery for the haemophilia carrier expecting an affected infant is Caesarean delivery. Haemophilia. 2010;16:420–4.
81. Huq FY, Kadir RA. Management of pregnancy, labour and delivery in women with inherited bleeding disorders. Haemophilia. 2011;17 Suppl 1:20–30.
82. Kadir RA, Economides DL, Braithwaite J, Goldman E, Lee CA. The obstetric experience of carriers of haemophilia. BJOG. 1997;104:803–10.

Inherited Bleeding Disorders in Pregnancy: Rare Coagulation Factor Defects

12

Marzia Menegatti, Simona Maria Siboni, and Flora Peyvandi

Abstract

Inherited deficiencies of plasma proteins involved in blood coagulation generally lead to lifelong bleeding disorders. Rare bleeding disorders (RBDs), discussed in this chapter, represent 3–5 % of all the inherited coagulation deficiencies, with prevalence ranging from approximately 1:500,000 to 1:2,000,000 in the general population. Patients affected with bleeding disorders present a wide spectrum of clinical symptoms that vary from a mild or moderate bleeding tendency to severe episodes. Women with inherited bleeding disorders are particularly disadvantaged since, in addition to suffering from general bleeding symptoms, they are also at risk of bleeding complications from regular haemostatic challenges: menstruation, pregnancy and childbirth. Moreover, affected women may experience reduced quality of life caused by limitations in activities and work, and the impact on their reproductive life. Management of women with RBDs is difficult because of considerable inter-individual variation. Furthermore, reliable information on clinical management is scarce, with only a few long-term prospective studies of large cohorts providing evidence to guide diagnosis and treatment.

Keywords

Women's health • Rare bleeding disorders • Inherited deficiencies • Bleeding symptoms • Pregnancy • Miscarriage • Post-partum haemorrhage • Laboratory diagnosis

M. Menegatti, PhD • F. Peyvandi, MD, PhD (✉)
Angelo Bianchi Bonomi, Hemophilia and Thrombosis Center, Fondazione IRCCS Ca' Granda Ospedale Maggiore Policlinico, Milan, Italy

Department of Pathophysiology and Transplantation, Università degli Studi di Milano and Luigi Villa Foundation, Milan, Italy
e-mail: flora.peyvandi@unimi.it

S.M. Siboni, MD, PhD
Angelo Bianchi Bonomi, Hemophilia and Thrombosis Center, Fondazione IRCCS Ca' Granda Ospedale Maggiore Policlinico, Milan, Italy

H. Cohen, P. O'Brien (eds.), *Disorders of Thrombosis and Hemostasis in Pregnancy: A Guide to Management*, DOI 10.1007/978-3-319-15120-5_12, © Springer-Verlag London 2015

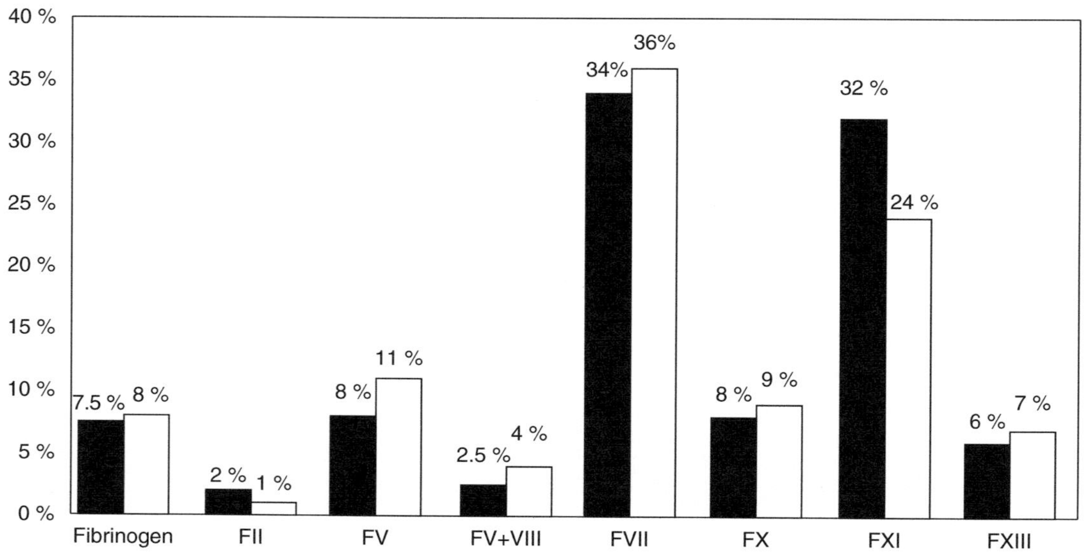

Fig. 12.1 Prevalence of RBDs according to WFH 2011 survey (www.wfh.org) (*closed bars*) and EN-RBD (www.rbdd.eu) (*open bars*)

12.1 Introduction

Inherited deficiencies of plasma proteins involved in blood coagulation generally lead to lifelong bleeding disorders, with severity directly proportional to the degree of factor deficiency (less factor/ more severe bleeding tendency). Hemophilia A and B are the most frequently inherited bleeding disorders and, together with von Willebrand disease (vWD), a defect of primary haemostasis associated with a secondary defect in coagulation factor VIII (FVIII), comprise 95–97 % of all the inherited deficiencies of coagulation factors. The remaining defects, named rare bleeding disorders (RBDs) represent 3–5 % of all the inherited coagulation deficiencies, with their prevalence ranging from approximately 1:500,000 to 1:2,000,000 in the general population [1]. The RBDs include the inherited deficiencies of fibrinogen, factor (F) II, FV, FV+FVIII, FVII, FX, FXI, and FXIII. They are usually transmitted as autosomal recessive traits, meaning that women represent about half of the affected patients. The prevalence of homozygous or double heterozygous patients, who generally carry the most severe form of the disease, is usually low in the general population [2]. However, in countries where consanguineous marriages are practiced such as Africa, India, and the Middle East, the number of affected patients seems 8–10-fold higher, representing a significant burden for public health, with greater demand for diagnosis and treatment [3]. Recent immigration from these countries to Europe has also increased the demand for diagnosis and treatment in this region of the world.

Information on the worldwide prevalence of RBDs can be derived from the data collected by the European Network of RBDs (EN-RBD: www.rbdd.eu) [4] and the World Federation of Hemophilia (WFH) global survey, showing that FVII and FXI deficiencies are the most prevalent RBDs representing 34 and 32 % of the total number of affected patients respectively, followed by the deficiencies of fibrinogen, FV and FX (7.5–8 %), FXIII (6 %), with the rarest disorders FII, and FV+FVIII deficiencies (2–2.5 %) (Fig. 12.1). Due to the rarity of RBDs, the available information on their clinical severity, laboratory diagnosis, and management, are still limited, because only a few centres follow and manage a significant number of patients. Accordingly, scientific reports are usually limited to small series of patients or single cases. Even the most reliable registries designed to gather detailed information are limited to single aspects of the disease (clinical or therapeutic) or to the analysis of a single RBD.

12.2 Classification of RBDs

Most RBDs are expressed phenotypically as a parallel reduction of plasma factors measured by functional assays and immunoassays (so-called type I deficiencies). Qualitative defects, characterized by normal, slightly reduced, or increased levels of factor antigen contrasting with much lower or undetectable functional activity (type II), are less frequent [2]. Regarding fibrinogen and prothrombin deficiency, quantitative defects are designated afibrinogenemia (as <0.2 g/L) or hypofibrinogenemia (0.2–1 g/L) and hypoprothrombinemia respectively (total absence of prothrombin is not compatible with life and no patient with <5 % of prothrombin level has been reported [5]). Qualitative defects are designated dysfibrinogenemia and dysprothrombinemia. A recently closed project, named "European Network of the Rare Bleeding Disorders (EN-RBD)", based on a cross-sectional study using data from 489 patients affected with different RBDs and registered in its database, evaluated the correlation between the coagulant residual plasma activity level and clinical bleeding severity [6]. Results of this data collection analysis showed the strongest association in fibrinogen, combined FV+FVIII, FX, and FXIII deficiencies, where patients with low coagulant activity levels had a higher occurrence of spontaneous major bleeding, while patients with sufficient factor activity remained asymptomatic. These observations helped to establish a new classification system with practical utility. A weaker association was present for FV and FVII deficiencies, while there was no association confirmed for FXI deficiency. From the data reported here, it seemed also clear that the minimum level to ensure complete absence of clinical symptoms is different for each disorder, leading to the conclusion that RBDs should not be considered as a single class of disorders, but instead that studies should focus on the evaluation of specific aspects of each single RBD.

12.3 Clinical Symptoms

Patients affected with RBDs present with a wide spectrum of clinical symptoms that vary from a mild or moderate bleeding tendency to severe bleeding episodes and with different patterns among RBDs. Mucosal bleeding is the most frequently reported symptom, whereas spontaneous life-threatening bleeding involving the central nervous system (CNS), gastrointestinal (GI), and musculoskeletal systems are relatively more frequent in patients with some specific deficiencies such as afibrinogenemia, severe FX or FXIII deficiency [2, 7–14]. A sign reported to be common to all RBDs is excessive bleeding at the time of surgical procedures [2, 7–14]. Women affected with RBDs are particularly disadvantaged because in addition to suffering from the common bleeding symptoms, they may also experience excessive monthly bleeding associated with menstruation. Menorrhagia, defined as blood loss of more than 80 mL per menstruation, is reported to be one of the most important symptoms in women affected with RBDs [15, 16]. Menstruation may be a source of inconvenience to women in general but is significantly more problematic for women affected with coagulation disorders who have excessive blood loss, which can have a major impact on their quality of life and employment. Many women do not go out at all during their periods, avoiding activities such as working, taking part in sports, traveling, and studying.

Menorrhagia is not the only gynaecological problem that women with RBDs are more likely to experience, they are also at risk of increased bleeding in conditions such as haemorrhagic ovarian cysts, endometriosis, endometrial hyperplasia, polyps, and fibroids [15]. Pregnancy and childbirth, two important stages in the life of a woman, pose particular clinical challenges in women with RBDs, since information about these issues is very scarce and limited to a few case reports. Pregnancy is accompanied by increased concentrations of fibrinogen, FVII, FVIII, FX, and von Willebrand factor (vWF), particularly marked in the third trimester [17–21]. At variance, FII, FV, FIX, and FXIII are relatively unchanged [17]. The active, unbound form of free protein S is decreased during pregnancy secondary to increased levels of its binding protein, the complement component C4b [20, 22]. Plasminogen activator inhibitor type 1 (PAI-1) levels are increased [23] (see Chap. 1 for further details). All of these changes contribute to the hypercoagulable state of pregnancy and, in women with RBDs, contribute to improved haemostasis. Despite improved haemostasis, however, women with factor deficiencies do not achieve the same factor levels as those of women without factor deficiencies [15], increasing the possibility of pregnancy loss or bleeding complications, especially if the defect is severe.

Detailed information about the pregnancy, pregnancy complications, and the management of women with RBDs is limited and often, apart from FXI deficiency [24, 25] (addressed in detail in Chap. 11), derived from small series or case reports. The authors are unaware of data reported in relation to pregnancy in women with FV + FVIII deficiency; the obstetric experience of women with FV deficiency could probably serve as a guide. In this chapter, a summary of the information currently available on complications of pregnancy in women with RBDs are reported.

12.3.1 Miscarriages

Miscarriage is common in the general population, with at least 12–13.5 % of recognized pregnancies resulting in spontaneous miscarriage [26, 27]. An increased risk of miscarriage and placental abruption resulting in recurrent foetal loss or premature delivery among women with afibrinogenemia [8, 28, 29] or FXIII deficiency [30, 31] has been reported. A study of the Scientific and Standardization Committee of the International Society on Thrombosis and Haemostasis (ISTH) reported a high incidence of spontaneous miscarriage (38 %) and also stillbirth in 15 women with 64 reported pregnancies fulfilling the criteria of familial dysfibrinogenemia and thrombosis not due to other causes [32]. It is generally believed that women with bleeding disorders are protected from miscarriage by the hypercoagulable state of pregnancy, but whether women with bleeding disorders other than familial dysfibrinogenaemia have an increased risk of miscarriage is unclear. Only two reports describe miscarriages: the first a case report of miscarriages in four out of eight pregnancies in a hypoprothrombinemic woman [33]; and the second, excessive bleeding after two early pregnancy losses in a series including ten pregnancies in four women affected with FVII deficiency [34]. Similarly, Kumar and Mehta reported four pregnancies in a woman with FX severe deficiency [35]: two pregnancies resulted in preterm labour and birth at 21 and 25 weeks' gestation (both babies died in the neonatal period). The mother was treated early in two subsequent pregnancies with regular FX replacement, and she delivered healthy babies at 34 and 32 gestational weeks of gestation. Whilst, prophylactic factor replacement therapy seemed to improve pregnancy outcome in this patient, other case reports have described successful term pregnancies in women with severe FX deficiency without antenatal prophylaxis [36, 37]. Further studies are needed to confirm whether inherited bleeding disorders, other than deficiency of fibrinogen or FXIII, are associated with a higher rate of miscarriage.

12.3.2 Bleeding During Pregnancy

Pregnancy is not contraindicated in patients with RBDs but requires a multidisciplinary approach for specialist management of affected women. As previously discussed, pregnancy is accompanied by increased concentrations of fibrinogen, FVII, FVIII, FX, and vWF, while FII, FV, and FIX are relatively unchanged, making women with RBDs at risk of bleeding during pregnancy. However, bleeding during pregnancy is a symptom reported in women with afibrinogenemia and severe FX deficiency [29, 35, 37, 38]. Siboni et al. collected information on menarche, bleeding during pregnancy and the postpartum period in 35 women affected with RBDs and 114 controls. These data showed bleeding during pregnancy in 21 % of patients vs 6 % of controls, however, this difference was not statistically significant P=0.11) [39]. Six successful pregnancies were achieved by afibrinogenemic women who received fibrinogen replacement therapy throughout pregnancy. Vaginal bleeding began at around 5 weeks' gestation in cases where replacement therapy was not commenced [40].

There is limited data on the changes of FXIII level during pregnancy, however it was recently confirmed that FXIII significantly reduces during gestation with a significant decrease in the third trimester [41]. In a recent systematic review by Sharief and Kadir on a total of 192 pregnancies women affected with FXIII-A and B deficiency, antepartum haemorrhage (APH: bleeding after 24 weeks gestation) occurred in five out of 65 at term pregnancies (7 %), in one case the woman was on prophylactic therapy (since the 32 week of gestation) [42]. Interestingly, patients affected with FXIII-B deficiency showed a higher frequency of APH (3/11, 27 %) compared to patients affected with FXIII-A deficiency (2/54, 4 %) [42]. Bleeding during early pregnancy was reported in one woman only [43].

12.3.3 Postpartum Hemorrhage (PPH)

PPH can be an anticipated problem in women with bleeding disorders. At the end of a normal pregnancy, an estimated 10–15 % of a woman's blood volume, or at least 750 mL/min, is lost through the uterus within the first few weeks after birth [44]. Normally after delivery of the baby and placenta, the uterine musculature or myometrium contracts around the uterine vasculature and the vasculature constricts in order to prevent exsanguination. Retained placental fragments and lacerations of the reproductive tract may also cause heavy bleeding, but the single most important cause of PPH is uterine atony [45].

Despite the critical role of uterine contractility in controlling postpartum blood loss, women with bleeding disorders are at an increased risk of PPH. There are multiple case reports and several case series documenting the incidence of PPH in women with bleeding disorders [24, 35, 46–48], but there are limited data that compare women with bleeding disorders to controls. PPH was found to be the most common obstetric complication occurring in 45 % (14/31 deliveries) among ten patients affected with hypofibrinogenemia [49], while a high incidence of postpartum thrombosis, predominantly venous, was noted among dysfibrinogenemic women (7/15, 47 %) [32]. PPH was also reported in 13 (76 %) of 17 deliveries among nine women with FV deficiency [50], which appears to be associated with an increased risk of developing this complication (especially in women with low FV activity levels). Although at a lower rate, PPH was also reported in patients with deficiencies of FVII [51], FX [52], or FXI [24]. Particularly interesting is the latter report of a large study of 164 pregnancies in 62 women with FXI deficiency (levels <17 IU/dL) showing that 69 % of the women never experienced PPH during 93 deliveries without any prophylactic cover with FXI replacement. The authors therefore argued that prophylactic treatment is not mandatory for these women, especially in the context of vaginal delivery (however, excessive bleeding at delivery did occur in around 20 % of deliveries not covered by replacement therapy).

The incidence of PPH in women with FXIII deficiency is not known, however primary PPH was reported in 16/65 (25 %) pregnancies in 12 women with FXIII-A and B deficiency; interestingly a higher frequency of PPH was observed in patients with FXIII-B deficiency compared to those affected with FXIII-A deficiency (82 % vs 13 %) [42]. Successful pregnancy in women with FXIII subunit A deficiency is generally achieved only with replacement therapy throughout pregnancy and at delivery [53]. No data are published on the rate of PPH in women affected with FII deficiency. Among all women, the median duration of bleeding after delivery is 21–27 days [54, 55], but coagulation factors, elevated during pregnancy, return to baseline within 14–21 days [56]. Therefore, there is a period of time, 2–3 weeks after delivery, when coagulation factors have returned to pre-pregnancy levels but women are still bleeding. Women with bleeding disorders are particularly vulnerable to delayed or 'secondary' PPH during this same period of time. The implication is that women with bleeding disorders may require prophylaxis and/or close observation for several weeks after delivery.

12.4 Laboratory Diagnosis

12.4.1 Phenotype Analysis

The combined performance of the screening coagulation tests, the prothrombin time (PT) and activated partial thromboplastin time (APTT), is usually applied to identify RBDs of clinically significant severity. A prolonged APTT with a normal PT is suggestive of FXI deficiency (after exclusion of FVIII, FIX, and FXII deficiencies). The reverse pattern (normal APTT and prolonged PT) is typical of FVII deficiency, whereas the prolongation of both tests directs further analysis towards identification of possible deficiencies of FX, FV, or prothrombin. The sensitivity of the PT and APTT to the presence of coagulation factor deficiencies is dependent on the test system employed [57, 58]. All coagulation tests that depend on the formation of fibrin as the end point are necessary to evaluate fibrinogen deficiency, hence, in addition to the PT and APTT, the thrombin time (TT) also has to be performed. These three tests show infinitely prolonged clotting times in the case of afibrinogenemia and results are variable in the case of hypodys- or dysfibrinogenemia. Specific assays of factor coagulant activity are necessary when the degree of prolongation of the global tests suggests the presence of clinically significant deficiencies. Factor antigen assays are not strictly necessary for diagnosis and treatment but are necessary to distinguish type I from type II deficiencies. However, these data are important in the characterisation of deficiency of fibrinogen or FII, where a normal antigen level associated with reduced activity (dysfibrinogenemia and dysprothrombinemia) is associated with higher risk of thrombosis.

The standard laboratory tests of haemostasis (PT, APTT, fibrinogen level, platelet count, bleeding time) are normal in FXIII deficiency. The diagnosis of FXIII deficiency is established by the demonstration of increased clot solubility in 5 M urea, dilute monochloroacetic acid, or acetic acid. However, this method is not quantitative and not standardized. The sensitivity of these assays mainly depends on the fibrinogen level, on the reagents used to trigger the coagulation of the plasma (thrombin and/or Ca^{2+}), on specific features of the solubilizing agent, and on the concentration of FXIII. In a UK National External Quality Assessment Scheme (NEQAS) study, 15 combinations of these variables were used among participant laboratories [59], and the clot solubility test detected only very severe FXIII deficiency (where the FXIII activity in the patient's plasma was significantly <5 %). If clot solubility in these reagents is found, a mixing study (FXIII activity determination on a mixture of patient and normal plasma) is needed to exclude the presence of a FXIII inhibitor. FXIII activity should also be determined quantitatively by a chromogenic assay that measures the incorporation of fluorescent or radioactive amines into proteins [60]. Specific ELISA tests have been developed to establish FXIII-A and FXIII-B antigen levels [61]. Diagnostic tests for RBDs may be ordered by a gynaecologist or the family physician, or alternatively, the woman may be referred directly to a specialist haemostasis centre. However, interpretation of abnormal or borderline results usually requires referral to a specialist haematology (or an internal medicine) consultant. These assays are routinely available in many coagulation laboratories in Europe and North America but are seldom carried out, so that proficiency and standardization may be limited.

12.4.2 Molecular Diagnosis

RBDs are usually due to DNA defects in genes encoding the corresponding coagulation factors [2]. Exceptions are the combined deficiencies of coagulation FV and FVIII and of vitamin-K-dependent proteins (FII, FVII, FIX, and FX) caused, respectively, by mutations in genes encoding proteins involved in the FV and FVIII intracellular transport mechanism (*LMAN1* and *MCFD2*) and in genes that encode enzymes involved in posttranslational modifications and in vitamin K metabolism (*GGCX* and *VKORC1*) [62–65]. The pattern of inheritance is usually autosomal recessive for all RBDs, except for FXI, where in some cases, missense mutations have been shown to exert a dominant negative effect through heterodimer formation between the mutant and wild-type polypeptides, resulting in a pattern of dominant transmission [66]. The identification of gene defects in patients with RBDs could represent the basis on which to carry out prenatal diagnosis in families that already have one affected child with a severe bleeding history. Molecular characterization and subsequent prenatal diagnosis gain importance particularly in developing countries, where patients with these deficiencies rarely survive beyond childhood and where management is still largely inadequate; therefore, prenatal diagnosis is an important option for the prevention of the birth of children affected with RBDs and severe bleeding manifestations, particularly in regions with low economic resources and a high rate of consanguineous marriages.

12.5 Therapeutic Management

Based on the observations detailed above, regular replacement therapy throughout pregnancy in order to maintain a minimum activity level is recommended in women with afibrinogenemia. In these women, replacement therapy should be commenced as soon as possible in pregnancy to reduce the probability of early fetal loss [40, 67, 68], and should be continued during labour and delivery to minimize the risk of bleeding complications. Thrombotic events have also been reported in patients with inherited afibrinogenemia [8], and so the risks of both bleeding and thrombosis should be considered and balanced during pregnancy. The management of women with hypofibrinogenemia should follow similar lines depending on the fibrinogen level, individual bleeding tendency, and family history, as well as previous obstetric history [69]. Thrombotic events during the puerperium have also been reported among women with hypofibrinogenemia [70], and here again the potential for thrombosis associated with replacement therapy must be carefully evaluated and balanced against the risk of bleeding. The management of pregnancy in women with dysfibrinogenemia needs to be individualized, taking into account the fibrinogen level and personal and family history of bleeding and thrombosis [67]. No specific treatment is required in asymptomatic women.

In view of the very limited available data, it is difficult to make recommendations for the obstetric management of women with prothrombin, FV, and FV + FVIII deficiencies. It is unknown whether or not prophylactic replacement therapy is required or not during pregnancy. However, women with prothrombin and FV deficiency, particularly those with low coagulant activity levels, appear to be at increased risk of PPH. Therefore, careful management of labour and the immediate postpartum period is necessary. As regards women with FV + FVIII deficiency, the obstetric experience of women with FV deficiency and carriers of haemophilia could probably serve as a useful guide.

A significant rise in the FVII level is observed during pregnancy in women with mild/moderate forms of FVII deficiency (heterozygotes) [34], but not in women with severe deficiency [48, 51, 71]. Therefore, in women with mild/moderate deficiency, in whom the FVII level may normalize at term, replacement therapy may not be required for labour and delivery. Women with severe deficiency or a positive bleeding history are more likely to be at risk of PPH; hence, prophylactic treatment is required for women with low FVII coagulant activity levels at term and/or a significant bleeding history [46, 51, 72, 73]. In women with FX deficiency, replacement therapy should be considered if bleeding occurs or if the patient is undergoing an invasive procedure. Women with severe deficiency and a history of adverse pregnancy outcome may benefit from replacement therapy during a subsequent pregnancy [67, 74]. Replacement therapy is also required to cover labour and delivery in these women to minimize the risk of bleeding complications [75, 76]. Treatment is not mandatory for women with FXI deficiency (addressed in detail in Chap. 11), especially with vaginal delivery [24]; however, due to the unpredictable bleeding tendency in FXI deficiency, especially during surgery, the decision whether or not to give prophylaxis during labour and delivery needs to be individualized and must take into consideration the FXI level, personal/family history of bleeding and thrombosis, and mode of delivery. In FXIII deficiency, replacement therapy should be commenced as early as possible in pregnancy to prevent fetal loss [43, 77]; the treatment should also be continued during labour and delivery to minimize the risk of bleeding complications. Higher FXIII levels may be required for delivery [78].

The management of women with inherited bleeding disorders during bleeding episodes or delivery remains a challenge due to the scant availability of specific evidence-based guidelines. However, consensus guidelines were developed by government agencies or haemophilia organizations and summarized in a review by James [79]. Table 12.1 details available recommendations for the obstetric management of women with inherited bleeding disorders [29, 80–82]. Moreover, focused data collection, such as that reported by Byams et al. within the Centers for Disease Control and Prevention surveillance program, may help in identifying risk factors and direct efforts to improve guidance on management for affected women [83].

Table 12.1 Available recommendations for the obstetric management of women with inherited bleeding disorders [29, 80–82]

a- and hypo-fibinogenemia	It is recommended to maintain fibrinogen levels ≥0.6 g/L, and ideally at >1.0 g/L throughout pregnancy to prevent early fetal loss and bleeding complications. A fibrinogen level of ≥1.5 g/L (ideally >2.0 g/L) is recommended to prevent placental abruption during labour and to prevent PPH in afibrinogenemia For women with hypofibrinogenemia, intrapartum replacement is required if the fibrinogen level is below 1.5 mg/dL and/or the woman has a significant bleeding history. Thrombosis events have been reported during the puerpuerium, hence postpartum management, including the use of postpartum prophylaxis, should take into account any personal and family history of bleeding and thrombosis
Dysfibrinogenemia	Women with dysfibrinogenemia are also at risk of both postpartum thrombosis and PPH. Postpartum management of these women should be individualized based on their fibrinogen level as well as personal and family history of bleeding and thrombosis
FII	Secondary PPH was reported in one pregnancy. Based on these limited data, it is difficult to make a recommendation for obstetric management. A prothrombin level of 20–30 IU/dL is believed to be required for normal hemostasis, and it is recommended that a prothrombin level of more than 25 IU/dL should be achieved during labour and delivery
FV	In women with partial deficiency and no history of bleeding, labour and delivery could be managed expectantly. Women with FV deficiency, especially those with low FV levels, appear to be at increased risk of PPH. Substitution therapy with FFP is recommended to raise FV level to above 15–25 %
FV + VIII	There are not enough data in relation to pregnancy in these women; the obstetric experience of women with FV deficiency and carriers of haemophilia could probably serve as a useful guide in these patients: during labour, virally inactivated FFP at an initial dose of 15–20 mL/kg should be used to maintain FV levels >15 IU/dL and recombinant FVIII concentrate should be used to maintain FVIII levels >50 IU/dL. If a Cesarean section is required, FV levels should be increased to >25 IU/dL and factor replacement should continue until wound healing has occurred
FVII	Women with low FVII levels or positive bleeding history are more likely to be at risk of PPH; therefore, prophylactic treatment is required for women with a FVII level of <10–20 %. rFVIIa (15–30 μg/kg) should be the treatment of choice
FX	Patients with severe FX deficiency (<1 %) tend to be the most seriously affected patients with RBDs; therefore, they may benefit from replacement therapy during pregnancy and to cover labour and delivery to minimize the risk of bleeding complications. In women with a FX level 10–20 % and no significant bleeding history, a conservative approach could be adopted
FXI	FXI concentrate has been associated with an increased risk of thrombosis, and therefore doses should not exceed 30 IU/kg (to maintain an FXI level no higher than 70 IU/dL). An antifibrinonlytic agent (tranexamic acid) should be given in the postpartum period to prevent PPH and can be administered for up to 2 weeks after delivery. However, it should not be given concomitantly with FXI concentrate in view of possible thrombogenicity In patients who have developed inhibitors to FXI, rVIIa has been successfully used to prevent bleeding during surgical procedures, although it is not currently licensed for this use
FXIII	FXIII concentrate is the treatment of choice (rather than FFP or cryoprecipitate), with a target FXIII level >10 IU/dL. This level can be achieved by administering 250 IU of FXIII concentrate weekly from pregnancy confirmation up until 22 weeks' gestation, and 500 IU weekly from 23 weeks onwards. At the onset of labour, an additional dose of 1,000 IU should be given to increase the FXIII level to >30 IU/dL. The incidence of PPH in women with FXIII deficiency is not known. Successful pregnancy in women with FXIII subunit A deficiency is generally only achieved with replacement therapy throughout pregnancy; a level >10–20 % during pregnancy should be considered

PPH primarily pulmonary hypertension, *RBD* rare bleeding disorder, *FFP* fresh frozen plasma

A peri-delivery plan should be discussed with the patient and documented. This should include advice on peridelivery analgesia, which should involve a pre-delivery anaesthetic consultation (see Chap. 21). The use of tranexamic acid and desmopressin should be considered in patients with a mild phenotype.

12.6 Multidisciplinary Clinics

The optimal management of women with an inherited coagulation defect is within specialist multidisciplinary clinics with a gynaecologist/obstetrician, haematologist and, when relevant, an anaesthetist. However, at present, few such clinics exist and these women are usually managed suboptimally in separate gynaecology and/or haematology clinics. The ideal multidisciplinary team should have an even broader representation of expertise and would include a haemostasis clinician, a laboratory haematologist, an obstetrician/gynaecologist, an anaesthetist, a family physician, a social worker, a pharmacist, and a biomedical scientist. The presence of a psychologist should also be taken into consideration on the basis of studies showing that health-related quality of life is impaired in women with menorrhagia in general and in those with inherited bleeding disorders [84].

12.7 Case Studies

Case Study 1
In 2005, a 25-year-old woman attended a Hemophilia and Thrombosis Centre having been diagnosed with severe FXIII deficiency (chromogenic activity <5 %) at birth after umbilical cord bleeding. She had experienced mild gum bleeding, recurrent bruising and hematomas after mild trauma, and one post-traumatic haemarthrosis of the ankle, requiring multiple plasma transfusions. In view of the recurrent hematomas, she was commenced on long-term prophylaxis with 1,500 IU plasma-derived human FXIII (pdFXIII) Fibrogammin-P (17 U/kg) by intravenous infusion every 5 weeks and has not had any further bleeding episodes on this regimen. The plasma FXIII activity levels before and after the pdFXIII infusion were approximately 2 and 52 %, respectively. When aged 32 years, she had an early fetal loss at 8 weeks gestation, unassociated with bleeding complications. During her second pregnancy, when aged 38 years, the prophylactic regimen was intensified to 1,500 IU every 3 weeks to prevent fetal loss. She did not experience any bleeding symptoms during pregnancy. She received 1,500 IU pdFXIII (16 U/kg) before elective Cesarean section at 38 weeks gestation when a healthy female infant, birth weight (BW) 2,700 g. The post-infusion plasma factor XIII level was not available. She had a primary postpartum haemorrhage (estimated blood loss 2,000 mL) associated with uterine atony occurred, and was therefore treated with uterine massage, oxytocin, foley catheter placement and red cell transfusion (2 units). One hour post-Cesarean section, the plasma FXIII chromogenic activity level was 21 %, requiring infusion of an additional 1,000 IU of pdFXIII. In the following days the haemoglobin stabilised and she had no further bleeding symptoms.

Case Study 2
In 2013, a 29-year-old woman attended a Hemophilia and Thrombosis centre with a previous diagnosis of dysfibrinogenemia (fibrinogen coagulant activity 0.5 g/L, antigen levels were not available). This diagnosis was made when she was aged 24 years, after an episode of bleeding during pregnancy, at 16 weeks gestation, because of placental abruption. She reported that she had been previously treated for a few weeks with subcutaneous enoxaparin 40 mg daily starting from the 25th week of gestation. She also reported an uncomplicated vaginal delivery at 38 weeks' gestation, with the birth weight (BW) of her female infant 2,630 g. She did not experience any additional bleeding episodes, although she reported a family history of thrombotic events. During her second pregnancy, when aged 27 years, she was treated with enoxaparin 40 mg daily starting from the 12th week of pregnancy. She had a vaginal delivery at 37 weeks' gestation with no complications, and her female infant's

BW 2,800 g. She came to specialist attention during her third pregnancy, at 7 weeks' gestation, when a diagnosis of hypofibrinogenemia was made: fibrinogen coagulant activity was 0.6 g/L and antigen levels 0.89 g/L. She was commenced on enoxaparin 20 mg daily during the first trimester of pregnancy, which was increased to 40 mg daily during the second and third trimesters. On the basis of her family history of thrombosis, fibrinogen concentrate was not administered prophylactically and was kept on standby. The enoxaparin was omitted when she went into labour at 38 weeks' gestation, and recommenced 12 h after delivery, continuing for 6 weeks postpartum. A healthy male infant (BW 3,850 g) was delivered by normal vaginal delivery. No bleeding or thrombotic complications were observed.

Key Learning Points

- In women who have a personal or family history of bleeding, further investigation should be considered.
- Inherited bleeding disorders should be considered in the differential diagnosis of all women presenting with menorrhagia or other gynaecological bleeding complications.
- Pregnancy is accompanied by increased concentrations of fibrinogen, FVII, FVIII, FX, and von Willebrand factor, while FII, FV, and FIX remain relatively unchanged. Despite improved haemostasis, women with coagulation factor deficiencies may not achieve the same factor levels as those of women without such defects, therefore the level of haemostatic factors should be monitored during each pregnancy.
- Miscarriage is common in the general population, with at least 12–13.5 % of recognized pregnancies resulting in pregnancy loss. An increased risk of miscarriage and placental abruption resulting in fetal loss or preterm delivery is reported in women with deficiency of fibrinogen or FXIII.
- Thrombotic events have been reported in patients with inherited fibrinogen deficiency, so the risks of bleeding and thrombosis should be considered and balanced throughout the pregnancy and puerperium, particularly in patients with dysfibrinogenemia. The antigen level of fibrinogen should be evaluated in addition to the activity level in order to ensure an accurate diagnosis.
- Women affected with RBDs may continue to bleed during the first 2–3 weeks after delivery, when coagulation factors return to pre-pregnancy levels. Women with bleeding disorders are particularly vulnerable to delayed or secondary PPH during this period, and may require prophylaxis and/or close observation for several weeks after delivery.

References

1. Mannucci PM, Duga S, Peyvandi F. Recessively inherited coagulation disorders. Blood. 2004;104:1243–52.
2. Tuddenham EGD, Cooper DN. The molecular genetics of haemostasis and its inherited disorders, Oxford monographs on medical genetics, No. 25. Oxford: Oxford Medical Publications; 1994.
3. Peyvandi F, Palla R, Menegatti M, Mannucci PM. Introduction: rare bleeding disorders: general aspects of clinical features, diagnosis, and management. Semin Thromb Hemost. 2009;35:349–55.
4. Peyvandi F, Palla R, Menegatti M. European registry of rare bleeding disorders. Hematology Education: the education programme for the annual congress of the European Hematology Association 2010;4:63–8.
5. Sun WY, Witte DP, Degen JL, et al. Prothrombin deficiency results in embryonic and neonatal lethality in mice. Proc Natl Acad Sci U S A. 1998;95:7597–602.
6. Peyvandi F, Palla R, Menegatti M, et al. Coagulation factor activity and clinical bleeding severity in rare bleeding disorders: results from the European Network of Rare Bleeding Disorders. J Thromb Haemost. 2012;10:615–21.
7. Lak M, Sharifian R, Peyvandi F, Mannucci PM. Symptoms of inherited factor V deficiency in 35 Iranian patients. Br J Haematol. 1998;103:1067–9.
8. Lak M, Keihani M, Elahi F, et al. Bleeding and thrombosis in 55 patients with inherited afibrinogenaemia. Br J Haematol. 1999;107:204–6.

9. Lak M, Peyvandi F, Ali Sharifian A, et al. Pattern of symptoms in 93 Iranian patients with severe factor XIII deficiency. J Thromb Haemost. 2003;1:1852–3.
10. Peyvandi F, Mannucci PM, Asti D, et al. Clinical manifestations in 28 Italian and Iranian patients with severe factor VII deficiency. Haemophilia. 1997;3: 242–6.
11. Peyvandi F, Mannucci PM, Lak M, et al. Congenital factor X deficiency: spectrum of bleeding symptoms in 32 Iranian patients. Br J Haematol. 1998;102: 626–8.
12. Peyvandi F, Tuddenham EG, Akhtari AM, et al. Bleeding symptoms in 27 Iranian patients with the combined deficiency of factor V and factor VIII. Br J Haematol. 1998;100:773–6.
13. Peyvandi F, Lak M, Mannucci PM. Factor XI deficiency in Iranians: its clinical manifestations in comparison with those of classic hemophilia. Haematologica. 2002;87:512–4.
14. Acharya SS, Coughlin A, Dimichele DM. Rare Bleeding Disorder Registry: deficiencies of factors II, V, VII, X, XIII, fibrinogen and dysfibrinogenemias. J Thromb Haemost. 2004;2:248–56.
15. James AH. More than menorrhagia: a review of the obstetric and gynaecological manifestations of bleeding disorders. Haemophilia. 2005;11:295–307.
16. Kadir RA, Economides DL, Sabin CA, et al. Frequency of inherited bleeding disorders in women with menorrhagia. Lancet. 1998;351:485–9.
17. Stirling Y, Woolf L, North WR, et al. Haemostasis in normal pregnancy. Thromb Haemost. 1984;52: 176–82.
18. Sanchez-Luceros A, Meschengieser SS, Marchese C, et al. Factor VIII and von Willebrand factor changes during normal pregnancy and puerperium. Blood Coagul Fibrinolysis. 2003;14:647–51.
19. Wickstrom K, Edelstam G, Lowbeer CH, et al. Reference intervals for plasma levels of fibronectin, von Willebrand factor, free protein S and antithrombin during third-trimester pregnancy. Scand J Clin Lab Invest. 2004;64:31–40.
20. Bremme KA. Haemostatic changes in pregnancy. Best Pract Res Clin Haematol. 2003;16:153–68.
21. Hellgren M, Blomback M. Studies on blood coagulation and fibrinolysis in pregnancy, during delivery and in the puerperium. Normal condition. Gynecol Obstet Invest. 1981;12:141–54.
22. Bremme K, Ostlund E, Almqvist I, et al. Enhanced thrombin generation and fibrinolytic activity in normal pregnancy and the puerperium. Obstet Gynecol. 1992;80:132–7.
23. Sie P, Caron C, Azam J, et al. Reassessment of von Willebrand factor (VWF), VWF propeptide, factor VIII: C and plasminogen activator inhibitors 1 and 2 during normal pregnancy. Br J Haematol. 2003;121: 897–903.
24. Salomon O, Steinberg DM, Tamarin I, et al. Plasma replacement therapy during labor is not mandatory for women with severe factor XI deficiency. Blood Coagul Fibrinolysis. 2005;16:37–41.
25. Myers B, Pavord S, Kean L, et al. Pregnancy outcome in Factor XI deficiency: incidence of miscarriage, antenatal and postnatal haemorrhage in 33 women with Factor XI deficiency. BJOG. 2007;114:643–6.
26. Everett C. Incidence and outcome of bleeding before the 20th week of pregnancy: prospective study from general practice. BMJ. 1997;315:32–4.
27. Nybo Andersen AM, Wohlfahrt J, Christens P, et al. Maternal age and fetal loss: population based register linkage study. BMJ. 2000;320:1708–12.
28. Evron S, Anteby SO, Brzezinsky A, et al. Congenital afibrinogenemia and recurrent early abortion: a case report. Eur J Obstet Gynecol Reprod Biol. 1985;19: 307–11.
29. Kobayashi T, Kanayama N, Tokunaga N, et al. Prenatal and peripartum management of congenital afibrinogenaemia. Br J Haematol. 2000;109:364–6.
30. Inbal A, Kenet G. Pregnancy and surgical procedures in patients with factor XIII deficiency. Biomed Prog. 2003;16:69–71.
31. Burrows RF, Ray JG, Burrows EA. Bleeding risk and reproductive capacity among patients with factor XIII deficiency: a case presentation and review of the literature. Obstet Gynecol Surv. 2000;55:103–8.
32. Haverkate F, Samama M. Familial dysfibrinogenemia and thrombophilia. Report on a study of the SSC Subcommittee on Fibrinogen. Thromb Haemost. 1995;73:151–61.
33. Catanzarite VA, Novotny WF, Cousins LM, Schneider JM. Pregnancies in a patient with congenital absence of prothrombin activity: case report. Am J Perinatol. 1997;14:135–8.
34. Kulkarni AA, Lee CA, Kadir RA. Pregnancy in women with congenital factor VII deficiency. Haemophilia. 2006;12:413–6.
35. Kumar M, Mehta P. Congenital coagulopathies and pregnancy: report of four pregnancies in a factor X-deficient woman. Am J Hematol. 1994;46:241–4.
36. Larrain C. Congenital blood coagulation factor X deficiency. Successful result of the use prothrombin concentrated complex in the control of caesarean section hemorrhage in 2 pregnancies. Rev Med Chil. 1994;122:1178–83.
37. Romagnolo C, Burati S, Ciaffoni S, et al. Severe factor X deficiency in pregnancy: case report and review of the literature. Haemophilia. 2004;10:665–8.
38. Greer IA, Lowe GD, Walker JJ, Forbes CD. Haemorrhagic problems in obstetrics and gynaecology in patients with congenital coagulopathies. Br J Obstet Gynaecol. 1991;98:909–18.
39. Siboni SM, Spreafico M, Calò L, et al. Gynaecological and obstetrical problems in women with different bleeding disorders. Haemophilia. 2009;15:1291–9.
40. Inamoto Y, Terao T. First report of case of congenital afibrinogenemia with successful delivery. Am J Obstet Gynecol. 1985;153:803–4.
41. Sharief LT, Lawrie AS, Mackie IJ, Smith C, Peyvandi F, Kadir RA. Changes in factor XIII level during pregnancy. Haemophilia. 2013;20(2):e144–8. doi:10.1111/hae.12345. Epub ahead of print.

42. Sharief LA, Kadir RA. Congenital factor XIII deficiency in women: a systematic review of literature. Haemophilia. 2013;19(6):e349–57.
43. Kobayashi T, Terao T, Kojima T, Takamatsu J, Kamiya T, Saito H. Congenital factor XIII deficiency with treatment of factor XIII concentrate and normal vaginal delivery. Gynecol Obstet Invest. 1990;29:235–8.
44. Ross M. Placental and fetal physiology. In: Gabbe S, Niebyl J, Simpson J, editors. Obstetrics: normal and problem pregnancies. New York: Churchill Livingstone; 2002. p. 37–62.
45. Benedetti T. Obstetrical hemorrhage. In: Gabbe S, Niebyl J, Simpson J, editors. Obstetrics: normal and problem pregnancies. New York: Churchill Livingstone; 2002. p. 503–38.
46. Fadel HE, Krauss JS. Factor VII deficiency and pregnancy. Obstet Gynecol. 1989;73:453–4.
47. Strickland DM, Galey WT, Hauth JC. Hypofibrinogenemia as a cause of delayed postpartum hemorrhage. Am J Obstet Gynecol. 1982;143:230–1.
48. Robertson LE, Wasserstrum N, Banez E, et al. Hereditary factor VII deficiency in pregnancy: peripartum treatment with factor VII concentrate. Am J Hematol. 1992;40:38–41.
49. Goodwin TM. Congenital hypofibrinogenemia in pregnancy. Obstet Gynecol Surv. 1989;44:157–61.
50. Noia G, De Carolis S, De Stefano V, et al. Factor V deficiency in pregnancy complicated by Rh immunization and placenta previa. A case report and review of the literature. Acta Obstet Gynecol Scand. 1997; 76:890–2.
51. Rizk DE, Castella A, Shaheen H, Deb P. Factor VII deficiency detected in pregnancy: a case report. Am J Perinatol. 1999;16:223–6.
52. Girolami A, Lazzarin M, Scarpa R, Brunetti A. Further studies on the abnormal factor X (factor X Friuli) coagulation disorder: a report of another family. Blood. 1971;37:534–41.
53. Ichinose A, Asahina T, Kobayashi T. Congenital blood coagulation factor XIII deficiency and perinatal management. Curr Drug Targets. 2005;6:541–9.
54. Edwards A, Ellwood DA. Ultrasonographic evaluation of the postpartum uterus. Ultrasound Obstet Gynecol. 2000;16:640–3.
55. Visness CM, Kennedy KI, Ramos R. The duration and character of postpartum bleeding among breast-feeding women. Obstet Gynecol. 1997;89:159–63.
56. Dahlman T, Hellgren M, Blombäck M. Changes in blood coagulation and fibrinolysis in the normal puerperium. Gynecol Obstet Invest. 1985;20:37–44.
57. Lawrie AS, Kitchen S, Purdy G, et al. Assessment of actin FS and actin FSL sensitivity to specific clotting factor deficiencies. Clin Lab Haematol. 1998;20:179–86.
58. Turi DC, Peerschke EI. Sensitivity of three activated partial thromboplastin time reagents to coagulation factor deficiencies. Am J Clin Pathol. 1986;85:43–9.
59. Jennings I, Kitchen S, Woods TAL, Preston FE. Problems relating to the laboratory diagnosis of factor XIII deficiency: a UK NEQAS study. J Thromb Haemost. 2003;1:2603–8.
60. Muszbek L, Bagoly Z, Cairo A, Peyvandi F. Novel aspects of factor XIII deficiency. Curr Opin Hematol. 2011;18(5):366–72.
61. Katona E, Haramura G, Karpati L, et al. A simple, quick one-step ELISA assay for the determination of complex plasma factor XIII (A2B2). Thromb Haemost. 2000;83:268–73.
62. Nichols WC, Seligsohn U, Zivelin A, et al. Mutations in the ER-Golgi intermediate compartment protein ERGIC-53 cause combined deficiency of coagulation factors V and VIII. Cell. 1998;93:61–70.
63. Zhang B, Cunningham MA, Nichols WC, et al. Bleeding due to disruption of a cargo-specific ER-to-Golgi transport complex. Nat Genet. 2003;34:220–5.
64. Mousallem M, Spronk HM, Sacy R, et al. Congenital combined deficiencies of all vitamin K-dependent coagulation factors. Thromb Haemost. 2001;86:1334–6.
65. Rost S, Fregin A, Ivaskevicius V, et al. Mutations in VKORC1 cause warfarin resistance and multiple coagulation factor deficiency type 2. Nature. 2004; 427:537–41.
66. Kravtsov DV, Wu W, Meijers JC, et al. Dominant factor XI deficiency caused by mutations in the factor XI catalytic domain. Blood. 2004;104:128–34.
67. Bolton-Maggs PH, Perry DJ, Chalmers EA, et al. The rare coagulation disorders – review with guidelines for management from the United Kingdom Haemophilia Centre Doctors' Organisation. Haemophilia. 2004;10:593–628.
68. Trehan AK, Fergusson IL. Congenital afibrinogenaemia and successful pregnancy outcome (case report). Br J Obstet Gynaecol. 1991;98:722–4.
69. Frenkel E, Duksin C, Herman A, Sherman DJ. Congenital hypofibrinogenemia in pregnancy: report of two cases and review of the literature. Obstet Gynecol Surv. 2004;59:775–9.
70. Dupuy E, Soria C, Molho P, et al. Embolized ischemic lesions of toes in an afibrinogenemic patient: possible relevance to in vivo circulating thrombin. Thromb Res. 2001;102:211–9.
71. Braun MW, Triplett DA. Case report: factor VII deficiency in an obstetrical patient. J Indiana State Med Assoc. 1979;72:900–2.
72. Eskandari N, Feldman N, Greenspoon JS. Factor VII deficiency in pregnancy treated with recombinant factor VIIa. Obstet Gynecol. 2002;99:935–7.
73. Jimenez-Yuste V, Villar A, Morado M, et al. Continuous infusion of recombinant activated factor VII during caesarean section delivery in a patient with congenital factor VII deficiency. Haemophilia. 2000; 6:588–90.
74. Nance D, Josephson NC, Paulyson-Nunez K, James AH. Factor X deficiency and pregnancy: preconception counselling and therapeutic options. Haemophilia. 2012;18:e277–85.
75. Konje JC, Murphy P, de Chazal R, et al. Severe factor X deficiency and successful pregnancy. Br J Obstet Gynaecol. 1994;101:910–1.
76. Bofill JA, Young RA, Perry Jr KG. Successful pregnancy in a woman with severe factor X deficiency. Obstet Gynecol. 1996;88:723.

77. Rodeghiero F, Castaman GC, Di Bona E, et al. Successful pregnancy in a woman with congenital factor XIII deficiency treated with substitutive therapy. Report of a second case. Blut. 1987;55:45–8.
78. Asahina T, Kobayashi T, Takeuchi K, Kanayama N. Congenital blood coagulation factor XIII deficiency and successful deliveries: a review of the literature. Obstet Gynecol Surv. 2007;62:255–60.
79. James AH. Guidelines for bleeding disorders in women. Thromb Res. 2009;123 Suppl 2:S124–8.
80. Kadir R, Chi C, Bolton-Maggs P. Pregnancy and rare bleeding disorders. Haemophilia. 2009;15:990–1005.
81. Pike GN, Bolton-Maggs PH. Factor deficiencies in pregnancy. Hematol Oncol Clin North Am. 2011;25(2):359–78, viii–ix. doi:10.1016/j.hoc.2011.01.007.
82. Peyvandi F, Garagiola I, Menegatti M. Gynecological and obstetrical manifestations of inherited bleeding disorders in women. J Thromb Haemost. 2011;9 Suppl 1:236–45.
83. Byams VR, Koudies PA, Kulkarni R, et al. Surveillance of female patients with inherited bleeding disorders in United States Haemophilia Treatment Centres. Haemophilia. 2011;17 Suppl 1:6–13.
84. von Mackensen S. Quality of life in women with bleeding disorders. Haemophilia. 2011;17 Suppl 1:33–7.

13 Inherited Bleeding Disorders in Pregnancy: Platelet Defects

Andrew D. Mumford and Amanda Clark

Abstract

Platelet function disorders (PFDs) include the severe bleeding disorders Glanzmann thrombasthenia (GT) and Bernard Soulier syndrome (BSS), and a heterogenous group of other non-severe phenotype platelet defects. GT and BSS confer significant risk of ante-partum and post-partum bleeding and may be complicated by alloimmunisation against platelet antigens, potentially causing maternal platelet refractoriness and fetal alloimmune thrombocytopenia. This chapter reviews the prevalence of bleeding in GT and BSS, and in non-severe PFDs. We describe the available therapies to prevent or treat obstetric bleeding in women with PFD and summarise current management strategies.

Keywords

Platelets • Bleeding • Platelet function disorders • Glanzmann thrombasthenia • Bernard Soulier syndrome

A.D. Mumford, MB ChB, PhD, FRCPath (✉)
School of Cellular and Molecular Medicine, University of Bristol, Bristol Royal Infirmary, Marlborough Street, Bristol BS2 8HW, UK
e-mail: a.mumford@bristol.ac.uk

A. Clark, BSc, MBBS, FRCPath
Department of Haematology, Bristol Haematology and Oncology Centre, University Hospitals Bristol NHS Foundation Trust, Horfield Road, Bristol BS2 8ED, UK
e-mail: amanda.clark@uhbristol.nhs.uk

13.1 Introduction

Platelets are anuclear cellular components of blood that are a critical component of primary hemostasis and support the activation of plasma coagulation factors to enable fibrin clot formation. Platelets also have pro-inflammatory and pro-proliferative activities and mediate vascular disorders such as atherothrombosis. In pregnancy, platelets are essential to maintain adequate hemostasis at delivery and contribute to the pathogenesis of vascular disorders such as preeclampsia and other microangiopathic coagulopathies.

Disorders of platelet number may give rise to significant maternal and fetal morbidity because

H. Cohen, P. O'Brien (eds.), *Disorders of Thrombosis and Hemostasis in Pregnancy: A Guide to Management*, DOI 10.1007/978-3-319-15120-5_13, © Springer-Verlag London 2015

of bleeding. This group of disorders are described elsewhere in this volume. Similar morbidity may arise from platelet function disorders (PFDs) which include rare heritable disorders such as Glanzmann thrombasthenia (GT) and Bernard-Soulier syndrome (BSS) which may be associated with severe bleeding in pregnancy. This group also includes non-severe PFDs which are heterogeneous and common disorders that may also be associated with adverse pregnancy outcomes. The non-severe PFDs often present significant difficulties in diagnosis and management.

This chapter provides a description of the expected changes in platelet function in normal and abnormal pregnancies and summarizes the key diagnostic features of the major platelet function disorders. A systematic review is presented of the worldwide experience of pregnancy in women with severe GT and BSS and non-severe PFDs and includes consensus guidance for optimum management.

13.2 Changes in Platelet Function in Normal Pregnancy

Platelet aggregation and ATP secretion in response to activating agonists have been shown to increase in women during normal pregnancy compared to nonpregnant controls [1–3]. This difference was most evident in the third trimester, but by 6–12 weeks after delivery, platelets from the pregnant and nonpregnant groups were indistinguishable [1, 2]. Increased platelet surface expression of the lysosome marker CD63 also increased during normal pregnancy both in non-stimulated and agonist-stimulated platelets [4, 5]. Similarly, the plasma concentrations of the soluble platelet activation markers β-thromboglobulin and soluble CD40 ligand increased during normal pregnancy [5, 6] suggesting an increase in basal activation of platelets *in vivo*. However, alternative markers of platelet activation, such as platelet binding of fibrinogen or markers of the open-conformation $\alpha_{IIb}\beta_3$ integrin, were shown not to increase in non-stimulated platelets during normal pregnancy [3, 5]. There was also no increase in the platelet surface expression of P-selectin which is a marker of platelet α-granule secretion [7, 8]. Other smaller studies have shown decreased platelet surface expression of P-selectin in response to agonist stimulation during pregnancy and lower plasma concentrations of β-thromboglobulin [9, 10].

Interpretation of these observational data is hampered by the limited sample sizes of the individual studies and by difficulties in standardization of platelet function assays between laboratories. However, taken together, these data suggest that normal pregnancy is associated with increased platelet responsiveness to activating stimuli but not necessarily an increase in basal platelet activation *in vivo*. This increase in responsiveness has been linked mechanistically to suppression of the cAMP pathway which normally inhibits platelet activation [3, 11], increased thromboxane A_2 synthesis [3], and increased mobilization of cytoplasmic Ca^{2+} [3] which have been observed consistently in platelets during normal pregnancy. The initiating stimulus for these changes is unknown.

13.3 Changes in Platelet Function in Abnormal Pregnancy

Pregnancy complicated by preeclampsia has been associated with increased expression of P-selectin and CD63 on non-stimulated and ADP-stimulated platelets compared to normotensive pregnancy controls [5, 8, 12]. Plasma concentrations of P-selectin [13] and soluble CD40 ligand [10, 14] also markedly increased supporting the notion that preeclampsia is associated with pathological platelet activation *in vivo*. In apparent conflict with this, platelets obtained from pregnant women with preeclampsia showed reduced aggregation responses to activating agonists compared to normotensive pregnancy controls [15, 16]. However, this apparent loss of function ex vivo may be a consequence of increased *in vivo* activation because of depletion or downregulation of activating receptors and signaling pathways. A similar phenomenon may be observed in other disorders such as the myeloproliferative disorders in which there is also increased platelet activation *in vivo*. Evidence for platelet activation *in vivo* during non-proteinuric hypertension during pregnancy is less compelling and contradictory [17].

13.4 Spectrum of Platelet Function Disorders

The heritable PFDs may be subclassified according to clinical severity into groups that comprise *severe GT and BSS* in which there are frequent or severe bleeding episodes and *non-severe PFDs* in which abnormal bleeding usually only follows trauma or surgery. Within the non-severe PFD group are some uncommon GT and BSS variants (e.g., type II GT, Bolzano BSS variant) in which bleeding is usually mild (Table 13.1).

Table 13.1 Classification of platelet function disorders

Severe phenotype platelet function disorders
Severe Glanzmann thrombasthenia
Severe Bernard-Soulier syndrome
Non-severe phenotype disorders
Defects in platelet aggregation or adhesion
Rare Glanzmann thrombasthenia variants (type II)
Rare Bernard-Soulier syndrome variants
Some "heterozygous" Bernard-Soulier syndrome variants
Defects of platelet receptors
Deficiency of receptors ADP ($P2Y_{12}$), thromboxane A_2, collagen (GPVI)
Defects in signal transduction
Thromboxane synthesis defect ("aspirin-like" defect) G-protein activation defect
Ca^{2+} mobilization defect
Integrin $\alpha_{IIb}\beta_3$ activation defect
Protein phosphorylation defects (e.g., protein kinase-θ defect)
Phosphatidylinositol metabolism defects (e.g., phospholipase C deficiency)
Defects in platelet secretion
Isolated δ-storage pool disease Combined αδ-storage pool disease
α-granule deficiency (e.g., Grey platelet syndrome)
Syndromic secretion defects (e.g., Hermansky-Pudlak syndrome)
Quebec platelet disorder
Miscellaneous disorders
Platelet procoagulant function disorder (Scott syndrome)

Modified from Refs. [18–20]

13.4.1 Severe Glanzmann Thrombasthenia

Severe GT is a rare autosomal recessive disorder caused by a quantitative deficiency of the platelet glycoprotein (GP) IIb-IIIa ($\alpha_{IIb}\beta_3$ integrin) which is the major platelet receptor of fibrinogen and other macromolecular adhesive proteins. Absence of functional GPIIb-IIIa results in a major defect in platelet-platelet aggregation and markedly impaired primary hemostasis [21]. Laboratory analysis of platelets shows markedly reduced or absent aggregation responses to all agonists except ristocetin. Flow cytometry shows markedly reduced or absent surface expression of GPIIb (CD41) and GPIIIa (CD61) [22]. The platelet count and morphology are normal. Affected individuals are homozygous or compound heterozygous for deleterious mutations in *ITGA2B* and *ITGB3* which encode GPIIb and GPIIIa, respectively [23].

Fetal intracranial hemorrhage before or during delivery is rare in severe GT. However, most affected children present before the age of 5 years with purpura, petechiae, or abnormal bruising [24]. Abnormal mucocutaneous bleeding persists through childhood, and gingival bleeding and severe epistaxis are common [24]. Menorrhagia is frequently severe in GT, and life-threatening bleeding has been reported at the menarche [25]. Other prominent symptoms include bleeding from the gastrointestinal and urinary tracts, prolonged surgical and traumatic bleeding, and oral bleeding after exfoliation of deciduous teeth [24].

13.4.2 Severe Bernard-Soulier Syndrome

Severe BSS is an autosomal recessive disorder caused by a quantitative deficiency of the platelet glycoprotein GPIb-IX-V complex. This complex is the major platelet receptor for von Willebrand factor (VWF) and mediates platelet adhesion to collagen in primary hemostasis. The GPIb-IX-V complex also facilitates platelet activation by thrombin and regulates pro-platelet formation by megakaryocytes. BSS patients have defective platelet adhesion but also thrombocytopenia with large circulating platelets [26].

Laboratory analysis of platelets in severe BSS shows failure of agglutination with ristocetin but normal aggregation with other activating agonists. Flow cytometry shows markedly reduced or absent platelet surface expression of the GPIb-IX-V complex. The platelet count is usually reduced and the mean platelet volume increased, but these features are highly variable among affected individuals [18, 22]. Severe BSS is associated with homozygous or compound heterozygous mutations in *GPIBA*, *GPIBB*, or *GP9* which encode components of GPIb and GPIX [27].

Severe BSS usually presents in early life with abnormal mucocutaneous or traumatic bleeding that is more severe than expected from the degree of thrombocytopenia. However, the clinical bleeding phenotype in BSS is variable. Some individuals with a marked deficiency of GPIb-IX-V present later in childhood or in early adulthood with abnormal bleeding after trauma or surgery or with prolonged bleeding at menarche [28].

13.4.3 Non-severe Platelet Function Disorders

Non-severe PFDs include some rare GT or BSS variants in which there is partial loss of glycoprotein function rather than absence of expression. Mild bleeding may also arise in some individuals who are "carriers" of severe BSS and who are heterozygous for mutations affecting GPIb-IX-V [29]. Otherwise, the non-severe PFDs comprise a heterogeneous group of defects of platelet surface receptors, signal transduction, and secretion pathway proteins [18–20] (Table 13.1). Laboratory tests of platelet function such as light transmission aggregation may show a wide range of abnormalities, and there is currently poor consensus about minimal diagnostic criteria for many disorders in this group [30]. Molecular genetic defects have been identified in only a small proportion of reported families [31].

By contrast to severe GT and BSS, the non-severe PFDs typically show a mild bleeding phenotype that often manifests in later childhood or adulthood with mucocutaneous bleeding and prolonged bleeding after trauma or surgery. Non-severe PFDs are prevalent in women with otherwise unexplained heavy menstrual bleeding [32, 33]. It is likely that the prevalence of this group of disorders is high and that many non-severe PFDs are not recognized. Some non-severe PFDs such as Hermansky-Pudlak syndrome are associated with syndromic feature (oculocutaneous albanism and nystagmus in the case of Hermansky Pudlak syndrome) which may aid clinical diagnosis [18].

13.5 Platelet Function Disorders and Pregnancy Outcomes

Data on pregnancy outcome in women with PFDs are sparse in the literature and comprise single case reports or single-center case series with small numbers of patients. Therefore, the absolute risk of adverse maternal and fetal outcomes is difficult to quantify because of reporting bias toward adverse outcomes. However, despite these limitations, it is clear that severe GT and BSS confer an increased maternal risk of postpartum hemorrhage (PPH) and increased fetal bleeding risk from fetal alloimmune thrombocytopenia. Reports of pregnancy outcomes for the non-severe PFDs are infrequent and contain anecdotal descriptions of adverse maternal outcomes because of bleeding.

13.5.1 Maternal Bleeding in Platelet Function Disorders

There are descriptions of clinical course and outcomes in approximately 40 pregnancies in women with severe GT [24, 34]. Abnormal bleeding before the onset of labor was described in approximately 50 % of the reports that documented the antenatal course in GT pregnancies and was usually mild. Bleeding episodes occurring throughout pregnancy included epistaxis, urinary tract bleeding, skin bruising, and gingival bleeding which are similar to bleeding symptoms in nonpregnant women with severe GT. Antenatal vaginal bleeding has been reported after vaginal examination [35] and in association with placenta previa [36].

The majority of pregnant women with severe GT received prophylaxis against PPH, usually with platelet transfusion and antifibrinolytics (see Sect. 13.7.3.1) as well as obstetric active management of the third stage of labour. However, despite these measures, PPH was reported in approximately 50 % of reported pregnancies in severe GT of which half occurred between 24 h and 2 weeks after delivery (namely 'secondary' PPH) [37]. Severe PPH has been reported after vaginal laceration during a forceps delivery [38] and after perineotomy [39]. There is a single report of hysterectomy that was performed during pregnancy for severe obstetric sepsis [40].

A systematic review has been performed of similar data available for approximately 30 pregnancies in women with BSS, including both severe and non-severe BSS variants [41]. Mild antenatal bleeding was reported in less than 15 % of all BSS pregnancies. However, primary PPH occurred in approximately 33 % and secondary PPH up to 6 weeks after delivery in approximately 40 % despite the widespread use of platelet transfusion as prophylaxis against PPH [41]. Cesarean hysterectomy for bleeding was reported in two pregnancies [42, 43].

Reports of maternal outcomes in women with non-severe PFDs include descriptions of primary PPH or bleeding at cesarean section in Hermansky-Pudlak syndrome [44, 45] and nonsyndromic δ-storage pool disease [46]. In a case series that reported seven women with non-severe PFDs, there was no abnormal maternal bleeding although most women received intrapartum platelet transfusion and oral antifibrinolytics [47].

13.5.2 Fetal Bleeding in Platelet Function Disorders

Severe GT and BSS and many other non-severe PFDs are autosomal recessive traits. Therefore, affected women are unlikely to carry an affected fetus unless from a consanguineous partner. In this circumstance, major fetal bleeding such as intracranial hemorrhage is rare although a single-center case series identified petechiae and scalp hematomas in approximately 25 % of neonates with severe GT who were delivered vaginally [48]. Some non-severe PFDs, including some BSS variants and storage pool disorders, show autosomal dominant inheritance. For these disorders, it is predicted that 50 % of fetuses from an affected mother will also have a non-severe PFD. Delivery of fetuses with autosomal dominant non-severe PFDs carries low risk of intracranial or other major bleeds [18].

13.5.3 Fetal Alloimmune Thrombocytopenia

Women with PFDs who have previously received donor platelets for the treatment of bleeding are at increased risk of developing alloantibodies against the human platelet antigen (HPA) or human leucocyte antigen (HLA) systems. This may be more common in women with severe GT or BSS because women with these disorders usually have frequent exposures to donor platelets [24, 28]. Absent expression of GPIIb-IIIa or GPIb/IX/V in severe GT or BSS may also promote alloantibody formation against HPA epitopes within these glycoproteins [41, 49]. Both HPA and HLA alloantibodies may cause refractoriness to further platelet transfusion and may jeopardize future treatment of bleeding.

Alloantibodies against GPIIb-IIIa and GPIb-IX-V may also cross the placenta and cause severe fetal thrombocytopenia through immune-mediated consumption of platelets in the fetal circulation. This has been associated with intracranial hemorrhage or other severe fetal bleeds in both severe GT [35, 49, 50] and BSS [43, 51] sometimes resulting in intrauterine or early postnatal death [43, 49, 52]. In most of the reported pregnancies with fetal alloimmune thrombocytopenia, the affected women had previously received platelet transfusions and had detectable alloantibodies against GPIIb-IIIa or GPIb-IX-V before pregnancy.

An anamnestic rise in the titer of alloantibodies against GPIIb-IIIa has also been reported during pregnancy in GT [35, 53] suggesting that exposure to fetal platelet antigens may also be a significant cause of alloimmunization in women with severe GT and BSS. Therefore, the absence of platelet alloantibodies at the start of pregnancy does not preclude alloimmunization later in pregnancy.

13.6 Approaches to Treatment or Prevention of Bleeding in Platelet Function Disorders

The choice of agent to treat or prevent bleeding in the PFDs during pregnancy requires evaluation of the site and severity of bleeding or anticipated bleeding. It is also essential to consider previous clinical responses to different agents. For platelet transfusion, the recoveries or corrected count increments following previous platelet transfusions should be calculated, and it should be determined whether platelet alloantibodies are present. The relative safety of different therapies should also be considered, particularly platelet transfusion which may carry particular hazards for pregnant women with PFDs.

In this section, the mode of action, indications, and safety of different pro-hemostatic agents are discussed. Management approaches are also suggested for the treatment or prevention of bleeding in nonpregnant and pregnant women. Specific measures to prevent or treat PPH are described in Sect. 13.7.3.

13.6.1 Local Measures and Antifibrinolytics

For minor mucocutaneous bleeds that occur commonly throughout pregnancy in severe GT and BSS, local measures and oral antifibrinolytics such as tranexamic acid, 1–1.5 g (or 15–25 μg/kg) tds for 5–7 days, may be sufficient [18, 54]. Local therapies such as topical thrombin or antifibrinolytics may also improve local hemostasis [55]. Intravenous preparations of tranexamic acid or the alternative antifibrinolytic ε-aminocaproic acid are available, but it should be emphasized that all antifibrinolytics are unsuitable for urinary tract bleeding because of the risk of ureteric obstruction with clot.

13.6.2 Desmopressin

Desmopressin (DDAVP; 1-deamino-8-D-arginine vasopressin) is a selective agonist of the endothelial V2 vasopressin receptor that stimulates release of VWF and tissue plasminogen activator (t-PA) and also causes plasma factor VIII activity to increase [56]. This agent promotes primary hemostasis in a variety of platelet function disorders [57] probably through an indirect VWF-mediated effect through activation of platelet GPIb-IX-V [56].

In women with non-severe PFDs outside of pregnancy, desmopressin 0.3 mg/kg in combination with antifibrinolytics may be sufficient for mild or moderate bleeding. This agent is usually administered by intravenous infusion or subcutaneous injection although a concentrated nasal spray preparation also enables home treatment by women with frequent minor bleeds or menorrhagia [18]. Since desmopressin has very little activity against the V1 vasopressin receptor, there is negligible vasoconstrictor or pro-oxytocic effect on uterine contraction [57]. Therefore, concerns that this agent might cause placental arterial insufficiency or preterm labor appear to be unfounded [58]. Instead, the clinical experience of desmopressin in women with diabetes insipidus [59] or von Willebrand disease [60] in pregnancy is favorable.

Desmopressin may therefore be considered as a pro-hemostatic agent throughout pregnancy for mild PFDs. In common with the use of this agent outside pregnancy, desmopressin may exert a potent antidiuretic effect [61]. Therefore, all pregnant women who receive desmopressin should be advised to avoid excessive fluid intake for 24 h after therapy. A significant clinical response to desmopressin is unlikely in severe GT or BSS, and even in mild PFDs, the clinical response is often unpredictable.

Laboratory testing of platelets after trial doses of desmopressin is uninformative, but a previous satisfactory clinical response to treatment may be helpful in predicting a good response in pregnancy. If a desmopressin infusion fails to control bleeding, then repeated treatment is unlikely to be successful because there is significant tachyphylaxis in the pro-hemostatic response [56].

13.6.3 Recombinant FVIIa

Recombinant FVIIa promotes hemostasis in severe GT and BSS by enhancing thrombin generation on the platelet surface which leads to increased platelet activation [62].

An international registry has reported the safe and effective use of rFVIIa as a pro-hemostatic therapy in GT outside of pregnancy [63]. Accordingly, rFVIIa is licensed by the European Medicines Agency for GT with antibodies to GPIIb-IIIa or HLA and with past or present refractoriness to platelet transfusion. There is also some favorable experience of rFVIIa in severe BSS [64], and it is now recommended that rFVIIa is considered either alone or in combination with platelet transfusion in both severe GT and BSS even if there are no alloantibodies or platelet refractoriness [18]. rFVIIa may have greater efficacy in severe GT and BSS if doses of at least 90 mg/kg bodyweight are given early after the start of bleeding or immediately before an invasive procedure such as chorionic villus sampling (CVS) or amniocentesis. It is also recommended that rFVIIa doses are repeated at 90–120-min intervals until hemostasis is achieved [18, 65]. rFVIIa has a good safety record in pregnancy and is an attractive treatment option in women with severe GT and BSS since it may avoid exposure to donor platelets. However, rFVIIa has been associated with venous thromboembolism and arterial thrombosis during "off-label" use for severe PPH in women without PFDs [66, 67]. Therefore, in women with other thrombosis risk factors, this agent should be used with caution.

13.6.4 Platelet Transfusion

Platelet transfusion is an alternative or adjunct to rFVIIa and anti fibrinolytics for the management of bleeding in severe GT and BSS and refractory bleeding in any PFD. Standard platelet components are now supplied in the UK either as a pooled product from the buffy coats of four whole blood donations or from a single donor prepared by apheresis [68]. For most bleeding episodes, one or two standard adult therapeutic doses, each of which contains $>240 \times 10^9$ platelets, will achieve initial hemostasis although further treatments may be necessary according to clinical response [18].

Platelet transfusion also confers risk of alloimmunization, allergy, and transfusion-transmitted infection, which in the UK includes the prion associated with variant Creutzfeldt-Jakob disease which is transmissible through cellular blood products [69]. These risks increase with multiple donor exposures, and so platelet transfusion in severe GT and BSS is now usually reserved for refractory bleeding or prevention of bleeding in high-risk surgical procedures. If platelet transfusion is unavoidable, then the incidence of alloimmunization in women with PFDs may be reduced by pre-storage leucodepletion of blood products, which is now performed on all the UK platelet components [70]. This risk may be reduced further by using HLA-selected platelets which is now the preferred component for all women with severe GT or BSS who require platelets [18, 54]. It should be emphasized that HLA-selected platelets will not prevent alloimmunization against HPA epitopes in severe GT or BSS. Random donor pool platelets may be the only available option for the emergency treatment of bleeding that is unanticipated.

In women who already have platelet alloantibodies detected by platelet immunofluorescence testing (PIFT), it is essential to define the specificity of the antibodies using a monoclonal antibody immobilization of platelet antigen (MAIPA) assay. If platelet transfusion is required, then HLA- or HPA- selected platelets should be supplied, and the platelet recovery or corrected count increment in response to each treatment episode should be documented [68]. Close liaison with a specialist transfusion laboratory is required.

13.7 Management of Pregnancy and Delivery

13.7.1 Preconception Counseling

Most women with severe GT or BSS will have received a diagnosis well before pregnancy and ideally, should undergo preconception counseling during which the risks of maternal PPH and alloimmunization are discussed. When a woman with severe GT or BSS is in a consanguineous partnership, the risk that the fetus may also have severe GT or BSS is significant. Therefore, counseling should include specific discussion of the lifelong impact of these disorders. It is preferable for preconception counseling to be performed after genetic diagnosis of severe GT or BSS in the maternal proband and after genetic testing of partners in consanguineous families. Antenatal diagnosis of severe GT or BSS should be considered, although chorionic villus sampling or amniocentesis requires pro-hemostatic therapy to prevent maternal bleeding, usually with platelet transfusion. The benefits and relative hazards of this approach should be considered carefully with the individual.

Diagnosis of the non-severe PFDs is also made in most affected women before pregnancy. Preconception counseling in these highly heterogeneous disorders should explore the fact that the prediction of maternal bleeding risk may be difficult and that the fetal risk of also having a PFD may be hard to estimate if the inheritance pattern in the affected family is unclear. For women who present during pregnancy with a family history of a non-severe PFD, attempts should be made to offer definitive diagnosis well before delivery. This will usually require a detailed symptomatic enquiry and laboratory testing of platelets. However, it should be recognized that changes in platelet responsiveness to laboratory agonists during pregnancy may hamper diagnosis, particularly if pregnancy is complicated by disorders such as preeclampsia. Molecular diagnosis in the non-severe PFDs is seldom possible since the genetic basis of these disorders is usually unknown.

13.7.2 General Measures

When pregnancy is confirmed, it is preferable that antenatal management occurs in a center with specific expertise in hemostatic disorders and with readily available access to platelets and other pro-hemostatic therapies. Close collaboration is required between hemostasis clinicians, obstetricians, anesthetists and neonatologists, and a written delivery plan should be generated and discussed with the family.

Previous reports of pregnancy in women with severe GT or BSS indicate that PPH may complicate both cesarean and vaginal delivery. It is therefore not currently possible to recommend the optimum mode of delivery. Since fetal intracranial hemorrhage in pregnancies complicated by maternal alloimmunization frequently antecedes delivery [49, 52], cesarean section will not guarantee against adverse fetal outcomes. However, many obstetricians prefer this route of delivery in women with alloantibodies in order to minimize the potential further risk of fetal bleeding during vaginal birth. Cesarean section can be performed for standard obstetric indications in all women with PFDs, and in situations where difficult instrumental delivery is anticipated, consideration should be given to performing cesarean section in preference [18, 41].

Regional analgesia is contraindicated in women with severe GT or BSS because of the difficulty in guaranteeing hemostasis with current therapies [18, 41]. Cesarean section in women with these severe disorders therefore requires general anesthesia. In women with non-severe PFDs, the contraindication to regional anesthesia is less absolute, and the risk of spinal hematoma must be weighed against the individual's risk of general anesthesia for cesarean section [47].

Delivery plans should include specific measures to ensure uterine contraction which is essential for peripartum hemostasis, especially in women with hemostatic disorders. The most widely used uterotonic syntometrin requires intramuscular injection and is therefore not ideal for most women with PFDs. However, intravenous oxytocin (10 IU) is equally effective and is a reasonable alternative in this circumstance. Misoprostol is another uterotonic that can be administered rectally, vaginally, orally (sublingual) or, at cesarean section, directly into the uterine cavity. During cesarean section or surgical repair of episiotomy or perineal trauma, there should be meticulous attention to surgical hemostasis.

13.7.3 Prevention and Treatment of Postpartum Hemorrhage

13.7.3.1 Severe Platelet Function Disorders

Since postpartum hemorrhage is a major hazard for women with severe GT or BSS, and pro-hemostatic therapy is required to minimize maternal risk. Platelet transfusion has been used widely in women with these disorders, usually in combination with antifibrinolytics [36, 41, 71]. rFVIIa has been also used in combination with platelet transfusion in GT [72, 73], but there is less published experience in severe BSS.

For vaginal delivery, it is currently recommended that rFVIIa with an oral antifibrinolytic is considered as a first-line agent for both severe GT and BSS. rFVIIa 90 μg/kg (early pregnancy weight) should be administered as soon as possible and repeated every 2 h for at least 3 doses or until hemostasis is secure. An alternative approach is to combine an oral antifibrinolytic with one or two adult therapeutic doses of HLA-selected platelets immediately before delivery and repeated if necessary according to clinical hemostasis. For refractory PPH, or if there are platelet alloantibodies, then rFVIIa in conjunction with HLA-selected platelets and an oral antifibrinolytic may be effective [49, 72, 74]. This combination of therapies should be considered in women with platelet alloantibodies even if platelet refractoriness has not been documented. Severe secondary PPH several weeks after delivery has been recognized in severe GT and BSS, even following apparently uncomplicated deliveries [24, 41]. Therefore, it is recommended that oral antifibrinolytics are continued weeks postpartum and that women are observed closely throughout weeks after the birth [18].

Cesarean section carries major bleeding risk in this group, and HLA-selected plate-lets are justified before and after delivery. All women require prolonged treatment with oral antifibrinolytics and careful inpatient observation for bleeding. rFVIIa should be considered as additional treatment if there is any clinical concern about the efficacy of platelet transfusion alone [18, 36]. Approaches such as uterine artery embolisation or hysterectomy may be necessary for uncontrolled PPH that is refractory to therapy or other conservative surgical measures [42, 43].

13.7.3.2 Non-severe Platelet Function Disorders

For the non-severe PFDs, the individual risk of PPH and the efficacy of different therapies are difficult to estimate before delivery. However, women who have a history before pregnancy of frequent or severe bleeding are anticipated to be a greater risk of PPH and to require pro-hemostatic therapy. In previous reports, oral antifibrinolytics, desmopressin, and platelet transfusion have been administered with variable success in preventing PPH [44, 46, 47].

For vaginal delivery in women with mild PFDs, careful observation may be adequate or oral antifibrinolytics alone may prevent PPH. However, in women with a more significant bleeding history, and particularly a previous history of PPH, desmopressin should be considered during the second stage of labor. Platelet transfusion may also be necessary if PPH occurs despite desmopressin. For cesarean section, most women require preoperative platelet transfusion with an oral antifibrinolytic repeated as necessary after delivery. There is limited experience of rFVIIa in mild platelet function disorders, and this agent should be considered only if there is refractory bleeding despite platelet transfusion [18].

13.7.4 Surveillance and Management of Alloantibody Formation

Maternal alloimmunization against HPA and HLA antigens is highly significant because of the associations with maternal refractoriness to platelet transfusion and with fetal thrombocytopenia and intracranial hemorrhage. Therefore, all women with severe GT or BSS, in which the risk of alloimmunization against clinically significant alloantigens is greatest, should be tested for anti-HPA and anti-HLA alloantibodies at the start of pregnancy and after any exposure to donor platelets during pregnancy (the reader should also refer to Chap. 16). Initial testing should be by PIFT, and the specificities of antibodies should be determined using a MAIPA assay. Testing should be repeated periodically through pregnancy even if there is no further exposure to donor platelets [18] because of the possibility of alloimmunization from fetal platelets crossing the placenta into the maternal circulation.

It should be recognized that there is little relationship between antibody specificity or titer, and the risk of fetal bleeding and that adverse fetal outcomes have been reported in pregnancies without demonstrable maternal alloantibodies [51]. However, a rising maternal alloantibody titer, platelet refractoriness, or a previous pregnancy complicated by fetal thrombocytopenia or intracranial hemorrhage should be considered as indications for intervention. Maternal intravenous immunoglobulin [51, 75], oral corticosteroids [43, 50], and plasma exchange or immunoabsorption [35, 75, 76] have been reported as successful interventions in this setting. Fetal cordocentesis to detect thrombocytopenia or to administer platelets or immunoglobulin may have benefit in neonatal alloimmune thrombocytopenia in women without PFDs [77]. However, in women with PFDs, cordocentesis confers additional bleeding risk in both the fetus (umbilical cord haematoma or haemorrhage can be fatal) and in the woman herself the needle passes through both the abdominal wall and the uterine wall. Therefore, the benefits of these fetal interventions remain uncertain, even in severe alloimmunization.

13.7.5 Measures to Minimize the Risk of Fetal Bleeding

For pregnancies in which the fetus is also at risk of a PFD or of neonatal thrombocytopenia, interventions during labor such as application of a fetal scalp electrode (FSE), fetal scalp, blood sampling (FBS), and instrumentation by vacuum (for example ventouse) or rotational forceps should be avoided. Ideally, a prolonged second stage of labor should also be avoided, but each case should be judged individually. If, for example, there is steady, albeit slow, progress in the second stage, waiting a little longer for normal delivery will be preferable to instrumental or cesarean delivery. After delivery, oral or intravenous rather than intramuscular vitamin K for the baby is preferred. The cord blood platelet count should be measured and a cranial ultrasound considered in all neonates at risk of thrombocytopenia. Cord blood may also be used to identify neonates who have inherited severe GT or BSS although platelet function and flow cytometry results should be interpreted with care because normal laboratory reference ranges differ markedly between neonates and older children or adults.

The management of bleeding in neonates who also have a PFD should be guided by the site and severity of bleeding. For significant bleeds, platelet transfusion using ABO and RhD identical, CMV screened and free of clinically significant irregular blood group antibodies may be required. For bleeding caused by fetal alloimmune thrombocytopenia, neonates should receive platelet transfusion matched according to the specificity of the maternal alloantibody. HLA-selected platelets should be considered if immediately available.

13.8 Case Studies

Case Study 1

A 24-year-old Pakistani woman presented at 8-week gestation in her first pregnancy. She had been diagnosed to have Bernard-Soulier syndrome at another center and gave a history of lifelong easy bruising, occasional prolonged epistaxis, and menorrhagia. She had previously received platelet transfusions before a dental extraction, after a traumatic skin bleed, and for prolonged bleeding after a previous miscarriage. Consistent with her previous diagnosis, repeat investigations showed that her platelets failed to agglutinate with ristocetin and failed to express GPIb-IX-V. A causative mutation was identified in the *GPIBA* gene, and this was also present in the woman's current partner. Antenatal diagnosis was declined. The platelet count was 105×10^9/l, and platelet alloantibodies against class II HLA epitopes were identified by MAIPA assay. Surveillance blood tests at 6 weekly intervals throughout pregnancy showed no change in the platelet count or maternal alloantibody titer. There was no abnormal antenatal bleeding.

The woman presented at 39 + 1 weeks in spontaneous labor. In accordance with the delivery plan, she received tranexamic acid 1 g every 6 h. Two adult doses of random donor pool platelets were moved from the blood transfusion laboratory to a platelet agitator within the delivery suite for use only in the event of uncontrolled bleeding. When cervical dilation has progressed to 5 cm, the woman received an intravenous infusion of rFVIIa 90 μg/kg and vaginal delivery proceeded without regional anesthesia. The delivery was not instrumented although an episiotomy was required that was repaired using local anesthetic. A second infusion of rFVIIa 90 μg/kg was given 30 min after delivery, and the woman received an intravenous syntocinon infusion. Postpartum blood loss was 500 mL. The neonate was well with no evidence of abnormal bleeding on clinical examination or by cranial ultrasound. Cord blood was obtained for flow cytometry and genetic testing and later confirmed that the neonate was unaffected with severe BSS.

Tranexamic acid 1 g every 6 h was continued after delivery, and mother and baby were observed in hospital for a further 7 days before discharge home with instructions to continue tranexamic acid for a further 3 weeks. At 22 days after delivery, the patient was readmitted with a 400-mL-secondary PPH that was managed by infusion of two adult doses of random donor pool platelets and rFVIIa 90 μg/kg. There was a satisfactory platelet recovery of 50 % at 1 h and 35 % at 24 h after transfusion. The rFVIIa infusion was repeated at 2, 4, and 6 h. There was no further bleeding, and mother and baby were discharged home after a further 7-day observation period in hospital.

Case Study 2

A 36-year-old Caucasian woman with a lifelong history of mild mucocutaneous bleeding and menorrhagia presented at 8-week gestation in her second pregnancy. There was a history of similar symptoms in her mother and older sister. During a previous evaluation as a teenager, she showed reduced platelet aggregation and absent ATP secretion in response to multiple platelet agonists and reduced platelet ADP consistent with a δ-storage pool disorder. Wisdom teeth extraction at 18 years was managed successfully with desmopressin. Her previous pregnancy at 32 years was managed at her local maternity unit and was uncomplicated. However, before delivery, she received a single adult dose of random donor pool platelets. Investigation by PIFT in her current pregnancy showed no platelet alloimmunization. Since her non-severe PFD was tracking in her family as an autosomal dominant trait, she was counseled that the fetus in her current pregnancy had a 50 % probability of a similar disorder and that delivery would be performed using standard hemostatic precautions.

At 32-week gestation, the woman developed persistent nose bleeds that initially responded to local compression and ice. However, at 33+2 weeks, she attended the maternity unit with persistent bleeding of 4 h duration. She was not hemodynamically compromised, and she was managed with oral tranexamic acid 1 g every 6 h and 0.3 μg/kg (pre-pregnancy weight) desmopressin by subcutaneous injection. There was a rapid resolution of bleeding, and the woman was observed in hospital overnight during which time she was instructed to avoid excessive fluid intake. The woman continued oral tranexamic acid at home.

She represented at 40 + 2 weeks in established second stage of labor. Oral tranexamic acid was continued, and she received a further dose of 0.3 μg/kg desmopressin. Uncomplicated vaginal delivery proceeded without regional anesthesia. After delivery, the woman received intravenous syntocinon. Blood loss after delivery was 150 mL, and the fetus was well with no clinical evidence of bleeding. The woman was discharged from hospital at 48 h after with instructions to continue oral tranexamic acid for 2 weeks.

Key Learning Points

- The obstetric management of all women with PFDs requires a multidisciplinary approach between hemostasis clinicians, obstetricians, anesthetists and neonatologists.
- Women with severe GT or BSS are at high risk of postpartum hemorrhage and require meticulous pro-haemostatic support with oral antifibrinolytics, rFVIIa, and/or HLA-selected platelet transfusions that should continue after delivery.
- Maternal alloimmunization against platelet antigens is common in severe GT and BSS and may cause maternal platelet refractoriness and fetal bleeding through alloimmune thrombocytopenia. All women with severe GT or BSS should be screened for platelet alloantibodies throughout pregnancy.
- The maternal and fetal risks of bleeding in non-severe PFDs vary markedly between affected women. Each pregnancy requires an individualized management plan based on the previous clinical severity of maternal bleeding and response to pro-hemostatic therapies.
- Delivery in all women with PFDs should be performed using careful hemostatic precautions and active management of the third stage of labor. Regional anesthesia is contraindicated in severe GT or BSS and should be considered cautiously in women with non-severe PFDs.

References

1. Morrison R, Crawford J, MacPherson M, Heptinstall S. Platelet behaviour in normal pregnancy, pregnancy complicated by essential hypertension and pregnancy-induced hypertension. Thromb Haemost. 1985;54:607–11.
2. Louden KA, Broughton Pipkin F, Heptinstall S, Fox SC, Mitchell JR, Symonds EM. A longitudinal study of platelet behaviour and thromboxane production in whole blood in normal pregnancy and the puerperium. Br J Obstet Gynaecol. 1990;97:1108–14.
3. Sheu JR, Hsiao G, Shen MY, Lin WY, Tzeng CR. The hyperaggregability of platelets from normal pregnancy is mediated through thromboxane A2 and cyclic AMP pathways. Clin Lab Haematol. 2002;24:121–9.
4. Bagamery K, Landau R, Kvell K, Graham J. Different platelet activation levels in non-pregnant, normotensive pregnant, pregnancy-induced hypertensive and pre-eclamptic women. A pilot study of flow cytometric analysis. Eur J Obstet Gynecol Reprod Biol. 2005;121:117–8.
5. Janes SL, Goodall AH. Flow cytometric detection of circulating activated platelets and platelet hyper-responsiveness in pre-eclampsia and pregnancy. Clin Sci (Lond). 1994;86:731–9.
6. Douglas JT, Shah M, Lowe GD, Belch JJ, Forbes CD, Prentice CR. Plasma fibrinopeptide A and beta-thromboglobulin in pre-eclampsia and pregnancy hypertension. Thromb Haemost. 1982;47:54–5.
7. Star J, Rosene K, Ferland J, DiLeone G, Hogan J, Kestin A. Flow cytometric analysis of platelet activation throughout normal gestation. Obstet Gynecol. 1997;90:562–8.
8. Harlow FH, Brown MA, Brighton TA, Smith SL, Trickett AE, Kwan YL, Davis GK. Platelet activation in the hypertensive disorders of pregnancy. Am J Obstet Gynecol. 2002;187:688–95.
9. Nicolini U, Guarneri D, Gianotti GA, Campagnoli C, Crosignani PG, Gatti L. Maternal and fetal platelet activation in normal pregnancy. Obstet Gynecol. 1994;83:65–9.
10. Oron G, Ben-Haroush A, Hod M, Orvieto R, Bar J. Serum-soluble CD40 ligand in normal pregnancy and in preeclampsia. Obstet Gynecol. 2006;107:896–900.
11. Horn EH, Cooper JA, Hardy E, Heptinstall S, Rubin PC. Longitudinal studies of platelet cyclic AMP during healthy pregnancy and pregnancies at risk of pre-eclampsia. Clin Sci (Lond). 1995;89:91–9.
12. Konijnenberg A, Stokkers EW, van der Post JA, Schaap MC, Boer K, Bleker OP, Sturk A. Extensive platelet activation in preeclampsia compared with normal pregnancy: enhanced expression of cell adhesion molecules. Am J Obstet Gynecol. 1997;176:461–9.
13. Halim A, Kanayama N, el Maradny E, Nakashima A, Bhuiyan AB, Khatun S, Terao T. Plasma P selectin (GMP-140) and glycocalicin are elevated in pre-eclampsia and eclampsia: their significances. Am J Obstet Gynecol. 1996;174:272–7.
14. Mellembakken JR, Solum NO, Ueland T, Videm V, Aukrust P. Increased concentrations of soluble CD40

ligand, RANTES and GRO-alpha in preeclampsia – possible role of platelet activation. Thromb Haemost. 2001;86:1272–6.

15. Norris LA, Gleeson N, Sheppard BL, Bonnar J. Whole blood platelet aggregation in moderate and severe pre-eclampsia. Br J Obstet Gynaecol. 1993;100:684–8.
16. Takeuchi T, Yoneyama Y, Suzuki S, Sawa R, Otsubo Y, Araki T. Regulation of platelet aggregation in vitro by plasma adenosine in preeclampsia. Gynecol Obstet Invest. 2001;51:36–9.
17. Ahmed Y, Sullivan MH, Elder MG. Detection of platelet desensitization in pregnancy-induced hypertension is dependent on the agonist used. Thromb Haemost. 1991;65:474–7.
18. Bolton-Maggs PH, Chalmers EA, Collins PW, Harrison P, Kitchen S, Liesner RJ, Minford A, Mumford AD, Parapia LA, Perry DJ, Watson SP, Wilde JT, Williams MD. A review of inherited platelet disorders with guidelines for their management on behalf of the UKHCDO. Br J Haematol. 2006;135:603–33.
19. Rao AK, Jalagadugula G, Sun L. Inherited defects in platelet signaling mechanisms. Semin Thromb Hemost. 2004;30:525–35.
20. Nurden P, Nurden AT. Congenital disorders associated with platelet dysfunctions. Thromb Haemost. 2008;99:253–63.
21. Plow EF, Pesho MM, Ma Y-Q. Integrin $\alpha_{IIb}\beta_3$. 2nd ed. Boston: Elsevier; 2007.
22. Kottke-Marchant K, Corcoran G. The laboratory diagnosis of platelet disorders. Arch Pathol Lab Med. 2002;126:133–46.
23. French DL. The molecular genetics of Glanzmann's thrombasthenia. Platelets. 1998;9:5–20.
24. George JN, Caen JP, Nurden AT. Glanzmann's thrombasthenia: the spectrum of clinical disease. Blood. 1990;75:1383–95.
25. Markovitch O, Ellis M, Holzinger M, Goldberger S, Beyth Y. Severe juvenile vaginal bleeding due to Glanzmann's thrombasthenia: case report and review of the literature. Am J Hematol. 1998;57:225–7.
26. Andrews RK, Berndt MC, Lopez JA. Platelets. London: Elsevier; 2007.
27. Kunishima S, Kamiya T, Saito H. Genetic abnormalities of Bernard-Soulier syndrome. Int J Hematol. 2002;76:319–27.
28. Lopez JA, Andrews RK, Afshar-Kharghan V, Berndt MC. Bernard-Soulier syndrome. Blood. 1998;91:4397–418.
29. Savoia A, Balduini CL, Savino M, Noris P, Del Vecchio M, Perrotta S, Belletti S. Poggi, iolascon A: autosomal dominant macrothrombocytopenia in Italy is most frequently a type of heterozygous Bernard-Soulier syndrome. Blood. 2001;97:1330–5.
30. Hayward CP, Pai M, Liu Y, Moffat KA, Seecharan J, Webert KE, Cook RJ, Heddle NM. Diagnostic utility of light transmission platelet aggregometry: results from a prospective study of individuals referred for bleeding disorder assessments. J Thromb Haemost. 2009;7:676–84.
31. Watson S, Daly M, Dawood B, Gissen P, Makris M, Mundell S, Wilde J, Mumford A. Phenotypic approaches to gene mapping in platelet function disorders – identification of new variant of P2Y12, TxA2 and GPVI receptors. Hamostaseologie. 2010;30:29–38.
32. Kouides PA, Kadir RA. Menorrhagia associated with laboratory abnormalities of hemostasis: epidemiological, diagnostic and therapeutic aspects. J Thromb Haemost. 2007;5 Suppl 1:175–82.
33. Philipp CS, Dilley A, Miller CH, Evatt B, Baranwal A, Schwartz R, Bachmann G, Saidi P. Platelet functional defects in women with unexplained menorrhagia. J Thromb Haemost. 2003;1:477–84.
34. Siddiq S, Clark A, Mumford A. A systematic review of the management and outcomes of pregnancy in Glanzmann thrombasthenia. Haemophilia. 2011;17: 858–69.
35. Vivier M, Treisser A, Naett M, Diemunsch P, Schmitt JP, Waller C, Tongio MM, Hemmendinger S, Lutz P. Glanzmann's thrombasthenia and pregnancy. Contribution of plasma exchange before scheduled cesarean section. J Gynecol Obstet Biol Reprod (Paris). 1989;18:507–13.
36. Bell JA, Savidge GF. Glanzmann's thrombasthenia proposed optimal management during surgery and delivery. Clin Appl Thromb Hemost. 2003;9:167–70.
37. Malhotra N, Chanana C, Deka D. Pregnancy in a patient of Glanzmann's thrombasthenia. Indian J Med Sci. 2006;60:111–3.
38. Caen JP, Castaldi PA, Leclerc JC, Inceman S, Larrieu MJ, Probst M, Bernard J. Congenital bleeding disorders with long bleeding time and normal platelet count I. Am J Med. 1966;41:4–26.
39. Cézar Alencar de Lima R, Ana Lúcia de Castro FM, Regina Amélia Lopes PA, Vitor Hugo de M, Madalena Maria Ferreira M, Eduardo Barçante R, Lúcia Jamille A, Darci Ribeiro da S. Glanzmann's thrombasthenia and pregnancy: a case report. J Bras Ginecol. 1998;108:375–8.
40. Heyes H, Scheck R, Rasche H. Obstetrical problems in patients with Glanzmann's thrombasthenia. A casuistic presentation (author's transl). Geburtshilfe Frauenheilkd. 1979;39:68–74.
41. Peitsidis P, Datta T, Pafilis I, Otomewo O, Tuddenham EG, Kadir RA. Bernard Soulier syndrome in pregnancy: a systematic review. Haemophilia. 2010; 16:584–91.
42. Michalas S, Malamitsi-Puchner A, Tsevrenis H. Pregnancy and delivery in Bernard-Soulier syndrome. Acta Obstet Gynecol Scand. 1984;63:185–6.
43. Fujimori K, Ohto H, Honda S, Sato A. Antepartum diagnosis of fetal intracranial hemorrhage due to maternal Bernard-Soulier syndrome. Obstet Gynecol. 1999;94:817–9.
44. Zatik J, Poka R, Borsos A, Pfliegler G. Variable response of Hermansky-Pudlak syndrome to prophylactic administration of 1-desamino 8D-arginine in subsequent pregnancies. Eur J Obstet Gynecol Reprod Biol. 2002;104:165–6.
45. Beesley RD, Robinson RD, Stewart TL. Two successful vaginal births after cesarean section in a patient with Hermansky-Pudlak syndrome who was treated with 1-deamino-8-arginine-vasopression during labor. Mil Med. 2008;173:1048–9.

46. Rahman SS, Myers JE, Gillham JC, Fitzmaurice R, Johnston TA. Post partum haemorrhage secondary to uterine atony, complicated by platelet storage pool disease and partial placenta diffusa: a case report. Cases J. 2008;1:393.
47. Chi C, Lee CA, England A, Hingorani J, Paintsil J, Kadir RA. Obstetric analgesia and anaesthesia in women with inherited bleeding disorders. Thromb Haemost. 2009;101:1104–11.
48. Awidi AS. Delivery of infants with Glanzmann thrombasthenia and subsequent blood transfusion requirements: a follow-up of 39 patients. Am J Hematol. 1992;40:1–4.
49. Leticee N, Kaplan C, Lemery D. Pregnancy in mother with Glanzmann's thrombasthenia and isoantibody against GPIIb-IIIa: is there a foetal risk? Eur J Obstet Gynecol Reprod Biol. 2005;121:139–42.
50. Kashyap R, Kriplani A, Saxena R, Takkar D, Choudhry VP. Pregnancy in a patient of Glanzmann's thrombasthenia with antiplatelet antibodies. J Obstet Gynaecol Res. 1997;23:247–50.
51. Uotila J, Tammela O, Makipernaa A. Fetomaternal platelet immunization associated with maternal Bernard-Soulier syndrome. Am J Perinatol. 2008;25:219–23.
52. Peng TC, Kickler TS, Bell WR, Haller E. Obstetric complications in a patient with Bernard-Soulier syndrome. Am J Obstet Gynecol. 1991;165:425–6.
53. Monrigal C, Beurrier P, Mercier FJ, Boyer-Neumann C, Gillard P. Glanzmann's thrombasthenia and pregnancy: a case and review of the literature. Ann Fr Anesth Reanim. 2003;22:826–30.
54. Alamelu J, Liesner R. Modern management of severe platelet function disorders. Br J Haematol. 2010;149: 813–23.
55. Bellucci S, Caen J. Molecular basis of Glanzmann's Thrombasthenia and current strategies in treatment. Blood Rev. 2002;16:193–202.
56. Kaufmann JE, Vischer UM. Cellular mechanisms of the hemostatic effects of desmopressin (DDAVP). J Thromb Haemost. 2003;1:682–9.
57. Mannucci PM. Desmopressin (DDAVP) in the treatment of bleeding disorders: the first 20 years. Blood. 1997;90:2515–21.
58. Cohen AJ, Kessler CM, Ewenstein BM. Management of von Willebrand disease: a survey on current clinical practice from the haemophilia centres of North America. Haemophilia. 2001;7:235–41.
59. Ray JG. DDAVP use during pregnancy: an analysis of its safety for mother and child. Obstet Gynecol Surv. 1998;53:450–5.
60. Mannucci PM. Use of desmopressin (DDAVP) during early pregnancy in factor VIII-deficient women. Blood. 2005;105:3382.
61. Nolan B, White B, Smith J, O'Reily C, Fitzpatrick B, Smith OP. Desmopressin: therapeutic limitations in children and adults with inherited coagulation disorders. Br J Haematol. 2000;109:865–9.
62. Hers I, Mumford A. Understanding the therapeutic action of recombinant factor VIIa in platelet disorders. Platelets. 2008;19:571–81.
63. Poon MC, D'Oiron R, Von Depka M, Khair K, Negrier C, Karafoulidou A, Huth-Kuehne A, Morfini M. Prophylactic and therapeutic recombinant factor VIIa administration to patients with Glanzmann's thrombasthenia: results of an international survey. J Thromb Haemost. 2004;2:1096–103.
64. Almeida AM, Khair K, Hann I, Liesner R. The use of recombinant factor VIIa in children with inherited platelet function disorders. Br J Haematol. 2003;121: 477–81.
65. Poon MC. The evidence for the use of recombinant human activated factor VII in the treatment of bleeding patients with quantitative and qualitative platelet disorders. Transfus Med Rev. 2007;21:223–36.
66. Alfirevic Z, Elbourne D, Pavord S, Bolte A, Van Geijn H, Mercier F, Ahonen J, Bremme K, Bodker B, Magnusdottir EM, Salvesen K, Prendiville W, Truesdale A, Clemens F, Piercy D, Gyte G. Use of recombinant activated factor VII in primary postpartum hemorrhage: the Northern European registry 2000–2004. Obstet Gynecol. 2007;110:1270–8.
67. Franchini M, Franchi M, Bergamini V, Montagnana M, Salvagno GL, Targher G, Lippi G. The use of recombinant activated FVII in postpartum hemorrhage. Clin Obstet Gynecol. 2010;53:219–27.
68. British Committee for Standards in Haematology, Blood Transfusion Task Force. Guidelines for the use of platelet transfusions. Br J Haematol. 2003;122: 10–23.
69. Ponte ML. Insights into the management of emerging infections: regulating variant Creutzfeldt-Jakob disease transfusion risk in the UK and the US. PLoS Med. 2006;3:e342.
70. Novotny VM. Prevention and management of platelet transfusion refractoriness. Vox Sang. 1999;76:1–13.
71. Dede M, Ural AU, Yenen M, Mesten Z, Baser I. Glanzmann's thrombasthenia in two pregnant females. Am J Hematol. 2007;82:330–1.
72. Kale A, Bayhan G, Yalinkaya A, Yayla M. The use of recombinant factor VIIa in a primigravida with Glanzmann's thrombasthenia during delivery. J Perinat Med. 2004;32:456–8.
73. Monte S, Lyons G. Peripartum management of a patient with Glanzmann's thrombasthenia using Thrombelastograph. Br J Anaesth. 2002;88:734–8.
74. Sugihara S, Katsutani S, Hyodo H, Hyodo M, Kudo Y, Fujii T, Kimura A. Postpartum hemorrhage successfully treated with recombinant factor VIIa in Glanzmann thromboasthenia. Rinsho Ketsueki. 2008; 49:46–50.
75. Peaceman AM, Katz AR, Laville M. Bernard-Soulier syndrome complicating pregnancy: a case report. Obstet Gynecol. 1989;73:457–9.
76. Ito K, Yoshida H, Hatoyama H, Matsumoto H, Ban C, Mori T, Sugiyama T, Ishibashi T, Okuma M, Uchino H, et al. Antibody removal therapy used successfully at delivery of a pregnant patient with Glanzmann's thrombasthenia and multiple anti-platelet antibodies. Vox Sang. 1991;61:40–6.
77. Birchall JE, Murphy MF, Kaplan C, Kroll H. European collaborative study of the antenatal management of feto-maternal alloimmune thrombocytopenia. Br J Haematol. 2003;122:275–88.

Acquired Bleeding Disorders in Pregnancy: Obstetric Hemorrhage

14

Sathana Ponnampalam, Sasha Wilson, and Asma Khalil

Abstract

Obstetric hemorrhage can be antepartum or postpartum, and may be life-threatening for the woman and (if antepartum) for her baby. Each has a variety of causes, and management is directed at identifying and dealing with the cause (usually by the obstetrician and midwife, at times supported by the interventional radiologist), while at the same time resuscitating the woman (by the anesthetist supported by the hematologist and blood transfusion laboratory). Major obstetric hemorrhage should be managed by a multidisciplinary team including these professionals but also important ancillary staff such as porters.

Keywords

Placenta praevia • Placental abruption • Postpartum hemorrhage • Massive obstetric hemorrhage • Transfusion

S. Ponnampalam, MB ChB (✉)
Department of Obstetrics and Gynaecology, National Women's Hospital, 94A Taylor Street, Blockhouse Bay, Auckland 0600, New Zealand
e-mail: write2sathana@gmail.com

S. Wilson, RGN
Haematology/Blood Transfusion, University College London Hospitals NHS Foundation Trust, Pathology Directorate, 3rd Floor Central, 250 Euston Rd, London NW1 2PG, UK
e-mail: sasha.wilson@uclh.nhs.uk

A. Khalil, MB BCh, MD, MRCOG, MSc, DFSRH
Department of Obstetrics and Gynaecology, St. George's Hospital, St George's Healthcare NHS Trust, Blackshaw Road, Tooting, London SW17 OQT, UK
e-mail: asmakhalil79@googlemail.com

14.1 Introduction

Obstetric hemorrhage encompasses both antepartum and postpartum hemorrhage and remains one of the leading causes of preventable maternal mortality, accounting for at least a quarter of maternal deaths worldwide [1]. The vast majority of obstetric hemorrhages occur postpartum. In the United Kingdom (UK), major obstetric hemorrhage occurs in around 3.7 per 1,000 births [2]; between the years 2006 and 2008 there were 9 maternal deaths as a direct result of hemorrhage, with a mortality rate of 0.39 per 100,000 [3]. Although mortality as a direct result of maternal hemorrhage appears to be falling in the UK [3],

H. Cohen, P. O'Brien (eds.), *Disorders of Thrombosis and Hemostasis in Pregnancy: A Guide to Management*, DOI 10.1007/978-3-319-15120-5_14, © Springer-Verlag London 2015

there is evidence to suggest that the incidence of obstetric hemorrhage is increasing in the western world [4].

14.2 Antepartum Hemorrhage

Antepartum hemorrhage (APH) is defined as bleeding from the genital tract in the second half of pregnancy (definitions in the literature vary, with the early threshold ranging from 20 to 28 weeks; bleeding earlier than this is termed 'threatened miscarriage') until the completion of the second stage of labour. It has an incidence of 2–5 % of all pregnancies [5].

14.2.1 Causes of Antepartum Haemorrhage

The causes of APH may be maternal or fetal [5, 6].

Maternal causes:

(a) Local causes

These include cervicitis, cervical polyps, cervical or vaginal infection, cervical ectropion, vaginal varicose veins, local trauma and rarely malignancy. APH due to local causes is generally minor and self-limiting.

(b) Placental causes include placental abruption and placenta previa.

(c) Systemic diseases

These result in bleeding as a result of maternal hematological disorders or coagulopathy such as von Willebrand disease and Hodgkin's lymphoma, and are a rare cause of APH.

Fetal causes

Vasa previa

APH of unknown origin

In around half of all cases of APH, the cause remains undetermined [7, 8]. Of those with a known cause, at least 90 % are placental in origin [7]. Most significant or life-threatening APH are a result of abnormal placental insertion or separation that will be addressed in this chapter.

14.2.2 Placenta Previa and Placenta Accreta, Increta and Percreta

Placenta previa occurs when the placenta is partially or completely inserted into the lower segment of the uterus. It is classified by ultrasound imaging as 'major' – when the placenta covers the internal cervical os partially or completely; or 'minor' when the placenta is low lying but not covering the os (<2 cm distance from the placental edge to the cervical os).

An abnormally adherent placenta is referred to as placenta accreta and this is further sub-classified based on the extent of myometrial infiltration. Placenta accreta is characterised by chorionic villi reaching the inner myometrial surface, placenta increta by villus infiltration of the myometrium and placenta percreta if it penetrates through the entire myometrium and serosa (and at times into an adjacent organ such as the bladder) [9, 10].

14.2.2.1 Epidemiology and Risk Factors

Placenta previa complicates 3–5 per 1,000 pregnancies at term [11] and placenta accreta 1 in 2,500 pregnancies [12]. Risk factors associated with placenta previa are summarised in Table 14.1 [5, 7, 13].

Approximately 10% of women with placenta previa will develop placenta accreta; the diagnosis of placenta accreta is virtually excluded in the absence of placenta previa, with an incidence of only 0.005 % [12]. Previous Cesarean section (CS) and increased maternal age are independent risk factors for developing placenta accreta [12]. The incidence of placenta accreta and the risk of

Table 14.1 Risk factors for placenta previa [5, 7, 13]

Maternal age over 40 years
Multiparity
Previous Cesarean section
Uterine scarring (previous myomectomy, uterine curettage)
Previous spontaneous or induced miscarriage
Cigarette smoking and use of drugs such as cocaine
Multiple pregnancies
Previous placenta previa

peripartum hysterectomy rises with the number of previous CS [14]. With the rising incidence of CS as well as steadily increasing average maternal age, the incidence of placenta previa/accreta and the associated complications are expected to rise.

14.2.2.2 Diagnosis

Current practice involves screening for low-lying placentas at the routine second trimester anatomy scan in order to predict the likelihood of placenta previa at delivery. If the placenta remains low lying in the third trimester, a transvaginal scan should be performed to confirm the diagnosis. Transvaginal sonography is deemed safe and more accurate in the diagnosis of placenta previa [15–18].

The majority of women in whom the placental edge reaches or overlaps the internal os in mid-pregnancy will not have placenta previa at term. 'Placental migration' is believed to occur in the second and third trimesters as the lower segment of the uterus develops. It is less likely to occur in cases where the placenta is posterior, in women who have had previous Cesarean section(s) and when the placenta completely or substantially overlaps the internal os [19–27].

Regardless of previous scan results, placenta previa should be suspected in any pregnant woman who presents with painless vaginal bleeding, particularly with a high presenting part or an abnormal fetal lie (because the placenta prevents the fetal presenting part, usually the head, from engaging into its mother's pelvis).

Women who have had a previous CS and have an anterior placenta or placenta previa are at significantly increased risk of placenta accreta. Clinical suspicion of placenta accreta may be confirmed by ultrasonography; when ultrasonography is equivocal, magnetic resonance imaging (MRI) may clarify the situation. Two recent meta-analyses suggest that ultrasound has a sensitivity of 80–90 % in the diagnosis of placenta accreta, with specificity of 95–97 % [28, 29]. One of these meta-analyses [29] also looked at MRI diagnosis; sensitivity for placenta accreta was 82 % with a specificity of 88 %. Definitive diagnosis, however, can be made only at the time of CS and by histopathological examination.

14.2.2.3 Presentation and Management

Women with placenta previa and/or accreta may be asymptomatic (i.e. with no history of APH) or symptomatic (i.e. present with vaginal bleeding).

Elective CS is recommended for women with placenta previa persisting at term. CS is usually performed at 38 weeks' gestation in cases with placenta previa and at 36–37 weeks in cases of placenta accreta, in order to minimise the risk of labour leading to bleeding prior to the booked CS date. Of course, if there is major APH prior to this, urgent delivery may be required, regardless of the gestation [20]. Evidence around the mode of delivery for women who have minor placenta previa is less clear. Women with a placental edge which lies less than 2 cm from the cervical os are likely to require delivery by CS. If the fetal head is engaged closer to term (as the lower segment continues to develop beyond 36 weeks), a transvaginal ultrasound scan is performed. If the leading placental edge is more than 2 cm from the internal os, the likelihood of achieving a vaginal delivery is at least 63 % [30]. The risk of postpartum hemorrhage (PPH) remains higher in this group of women, so should be anticipated and managed accordingly.

The management of women who present with bleeding depends on the extent of bleeding and fetal maturity. All women should have a full blood count (FBC) and 'group and save' on admission. Corticosteroids should be administered in women less than 35 weeks' gestation to improve fetal lung maturity in the event of threatened preterm delivery [31]. All RhD (Rhesus) negative women should have estimation of fetal maternal hemorrhage by the Kleihauer-Betke test or flow cytometry, and receive prophylactic anti-D immunoglobulin intramuscularly (IM) [32]. Women who present with massive ongoing bleeding will require urgent surgical intervention following hemodynamic stabilisation. Women that are stable at presentation (i.e. no maternal or fetal compromise) with a self-limiting episode of painless unprovoked bleeding can be managed conservatively. However, they are thought to be at high risk of further sudden unprovoked bleeding, so are routinely admitted for 24–48 h following cessation of bleeding.

The use of tocolytics [33–37] or cervical cerclage [38, 39] to treat women who bleed with placenta previa has been investigated; their use remains controversial and is not recommended for routine clinical use.

In the past it was recommended that women with major previa who had previously bled should receive in-patient care from approximately 34 weeks of gestation [40]. There is, however, no clear evidence to suggest an association between the extent of placenta previa and the likelihood of bleeding or the requirement for urgent delivery [22, 25]; the risk of bleeding and need for in-patient management should be assessed on an individual basis. All women with a risk of major APH should be advised to remain close to the recommended hospital for delivery for the duration of the third trimester.

As a minimum requirement, a consultant obstetrician and consultant anaesthetist should be present on site when women with a placenta previa undergo CS. All women should have a baseline FBC and four units of red cells cross-matched. The Royal College of Obstetricians & Gynaecologists' (RCOG) guideline [25] suggests that prophylactic steroids for fetal lung maturation should be given prior to any elective CS performed up to 38+6 weeks' gestation. Prior to delivery a consultant led discussion regarding the delivery, risk of significant hemorrhage, indications for transfusion and the possibility of peripartum hysterectomy should be held and documented clearly.

In cases of confirmed or suspected placenta accreta a consultant obstetrician and anaesthetist should be present and directly supervising delivery. The procedure is ideally planned ahead, involving a multidisciplinary team (including haematologist, interventional radiologist, intensive care staff, and blood transfusion laboratory staff), with blood and blood components available on standby. Discussion regarding the significant risk of peripartum hemorrhage, anticipated skin and uterine incisions and possible interventions including conservative management, use of cell salvage, interventional radiology and the possibility of hysterectomy should be discussed with the woman and documented clearly in both the notes and consent form.

When placenta accreta is suspected antenatally, the surgical avoidance of the placental site and non-separation of the placenta is thought to be associated with reduced maternal mortality by reducing the risk of bleeding [25, 41]. Data from observational studies support avoiding the placenta and leaving it attached, or proceeding with peripartum hysterectomy [41–43] in cases of placenta percreta.

The risk of massive PPH is 12 times greater in women with placenta previa [40]. This is mainly because the lower segment of the uterus (where the placenta was implanted) contracts less efficiently than the upper segment (the usual site of placental implantation), leading to continued bleeding from the placental bed vessels. The rate of peripartum hysterectomy is also increased, particularly if the woman has had a previous CS.

Leaving the placenta adherent may reduce intra-operative bleeding but is associated with an increased risk of postpartum bleeding and infection. Prophylactic antibiotics may be considered postpartum. Prophylactic arterial embolisation or methotrexate have not been shown to reduce the risk of these complications and are therefore not routinely recommended [25].

If the placenta separates, it should be delivered. Subsequent hemorrhage must be anticipated and managed appropriately. Partial separation of the placenta is also possible and adherent portions may be left attached. Massive hemorrhage is highly likely in this situation and timely and appropriate management is essential [12, 44].

14.2.3 Placental Abruption

Placental abruption is defined as the partial or complete separation of the placenta prior to the delivery of the fetus [45].

14.2.3.1 Incidence and Risk Factors

Fewer than 1 in 100 pregnancies are complicated by placental abruption at term [46]. The occurrence is significantly higher in preterm pregnancies, affecting around 5 % of preterm deliveries [47]. Risk factors for placental abruption are summarised in Table 14.2 [47–56].

Table 14.2 Risk factors for placental abruption [50–58]

Prior history of abruption (15–20 fold increase in risk) [53, 59]
Advanced maternal age
Multiparity
Cigarette smoking
Recreational drug use
Multiple pregnancy
Pre-eclampsia
Chronic hypertension
Gestational hypertension
Premature rupture of membranes
Oligohydramnios
Chorioamnionitis

Placental abruption is also associated with trauma [57], CS for first birth (compared to vaginal first birth) [56, 57], vaginal bleeding in early pregnancy [58, 59], thrombophilias [60, 61] and raised second trimester alpha-fetoprotein [62].

14.2.3.2 Diagnosis

The diagnosis of placental abruption is made clinically. The classic symptoms are abdominal pain and vaginal bleeding. In practice, there is a wide spectrum of clinical presentations ranging from asymptomatic or minor bleeding to massive abruption leading to fetal demise and/or severe maternal morbidity. Placental abruption may also present as idiopathic preterm labour. On examination, the uterus is often tender and may be hard ('woody') on palpation. There may be evidence of acute fetal hypoxia on fetal monitoring. In cases of concealed abruption women may present with hypovolemic shock or abnormal bleeding secondary to disseminated intravascular coagulation (DIC) as a result of concealed hemorrhage.

A range of ultrasonographic appearances of placental abruption have been described [63–66]. The diagnosis of abruption is highly likely when the possibility of placental abruption is suggested by ultrasound. A seemingly normal ultrasound scan does not, however, exclude the diagnosis of placental abruption; by the time an abruption is apparent on ultrasound scan, it is usually clinically obvious.

14.2.3.3 Management

The management of placental abruption depends on the gestation, the presentation and degree of fetal and/or maternal compromise. All women who present with suspected placental abruption should have an FBC, coagulation studies and group and save on admission. Blood should be crossmatched when there is evidence of significant bleeding. Corticosteroids should be administered to women less than 35 weeks' gestation in view of the increased risk of preterm delivery [31] and all RhD negative women should have estimation of fetal maternal hemorrhage by the Kleihauer-Betke test or flow cytometry, and receive prophylactic anti-D immunoglobulin IM [32].

Prompt delivery is indicated in women who present with placental abruption at or near term with a live fetus. If there is no evidence of fetal or maternal compromise, conservative management with the aim of vaginal delivery is appropriate and these women often labour and deliver quickly. Both the fetus and mother should be monitored closely during labour and, should there be any evidence of fetal or maternal compromise, delivery should be expedited.

Conservative management is appropriate in those who present with partial abruption in preterm pregnancies (between 20 and 34 weeks' gestation) when the status of both the mother and fetus is reassuring. This is appropriate given that preterm birth is the leading cause of perinatal mortality in cases of placental abruption. If there is evidence of fetal or maternal compromise in pregnancies greater than 24 weeks' gestation; delivery is indicated.

In women who present with severe abruption with fetal demise at any gestation, it is reasonable to aim for a vaginal delivery, as long as the mother is stable and there are no contraindications to vaginal delivery. If the labour fails to progress as expected, if the mother is unstable or there is clinical evidence of significantly worsening coagulopathy, Cesarean delivery is indicated. Fetal compromise alone is not an indication to expedite delivery if the fetus is not viable (i.e. less than 24 weeks' gestation) and conservative management may be considered in these cases if the mother's condition allows.

When placental abruption is discovered incidentally on ultrasound scan, a thorough history and examination should be sought including identification of predisposing factors. Management should be individually tailored, taking into account the gestational age as well as fetal and maternal well-being.

Significant PPH is 13 times more common in women with placental abruption [40]. This is because they may have already developed coagulopathy by the time the baby is delivered. Furthermore, they may have a Couvelaire uterus; this is when blood tracks into the myometrium, making it 'woody' so that it contracts poorly after delivery, leading to prolonged bleeding from the placental bed. These women are also at significant risk of developing hypovolemic shock and renal failure.

All women who are admitted with placental abruption associated with major hemorrhage should be managed as detailed below. Principles of management include careful clinical monitoring with regular assessment including fluid balance and blood tests to check FBC, renal function, and coagulation screen plus fibrinogen. Blood and blood volume should be appropriately replaced, and coagulopathy and thrombocytopenia corrected. Management should involve a multidisciplinary team including a haematologist, interventional radiologist, intensive care staff, laboratory staff, and blood bank.

14.2.4 Vasa Previa

Vasa previa is a condition in which the fetal blood vessels traverse the fetal membranes of the lower segment of the uterus below the presenting part, unsupported by the umbilical cord or placental tissue [67]. Vasa previa has an estimated incidence of 1 in 2,000–5,000 deliveries [67, 68]. Associated risk factors are summarised in Table 14.3 [67–74].

Table 14.3 Risk factors for vasa previa [10, 70–75]

A low-lying placenta in the second trimester
Accessory placental lobes
Multiple pregnancy
Pregnancies resulting from *in vitro* fertilization
Velamentous cord insertion

14.2.4.1 Diagnosis

In the absence of any signs or symptoms, vasa previa may be found incidentally on digital vaginal examination [75] or at a routine antenatal ultrasound scan. More often the diagnosis is confirmed following delivery of placenta.

The possibility of vasa previa, though rare, should always be borne in mind when a woman presents with vaginal bleeding, particularly if associated with rupture of the membranes and there is evidence of of fetal compromise. Immediate delivery should be arranged without delaying management to confirm the diagnosis.

Several tests may differentiate between fetal and maternal blood [76–79]. These include the Kleihauer-Bekte test, the Apt test and hemoglobin electrophoresis. Their use is not usually practical in this situation given the invariable urgency for delivery. A bedside test using sodium hydroxide has been described by Lindqvist and Glen which may be useful in the setting of vasa previa but it needs further evaluation [80].

Vasa previa can be diagnosed antenatally with expert ultrasonography. Although specificity is good, the sensitivity cannot be determined owing to the low prevalence of this condition [81–88]. Several groups advocate screening with Doppler ultrasound for those at increased risk of developing vasa previa [10, 89–91], but this approach is not universally accepted as the test does not fulfil the requirements of a screening test; there remains insufficient information on the case definition, natural history and epidemiology of the condition. Moreover, if vasa previa is diagnosed, there is no consensus on appropriate management.

14.2.4.2 Management

There is currently no agreed management pathway for those with vasa previa diagnosed antenatally [87, 92]. If a woman presents with bleeding with a confirmed diagnosis of vasa previa, an urgent CS should be performed. In women who have confirmed vasa previa at term, an elective

CS should be carried out at 39 weeks' gestation, though some recommend earlier delivery [93]. In utero laser ablation of aberrant vessels has been reported in a few case reports [94].

14.3 Postpartum Haemorrhage

Postpartum hemorrhage is the commonest form of obstetric hemorrhage. There is currently no single globally agreed definition for PPH, hence various definitions exist [95]. Traditionally, PPH is defined as blood loss from the genital tract more than 500 mL occurring after delivery until 12 weeks after birth [96]. At CS, PPH has traditionally been defined as blood loss greater than 1,000 mL [97]. Primary PPH is that occurring within the first 24 h of delivery, though usually occurs shortly after birth. Secondary PPH is hemorrhage which occurs more than 24 h but before 12 weeks after delivery [95]. PPH can be minor (500–1,000 mL) or major (more than 1,000 mL). Major PPH may be further sub-classified into moderate (1,000–2,000 mL) or severe (more than 2,000 mL) [40].

14.3.1 Incidence and Risk Factors

Varying incidences of PPH are described in the literature, partly as a result of the lack of a universal definition and partly due to inaccuracy in estimates of blood loss [98]. Although an incidence of between 3 and 6 % has been reported based on hospital discharge data in the United States, Canada and Australia [99–101], up to 15 % women are reported to suffer from excessive bleeding following delivery [102]. There were 5 deaths as a direct result of PPH reported in the 2006–2008 triennium in the UK [3]. Although mortality rates as a result of PPH may be declining in the UK (there were 9 deaths related to PPH in the previous (2003–2005) triennium), the incidence of PPH is increasing in the western world in general [4].

PPH results from abnormalities in four processes – uterine contraction, retained products of conception, genital tract trauma and coagulation abnormalities. These are often referred to as the "four T's"- Tone, Tissue, Trauma and Thrombin [102]. Of these, the most common cause of PPH is uterine atony, accounting for over 70 % of PPH [98]. The risk factors for PPH can be antenatal or intrapartum and are summarised in Table 14.4 [103–107].

Table 14.4 Risk factors for postpartum haemorrhage (PPH) [106–110]

Antenatal
Previous PPH
Asian ethnicity
Obesity (BMI > 35 kg/m^2)
Pre-eclampsia/gestational hypertension
Anaemia (<9 g/dL)
Multiple pregnancy
Polyhydramnios
Placenta previa
Known or suspected placenta abruption
Age over 40 years
Grand multiparity (≥5 deliveries)
Underlying bleeding disorders
Intrapartum
Induction of labor
Cesarean delivery (elective or emergency)
Retained placenta
Mediolateral episiotomy
Assisted vaginal delivery
Intrapartum pyrexia
Prolonged labor > 12 h
Large for gestational age infant > 4kg

14.3.2 Prevention

Although women with risk factors are more likely to experience PPH, unfortunately most cases of PPH occur in women who do not have any identifiable risk factors. Prevention begins with assessment and identification of risk factors, and women at high risk should be advised to deliver at a centre with adequate obstetric and hematological facilities.

Modifiable risk factors such as anemia should be addressed antenatally. Women at significantly increased risk of major PPH, such as those with placenta accreta or with a history of bleeding disorders, should ideally have a planned delivery at a centre where specialised obstetric, hematology and anesthetic services, as well as intensive care, blood transfusion laboratory, and pharmacy services are available. In cases where significant hemorrhage is expected an individualised management plan for delivery and blood component replacement should be drawn up prior to delivery.

Active management of the third stage of labour includes the use of a uterotonic drug, early clamping of the umbilical cord and controlled traction for the delivery of the placenta [108], and has been shown to reduce blood loss as well as the incidence of moderate and severe PPH [108, 109] compared to allowing a physiological third stage of labour.

The uterotonic of choice for routine prophylaxis in women with no risk factors for PPH is oxytocin (5 or 10 units by IM injection) [40]. Five units of slow intravenous injection is recommended in women who deliver by CS [110]. Syntometrine (oxytocin-ergometrine) may be used in the absence of hypertension or severe cardiac disease, as it has been shown to further reduce minor PPH when compared with oxytocin alone; however, there is a fivefold increase in side-effects of nausea, vomiting and increased blood pressure when ergometrine is used [111]. Oral misoprostol may also be used for active management of the third stage; however, it is not as effective as oxytocin and may be of benefit in community or resource poor settings where there is not ready access to the injectable oxytocics (oxytocin and ergometrine) [112, 113].

14.3.3 Management of Primary Postpartum Haemorrhage

14.3.3.1 General Measures

Analysis by CMACE shows that the management of fatal cases was often suboptimal with underestimation of the degree of hemorrhage and poor team working, and the CMACE team emphasise the need for the following: (a) clear local policies; (b) training of front-line staff; (c) multidisciplinary team working; (d) regular 'fire drills'; and (e) excellent communication with the blood transfusion laboratory [3].

The RCOG has identified four components to be initiated and simultaneously progressed in the management of PPH. These include communication, resuscitation, monitoring and intervention [40].

A rapid clinical response with an appropriate multi-disciplinary approach is essential in order to reduce the morbidity and prevent mortality associated with PPH. For minor PPH (500–1,000 mL with no clinical evidence of shock) the charge midwife and first-line obstetric and anesthetic staff should be informed. In cases of major bleeding (blood loss >1 L, with ongoing bleeding and/or clinical shock) the on-call consultant obstetrician and anesthetist should be called and the consultant hematologist, blood transfusion laboratory and porters (for delivery of blood samples and components/products) should be alerted and involved early in the management.

Initial resuscitation should be tailored to the degree of clinical shock. Resuscitation in the management of all PPH should begin with the simple 'ABC' ('airway, breathing, circulation') approach. Administration of high flow oxygen is recommended regardless of oxygen saturation [40]. At least one large bore (14G) intravenous cannula should be inserted and a crystalloid infusion commenced in the first instance when dealing with what appears to be minor PPH.

In cases where a minor bleed progresses to meet the definition of major PPH (blood loss of >1 L, ongoing bleeding and/or clinical signs of shock), the woman should have two 14G intravenous cannulae and should be repositioned to remain supine. Fluid resuscitation should begin immediately and transfusion should be sought as soon as possible. Up to 3.5 L of rapid warmed clear fluids may be infused until red cells are available. If crossmatched red cells are unavailable by the time 3.5 L of clear fluids have been infused, ABO and Rh group specific or, if the group is unknown, O RhD negative red cells may be given.

The trigger for activating a massive obstetric haemorrhage (MOH) protocol must be clearly defined in all institutions, and in most is an estimated blood loss of 1,000–1,500 mL [113]. Key principles of an MOH are: first, that the blood transfusion laboratory staff and a senior hematologist should be contacted immediately when the MOH protocol is activated; and secondly, locally agreed protocols should enable red cells, FFP, cryoprecipitate and platelets to be issued at the earliest possible opportunity, without the initial approval of a hematologist.

The goals in the management of massive hemorrhage are to maintain a haemoglobin above 80 g/L, a platelet count of >50 g × 10^9/L (with a platelet transfusion trigger of 75 to provide a margin of safety), prothrombin time (PT) and activated partial thromboplastin time (APTT) less than 1.5 times the mean control level, and fibrinogen greater than 1 g/L [114, 115].

The following general principles should be observed:

- Inadequate volume replacement, acidosis and hypothermia increase the risk of DIC. The woman should be kept warm and blood components transfused using a validated blood warmer; hypothermia will exacerbate coagulopathy.
- Hypothermia adversely affects hemostasis on several levels: platelet function, the coagulation cascade and fibrinolytic system.
- Rapid infusion of blood components/products, particularly fresh frozen plasma (FFP) and platelets which contain citrate as the anticoagulant, will lower ionised calcium and reduce cardiac contractility/lower blood pressure; the calcium should be corrected if indicated. Hypocalcemia is unlikely to occur when less than 1.5 × blood volume is replaced. Citrate toxicity is more likely in the hypothermic patient due to impaired citrate metabolism.
- Hyperkalemia is possible in massive transfusion due to the concentration of potassium in stored red cells as they near expiry; this is usually a problem only if the woman has coexisting renal or hepatic disease but may be exacerbated by hypothermia [115–117].

An FBC and group and screen must be obtained in all women with even a minor PPH. A coagulation screen, fibrinogen and baseline liver and renal function tests should be obtained if massive hemorrhage is anticipated, and the pulse and blood pressure monitored every 15 min until stabilised. In cases of massive hemorrhage, continuous pulse, blood pressure and respiratory rate monitoring should be commenced. An indwelling catheter should be inserted to monitor hourly urine output.

14.3.4 Obstetric Management

In tandem with resuscitation efforts, the cause of the PPH must be sought (considering the four T's); extra-genital bleeding (such as splenic rupture or sub-capsular liver rupture) is rare but should be borne in mind.

Uterine atony is the commonest cause of primary PPH and it is best to administer further uterotonics (see below) while other possible causes for the PPH are being sought. Non-pharmacological measures are traditionally used as the first line management while these further uterotonics are being prepared. These include fundal massage, bimanual uterine compression and the emptying of the bladder in order to stimulate uterine contractions.

The pharmacological means of managing uterine atony are as follows [40]:

1. 5 Units of oxytocin by slow intravenous injection (IVI)
2. Ergometrine 0.5 mg by IM injection (contraindicated in hypertension or severe cardiac disease)
3. Oxytocin infusion (40 units in 500 mL Hartmann's solution at 125 mL/h)
4. Carboprost [0.25 mg = 250 mcg, IM or intramyometrially (easier to achieve at the time of CS), repeated at 15 min intervals to a maximum of 6 doses]. Contraindicated in women with asthma as it may cause severe bronchospasm.
5. Misoprostol 800 micrograms rectally.

If bleeding persists in spite of these initial measures, the woman should be transferred to the operating theatre for examination under anesthesia so that a more thorough, controlled assessment for retained products and genital tract trauma can be made, and treatment carried out, if indicated. If bleeding continues despite pharmacological therapy, surgical therapy is warranted. There is limited evidence with regards to the most effective techniques in this situation: surgical techniques, radiological interventions or other hemostatic medical therapies. The available guidelines and recommendations are based on observational data and consensus only.

If the bleeding is perceived to be mainly or only from uterine atony, the first line surgical therapy is balloon tamponade. This technique has superseded the more traditional uterine packing. Several types of balloon catheters have been described such as the urological Rusch balloon [118], Foley catheter [119], Bakri balloon [120], Sengstaken–Blakemore esophageal catheter [121] and a condom catheter [122]. An 87 % success rate (defined as avoidance of hysterectomy) has been described in a series of 53 women who underwent balloon tamponade for the management of PPH [123].

Uterine hemostatic brace suturing is the next line of surgical management for atonic bleeding. Data from observational studies have shown that hemostatic brace suturing can successfully prevent hysterectomy in up to 81 % of cases [123]. Several variations of compression sutures have been described, the best known of which was described by B-Lynch in 1997 [124]. In the absence of comparative data, no particular method is thought to be superior.

Selective arterial embolisation may also be utilised to manage PPH, if onsite interventional radiology services are available; success rates of 75–100 % have been reported [123, 125, 126].

Step-wise ligation of uterine or internal iliac arteries has also been utilised [127]. The available evidence suggests that balloon tamponade and hemostatic suturing may be more effective. Lack of comparative studies means that one surgical technique cannot be strongly recommended above another. The appropriate surgical management will depend at least in part on the expertise and experience of the available staff.

Aortic compression may be used as a temporary means of hemostasis while awaiting surgical support or to allow resuscitation. The decision for hysterectomy as a life saving measure in the treatment of PPH should be made by a consultant and ideally discussed with and performed with a second consultant.

14.3.5 Causes and Management of Secondary Postpartum Hemorrhage

Secondary PPH typically occurs 10–14 days after the birth, and causes include retained products of conception and infection (endometritis). Endometritis may be managed with antibiotics. In case of excessive or ongoing bleeding, surgical management is warranted regardless of ultrasound findings. The decision for surgical management should involve a consultant, given the high risk of uterine perforation in this situation (because the uterine cavity is still large and the myometrium very soft).

14.3.6 Hematological Management of Postpartum Hemorrhage

During massive obstetric hemorrhage, blood loss >40 % of the patient's estimated blood volume (EBV) is immediately life threatening. Clear communication, cooperation & effective team working by all members of the multidisciplinary team are a priority and essential for optimal clinical management of the patient. Early recognition of the deteriorating patient and the activation of a locally agreed 'massive obstetric hemorrhage protocol' at the appropriate point are essential.

The priorities from a haematological perspective are [114, 115]:

- To maintain tissue/organ perfusion and oxygenation by restoration of blood volume and hemoglobin, through rapid provision of red cells.
- To maintain hemostasis through the appropriate use of additional blood components, to correct resultant coagulopathy and thrombocytopenia.
- To control ongoing bleeding ensuing from obstetric, surgical origins and/or abnormal systemic hemostasis.

Initial assessment is a combination of clinical signs and estimation of blood loss, with reference to baseline and ongoing hematology results (when available); non-visible blood loss (for example intra-peritoneal bleeding from a uterine rupture or bleeding into the broad ligament from cervical or uterine trauma) may be difficult to quantify. Empiric use of blood components may be required whilst awaiting coagulation results.

14.4 Massive Obstetric Hemorrhage (MOH) Protocols

Massive blood loss is normally defined as the loss of one blood volume in 24 h. An alternative definition which may be more useful in an acute situation is loss of 50 % of total blood volume in 3 h or >150 mL/min [40, 114, 115].

Estimated blood volume: pregnant women at term have an approx EBV of 100 mL/kg, when allowing for physiological increase. A pregnant woman weighing 70 kg at delivery would have an EBV of 7,000 mL; a loss of 20 % blood volume would be approximately 1,500 mL and a loss of 40 %, approximately 2,800 mL, and will require rapid access to red cell transfusion [40].

Many women will be able to tolerate an estimated blood loss between 500 and 1,500 mL without requiring blood component transfusion, provided they have had adequate fluid resuscitation. Consideration should be given to the patient's underlying condition (e.g. respiratory/cardiac status), body weight & baseline hemoglobin. Reliable estimation of blood loss is extremely difficult and blood loss is frequently underestimated; if a woman is showing clinical signs of shock during massive obstetric haemorrhage (MOH), with ongoing blood loss, the MOH protocol should be activated to mobilise additional resources. Many institutions define the trigger for activation of an MOH protocol as an estimated blood loss of between 1,000 and 1,500 mL [113].

Successful management of PPH will require the involvement of clinicians, departments and personnel not present at the site of hemorrhage:

- Robust systems must be in place to improve outcomes for women: effective local protocols must be developed in consultation with all the departments and people involved in the care of women during an MOH [127].
- There must be an explicit and well understood phrase used for the activation of an MOH protocol, for example 'massive obstetric hemorrhage' 'location and contact number'[128].
- During an MOH a nominated clinician should be responsible for coordinating communications with laboratory staff, hematologists and personnel transporting blood components/products, for the duration of the emergency. The rapid provision of red cells and other blood components is critical and the importance of effective communication cannot be over-emphasised.
- Blood transfusion laboratory staff and a senior hematologist should be contacted immediately when the MOH protocol is activated.
- Locally agreed protocols should enable red cells, FFP, cryoprecipitate and platelets to be issued at the earliest possible opportunity, without the initial approval of a hematologist.
- Protocols may define a 'hemorrhage pack' containing red cells and blood components that can be requested on the activation of the MOH procedure to facilitate rapid access to appropriate components.
- All members of the multidisciplinary team who may be involved in an MOH should be familiar with the agreed protocol and know where to locate it; this should be supported by regular training, education and drills to practice and test the effectiveness of the procedure [127, 128].
- Straightforward algorithms describing the key steps within the local protocol and system for communication during PPH should be available in all relevant clinical areas.

14.4.1 Blood Transfusion: Laboratory Testing and General Principles

Blood transfusion:

- Patient blood samples used for crossmatching (current practice is to undertake a group and antibody screen, and electronic issue) should be no more than 7 days old [40, 129, 130]. Red cell alloimmunisation is most likely to occur in the last trimester of pregnancy [40, 129]. If blood transfusion is anticipated or required, a sample must be sent to the blood transfusion laboratory.

- If immediate transfusion of emergency group O RhD negative blood is required, the group and screen/crossmatch sample must be taken before administration of emergency blood.
- When a woman has clinically significant atypical red cell antibodies, antigen negative blood may be indicated and this may necessitate additional testing in the blood transfusion laboratory. If a delay in obtaining fully compatible antigen negative red cells would be immediately life-threatening, transfusion of emergency group O RhD negative or ABO compatible serologically least incompatible blood should be undertaken with caution and advice from a senior hematologist sought. Many red cell antibodies have the potential to cause immediate or delayed hemolytic transfusion reactions; strategies to mitigate the immunological response should be considered [129, 131].
- The risk of a hemolytic transfusion reaction following the transfusion of emergency uncrossmatched group O RhD negative blood has been reported to be as high as 5 %. However, reports in the literature on the experience in trauma patients suggest much lower complication rates [117, 132, 133].
- Only K (Kell) negative red cells should be used for transfusion in women of childbearing age unless they are known to be K positive. Red cells provided to obstetric units by transfusion laboratories should be K negative as standard [40, 117, 134].
- Cytomegalovirus (CMV) seronegative red cells & platelets should be provided for elective transfusions in pregnancy for CMV seronegative women or where the CMV status is unknown. Urgent transfusion should not be delayed if CMV seronegative components are not immediately available, and leucodepleted components (standard in the UK) may be used in an emergency to avoid delay. Primary infection with CMV in seronegative women during pregnancy is a risk for the fetus and transfusion transmitted infection should be avoided when possible; this is particularly relevant in APH when the baby is still in utero. The risk of transmission is low where cellular blood products have been leucodepleted; this is standard in the UK. Blood component/product transfusion should not be delayed in hemorrhage if CMV seronegative products are not available [40, 114, 130].
- When women with placenta previa are hospitalised or approaching the delivery date, consideration should be given to ensuring that 4 units of crossmatched red cells are available in the hospital issue refrigerator or labour ward blood refrigerator. In this case, it is important to liaise with the blood transfusion laboratory; repeat group and screen samples should be sent on a weekly basis and there should be a planned agreement with the laboratory to replace red cells every 7 days until the woman has delivered.

14.4.2 Hematology and Coagulation: Investigations and General Principles

- Baseline samples for FBC, coagulation screen, i.e. PT, APTT and fibrinogen should routinely be sent from all patients at the beginning of a PPH. The results may not be available in time to influence initial management in a rapidly evolving clinical situation, but the baseline may help to inform later decisions regarding ongoing blood component/product usage and may identify any abnormal results present at the start.
- Coagulation tests (at a minimum PT, APTT and fibrinogen) and FBC should be performed at regular intervals: every 4 h or after each batch of components/products has been transfused. Ongoing platelet counts and coagulation results should be used as a guide and interpreted in conjunction with the patient's clinical condition [114].
- Near-patient testing, routinely FBC and INR, should be utilised by trained operators where

available. A Cochrane database systematic review concluded that there is an absence of evidence that thromboelastography (TEG) or thromboelastometry (ROTEM) improves morbidity or mortality in patients with severe bleeding. Application of a TEG or ROTEM guided transfusion strategy seems to reduce the amount of bleeding but whether this has implications for the clinical condition of patients remains uncertain [116]. Karlsson et al reported that the TEG provides faster results; however laboratory analyses found greater differences in coagulation variables, which correlated better with estimated blood loss [135].

- When a woman is identified during the antenatal period as being at high risk of PPH, every effort should be made to optimise her hemoglobin prior to delivery; iron status (iron deficiency being the most common cause of anemia in pregnancy) as well as levels of B12 and folate should be reviewed on a regular basis, and supplementation prescribed as indicated. Oral iron replacement is appropriate for most patients, but intravenous iron (after the first trimester) may produce a more rapid response and should be used in women intolerant of oral iron. As most cases of PPH occur in women who do not have any identifiable risk factors, the identification and correction of anemia in pregnancy, which avoids unnecessary blood transfusion, should be universal.
- When the woman has a coexisting bleeding disorder such as von Willebrand disease, thrombocytopenia, a platelet function defect or coagulation factor deficiency, a specific plan for management and follow-up will be required. This should be prepared in consultation with a consultant hematologist who specialises in disorders of hemostasis (see Chaps. 11, 12, 13, and 16).

14.4.3 Blood Component/Product Transfusion

The evidence base to guide transfusion practice in MOH is not currently supported by data from randomised controlled trials or well controlled clinical studies; recent changes in transfusion practice have predominantly arisen from the literature in relation to the management of hemorrhaging trauma patients and expert opinion. Recommendations advocating early transfusion of blood products to increase hemoglobin and correct coagulopathy/thrombocytopenia would appear to translate to the obstetric setting. Obstetric hemorrhage is often complicated by DIC, as a result of the pre-existing physiological activation of the hemostatic system in pregnancy, and clinicians managing these patients should be aware of this. Profound hypofibrinogenemia is not uncommon in this setting, and careful monitoring for this and appropriate management is of critical importance [114, 115, 130, 136, 137]. The decrease in fibrinogen does appear to be the most useful marker of developing hemostatic impairment and an early predictor of the severity of PPH, with a positive predictive value of a fibrinogen concentration ≤2 g/L for severe PPH of 100 % [138, 139].

Blood components must be transfused using an administration set with a built-in screen filter and platelets must be transfused using a new sterile line that should not be used for subsequent red cell transfusion. Each component should be stored correctly prior to transfusion to ensure optimal functioning and reduce the risk of adverse effects due to inappropriate temperature control [114, 130].

Massive transfusion of blood components increases the risk of adverse reactions. As detailed in the reports from the Serious Hazards of Transfusion (SHOT) and other national hemovigilance schemes [140], anaphylactic reactions and transfusion related acute lung injury (TRALI) are both more likely with plasma-containing components. Careful identification of the patient prior to administration of blood components is essential to prevent acute hemolytic transfusion reactions due to ABO incompatibility. The Department of Health 'Never Events 2013/14 update' lists the inadvertent transfusion of ABO incompatible components where death or serious harm resulted, and the misidentification of patients as two serious, preventable errors [141].

Transfusion-associated circulatory overload (TACO), a major cause of transfusion-associated major morbidity, may occur following MOH. Contributory factors for TACO in this scenario are difficulties in estimating actual blood loss, particularly because of the changing blood volume, and circulatory capacity. There may also be a failure to recognise TACO in obstetric patients who, as young individuals, are often considered to be 'immune' to TACO. A good quality echocardiogram to assess cardiac function during MOH will aid assessment; however, this may be difficult to achieve during the emergency situation [142]. SHOT has also highlighted that delayed or under-transfusion in patients with major hemorrhage can lead to potentially avoidable major morbidity and mortality [143].

14.4.3.1 Red Cells

Early transfusion of red cells in the hemorrhaging patient is recommended, in preference to prolonged fluid volume resuscitation, for the provision of oxygen to tissues and to contribute to hemostasis though the effect on platelet margination and function [130, 137]. In uncontrolled hemorrhage, aggressive fluid volume administration could exacerbate bleeding and increase the risk of mortality [133].

The aim should be to maintain hemoglobin >70–90 g/L; one unit of blood will increase haemoglobin by approximately 1 g/dL. Where an accurate hemoglobin result is available to guide decision making in early PPH, red cell transfusion is almost always indicated when the hemoglobin falls below 60 g/L [40, 117].

Hemoglobin/hematocrit levels in acute massive blood loss may not immediately reflect the level of blood loss and ability to deliver oxygen, due to their strong correlation with plasma volume, and can fall rapidly during fluid resuscitation [140].

Uncrossmatched group O RhD negative red cells should be transfused if blood transfusion is required immediately. When a blood transfusion laboratory is in receipt of a group and screen sample, group specific compatible red cells can generally be provided within 10 min plus transport time. If the woman has a positive antibody screen or a history of atypical red cell antibodies, a full serological crossmatch will be required and the availability of fully compatible red cells will depend on the antibody/antibodies present; in this situation red cell transfusion should be discussed with a hematologist.

Red cells transfused from salvaged blood does not contain platelets or clotting factors as these are removed in the washing process which leaves the red cells suspended in normal saline.

14.4.3.2 Fresh Frozen Plasma and Cryoprecipitate

Optimally, transfusion of FFP should be guided by laboratory results but in massive PPH, by the time the results become available, they may not accurately reflect the current clinical situation. When bleeding is uncontrolled, empirical transfusion may be indicated, if coagulopathy is suspected clinically.

Early FFP transfusion may be required (>0.5 EBV blood loss) in uncontrolled MOH when there has been significant fluid resuscitation. Dilution with red cell transfusion and blood volume expanders further reduces coagulation factor levels.

The starting volume for FFP transfusion is 12–15 mL/kg which equates to approximately 4 units in an average sized adult. When results are available, FFP transfusion is indicated when the PT or APTT are greater than 1.5 times the mean normal range, due to an increased risk of microvascular bleeding [40, 114].

Fibrinogen deficiency may develop when >1 EBV is replaced, and generally the threshold for fibrinogen replacement is a fibrinogen level of <1.0 g/dL [114]. However, given the higher levels of fibrinogen at term in pregnant women, and that a fibrinogen level below 2 g/L is a predictor of severe PPH [138], fibrinogen deficiency should be corrected with cryoprecipitate if the fibrinogen level remains below 2 g/L following FFP transfusion [144]. Cryoprecipitate contains a higher concentration of fibrinogen than FFP, typically around 15 g/L [145]. The recommended adult therapeutic dose is two pools of five units (or one unit per 5–10 kg body weight), which will generally raise the plasma fibrinogen by about 1 g/L [130].

Formulae to guide the ratio of FFP to red cell transfusion in hemorrhage are not supported by sufficiently robust evidence to provide definitive recommendations. Transfusion of 4 units of FFP to every 6 units of red cells may be used as a practical guideline (RCOG). Resuscitation using a 1:1 ratio of red cells:FFP has been increasingly reported in the literature following military experience of major trauma management in Iraq and translation of this practice to civilian trauma units, and there are some reports of this formula being employed in the obstetric setting. Survivorship bias in the patient outcome data for trauma patients receiving 1:1 red cells:FFP may be a factor when interpreting available retrospective studies [133, 136] and interim results from a prospective study published in 2011 suggest that a 1:1 ratio of red cells:FFP did not confer any additional advantage over ratios of 1:2–3:4 [146]. While there may be similarities in the management of the hemorrhaging patient across the specialities, the response of the obstetric patient may be influenced by pregnancy-related changes in coagulation and fibrinolysis, so direct comparison to transfusion strategies in multiple trauma patients cannot be assumed.

Both FFP and cryoprecipitate should be transfused as soon as possible after being issued by the Blood Transfusion laboratory. At room temperature both must be transfused within 4 h of being defrosted. After defrosting, FFP can be placed in a blood fridge for up to 24 h if not required immediately, but cryoprecipitate must remain at room temperature.

14.4.3.3 Fibrinogen Concentrate

Human fibrinogen concentrate is available and has some advantages over cryoprecipitate in that it can be stored at room temperature, does not have the short expiry time following defrosting and can be given in just a few minutes. Reports in the literature suggest that correction of hypofibrinogenemia can be achieved rapidly and case studies suggest favourable outcomes in MOH. Further well designed clinical trials are required to fully establish a favourable safety profile and improved outcomes when compared to cryoprecipitate transfusion before routine use as the standard treatment for hypofibrinogenemia in PPH can be recommended [147, 148]. The FIB-PPH (fibrinogen concentrate as initial treatment for postpartum hemorrhage) trial has investigated if early treatment with fibrinogen concentrate reduces the need for blood transfusion in women suffering severe PPH. In this randomised placebo-controlled double-blind multicentre trial (results awaited) (www.clinicaltrials.gov: NCT01359878), women with primary PPH were randomly allocated to either early treatment with 2 g fibrinogen concentrate or 100 mL isotonic saline (placebo). The primary outcome was the need for blood transfusion [149].

14.4.3.4 Platelets

The aim is to maintain the platelet count $>75\times10^9$/L, but $>100\times10^9$/L if the woman has abnormal platelet function. One pack of platelets should be requested initially and ongoing platelet requirements should be discussed with a hematologist. A platelet count of $<50\times10^9$/L should be anticipated after approximately 2 blood volumes have been replaced but there will be differences between individuals [114, 150]. In massive uncontrolled PPH, platelet counts should be interpreted in conjunction with the patient's clinical condition. Many hospital laboratories do not hold a stock of platelets for emergency use and therefore the need should be anticipated early and communicated to the local laboratory so they can be obtained from the blood transfusion service. Platelets should be Rh compatible but if only RhD positive platelets are available for transfusion to a RhD negative woman, 250 IU of anti-D immunoglobulin should be administered in addition to routine postnatal prophylaxis [40, 151].

14.4.4 Recombinant Factor VIIa

Recombinant Factor VIIa may be considered if there is ongoing massive blood loss, where appropriate blood/blood component management and clinical interventions have failed to control bleeding. Its use may also be an option in major PPH when the woman is refusing blood component transfusion. The use of recombinant factor

VIIa should be discussed with a consultant hematologist who specialises in hemostasis or transfusion. There is an increased risk of thrombotic episodes following administration and, given that there is already a higher risk of thromboembolism in pregnancy, the risk versus benefit ratio will need to be carefully considered. PPH is not a licensed indication for the use of recombinant factor VIIa and in the US the FDA has published a warning regarding the risk of serious thrombotic adverse events when used outside labelled indications [152, 153].

14.4.5 Tranexamic Acid

Administration of the antifibrinolytic drug tranexamic acid may contribute to reducing blood loss in PPH but good quality clinical evidence demonstrating a clear clinical benefit is not available [154]. Results from the CRASH-2 trial of tranexamic acid showing a reduction in the risk of death due to bleeding in trauma patients provide grounds for optimism that tranexamic acid may be useful in women with PPH. This is being addressed in the ongoing WOMAN (WOrld Maternal ANtifibrinolytic) Trial, an international, randomised, double-blind, placebo controlled trial in 15,000 women which aims to determine the effect of early administration of tranexamic acid on mortality, hysterectomy and other morbidities (surgical interventions, blood transfusion, risk of non-fatal vascular events) in women with clinically diagnosed PPH (http://www.thewomantrial.lshtm.ac.uk; ISRCTN76912190).

14.4.6 Intraoperative Cell Salvage

The use of intraoperative cell salvage (ICS) by teams experienced in the technique reduces exposure to donor red cells and can be life-saving, especially in women who decline allogeneic blood transfusion. ICS in obstetrics is endorsed by the National Institute for Health and Care Excellence (NICE). Salvaged blood should be transfused through a leucodepletion filter [116, 131].

14.4.7 Blood Refusal

The small risk of MOH should be discussed during the antenatal period with any woman stating her intention to refuse blood component transfusion. Antenatal hemoglobin optimization is particularly important in this patient group. A documented plan for the management of PPH should be agreed with the woman and relevant members of the multidisciplinary team. Cell salvage is often acceptable to women who refuse blood products. Acceptable treatments should be discussed and clearly documented; some Jehovah's Witness patients will, for example, accept human derived coagulation factors such as fibrinogen concentrate and cryoprecipitate as they are not considered to be primary blood components and therefore a matter for the individual's conscience. Recombinant factor VIIa may be considered (see above).

14.4.8 Post-hemorrhage Care

If the woman has a hemoglobin of less than 7–8 g/L when she is stable post-hemorrhage and no longer bleeding, the decision to transfuse further red cells should be made on an individual basis; if the woman is asymptomatic with no other co-existing conditions that might indicate a lower threshold for red cell transfusion, there may be no benefit in blood transfusion [40]. Assessment of the woman's hematinic status should be undertaken and supplementation to replace iron stores may be indicated.

PPH and blood transfusion are risk factors for venous thromboembolism so, when the risk of further significant bleeding has subsided and the hemostasis parameters return to normal, if there are additional risk factors, pharmacological prophylaxis with low molecular weight heparin may be initiated. Patients should wear graduated compression stockings to reduce the risk of lower limb deep venous thrombosis [116].

14.5 Case Study

A 36 years old female, gravida 8, Para 7, with a history of 5 previous Cesarean sections (CS), had a routine ultrasound scan which suggested anterior placenta previa accreta. She had a planned CS at 37+3 weeks' gestation. A multidisciplinary team meeting was held prior to the CS. At CS there were urologists and interventional radiologists on standby. The ureters were stented prior to the Cesarean procedure. A MOH pack was on standby in theatre prior to CS (included 4 units of RBC, 4 units of FFP and 2 pools of cryoprecipitate). The CS, undertaken by a consultant obstetrician, was difficult: there were dense omental adhesions to the anterior abdominal wall, uterus and bladder, and very difficult access to the abdomen and uterus. The rectus on the right was divided laterally to improve access. Good access was finally obtained before a uterine incision was made, cognizant of the possibility that emergency hysterectomy was likely to be necessary soon after delivery of the baby. The bladder was densely adherent to anterior uterus, with a very vascular junction between the bladder and uterus – this was not disturbed prior to delivery. Once the baby was delivered, there was massive hemorrhage from the lower uterus/placental bed. The estimated blood loss (EBL) was 3 L within 3 min. As agreed in advance with the patient, the obstetrician proceeded to emergency hysterectomy without delay (as her family was completed). The hysterectomy (with ovarian conservation) was difficult as expected, due to adhesions. During hysterectomy, she received repeated doses of uterotonic medication (oxytocin IV boluses and infusion; misoprostol rectally; carboprost intramyometrially), but this had little effect in controlling the bleeding. The total EBL was 25 L. She was resuscitated with the following: IV crystalloids; red cells (37 units); FFP (28 units); cryoprecipitate (10 pools); platelets (7 packs). There was no clinical or hematological evidence of DIC at any stage.

She spent 24 h in the intensive care unit. One unit of red cells was transfused. Twelve hours post-operatively. She made a speedy recovery.

Key Learning Points

- All hospitals should have a protocol for the management of massive obstetric hemorrhage (MOH), supported by regular training, education and drills. The rapid provision of red cells and other blood components is critical and the importance of effective communication cannot be over-emphasised. A nominated clinician should be responsible for coordinating communications with laboratory staff, hematologists and personnel transporting blood components, for the duration of the emergency.
- Accurate assessment of blood loss is very challenging and blood loss is typically underestimated. If crossmatched red cells are unavailable by the time 3.5 L of clear fluids have been infused, uncrossmatched ABO and RhD group specific blood or O RhD negative blood should be given.
- The goals in the management of MOH are to maintain a haemoglobin above 80 g/L, a platelet count of >50 g×10^9/L (with a platelet transfusion trigger of 75 to provide a margin of safety), prothrombin time (PT) and activated partial thromboplastin time (APTT) less than 1.5 times the mean control level and fibrinogen greater than 1 g/L. Regular assessment of hematological and coagulation parameters is required.
- Obstetric haemorrhage is often complicated by DIC, as a result of the preexisting physiological activation of the hemostatic system in pregnancy, and clinicians managing these patients

should be aware of this. Profound hypofibrinogenaemia is not uncommon in this setting, and careful monitoring for this and appropriate management is of critical importance. The decrease in fibrinogen does appear to be the most useful marker of developing hemostatic impairment, with a fribrinogen concentration ≤2 g/L an early predictor of severe PPH. Fibrinogen deficiency should be corrected with cryoprecipitate if the fibrinogen level remains below 2 g/L following FFP transfusion.

- Inadequate volume resuscitation, acidosis and hypothermia increase the risk of DIC. The woman should be kept warm and blood components transfused using a validated blood warmer.
- Massive transfusion of blood components increases the risk of adverse reactions such as anaphylactic reactions, transfusion-related acute lung injury and transfusion-associated circulatory overload. Acute haemolytic transfusion reactions secondary to ABO incompatibility may arise as a result of misidentification of the patient. It is important to remain cognisant that delayed or under transfusion in patients with major haemorrhage can lead to potentially avoidable major morbidity and mortality.

References

1. Khan KS, Wojdyla D, Say L, Gulmezoglu AM, Van Look PF. WHO analysis of causes of maternal death: a systematic review. Lancet. 2006;367(9516):1066–74.
2. Brace V, Kernaghan D, Penney G. Learning from adverse clinical outcomes: major obstetric haemorrhage in Scotland, 2003–05. BJOG. 2007;114(11):1388–96.
3. Cantwell R, Clutton-Brock T, Cooper G, Dawson A, Drife J, Garrod D, et al. Saving mothers' lives: reviewing maternal deaths to make motherhood safer: 2006–2008. The eighth report of the confidential enquiries into maternal deaths in the United Kingdom. BJOG. 2011;118 Suppl 1:1–203.
4. Knight M, Callaghan WM, Berg C, Alexander S, Bouvier-Colle MH, Ford JB, et al. Trends in postpartum hemorrhage in high resource countries: a review and recommendations from the International Postpartum Hemorrhage Collaborative Group. BMC Pregnancy Childbirth. 2009;9:55.
5. Sinha P, Kuruba N. Ante-partum haemorrhage: an update. J Obstet Gynaecol. 2008;28(4):377–81.
6. Chamberlain G. ABC of antenatal care. Antepartum haemorrhage. BMJ. 1991;302(6791):1526–30.
7. Mukherjee S, Bhide A. Antepartum haemorrhage. Obstet Gynaecol Reprod Med. 2008;18(12):335–9.
8. Ngeh N, Bhide A. Antepartum haemorrhage. Curr Obstet Gynaecol. 2006;16:79–83.
9. Armstrong CA, Harding S, Matthews T, Dickinson JE. Is placenta accreta catching up with us? Aust N Z J Obstet Gynaecol. 2004;44(3):210–3.
10. Oyelese Y, Smulian JC. Placenta previa, placenta accreta, and vasa previa. Obstet Gynecol. 2006;107(4):927–41.
11. Iyasu S, Saftlas AK, Rowley DL, Koonin LM, Lawson HW, Atrash HK. The epidemiology of placenta previa in the United States, 1979 through 1987. Am J Obstet Gynecol. 1993;168(5):1424–9.
12. Miller DA, Chollet JA, Goodwin TM. Clinical risk factors for placenta previa-placenta accreta. Am J Obstet Gynecol. 1997;177(1):210–4.
13. Faiz AS, Ananth CV. Etiology and risk factors for placenta previa: an overview and meta-analysis of observational studies. J Matern Fetal Neonatal Med. 2003;13(3):175–90.
14. Silver RM, Landon MB, Rouse DJ, Leveno KJ, Spong CY, Thom EA, et al. Maternal morbidity associated with multiple repeat cesarean deliveries. Obstet Gynecol. 2006;107(6):1226–32.
15. Smith RS, Lauria MR, Comstock CH, Treadwell MC, Kirk JS, Lee W, et al. Transvaginal ultrasonography for all placentas that appear to be low-lying or over the internal cervical os. Ultrasound Obstet Gynecol. 1997;9(1):22–4.
16. Lauria MR, Smith RS, Treadwell MC, Comstock CH, Kirk JS, Lee W, et al. The use of second-trimester transvaginal sonography to predict placenta previa. Ultrasound Obstet Gynecol. 1996;8(5):337–40.
17. Leerentveld RA, Gilberts EC, Arnold MJ, Wladimiroff JW. Accuracy and safety of transvaginal sonographic placental localization. Obstet Gynecol. 1990;76(5 Pt 1):759–62.
18. Sherman SJ, Carlson DE, Platt LD, Medearis AL. Transvaginal ultrasound: does it help in the diagnosis of placenta previa? Ultrasound Obstet Gynecol. 1992;2(4):256–60.
19. Becker RH, Vonk R, Mende BC, Ragosch V, Entezami M. The relevance of placental location at 20–23 gestational weeks for prediction of placenta previa at delivery: evaluation of 8650 cases. Ultrasound Obstet Gynecol. 2001;17(6):496–501.

20. Dashe JS, McIntire DD, Ramus RM, Santos-Ramos R, Twickler DM. Persistence of placenta previa according to gestational age at ultrasound detection. Obstet Gynecol. 2002;99(5 Pt 1):692–7.
21. Ghourab S, Al-Jabari A. Placental migration and mode of delivery in placenta previa: transvaginal sonographic assessment during the third trimester. Ann Saudi Med. 2000;20(5-6):382–5.
22. Love CD, Fernando KJ, Sargent L, Hughes RG. Major placenta praevia should not preclude outpatient management. Eur J Obstet Gynecol Reprod Biol. 2004;117(1):24–9.
23. Mustafa SA, Brizot ML, Carvalho MH, Watanabe L, Kahhale S, Zugaib M. Transvaginal ultrasonography in predicting placenta previa at delivery: a longitudinal study. Ultrasound Obstet Gynecol. 2002;20(4):356–9.
24. Oppenheimer L, Holmes P, Simpson N, Dabrowski A. Diagnosis of low-lying placenta: can migration in the third trimester predict outcome? Ultrasound Obstet Gynecol. 2001;18(2):100–2.
25. Royal College of Obstetricians and Gynaecologists. Placenta praevia, placenta praevia accreta and vasa praevia: diagnosis and management, Green-top guideline, vol. 272011. London: RCOG Press; 2011.
26. Taipale P, Hiilesmaa V, Ylostalo P. Transvaginal ultrasonography at 18–23 weeks in predicting placenta previa at delivery. Ultrasound Obstet Gynecol. 1998;12(6):422–5.
27. Zlatnik MG, Cheng YW, Norton ME, Thiet MP, Caughey AB. Placenta previa and the risk of preterm delivery. J Matern Fetal Neonatal Med. 2007;20(10):719–23.
28. D'Antonio F, Iacovella C, Bhide A. Prenatal identification of invasive placentation using ultrasound: systematic review and meta-analysis. Ultrasound Obstet Gynecol. 2013;42(5):509–17.
29. Meng X, Xie L, Song W. Comparing the diagnostic value of ultrasound and magnetic resonance imaging for placenta accreta: a systematic review and meta-analysis. Ultrasound Med Biol. 2013;39(11):1958–65 [Comparative Study Meta-Analysis Research Support, Non-U.S. Gov't Review].
30. Bhide A, Perfumo F, Moore J, Hollis B, Thilaganathan B. Placental edge to internal os distance in the late third trimester and mode of delivery in placenta praevia. BJOG. 2003;110:860–4.
31. Gynaecologists RCoOa. Antenatal corticosteroids to reduce neonatal morbidity (Green-top guideline no. 7). London: RCOG; 2010.
32. Royal College of Obstetricians and Gynaecologists. The use of anti-D immunoglobulin for Rhesus D prophylaxis, Green-top guideline, vol. 22. London: RCOG Press; 2011.
33. Cotton DB, Read JA, Paul RH, Quilligan EJ. The conservative aggressive management of placenta previa. Am J Obstet Gynecol. 1980;137(6):687–95 [Comparative Study Research Support, U.S. Gov't, P.H.S.].
34. Besinger RE, Moniak CW, Paskiewicz LS, Fisher SG, Tomich PG. The effect of tocolytic use in the management of symptomatic placenta previa. Am J Obstet Gynecol. 1995;172(6):1770–5; discussion 5–8. [Clinical Trial Controlled Clinical Trial].
35. Sharma A, Suri V, Gupta I. Tocolytic therapy in conservative management of symptomatic placenta previa. Int J Gynaecol Obstet. 2004;84(2):109–13 [Clinical Trial Randomized Controlled Trial].
36. Towers CV, Pircon RA, Heppard M. Is tocolysis safe in the management of third-trimester bleeding? Am J Obstet Gynecol. 1999;180(6 Pt 1):1572–8.
37. Magann EF, Johnson CA, Gookin KS, Roberts WE, Martin RW, Morrison JC. Placenta praevia: does uterine activity cause bleeding? Aust N Z J Obstet Gynaecol. 1993;33(1):22–4 [Research Support, Non-U.S. Gov't].
38. Cobo E, Conde-Agudelo A, Delgado J, Canaval H, Congote A. Cervical cerclage: an alternative for the management of placenta previa? Am J Obstet Gynecol. 1998;179(1):122–5 [Clinical Trial Randomized Controlled Trial].
39. Neilson JP. Interventions for suspected placenta praevia. Cochrane Database Syst Rev. 2003;(2):CD001998.
40. Royal College of Obstetricians and Gynaecologists. Prevention and management of postpartum haemorrhage, Green-top guideline, vol. 52. London: RCOG Press; 2009.
41. Wong HS, Hutton J, Zuccollo J, Tait J, Pringle KC. The maternal outcome in placenta accreta: the significance of antenatal diagnosis and non-separation of placenta at delivery. N Z Med J. 2008;121(1277): 30–8.
42. Eller AG, Porter TF, Soisson P, Silver RM. Optimal management strategies for placenta accreta. BJOG. 2009;116(5):648–54.
43. Timmermans S, van Hof AC, Duvekot JJ. Conservative management of abnormally invasive placentation. Obstet Gynecol Surv. 2007;62(8): 529–39.
44. ACOG committee opinion. Placenta accreta. Number 266, January 2002. American College of Obstetricians and Gynecologists. Int J Gynaecol Obstet. 2002;77(1):77–8.
45. Ananth CV, Oyelese Y, Yeo L, Pradhan A, Vintzileos AM. Placental abruption in the United States, 1979 through 2001: temporal trends and potential determinants. Am J Obstet Gynecol. 2005;192(1):191–8.
46. Ananth CV, Berkowitz GS, Savitz DA, Lapinski RH. Placental abruption and adverse perinatal outcomes. JAMA. 1999;282:1646–51.
47. Sheiner E, Shoham-Vardi I, Hadar A, Hallak M, Hackmon R, Mazor M. Incidence, obstetric risk factors and pregnancy outcome of preterm placental abruption: a retrospective analysis. J Matern Fetal Neonatal Med. 2002;11:34–9.
48. Ananth CV, Oyelese Y, Srinivas N, Yeo L, Vintzileos AM. Preterm premature rupture of membranes, intrauterine infection, and oligohydramnios: risk

factors for placental abruption. Obstet Gynecol. 2004;104:71–7.
49. Ananth CV, Savitz DA, Luther ER. Maternal cigarette smoking as a risk factor for placental abruption, placenta previa, and uterine bleeding in pregnancy. Am J Epidemiol. 1996;144:881–9.
50. Ananth CV, Savitz DA, Williams MA. Placental abruption and its association with hypertension and prolonged rupture of membranes: a methodologic review and meta-analysis. Obstet Gynecol. 1996;88:309–18.
51. Ananth CV, Savitz DA, Bowes Jr WA, Luther ER. Influence of hypertensive disorders and cigarette smoking on placental abruption and uterine bleeding during pregnancy. Br J Obstet Gynaecol. 1997;104: 572–8.
52. Ananth CV, Smulian JC, Demissie K, Vintzileos AM, Knuppel RA. Placental abruption among singleton and twin births in the United States: risk factor profiles. Am J Epidemiol. 2001;153:771–8.
53. Kramer MS, Usher RH, Pollack R, Boyd M, Usher S. Etiologic determinants of abruptio placentae. Obstet Gynecol. 1997;89:221–6.
54. Oyelese Y, Ananth CV. Placental abruption. Obstet Gynecol. 2006;108:1005–16.
55. Sheiner E, Shoham-Vardi I, Hallak M, Hadar A, Gortzak-Uzan L, Katz M, Mazor M. Placental abruption in term pregnancies: clinical significance and obstetric risk factors. J Matern Fetal Neonatal Med. 2003;13:45–9.
56. Toivonen S, Heinonen S, Anttila M, Kosma VM, Saarikoski S. Obstetric prognosis after placental abruption. Fetal Diagn Ther. 2004;19:336–41.
57. ACOG educational bulletin. Obstetric aspects of trauma management. Number 251, September 1998 (replaces Number 151, January 1991, and Number 161, November 1991). American College of Obstetricians and Gynecologists. Int J Gynaecol Obstet. 1999;64(1):87–94 [Guideline Practice Guideline].
58. Ananth CV, Oyelese Y, Prasad V, Getahun D, Smulian JC. Evidence of placental abruption as a chronic process: associations with vaginal bleeding early in pregnancy and placental lesions. Eur J Obstet Gynecol Reprod Biol. 2006;128(1–2): 15–21.
59. Weiss JL, Malone FD, Vidaver J, Ball RH, Nyberg DA, Comstock CH, et al. Threatened abortion: a risk factor for poor pregnancy outcome, a population-based screening study. Am J Obstet Gynecol. 2004;190(3):745–50.
60. Goddijn-Wessel TA, Wouters MG, van de Molen EF, Spuijbroek MD, Steegers-Theunissen RP, Blom HJ, et al. Hyperhomocysteinemia: a risk factor for placental abruption or infarction. Eur J Obstet Gynecol Reprod Biol. 1996;66(1):23–9.
61. Kupferminc MJ, Eldor A, Steinman N, Many A, Bar-Am A, Jaffa A, et al. Increased frequency of genetic thrombophilia in women with complications of pregnancy. N Engl J Med. 1999;340(1):9–13.
62. Katz VL, Chescheir NC, Cefalo RC. Unexplained elevations of maternal serum alpha-fetoprotein. Obstet Gynecol Surv. 1990;45(11):719–26.
63. Glantz C, Purnell L. Clinical utility of sonography in the diagnosis and treatment of placental abruption. J Ultrasound Med. 2002;21(8):837–40.
64. Jaffe MH, Schoen WC, Silver TM, Bowerman RA, Stuck KJ. Sonography of abruptio placentae. AJR Am J Roentgenol. 1981;137(5):1049–54.
65. Nyberg DA, Cyr DR, Mack LA, Wilson DA, Shuman WP. Sonographic spectrum of placental abruption. AJR Am J Roentgenol. 1987;148(1):161–4.
66. Nyberg DA, Mack LA, Benedetti TJ, Cyr DR, Schuman WP. Placental abruption and placental hemorrhage: correlation of sonographic findings with fetal outcome. Radiology. 1987;164(2): 357–61.
67. Oyelese KO, Turner M, Lees C, Campbell S. Vasa previa: an avoidable obstetric tragedy. Obstet Gynecol Surv. 1999;54(2):138–45.
68. Lee W, Lee VL, Kirk JS, Sloan CT, Smith RS, Comstock CH. Vasa previa: prenatal diagnosis, natural evolution, and clinical outcome. Obstet Gynecol. 2000;95(4):572–6.
69. Francois K, Mayer S, Harris C, Perlow JH. Association of vasa previa at delivery with a history of second-trimester placenta previa. J Reprod Med. 2003;48(10):771–4.
70. Nomiyama M, Toyota Y, Kawano H. Antenatal diagnosis of velamentous umbilical cord insertion and vasa previa with color Doppler imaging. Ultrasound Obstet Gynecol. 1998;12(6):426–9.
71. Paavonen J, Jouttunpaa K, Kangasluoma P, Aro P, Heinonen PK. Velamentous insertion of the umbilical cord and vasa previa. Int J Gynaecol Obstet. 1984;22(3):207–11.
72. Quek SP, Tan KL. Vasa praevia. Aust N Z J Obstet Gynaecol. 1972;12(3):206–9.
73. Schachter M, Tovbin Y, Arieli S, Friedler S, Ron-El R, Sherman D. In vitro fertilization is a risk factor for vasa previa. Fertil Steril. 2002;78(3): 642–3.
74. Sepulveda W, Rojas I, Robert JA, Schnapp C, Alcalde JL. Prenatal detection of velamentous insertion of the umbilical cord: a prospective color Doppler ultrasound study. Ultrasound Obstet Gynecol. 2003;21(6):564–9.
75. Young M, Yule N, Barham K. The role of light and sound technologies in the detection of vasa praevia. Reprod Fertil Dev. 1991;3(4):439–45.
76. Apt L, Downey Jr WS. Melena neonatorum: the swallowed blood syndrome; a simple test for the differentiation of adult and fetal hemoglobin in bloody stools. J Pediatr. 1955;47(1):6–12.
77. Jones KP, Wheater AW, Musgrave W. Simple test for bleeding from vasa praevia. Lancet. 1987;2(8573): 1430–1.
78. Kleihauer E, Braun H, Betke K. Demonstration of fetal hemoglobin in erythrocytes of a blood smear. Klin Wochenschr. 1957;35(12):637–8.

79. Ogita S, Ishiko O, Matsumoto M, Hasegawa H, Sugawa T. A simplified method for measuring fetal hemoglobin. Obstet Gynecol. 1976;48(2):237–8.
80. Lindqvist PG, Gren P. An easy-to-use method for detecting fetal hemoglobin–a test to identify bleeding from vasa previa. Eur J Obstet Gynecol Reprod Biol. 2007;131(2):151–3.
81. Baschat AA, Gembruch U. Ante- and intrapartum diagnosis of vasa praevia in singleton pregnancies by colour coded Doppler sonography. Eur J Obstet Gynecol Reprod Biol. 1998;79(1):19–25 [Case Reports].
82. Baulies S, Maiz N, Munoz A, Torrents M, Echevarria M, Serra B. Prenatal ultrasound diagnosis of vasa praevia and analysis of risk factors. Prenat Diagn. 2007;27(7):595–9.
83. Catanzarite V, Maida C, Thomas W, Mendoza A, Stanco L, Piacquadio KM. Prenatal sonographic diagnosis of vasa previa: ultrasound findings and obstetric outcome in ten cases. Ultrasound Obstet Gynecol. 2001;18(2):109–15.
84. Fung TY, Lau TK. Poor perinatal outcome associated with vasa previa: is it preventable? A report of three cases and review of the literature. Ultrasound Obstet Gynecol. 1998;12(6):430–3 [Case Reports Review].
85. Gagnon R, Morin L, Bly S, Butt K, Cargill YM, Denis N, et al. Guidelines for the management of vasa previa. J Obstet Gynaecol Can. 2009;31(8):748–60 [Practice Guideline Research Support, Non-U.S. Gov't Review].
86. Gianopoulos J, Carver T, Tomich PG, Karlman R, Gadwood K. Diagnosis of vasa previa with ultrasonography. Obstet Gynecol. 1987;69(3 Pt 2):488–91 [Case Reports].
87. Nelson LH, Melone PJ, King M. Diagnosis of vasa previa with transvaginal and color flow Doppler ultrasound. Obstet Gynecol. 1990;76(3 Pt 2):506–9.
88. Oyelese Y, Catanzarite V, Prefumo F, Lashley S, Schachter M, Tovbin Y, et al. Vasa previa: the impact of prenatal diagnosis on outcomes. Obstet Gynecol. 2004;103(5 Pt 1):937–42 [Comparative Study Multicenter Study].
89. Derbala Y, Grochal F, Jeanty P. Vasa previa. J Prenat Med. 2007;1:2–13.
90. Daly-Jones E, John A, Leahy A, Mckenna C, Sepulveda W. Vasa praevia; a preventable tragedy. Ultrasound. 2008;16:8–14.
91. Al-Khaduri M, Kadoch IJ, Couturier B, Dube J, Lapensee L, Bissonnette F. Vasa praevia after IVF: should there be guidelines? Report of two cases and literature review. Reprod Biomed Online. 2007;14(3):372–4.
92. UK National Screening Committee. The UK NSC policy on placenta praevia screening in pregnancy. Accessed Aug 2013.
93. Oleyese Y, Spong C, Fernandez MA, McLaren RA. Second trimester low-lying placenta and in-vitro fertilization? Exclude vasa previa. J Matern Fetal Med. 2000;9:370–2.
94. Quintero RA, Kontopoulos EV, Bornick PW, Allen MH. In utero laser treatment of type II vasa previa. J Matern Fetal Neonatal Med. 2007;20:847–51.
95. Rath WH. Postpartum hemorrhage-update on problems of definitions and diagnosis. Acta Obstet Gynecol Scand. 2011;90:421–8.
96. WHO recommendations for the prevention and treatment of postpartum haemorrhage. 2012. http://www.who.int/reproductivehealth/publications/maternal_perinatal_health/9789241548502/en/. World Health Organisation.
97. Pahlavan P, Nezhat C. Hemorrhage in obstetrics and gynecology. Curr Opin Obstet Gynecol. 2001;13(4):419–24.
98. Oyelese Y, Ananth CV. Postpartum hemorrhage: epidemiology, risk factors, and causes. Clin Obstet Gynecol. 2010;53(1):147–56.
99. Ford JB, Roberts CL, Simpson JM, Vaughan J, Cameron CA. Increased postpartum hemorrhage rates in Australia. Int J Gynaecol Obstet. 2007;98(3): 237–43.
100. James AH, Paglia MJ, Gernsheimer T, Grotegut C, Thames B. Blood component therapy in postpartum hemorrhage. Transfusion. 2009;49(11):2430–3.
101. Joseph KS, Rouleau J, Kramer MS, Young DC, Liston RM, Baskett TF. Investigation of an increase in postpartum haemorrhage in Canada. BJOG. 2007;114(6):751–9.
102. Schuurmans N, MacKinnon C, Lane C, Etches D. Prevention and management of postpartum haemorrhage: SOCG clinical practice guidelines no. 88. J Obstet Gynaecol Can. 2000;22(4):271–81.
103. Al-Zirqi I, Vangen S, Forsen L, Stray-Pedersen B. Prevalence and risk factors of severe obstetric haemorrhage. BJOG. 2008;115(10):1265–72.
104. Bateman BT, Berman MF, Riley LE, Leffert LR. The epidemiology of postpartum hemorrhage in a large, nationwide sample of deliveries. Anesth Analg. 2010;110(5):1368–73.
105. Combs CA, Murphy EL, Laros Jr RK. Factors associated with postpartum hemorrhage with vaginal birth. Obstet Gynecol. 1991;77(1):69–76.
106. Stones RW, Paterson CM, Saunders NJ. Risk factors for major obstetric haemorrhage. Eur J Obstet Gynecol Reprod Biol. 1993;48(1):15–8.
107. Tsu VD. Postpartum haemorrhage in Zimbabwe: a risk factor analysis. Br J Obstet Gynaecol. 1993; 100(4):327–33.
108. Prendiville WJ, Elbourne D, McDonald S. Active versus expectant management in the third stage of labour. Cochrane Database Syst Rev. 2000;(2): CD000007.
109. Cotter AM, Ness A, Tolosa JE. Prophylactic oxytocin for the third stage of labour. Cochrane Database Syst Rev. 2001;(4):CD001808.
110. National Institute for Health and Care Excellence. Caesarean section NICE guidelines (CG132). London: RCOG Press; 2011.
111. McDonald SJ, Abbott JM, Higgins SP. Prophylactic ergometrine-oxytocin versus oxytocin for the third

stage of labour. Cochrane Database Syst Rev. 2004;(1):CD000201.
112. Gulmezoglu AM, Forna F, Villar J, Hofmeyr GJ. Prostaglandins for prevention of postpartum haemorrhage. Cochrane Database Syst Rev. 2007;(3): CD000494.
113. B-Lynch C, Keith LG, Lalonde AB, Koroshi M, editors. A textbook of postpartum hemorrhage. Duncow: Sapiens Publishing; 2006.
114. Gynaecologists RCoOa. Blood transfusions in obstetrics, Green-top guideline, vol. 47. London: RCOG Press; 2007; minor revisions 2008.
115. Stainsby D, MacLennan S, Thomas D, Isaac J, Hamilton PJ. Guidelines on the management of massive blood loss. Br J Haematol. 2006;135(5): 634–41.
116. Afshari A, Wikkelso A, Brok J, Moller AM, Wetterslev J. Thrombelastography (TEG) or thromboelastometry (ROTEM) to monitor haemotherapy versus usual care in patients with massive transfusion. Cochrane Database Syst Rev. 2011;16(3), CD007871.
117. Fuller AJ, Bucklin B. Blood component therapy in obstetrics. Obstet Gynecol Clin North Am. 2007;34(3):443–58, xi. [Review].
118. Keriakos R, Mukhopadhyay A. The use of the Rusch balloon for management of severe postpartum haemorrhage. J Obstet Gynaecol. 2006;26(4):335–8.
119. Ikechebelu JI, Obi RA, Joe-Ikechebelu NN. The control of postpartum haemorrhage with intrauterine Foley catheter. J Obstet Gynaecol. 2005;25(1): 70–2.
120. Bakri YN, Amri A, Abdul Jabbar F. Tamponade-balloon for obstetrical bleeding. Int J Gynaecol Obstet. 2001;74(2):139–42.
121. Chan C, Razvi K, Tham KF, Arulkumaran S. The use of a Sengstaken-Blakemore tube to control postpartum hemorrhage. Int J Gynaecol Obstet. 1997;58(2):251–2.
122. Akhter S, Begum MR, Kabir Z, Rashid M, Laila TR, Zabeen F. Use of a condom to control massive postpartum hemorrhage. MedGenMed. 2003;5(3):38.
123. Lennox C, Marr L. Scottish confidential audit of severe maternal morbidity. 9th Annual Report (Data from 2011). Healthcare Improvement Scotland. 2013. Available online – http://www.scottishpatientsafetyprogramme.scot.nhs.uk/Media/Docs/MCQIC/Maternity%20Care/2013-08-09%20Final%209th%20annual%20SCASMM%20report.pdf.
124. B-Lynch C, Coker A, Lawal AH, Abu J, Cowen MJ. The B-Lynch surgical technique for the control of massive postpartum haemorrhage: an alternative to hysterectomy? Five cases reported. Br J Obstet Gynaecol. 1997;104(3):372–5.
125. Wee L, Barron J, Toye R. Management of severe postpartum haemorrhage by uterine artery embolization. Br J Anaesth. 2004;93(4):591–4.
126. Dildy 3rd GA. Postpartum hemorrhage: new management options. Clin Obstet Gynecol. 2002;45(2): 330–44.
127. Joshi VM, Otiv SR, Majumder R, Nikam YA, Shrivastava M. Internal iliac artery ligation for arresting postpartum haemorrhage. BJOG. 2007;114(3):356–61.
128. National Patient Safety Agency. Rapid response report: the transfusion of blood and blood components in an emergency. United Kingdom; 2010.
129. Milkins C, Berryman J, Cantwell C, Elliott C, Haggas R, Jones J, et al. Guidelines for pre-transfusion compatibility procedures in blood transfusion laboratories. British Committee for Standards in Haematology. Transfus Med. 2013;23(1):3–35 [Practice Guideline].
130. United Kingdon Blood Service. Effective transfusion in obstetrics practice. In: Norfolk D, editor. Handbook of transfusion medicine. 5th ed. London: The Stationery Office; 2013. p. 107–13
131. Win N. High titre Anti-A/B testing of donors within NHS Blood and Transplant (NHSBT). London: NBS; 2011 [cited 2012 November 28]; Available from: http://hospital.blood.co.uk/library/pdf/INF178.pdf.
132. Dutton RP, Shih D, Edelman BB, Hess J, Scalea TM. Safety of uncrossmatched type-O red cells for resuscitation from hemorrhagic shock. J Trauma. 2005;59(6):1445–9.
133. Murthi SB, Dutton RP, Edelman BB, Scalea TM, Hess JR. Transfusion medicine in trauma patients. Expert Rev Hematol. 2008;1(1):99–109 [Review].
134. Chandrasekar A, Morris KG, Tubman TR, Tharma S, McClelland WM. The clinical outcome of non-RhD antibody affected pregnancies in Northern Ireland. Ulster Med J. 2001;70(2):89–94.
135. Karlsson O, Jeppsson A, Hellgren M. Major obstetric haemorrhage: monitoring with thromboelastography, laboratory analyses or both? Int J Obstet Anesth. 2014;23(1):10–7 [Observational Study Research Support, Non-U.S. Gov't].
136. Dzik WH, Blajchman MA, Fergusson D, Hameed M, Henry B, Kirkpatrick AW, et al. Clinical review: Canadian National Advisory Committee on Blood and Blood Products–Massive transfusion consensus conference 2011: report of the panel. Crit Care. 2011;15(6):242 [Consensus Development Conference Research Support, Non-U.S. Gov't Review].
137. McLintock C, James AH. Obstetric hemorrhage. J Thromb Haemost. 2011;9(8):1441–51 [Review].
138. Charbit B, Mandelbrot L, Samain E, Baron G, Haddaoui B, Keita H, et al. The decrease of fibrinogen is an early predictor of the severity of postpartum hemorrhage. J Thromb Haemost. 2007;5(2):266–73 [Research Support, Non-U.S. Gov't].
139. de Lloyd L, Bovington R, Kaye A, Collis RE, Rayment R, Sanders J, et al. Standard haemostatic tests following major obstetric haemorrhage. Int J Obstet Anesth. 2011;20(2):135–41.
140. Knowles SM, Cohen H. The 2010 annual SHOT report: the Serious Hazards of Transfusion (SHOT) Steering Group; 2011.
141. NHS Department of Health/Patient Safety and Investigations. Transfusion of ABO-incompatible

blood components; 2012 (The "never events" list 2012/2013): Available from: https://www.gov.uk/government/uploads/system/uploads/attachment_data/file/142013/Never_events_201213.pdf.
142. Contreas C, editor. ABS of transfusion. 4th ed. Chichester: Wiley-Blackwell/BMJ Books; 2009.
143. Bolton-Maggs PHB, Cohen H. The 2011 annual SHOT report: the Serious Hazards of Transfusion (SHOT) Steering Group; 2012.
144. Ahonen J, Stefanovic V, Lassila R. Management of post-partum haemorrhage. Acta Anaesthesiol Scand. 2010;54(10):1164–78 [Review].
145. Sorensen B, Bevan D. A critical evaluation of cryoprecipitate for replacement of fibrinogen. Br J Haematol. 2010;149(6):834–43 [Evaluation Studies Research Support, Non-U.S. Gov't].
146. Davenport R, Curry N, Manson J, De'Ath H, Coates A, Rourke C, et al. Hemostatic effects of fresh frozen plasma may be maximal at red cell ratios of 1:2. J Trauma. 2011;70(1):90–5; discussion 5–6. [Research Support, Non-U.S. Gov't].
147. Rahe-Meyer N, Sorensen B. For: fibrinogen concentrate for management of bleeding. J Thromb Haemost. 2011;9(1):1–5 [Research Support, Non-U.S. Gov't].
148. Bell SF, Rayment R, Collins PW, Collis RE. The use of fibrinogen concentrate to correct hypofibrinogenaemia rapidly during obstetric haemorrhage. Int J Obstet Anesth. 2010;19(2):218–23 [Case Reports].
149. Wikkelsoe AJ, Afshari A, Stensballe J, Langhoff-Roos J, Albrechtsen C, Ekelund K, et al. The FIB-PPH trial: fibrinogen concentrate as initial treatment for postpartum haemorrhage: study protocol for a randomised controlled trial. Trials. 2012;13:110 [Multicenter Study Randomized Controlled Trial Research Support, Non-U.S. Gov't].
150. Hiippala ST, Myllyla GJ, Vahtera EM. Hemostatic factors and replacement of major blood loss with plasma-poor red cell concentrates. Anesth Analg. 1995;81(2):360–5.
151. Qureshi H, Massey E, Kirwan D, Davies T, Robson S, White J, et al. BCSH guideline for the use of anti-D immunoglobulin for the prevention of haemolytic disease of the fetus and newborn. Transfus Med. 2014;24(1):8–20.
152. Logan AC, Goodnough LT. Recombinant factor VIIa: an assessment of evidence regarding its efficacy and safety in the off-label setting. Hematology Am Soc Hematol Educ Program. 2010;2010:153–9 [Review].
153. Phillips LE, McLintock C, Pollock W, Gatt S, Popham P, Jankelowitz G, et al. Recombinant activated factor VII in obstetric hemorrhage: experiences from the Australian and New Zealand Haemostasis Registry. Anesth Analg. 2009;109(6):1908–15. [Research Support, Non-U.S. Gov't].
154. Ferrer P, Roberts I, Sydenham E, Blackhall K, Shakur H. Anti-fibrinolytic agents in post partum haemorrhage: a systematic review. BMC Pregnancy Childbirth. 2009;9:29 [Review].

15 Thrombocytopenia in Pregnancy: Gestational Thrombocytopenia and Immune Thrombocytopenic Purpura

Stavroula Tsiara, Catherine Nelson-Piercy, and Nichola Cooper

Abstract

The management of immune thrombocytopenic purpura (ITP) during pregnancy can be challenging. The diagnosis and distinction between gestational thrombocytopenia and ITP is important and requires assessment of the timing and degree of thrombocytopenia. Exclusion of thrombocytopenia of another origin and of secondary causes of ITP is also vital before embarking on treatment, and current therapeutic options are discussed in this chapter. The mode of delivery should be based on obstetric indications. Fetal scalp blood sampling is not recommended as the incidence of neonatal bleeding remains low, but an umbilical cord-derived blood count should be taken at birth. In babies who are thrombocytopenic, intravenous immunoglobulin treatment is recommended and platelet counts should be repeated daily until normalized.

Keywords

Gestational thrombocytopenia • Immune thrombocytopenic purpura • Corticosteroids • Intravenous immunoglobulin

S. Tsiara, MB ChB, MD, PhD, FRCP (✉)
Department of Internal Medicine,
University Hospital of Ioannina,
University Campus, Stavros Niarchos Av,
Ioannina 45 500, Greece
e-mail: stsiara@cc.uoi.gr

C. Nelson-Piercy, MBBS, MA, FRCP, FRCOG
Women's Health Academic Centre,
Guy's & St Thomas' Foundation Trust and Imperial College Healthcare Trust, St Thomas' Hospital,
Westminster Bridge Road, London SE17EH, UK
e-mail: catherine.nelson-piercy@gstt.nhs.uk

N. Cooper, MB ChB, MA, MD, FRCP, FRCPath
Centre for Haematology, Faculty of Medicine,
Hammersmith Campus, Imperial College Healthcare NHS Trust, Du Cane Road, London W12 0HS, UK
e-mail: n.cooper@imperial.ac.uk

15.1 Introduction

The most common isolated disorder of platelets observed during pregnancy is thrombocytopenia. This abnormality is of particular interest because it can affect both mother and fetus, causing maternal and neonatal hemorrhagic complications. Although the majority of women have normal platelet counts during pregnancy, there is frequently a slight platelet fall, particularly during the third trimester, with platelet counts fluctuating from 109 to 341×10^9/L [1–4] This mild thrombocytopenia reflects a benign condition called incidental or gestational thrombocytopenia (GT) [3, 4]. Other causes of isolated

H. Cohen, P. O'Brien (eds.), *Disorders of Thrombosis and Hemostasis in Pregnancy: A Guide to Management*, DOI 10.1007/978-3-319-15120-5_15, © Springer-Verlag London 2015

thrombocytopenia during pregnancy include immune thrombocytopenia (ITP); pre-eclampsia; hemolysis, elevated liver enzymes, low platelets (HELLP) syndrome; disseminated intravascular coagulation (DIC); microangiopathic hemolytic anemias (MAHA), including hemolytic uremic syndrome (HUS) and thrombotic thrombocytopenic purpura (TTP); antiphospholipid syndrome (APS); sepsis; HIV or malaria infection; thrombocytopenia induced by drugs (e.g. unfractionated heparin); type IIbIIB von Willebrand disease; and the congenital thrombocytopenias [3–6].

Following the widespread use of automatic hematologic counters, another cause of apparent thrombocytopenia has emerged: spurious thrombocytopenia or "pseudothrombocytopenia." This *in vitro* phenomenon, which is not of clinical significance, occurs when EDTA (ethylenediaminetetraacetic acid) is used as the anticoagulant for blood collection. Platelets agglutinate or form clumps and the real platelet number cannot be recognized by the automatic analyzer. This phenomenon is related to the activation of certain platelet membrane glycoprotein receptors and occurs only *ex vivo* when platelets are exposed to the EDTA. For the exclusion of spurious thrombocytopenia related to EDTA, blood must be collected in tubes containing sodium citrate or heparin as the anticoagulant, although these anticoagulants may also induce platelet clumping.

Another type of spurious thrombocytopenia is satellitism, when platelets form rosettes around white blood cells and cannot be accurately counted. Also, when there are large platelets in the circulation, they may be misdiagnosed as red cells by the automatic analyzer. In all thrombocytopenic patients, a careful examination of a blood smear is the best method to exclude misleading conditions in order to avoid unnecessary investigation and treatment [3–7].

15.2 Gestational Thrombocytopenia

Gestational thrombocytopenia was first described by Burrows and Kelton in 1988 and reflects a condition that occurs during the second and third trimesters of pregnancy [3–6, 8, 9]. In patients with GT, the antenatal booking platelet count is normal and, in the majority, the platelet count is mildly decreased to between 100 and 150×10^9/L. In rare cases, the platelet count might fall below 80×10^9/L [2–6]. The low platelet count usually returns to normal within 12 weeks of delivery [8, 9]. Differences in the timing of the platelet fall and the degree of thrombocytopenia, shown in Table 15.1, help to differentiate between GT and ITP [10]. Overall, when isolated mild thrombocytopenia appears in the last trimester of pregnancy, it is most commonly due to GT or pre-eclampsia, rather than to ITP or other causes of thrombocytopenia [3–6, 10]. Similarly, the platelet count on the day of delivery is significantly higher in patients with GT, relative to that of patients with ITP [10].

Table 15.1 Variables significantly differentiating gestational thrombocytopenia (GT) and immune thrombocytopenia (ITP) [10]

Variable	GT	ITP
Gestational age at diagnosis (weeks)	32.8 ± 7.6	20.1 ± 11.1
Gestational age when platelet count counts at nadir (weeks)	35.7 ± 5.5	27.0 ± 11.2
Platelet count at diagnosis ($\times 10^9$/L)	71.3 ± 19.2	40.0 ± 25.5
Platelet count at nadir ($\times 10^9$/L)	58.6 ± 24.1	24.3 ± 15.5
Platelet count on day of delivery ($\times 10^9$/L)	70.1 ± 28.2	37.3 ± 24.0
Platelet count on day 3 postpartum day 3 ($\times 10^9$/L)	100.9 ± 1.6	81.9 ± 26.3

The incidence of GT has been investigated by several authors. In two population studies, one including almost 7,000 and the other over 4,000 women, the rate of GT was 10.9 and 5.9 %, respectively, while in another study it was estimated at 5.4 % [2–6, 8]. Although the pathogenesis of this phenomenon is unknown, it has been proposed that thrombocytopenia results from the relative hemodilution that occurs in pregnancy in combination with the capture and destruction of platelets in the placental bed [11]. Women with GT are usually asymptomatic and do not have a history of previous thrombocytopenia, although if they have previously been pregnant, are likely also to have had GT in the previous pregnancy. The diagnosis is usually made when a low platelet count is discovered incidentally on routine laboratory testing during the second or third trimester, or when delivery is imminent [2–6]. Other hematological and biochemical parameters are usually normal [2–6].

In the majority of women with GT, pregnancy and the peripartum period are uneventful, and there are no complications for either mother or baby related to the low platelet count [2–6, 9]. The risk of developing a low platelet count in neonates of mothers with GT has been determined from cord blood samples and was found to be 4 %, similar to that observed in infants born to women with a normal platelet count [2–6]. However, in a prospective study of cord blood platelet counts in women with thrombocytopenia, 7 of 33 (21 %) babies of mothers with GT had low platelet counts (none of the babies had sepsis). The neonates' platelet counts ranged from 58 to 144×10^9/L, and none required treatment. The authors recommended that for every baby born to a mother with a pregnancy-associated thrombocytopenia, even in the case of confirmed GT, platelet count in cord blood should be checked [12]. Although GT is a benign condition, platelet counts should be monitored during pregnancy in order to detect any sudden decline with the potential for subsequent hemorrhagic manifestations [2–6].

15.3 Immune Thrombocytopenic Purpura (ITP): Definition

Immune thrombocytopenic purpura is an acquired disorder of platelet number that is characterized by immune-mediated platelet destruction [2–6, 13].

The disease is usually benign with the majority of patients being asymptomatic [3–6]. It is not infrequent in women of childbearing age, although the prevalence increases with age [14–16]. The main clinical feature of the disease is hemorrhagic manifestations ranging from mild cutaneous bleeding lesions such as petechiae and ecchymoses to, rarely, severe intracranial hemorrhage [2, 13, 17, 18]. Although in children the disease is usually self-limiting, in adults it usually runs a relapsing-remitting course [2, 17, 18].

15.4 ITP: Terminology and Classification

An international working group on ITP stipulated that its diagnosis requires a platelet count lower than 100×10^9/L [18] and that the thrombocytopenia should be isolated, with an otherwise normal full blood count, peripheral blood smear and biochemical indices [18]. Additionally, on clinical examination there should be no pathological features indicative of an underlying disease that could precipitate thrombocytopenia [18]. In borderline conditions, when the platelet count ranges between 100 and 150×10^9/L, patients have a low probability (6.9 %) of developing more profound thrombocytopenia and hemorrhagic complications [18]. These patients should be regularly monitored but they do not usually need treatment [18–20]. ITP is termed 'persistent' when it lasts between 3 and 12 months, and 'chronic' when low platelet counts are observed for more than 12 months [18]. It is very important to distinguish between primary and secondary ITP [18]. Secondary ITP has a different natural history and usually resolves when the underlying condition is treated [18].

The same definitions should be applied to pregnant women with ITP [21].

15.5 ITP: Epidemiology

The incidence of ITP is not well defined. In a study based on the UK General Practice Research Database, the incidence of ITP in the general population has been determined as 3.9 cases/100,000 person-years. The incidence of ITP in women ranges from 3.7 cases/100,000 person-years in those under 18 years to 3.8 between 18 and 64 years and 7.1 in women above 65 years [14–16].

During pregnancy, determination of the incidence of ITP is even more challenging because of the difficulty in distinguishing ITP from other causes of thrombocytopenia, including GT [2–6]. Some authors estimate the prevalence of ITP as approximately 1–5 cases/10,000 pregnancies, whereas the prevalence of GT in the same population is 100 times greater [2–6, 22–24]. Other investigators estimated that ITP occurs in 1/1,000–1/10,000 pregnant women [2–6, 14, 21–23]. In a Korean study, among 31,309 women who were reviewed, 25 (0.07 %) were diagnosed with ITP and 33 (0.1 %) were diagnosed with GT [10].

Similar results were obtained from a study that enrolled 62,441 pregnant women: The diagnosis of ITP was established in 55 women (0.08 %), 24 of whom had a previous history of ITP [25].

15.6 ITP: Pathophysiology

Although the underlying pathophysiological disorder in ITP remains unknown, several studies convincingly demonstrate an altered immune response, as reviewed by Cines and Mc Millan [26]. The major feature of ITP has been considered to be the production of anti-platelet antibodies (IgG or IgM) by activated B lymphocytes. The target of these antibodies is most frequently platelet membrane glycoproteins GPIIb/IIa and Ib/IX [26, 27], although other platelet membrane glycoprotein antibodies have also been described [26, 27]. Immune complexes containing platelets coated by antiplatelet antibodies are cleared by the Fcg receptors of the mononuclear cells in the reticuloendothelial system [28]. These cells are located primarily in the spleen but also in other organs such as the liver and bone marrow [28, 29]. Specific genetic polymorphisms of the Fcg receptors have been observed in patients with ITP, which may result in enhanced clearance of the antibody-coated platelet [27–31]. Although antiplatelet antibodies had been considered the hallmark of ITP, they have characteristically been difficult to measure and it is clear that T lymphocytes contribute to, if not initiate, ITP pathogenesis [26, 29, 32–34]. A number of studies have described polarization of T helper cells toward the Th1 immune response with an increase in the production of IL-2, IFN-g, and TNF-a [26, 29, 32–34]. This response activates cytotoxic, inflammatory and delayed hypersensitivity reactions [26, 29, 32–34]. In contrast, there is a reduction in Th2 response cells that produce IL-4, IL-5, IL-6, IL-9, IL-10, and IL-13 cytokines [26, 28, 29, 31–34]. Activated T cells not only increase the biogenesis of B cells producing antiplatelet antibodies but also show direct CD8-mediated cytotoxicity against platelets and megakaryocytes in some patients with ITP [32, 35]. More recently, regulatory T cells have been found.to be decreased in both number and functional activity when compared to those in healthy individuals, indicating loss of immune tolerance [36, 37]. Ongoing interaction between B cells and T cells is also suggested by elevated CD40 and CD40L (CD154) on the surface of B and T cells. Increased levels of CD154 were also found on the platelet surface in patients with ITP, suggesting that *in vivo* activation of autoreactive B lymphocytes may be driven by platelets [38].

There are also signals that impaired thrombopoiesis contributes to the thrombocytopenia in ITP [21, 26, 29, 39]. Platelet survival studies have revealed a low or inappropriately normal (rather than increased as a response to thrombocytopenia) production of platelets in patients with ITP [21, 26, 29, 39, 40]. Electron microscope images and *in vitro* studies suggest increased apoptotic indices and poor differentiation, presumably driven by antiplatelet antibodies directed at the megakaryocytes [41]. In addition, it has been reported that, in bone marrow biopsy specimens from ITP patients, there is an increased proportion of megakaryocytes with activated caspase-3, reflecting a direct effect of B and T cells on megakaryocytes [42].

Moreover, thrombopoietin, the growth factor for megakaryocytes and platelets, is inappropriately low for the platelet count when compared to the thrombopoietin levels in patients with thrombocytopenia due to other causes such as aplastic anemia [21].

Although in the majority of patients with ITP the precipitating cause remains obscure, it has been observed that viral and bacterial infections may initiate the condition [26, 29, 43]. Viruses may cause secondary ITP, inducing loss of immune tolerance, a decrease in T helper cells, direct proliferation of B cells leading to increased antibody production, and macrophage activation which contributes to the disease severity [26, 29]. Bacterial infections, such as H. pylori infection, are also implicated in the pathogenesis of ITP, and eradication therapy can result in prolonged remissions [43]. In this situation ITP may be caused by molecular mimicry where, instead of additional production of antibodies against H. pylori, there is antibody production to self. Moreover, alterations in the cytokine milieu stimulate B cell activation and loss of immune tolerance [26, 29, 43].

Overall, it is clear that ITP is characterized by pathogenetic diversity. Several factors can provoke the initiation of the disease and contribute to thrombocytopenia. This pathogenetic diversity observed in ITP leads to similar variability in the clinical expression of the disease. The variation observed in the clinical picture is irrespective of the severity of thrombocytopenia and the presence of antiplatelet antibodies [17].

Better understanding of the pathogenesis of the disease will hopefully lead to treatments targeted at many of these pathophysiological alterations, and amelioration of the hemorrhagic tendency [29].

15.7 ITP: Clinical Features and Differential Diagnosis

As also occurs in the general population with ITP, pregnant women with ITP may present with hemorrhagic manifestations of variable severity, or thrombocytopenia might be an incidental finding on routine laboratory testing. There may be a preceding history of ITP with or without treatment [2–6, 13, 44].

Women with a history of previous ITP may present with an exacerbation during any trimester, or the disease may remain quiescent [3–6]. As in the non-pregnant population, the diagnosis of ITP is one of exclusion [17, 22, 45]. In accordance with the International Consensus Report guidance on the diagnosis and treatment of ITP, it is important that other causes of maternal thrombocytopenia during pregnancy should be excluded [13, 17].

Table 15.2 Causes of thrombocytopenia exclusively associated with pregnancy

Gestational thrombocytopenia
Pre-eclampsia
HELLP syndrome
Obstetric hemorrhage
Acute fatty liver of pregnancy

HELLP hemolysis, elevated liver enzymes, and low platelets

Table 15.3 Causes of thrombocytopenia not necessarily associated with pregnancy

Spurious – EDTA-dependent platelet agglutination
Drug-related thrombocytopenia (e.g., unfractionated heparin)
Thrombotic microangiopathies (HUS, TTP, DIC)
SLE and antiphospholipid syndrome
Autoimmune diseases (autoimmune hepatitis, Crohn's disease, thyroiditis)
Nutritional deficiencies (folate and B12 deficiency)
Lymphoproliferative diseases (CLL and lymphomas)
Infections (HIV, HCV, H. Pylori)
Immunodeficiencies (common variable immunodeficiency, IgA deficiency)
Nutritional deficiencies (folate and B12 deficiency)
Concurrent bone marrow disorders
Congenital platelet disorders
Type II von Willebrand Disease (IIB vWD)
Hypersplenism

HUS hemolytic uremic syndrome, *TTP* thrombotic thrombocytopenic purpura, *DIC* disseminated intravascular coagulopathy, *SLE* systemic lupus erythematosus, *CLL* chronic lymphocytic leukaemia, *HIV* human immunodeficiency virus, *HCV* hepatitis C virus

In Table 15.2, the causes of thrombocytopenia associated only with pregnancy are shown. Thrombocytopenic conditions not necessarily associated with pregnancy are listed in Table 15.3 and laboratory investigations that should be performed in pregnant women with suspected ITP for the exclusion of underlying diseases are shown in Table 15.4. Serum antiplatelet antibodies cannot clearly establish the diagnosis of ITP because they lack specificity. During pregnancy, they are equally uninformative and they do not predict the risk of maternal or fetal hemorrhage [17, 44]. In a study including 6,770 pregnant women, 566 of whom had thrombocytopenia, anti-platelet antibodies

Table 15.4 Investigation of suspected immune thrombocytopenic purpura (ITP)

Full blood count and peripheral blood film
Coagulation screen (PT, APTT, fibrinogen)
Liver function tests
Antinuclear antibodies (ANA), anti-DNA and ENA
Blood RhD group (if anti-D contemplated)
HIV and HCV
Antiphospholipid antibodies (lupus anticoagulant, anticardiolipin and anti-beta 2 glycoprotein 1 antibodies)

PT prothrombin time, *APTT* activated partial thromboplastin time, *HIV* human immunodeficiency virus, *HCV* hepatitis C virus

detected using the monoclonal antibody-specific immobilization of platelet antigens assay (MAIPA), were identified in 6.7 % of thrombocytopenic women; this was no different to the incidence of detection of antibodies in non-thrombocytopenic women [46]. Other investigators found that antiplatelet antibodies were evident at a similar rate of 20.8 % of pregnant patients with ITP and 16.7 % of those with GT [10]. Similarly inconclusive results have been reported in other studies [8, 25]. In this context, the International Consensus Report does not recommend serum antiplatelet antibody testing as is not considered to be a valuable method to establish the diagnosis of ITP in pregnancy [13, 17]. Similarly, bone marrow examination is not necessary for the confirmation of ITP in pregnancy, unless there are clinical or laboratory indications of another underlying hematological disease [13, 17]. In patients who fail to respond to conventional therapeutic strategies, or when splenectomy is planned for curative purposes, bone marrow aspiration and biopsy should be considered [13, 17].

15.8 ITP: Risks of ITP During Pregnancy

Although sometimes difficult to achieve, it is critical to determine the cause of thrombocytopenia, because women with GT usually have an uneventful pregnancy and peripartum period. In contrast, women with ITP sometimes develop severe thrombocytopenia and experience hemorrhagic complications during delivery and postpartum, and require more careful monitoring [2, 13, 17]. The platelet count is an important predictor of hemorrhage in these patients [2, 13, 17].

The risk of significant hemorrhage is related to the severity of the thrombocytopenia and the gestational age at the time of diagnosis of ITP [2, 13, 17]. Women with thrombocytopenia also have a higher rate of non-hemorrhagic maternal and fetal complications. In one study which compared 199 pregnant women with thrombocytopenia due to a variety of causes (mainly GT and to a lesser extent ITP, pre-eclampsia, DIC, HELLP syndrome, and antiphospholipid syndrome APS), to 201 women with normal platelet counts, the following complications were significantly more common ($p<0.001$) in the thrombocytopenia group: preterm delivery (<37 weeks), placental abruption, intrauterine growth restriction ($p<0.003$), stillbirth, need for induction of labor, low neonatal Apgar scores (<7) at 1 and 5 min, and need for blood or blood component transfusion in the mother [11].

15.9 ITP: Management During Pregnancy

The management of ITP in pregnancy should be undertaken within a multidisciplinary setting with close liaison between obstetricians, haematologists, anesthetists and neonatologists. Management is based on the estimated risk of significant maternal hemorrhage [2, 13, 17, 47]. As the platelet count usually declines during the third trimester, careful monitoring is required to ensure that it is adequate around the time of delivery [2, 13, 17]. The frequency of platelet count determination is based on the absolute number of platelets and the gestation [13, 17].

In patients with secondary ITP because of hepatitis C (HCV) infection, antiviral therapy should be considered. However, the platelet count should be closely monitored because of the risk of worsening thrombocytopenia attributable to interferon. For patients with HIV-associated ITP, treatment of the HIV infection with antiviral therapy should be considered before other treatment options unless the patient has clinically significant bleeding complications. *H pylori* eradication therapy should be administered to patients found to have this infection [11].

Women with ITP should receive preconception counseling. Counseling of ITP patients considering pregnancy should address safety of mother and fetus, outcomes of worsening maternal disease, and risks of pregnancy itself [17].

15.10 ITP: Indications for Treatment

Throughout the first and the second trimesters, treatment for ITP is not indicated unless:

- Hemorrhagic manifestations are evident
- The platelet count is lower than $20–30 \times 10^9$/L
- There is a need to increase the platelet count to a level safe for an invasive procedure such as amniocentesis

During the second and the third trimesters or when delivery is imminent, the platelet count should exceed 20×10^9/L [2, 17, 48, 49]. There are some variations in guidance on platelet count thresholds around delivery, summarized here. The 2010 International Consensus Report states that hematologists believe that the platelet count considered safe for Cesarean section (CS) is at least 50×10^9/L (which is therefore also required for vaginal delivery as emergency CS may be required); and that obstetric anesthetists generally recommend a platelet count of at least 75×10^9/L for spinal or epidural anesthesia. The authors of the 2011 American Society of Hematology (ASH) guidelines state that they found no evidence has been found to support specific platelet count thresholds that are 'safe' in the antenatal or peripartum periods [1, 17, 48, 49].

15.11 ITP: Recommended Medical Treatment

Therapeutic options used for the treatment of ITP in pregnancy are similar to those used outside of pregnancy [2, 13, 17]. Drugs of choice for first-line treatment are corticosteroids and intravenous immunoglobulin (IVIg). There is also limited evidence supporting the use of intravenous (IV) anti-RhD immunoglobulin (anti-D) [2, 13, 50]. Splenectomy, azathioprine, or combinations of the first-line treatment options mentioned above can be used in unresponsive or relapsing patients [2, 13, 17].

Other therapeutic modalities such as rituximab, vinca alkaloids, danazol, recombinant thrombopoietin receptor agonists, and immunosuppressive drugs should generally be avoided during pregnancy because of lack of evidence of benefit and the risks of possible harmful effects on the fetus [17].

15.11.1 Corticosteroids

Prednisolone is the most commonly used therapy in both pregnant and non-pregnant patients [2, 13, 17]. Although the standard therapy for ITP is oral administration of prednisolone in a dose of 0.5–1 mg/kg/day [2, 13, 17], during pregnancy a lower dose, such as 10–20 mg a day, is frequently used [17]. Prednisolone is extensively metabolized in the placenta with only 10 % reaching the fetus, so is considered safe for both mother and fetus [4, 13, 17].

Concerns about the use of steroids include hypertension, hyperglycemia, osteoporosis, excessive weight gain and psychosis in the mother. If higher doses are used for initial therapy, the dose should be carefully tapered to the minimum required for maintaining a safe count for delivery [2, 22, 51].

Corticosteroid administration has been described in an observational study including 110 women, 37 of whom required therapy [24]. Prednisone alone was administered in eight patients, and in seven the drug was administered in combination with IVIg [24]. Treatment was effective in increasing the platelet count, but the increase was transient. No severe side-effects were observed [24]. In another study in 284 pregnant women, 94 required therapy. Eighty-five patients received corticosteroids in various dose regimens [52]. Women treated with doses exceeding 15 mg/day delivered infants with abnormal body weight, either small or large for dates ($p=0.017$) [52]. Although corticosteroids are considered safe therapy for the fetus, a slightly increased incidence of fetal death and congenital abnormalities ($p=0.043$) was observed in one group of patients treated with larger doses (exceeding 15 mg/day) compared with the non-treated patients [52]. It seems sensible, therefore, that the lowest dose of steroids required to maintain a "safe" platelet count should be used [24, 44, 52].

Platelet counts should be carefully monitored during pregnancy and after delivery, particularly during the phase of dose tapering, to avoid a rapid fall in levels [17].

15.11.2 Intravenous Immunoglobulin (IVIg)

When corticosteroid therapy is ineffective, or has unacceptable side effects, or high dose and prolonged duration of therapy is required to achieve an adequate platelet count, IVIg should be considered as an alternative [50, 53, 54]. As second-line treatment after steroid failure, IVIg should be administered when the platelet count falls below 10×10^9/L. IVIg should be administered, alone or in combination with corticosteroid, whenever a rapid rise in platelet count is needed, such as when the platelet count is $10–30\times10^9$/L and there is active bleeding, or in asymptomatic women with a platelet count $10–30\times10^9$/L when delivery is imminent [17, 22, 48].

There are no studies comparing the safety and efficacy of prednisolone and IVIg [53, 54]. However, data from observational studies on the administration of IVIg during pregnancy show that response rates are similar to those in the non-pregnant population, with an excellent safety profile for both mother and fetus [50, 53]. Although the response rate in pregnancy exceeds that with corticosteroids, with an increase in the platelet count of up to 80 %, the effect is usually transient [53].

The mode of activity of IVIg in ITP is complicated and relates to increased expression of the inhibitory receptor FcRIIb, possibly just from the activity of a small fraction of the IVIg used [50, 55]. IVIg recipients are more likely to attain a platelet increase within 24 h at a dose of 1 g/kg (1–2 infusions over 2 days) compared with the historical treatment regimen (0.4 g/kg/day over 5 days) [56]. The ASH guidelines suggest that, if IVIg is used, the dose should initially be 1 g/kg as a one-time dose. This dosage may be repeated if necessary [49]. A small number of patients who fail to respond to this dose may respond to a second infusion [17, 50]. If patients do not tolerate this large volume of infusion, smaller doses given over a number of days may be administered [50]. The infusion may be repeated if necessary to prevent hemorrhage and maintain platelet counts at a level safe for delivery [50].

Although generally well tolerated, IVIg causes adverse effects in approximately 5 % of patients; these include headaches, chills, myalgia, arthralgia, and back pain [17]. Headaches can be severe with acute aseptic meningitis occurring within 72 h of administration in a minority of individuals. If side-effects occur during treatment, the infusion should be slowed or stopped to alleviate symptoms. If symptoms are anticipated, the patient may take antihistamines and/or intravenous hydrocortisone to prevent a reaction. More serious adverse events such as intravascular hemolysis, renal failure, stroke, and myocardial infarction are very rare [17]. IVIg undergoes a very rigorous production process, and transmission of viruses through IVIg has not been reported since the hepatitis C transmission reported in the 1990s [17].

15.11.3 Intravenous Anti-RhD Immunoglobulin (IV Anti-D)

Although intravenous anti-RhD immunoglobulin (IV anti-D) is widely used in patients with ITP, there are few published series describing its use during pregnancy [31, 50, 57, 58]. It has been administered for ITP in pregnancy, either alone or in combination with other therapies, when an immediate rise in platelet count is required [50, 57–59]. In a small study including ten pregnant women with ITP, IV anti-D was administered during the second and the third trimesters [57]. Many of the women were taking concomitant therapy and received the drug in an attempt to increase the platelet count. In all patients, the platelet count increased above 30×10^9/L without severe side-effects [57, 58]. There were no adverse events in the neonates. In particular, none of the neonates became anemic or jaundiced even though the direct antiglobulin test (DAT) was positive in 3 of the 7 RhD (Rhesus D) positive newborns [58]. Intravenous anti-D was also administered to a woman resistant to treatment with steroids and IVIg. She achieved a platelet count of $>40\times10^9$/L and had an uneventful vaginal delivery [60]. The platelet count remained high 1 week postpartum [60].

The International Consensus Recommendations suggest that anti-D may be administered during the second and the third trimesters in doses of 50–75 mg/kg, as a second-line therapy (evidence level IIb) [17]. However, monitoring of the neonate for jaundice, anemia, and a positive DAT is required [17, 59, 60].

The mode of action of IV anti-D immunoglobulin is different to that of IVIg. Following administration, anti-D-coated red blood cell complexes saturate Fcγ receptor sites on macrophages, resulting in preferential destruction of red blood cells (RBCs), therefore sparing antibody-coated platelets [31, 50, 61]. Anti-D immunoglobulin is generally ineffective in RhD positive or splenectomized patients and responses can vary; patients with HIV have a better and longer-lasting response to anti-D immunoglobulin than to IVIg [17, 31, 50, 61]. Anti-D does not work through the inhibitory FcRIIb receptor but through the activating receptors [31, 61, 62].

Like IVIg, IV anti-D is usually well tolerated. As the mode of action relates to the destruction of antibody-coated red blood cells, a fall in hemoglobin is usually seen, with a median fall of 1.5 g/dL [17, 50]. However, most individuals recover their hemoglobin levels well and only infrequently do patients develop significant anemia [17, 50, 61]. Shivers and shakes, which can accompany the infusion, are ameliorated by the use of antihistamines, paracetamol, and prednisolone premedication [17, 50]. Much more rarely, intravascular hemolysis has been reported, although not during pregnancy [17, 50]. The cases described were almost exclusively associated with another comorbidity, and it is recommended that IV anti-D is avoided during episodes of sepsis or if there is overt evidence of hemolysis or a positive DAT [17].

Anti-D immunoglobulin may not be available in all countries, and in June 2009, the European Medicines Agency was formally notified by Cangene Europe Ltd of its decision to withdraw all its applications and all marketing authorizations for their anti-D immunoglobulin product WinRho SDF.

15.12 ITP: Second-Line Treatment Options

As in non-pregnant individuals, combinations of first-line therapeutic options or splenectomy are appropriate in severely thrombocytopenic patients, in patients with hemorrhage, or prior to delivery (evidence level IV) [17].

15.12.1 Splenectomy

Splenectomy is a technically difficult procedure in pregnancy, particularly after the 20th week, and carries an increased risk of pregnancy loss [2, 17]. Hence, it is reserved for patients with disease resistant to other therapeutic options. It may be performed during the second or third trimesters, preferably using a laparoscopic technique [17].

The benefit of lifelong antibiotic prophylaxis in splenectomized patients with ITP is unproven, with the risk of late infection low, and therefore no consensus has been reached. A practical policy is for splenectomized patients to have a home supply of antibiotics for use in case of a febrile illness (appropriate agents include amoxicillin or clarithromycin). Patients should be educated about the risk of postsplenectomy infection, including the need to go to the emergency department if fever higher than 101 °F (38 °C) occurs [17, 63]. During pregnancy it is probably prudent to administer prophylactic antibiotics (e.g. Penicillin V 250 mg b.d.) to asplenic patients.

15.12.2 Use of Rituximab in Pregnancy

Rituximab has been given during pregnancy for a variety of indications including ITP, autoimmune hemolytic anemia, and thrombotic thrombocytopenic purpura, and to treat lymphoma [17, 64]. A summary of eight case reports of rituximab given during pregnancy described no adverse events for the fetus or the neonate, despite passage of rituximab across the placenta [65]. Rituximab was given at all stages of gestation (from week 1 to 34), and in this series, three babies were delivered prematurely (at 30, 33 and 35) with no adverse events reported [65]. B cells were depleted in four of five babies who were tested and normalized in at least one of these cases (the tests in the remaining patients were not reported) [65]. One additional child had normal levels of B cells 1 month after birth, when the mother had been treated at 21 weeks [65]. Vaccination titers were adequate in the four babies that were assessed, and immunoglobulin levels were appropriate in three children. One child, whose mother had received rituximab between 30 and 34 weeks' gestation, had low immunoglobulin levels at 1–2 months, but with partial recovery by 6 months [65]. No infectious complications were reported [65]. Although not recommended during pregnancy and not licensed for use in ITP, rituximab can be considered in refractory cases and may be safer than splenectomy and other immunosuppressive agents [17]. Although there have been reports of increased infections and rare cases of progressive multifocal leukoencephalopathy (PML) following rituximab, this appears to be more frequent in patients receiving treatment for lymphoproliferative disorders or SLE and has only very rarely been reported in adults with ITP treated with rituximab [66].

15.12.3 Other Immunosuppressive Agents

As a general rule, immunosuppressive or cytotoxic agents should be avoided during pregnancy [17]. However, there are reports that come mainly from the use of azathioprine in patients with inflammatory bowel disease, lupus, and transplant recipients [17]. In these cases, the drug has been proved safe for the fetus and the mother and may safely be administered during pregnancy in all three trimesters (evidence level III) [17].

Although cyclosporine A appears safe for the fetus, it is not recommended for the treatment of ITP in pregnancy [17]. Vincristine and cyclophosphamide have been used to treat pregnant women with lymphomas and cancer; however, their use should generally be avoided especially during the first trimester [17, 59], because of potential teratogenicity. The same applies to mycophenolate mofetil (MMF), which at progressively increasing doses (250 mg up to optimally 1,000 mg/day twice a week over 3 weeks) produced a platelet increase in 39 % of patients with refractory ITP, but this rise was not sustained [67]. In a retrospective study, the overall response rate was 78 % (major response, >80 × 109/L; and moderate response, 30–80 × 109/L at 3 months) [68].

15.12.4 TPO-Receptor Agonists: Romiplostim and Eltrombopag

Thrombopoietin (TPO) is the primary factor regulating platelet production, and several TPO-receptor agonists have been developed that activate the TPO receptor and increase platelet production [69–73]. Two agents, romiplostim and eltrombopag, are FDA- and EMA-approved for the treatment of ITP. These are the only treatments for refractory ITP that have been shown in randomized controlled trials to be effective. They are indicated for adult chronic immune ITP splenectomized patients who are refractory to other treatments (e.g. corticosteroids, immunoglobulins). Animal studies have shown reproductive toxicity and it is unknown whether these agents are secreted into human breastmilk; they are therefore not recommended during pregnancy or lactation [74, 75]. Romiplostim has been reported to successfully treat severe thrombocytopenia in a pregnant patient with systemic lupus erythematosus, presenting with major bleeding at 27 weeks. She was resistant to most treatment modalities, including steroids, intravenous immunoglobulin (IVIg), rituximab, IV cyclophosphamide and eltrombopag. She responded to romiplostim with normalization of her platelet count, which enabled her to be delivered safely at 34 weeks of gestation [76].

15.12.5 Platelet Transfusions

Prophylactic platelet transfusions are not generally indicated in the management of ITP [17]. Transfused platelets are cleared by the macrophages soon after infusion. Platelets should be infused only in cases of severe hemorrhage or immediately before the delivery, regional anesthesia, or other invasive procedures in thrombocytopenic women, in whom other treatment options have failed [17].

15.13 ITP: Mode of Delivery

Although moderate thrombocytopenia ($<50\times10^9$/L) may occur in approximately 10 % of neonates [13, 24], intracranial hemorrhage occurs in only 0–1.5 % of newborns with thrombocytopenia [4, 9, 17, 23, 24, 52, 77–79]. Data from retrospective reports and small studies including 608 pregnant women with thrombocytopenia (most of whom had ITP) showed that 417 (68.5 %) had a vaginal birth and 191 (31.5 %) had Cesarean section [8, 10, 24, 44, 52, 54]. Patients who underwent Cesarean section had more peri-operative complications, mainly at the site of surgical incisions [8, 10, 25, 44, 54]. Although there was evidence that uncomplicated vaginal delivery was safer for the woman, mild hemorrhagic complications such as soft tissue hematomas, were observed [3–6, 8, 10, 25, 44, 52, 54].

Given the low incidence of hemorrhagic complications in the newborn, current guidance suggests that the mode of delivery should be based on obstetric indications and not determined in relation to the platelet count. Platelet counts of at least 50×10^9/L are considered safe for vaginal delivery or Cesarean Section. There is no evidence that Cesarean section is safer for the fetus with thrombocytopenia than uncomplicated vaginal delivery (which is usually safer for the mother) [13, 17, 49].

15.14 ITP: Anesthetic Options

The reader should also refer to Chap. 21 on peri-delivery analgesia and anesthesia. BCSH guidelines (2003, now archived) suggested that the safe platelet count for regional/neuraxial anesthesia is 80×10^9/L [2]. However, the current trend is towards acceptance of a lower threshold [48]. In a study including 80 women with platelet counts lower than 100×10^9/L during the peripartum period, 52 received epidural anesthesia and 28 did not [48]. In this series, although platelet count was lower than 100×10^9/L, no hemorrhagic complications or neurological sequelae were seen [48]. Although there are insufficient data to indicate a safe platelet count required for these procedures, the International Consensus Report from 2010 states that a small consensus of obstetric anesthetists agree that the minimum platelet count required is 50×10^9/L, in the absence of bruising, bleeding history and recent anticoagulation. The international normalized ratio (INR) and the activated partial thromboplastin time (APTT) test should be within normal limits (evidence grade IV) [17].

15.15 Venous Thromboembolism

Some patients with ITP in pregnancy may be at increased risk of venous thromboembolism (VTE) because of associated APS, or as a result of other patient- or pregnancy-related factors. All patients should be assessed for their risk of VTE and managed accordingly (see Chap. 3), taking into account the level of thrombocytopenia.

Pregnant women with thrombocytopenia and APS associated with obstetric morbidity such as recurrent miscarriage or a history of previous or current thrombosis, should receive low dose aspirin (LDA) and low molecular weight heparin (LMWH). In these patients, platelet counts should be closely monitored; a platelet count $>50\times10^9$/L is considered safe for anticoagulation and LDA.

15.16 ITP: Management of Fetal and Neonatal Thrombocytopenia

15.16.1 Risk of Fetal and Neonatal Thrombocytopenia

One major concern in managing ITP during pregnancy is the risk of severe thrombocytopenia and intracranial hemorrhage in the newborn. The incidence of severe thrombocytopenia in the newborn of mothers with ITP is very low. Several studies show that the incidence of severe neonatal thrombocytopenia (platelet count lower than 50×10^9/L) ranges from 9 to 15 % [4, 17, 23, 52, 77–79]. Retrospective studies including 1,109 newborns in total show that 119 (10 %) had a platelet count lower than 50×10^9/L [8, 11, 24, 25, 44, 46, 52, 54, 78, 79]. Hemorrhagic complications have been observed in 0–1.5 % of the neonates with thrombocytopenia [9, 11, 18, 25, 44, 46, 52, 54, 59, 78, 79]. The risk of severe intracranial hemorrhage in these studies is quoted as less than 1 % [78].

Moreover, it is clear that the majority of hemorrhagic complications in the newborn where the mother has ITP occur postpartum (as opposed to intrapartum), when the neonatal platelet count is at its nadir, between the second and fifth day of life. The risk remains high until platelet counts begins to rise; this usually occurs by the seventh day of life [17, 59, 78].

15.16.2 Assessment of the Neonatal Platelet Count

Although neonatal thrombocytopenia and related hemorrhagic complications are rare, it is well documented that infants born to mothers with ITP are at greater risk of severe bleeding compared to other babies [9, 22, 24, 54, 59, 78, 79]. At delivery, umbilical cord blood (which is fetal blood) should be taken for a platelet count. If the baby is thrombocytopenic (platelet count lower than 50×10^9/L), daily monitoring is recommended and the neonate should undergo evaluation for evidence of intracranial hemorrhage with transcranial ultrasound [13, 17, 22].

Several attempts have been made to predict which neonates will be born with a low platelet count. Circulating maternal antiplatelet antibodies and maternal platelet count do not predict the risk of neonatal thrombocytopenia [46]. One report indicates that women with a pre-gestational history of ITP and a previous thrombocytopenic infant are more likely to deliver a neonate with a low platelet count [59]. Additionally, a history of severe maternal disease requiring splenectomy during pregnancy is another risk factor for neonatal thrombocytopenia [59].

15.16.3 Fetal Blood Sampling

Since maternal characteristics have been proven to be unreliable in predicting the platelet count in the newborn, direct platelet count determination before delivery by fetal blood sampling was previously employed. The methods used were fetal scalp sampling and umbilical cord blood sampling. However, fetal scalp blood sampling can be technically difficult and is not accurate, usually underestimating the platelet count because platelets may form *in vitro* microaggregates [9, 24, 59, 78, 79]. Although *in utero* umbilical cord blood sampling is a reliable method for the assessment of the fetal platelet count, it carries an increased risk of fetal morbidity and a 1–2 % risk of fetal death. It may cause cord hematoma or hemorrhage or scalp hemorrhage, such that immediate Cesarean Section is necessary or indeed the pregnancy is lost. These risks are unacceptably higher than the risk of neonatal mortality observed in ITP and outweigh the benefits of determining the fetal platelet count;

therefore, attempts to determine platelet count before delivery are not recommended [9, 17, 24, 59, 78, 79]. Furthermore, procedures should be avoided that are associated with an increased risk of intracranial hemorrhage, or scalp hemorrhage or hematoma in the neonate; such procedures include application of a fetal scalp electrode, fetal scalp blood sampling, ventouse delivery, and rotational forceps [17].

15.16.4 Platelet Monitoring in the Neonate

The majority of infants born to mothers with ITP have satisfactory platelet counts at birth. However, during the first week of life, the platelet count may fall [3–6], usually reaching a nadir on the second or the third day postpartum [3–6]. Hemorrhagic complications are rare, but when they occur, it is most commonly during these days [3–6]. It is therefore recommended that all thrombocytopenic neonates born to mothers with ITP should have daily monitoring of their platelet count, until the thrombocytopenia resolves [2, 13, 17].

15.16.5 Treatment of the Thrombocytopenic Neonate

Although treatment of infants with a low platelet count is rarely required, the newborn with clinical evidence of hemorrhage and/or a platelet count less than 20×10^9/L should be treated [2, 13, 17]. The treatment of choice is IVIg 1 g/kg in repeated doses, if necessary [42]. The administration of IVIg usually produces a rapid response [17].

Hitherto, corticosteroid administration in addition to IVIg has been suggested [13, 45]. However, current guidance states that when life-threatening neonatal hemorrhage occurs and/or the central nervous system is involved, the infant should receive combined treatment with platelet transfusions and IVIg according to the International Consensus Report guidance [17].

Conclusions

The management of ITP during pregnancy can be challenging. The diagnosis of and distinction between GT and ITP is important, particularly because of the different implications for the fetal/neonatal platelet count, and requires assessment of the timing and degree of thrombocytopenia. Exclusion of thrombocytopenia of another etiology, and of secondary causes of ITP, is also vital before embarking on treatment.

In those patients who require treatment to bring the platelet count up to a level considered safe for pregnancy or delivery, options are limited. If possible, treatment should be restricted to low doses of steroids, and prednisolone 20 mg/day may be sufficient to maintain an adequate platelet count without causing excessive side-effects. IVIg is generally well tolerated and can be used when low doses of steroids are ineffective, not sufficient, or poorly tolerated. The use of IV anti-D, whilst not supported by robust evidence, appears safe during pregnancy with little ill effect on the fetus, although further studies are warranted.

Rituximab, although not recommended during pregnancy and not licensed for use in ITP, has been used during pregnancy with no ill effects on the fetus described so far. The data are limited; nevertheless, this may prove safer than other second-line therapies, although careful follow-up and safety data are required. Azathioprine may be useful on occasion, and the TPO-receptor agonists, although not recommended, may have a potential role in severe refractory thrombocytopenia during pregnancy.

Finally, the mode of delivery should be based on obstetric indications and not determined in relation to the platelet count. A platelet count of at least 50×10^9/L is required for safe delivery, and a platelet count of at least 75×10^9/L in generally considered safe for spinal or epidural anesthesia (although a lower threshold may be adequate). Fetal blood sampling is not recommended as the incidence of neonatal bleeding complications remains low, but a cord-derived blood count should be taken at birth. In babies that are thrombocytopenic (platelets $<50\times10^9$/L), IVIg treatment is recommended and platelet count should be repeated daily until it normalizes.

15.17 Case Study

A 31 year old woman was referred for a hematological opinion in her second pregnancy. She had become thrombocytopenic in her first pregnancy at 40 weeks' gestation when the platelet count was 60×10^9/L. The cord blood platelet count was unknown but her son had no complications. Her platelets subsequently remained at approximately 40×10^9/L without any bleeding manifestations, and she did not receive any specific therapy. During her second pregnancy, the platelet count was 31×10^9/L at 8 weeks' gestation with a raised immature platelet fraction. She had minor vaginal bleeding but no bleeding from other sites. Prednisolone 40 mg daily was started, with omeprazole cover, and she received a course of eradication therapy for H. pylori. Hepatitis C and HIV status were negative. Screening for antiphospholipid antibodies was negative. Her platelet count rose to 87×10^9/L on the prednisolone, then gradually fell to 14×10^9/L at 14 weeks' gestation, associated with minor oromucosal bleeding. IVIg 1 g/kg was added, and the platelet count increased to 160×10^9/L, followed by stabilization at $30–40\times10^9$/L. Azathioprine was started and uptitrated to a dose of 150 mg daily. The prednisolone was reduced to 20 mg daily. Regular monitoring demonstrated normoglycemia and she remained normotensive. Induction of labor was planned for 38 weeks' gestation. From 36 weeks she received weekly IVIg 0.4 g/kg. Her platelet count rose to 90×10^9/L, and was 83×10^9/L pre-induction. She had an uncomplicated normal vaginal birth of a healthy male infant, birth weight 3.60 kg. She did not wish to have regional analgesia although it was offered. The cord blood platelet count was normal. The baby was assessed by the neonatologists, and received intramuscular vitamin K.

Key Learning Points

- The diagnosis of and distinction between GT and ITP is important, particularly because of the different implications for the fetal/neonatal platelet count, and requires assessment of the timing and degree of thrombocytopenia.
- Exclusion of thrombocytopenia of another etiology and of secondary causes of ITP is vital before embarking on treatment.
- If possible, treatment should be restricted to low doses of steroids, and prednisolone 20 mg/day may be sufficient to maintain an adequate platelet count without causing excessive side-effects.
- IVIg is generally well tolerated and can be used when low doses of steroids are ineffective, not sufficient, or poorly tolerated.
- The use of IV anti-D, Rituximab and Azathioprine may be useful on occasion, and the TPO-receptor agonists, although not recommended, may have a potential role in severe refractory thrombocytopenia during pregnancy.
- The mode of delivery should be based on obstetric indications and not determined in relation to the platelet count.
- A platelet count of at least 50×10^9/L is required for safe delivery, and a platelet count of at least 75×10^9/L in generally considered safe for spinal or epidural anesthesia, (although a lower threshold may be adequate).
- Fetal blood sampling is not recommended as the incidence of neonatal bleeding remains low, but a cord-derived blood count should be taken at birth.
- In babies that are thrombocytopenic (platelets $<50\times10^9$/L), IVIg treatment is recommended and platelet counts should be repeated daily until normalized.

References

1. Boehlen F, Hohlfeld P, Extermann P. Platelet count at term pregnancy: a reappraisal of the threshold. Obstet Gynecol. 2000;95:29–33.
2. British Committee for Standards in Haematology General Haematology Task Force. Guidelines for the investigation and management of Idiopathic Thrombocytopenic Purpura in adults, children and in pregnancy. Br J Haematol. 2003;120:574–96.
3. Burrows RF. Platelet disorders in pregnancy. Curr Opin Obstet Gynecol. 2001;13:115–9.
4. Burrows RF, Kelton JG. Incidentally detected thrombocytopenia in healthy mothers and their infants. N Engl J Med. 1988;319:142–5.
5. Burrows RF, Kelton JG. Thrombocytopenia at delivery: a prospective survey of 6715 deliveries. Am J Obstet Gynecol. 1990;162:731–4.
6. Burrows RF, Kelton JG. Fetal thrombocytopenia and its relation to maternal thrombocytopenia. N Engl J Med. 1993;329:1463–6.
7. Zandecki M, Genevieve F, Gerard J, Gordon A. Spurious counts and spurious results on haematology analysers: a review. Part I: platelets. Int J Lab Hematol. 2007;29(1):4–20.
8. Sainio S, Kekomaki R, Riikonen S, Teramo K. Maternal thrombocytopenia at term: a population based study. Acta Obstet Gynecol Scand. 2000;79: 744–9.
9. Win N, Rowley M, Pollard C, Beard J, Hambley H, Booker M. Severe gestational (incidental) thrombocytopenia: to treat or not to treat. Hematology. 2005;10:69–72.
10. Kwon JY, Shin JC, Lee JW, Lee JK, Kim SP, Rha JG. Predictors of idiopathic thrombocytopenic purpura in pregnant women presenting with thrombocytopenia. Int J Gynecol Obstet. 2006;96:85–8.
11. Parnas M, Sheiner E, Shoham-Vardi I, Burnstein E, Yermiahu T, Levi I, Holcberg G, Yerushalmi R. Moderate to severe thrombocytopenia during pregnancy. Eur J Obstet Gynecol Reprod Biol. 2006;128:163–8.
12. Pourrat O, Valère G, Pierre F. Is incidental gestational thrombocytopaenia really always safe for the neonate? J Obstet Gynaecol. 2014;15:1–2. doi:10.3109/01443615.2014.915293.
13. The American Society of Hematology ITP Practice Guideline Panel. Diagnosis and treatment of idiopathic thrombocytopenic purpura: recommendations of the American Society of Hematology. Ann Intern Med. 1997;126:319–26.
14. Abrahamson PE, Hall SA, Feudjo-Tepie M, Mitrani-Gold FS, Logie J. The incidence of idiopathic thrombocytopenic purpura (ITP) among adults: a population based study and literature review. Eur J Haematol. 2009;83(2):83–9.
15. Frederiksen H, Schmidt K. The incidence of idiopathic thrombocytopenic purpura increases with age. Blood. 1999;94(3):909–13.
16. Schoonen WM, Kucera G, Coalson J, Li L, Rutstein M, Mowat F. Epidemiology of immune thrombocytopenic purpura in the General Practice Research Database. Br J Haematol. 2009;145:235–44.
17. Provan D, Stasi R, Newland AC, Blanchette VS, Bolton-Maggs P, Bussel JB, et al. International consensus report on the investigation and management of primary thrombocytopenia. Blood. 2010;115:168–86.
18. Rodeghiero F, Stasi R, Gernsheimer T, Michel M, Provan D, Arnold D, Bussel J, Cines D, Chong B, Cooper N, Godeau B, Lechner K, Mazzucconi MG, Mc Millan R, Sanz M, Imbach P, Blanchette V, Kuhne T, Ruggeri M, George JN. Standardization of terminology, definitions and outcome criteria in immune thrombocytopenic purpura of adults and children: report from an international working group. Blood. 2009;113:2386–93.
19. Stasi R, Stipa E, Masi M, Cecconi M, Scimo MT, Oliva F, Sciarra A, Perroti AP, Adomo G, Amadori S, Papa G. Long-term observation of 208 adults with chronic idiopathic thrombocytopenic purpura. Am J Med. 1995;98:436–42.
20. Stasi R, Amadori S, Osborn J, Newland AC, Provan D. Long term outcome of otherwise healthy individuals with incidentally discovered thrombocytopenia. PLoS Med. 2006;3:e24.
21. Kosugi S, Kurata Y, Tomiyama Y. Circulating thrombopoietin levels in chronic idiopathic thrombocytopenic purpura. Br J Haematol. 1996;93:704–6.
22. Gernsheimer T, Mc Crae KR. Immune thrombocytopenic purpura in pregnancy. Curr Opin Hematol. 2007;14:574–80.
23. Mc Crae KR, Samuels P, Schreiber AD. Pregnancy-associated thrombocytopenia: pathogenesis and management. Blood. 1992;80:2697–714.
24. Webert KE, Mittal R, Sigouin C, Heddle N, Kelton JG. A retrospective 11 year analysis of obstetric patients with idiopathic thrombocytopenic purpura. Blood. 2003;102:4306–11.
25. Sainio S, Joutsi L, Jarvenpaa AL, Kekomaki R, Koistinen E, Riikonen S, Teramo K. Idiopathic thrombocytopenic purpura in pregnancy. Acta Obstet Gynecol Scand. 1998;77:272–7.
26. Cines DB, Millan M. Pathogenesis of chronic immune thrombocytopenic purpura. Curr Opin Hematol. 2007;14(5):511–4.
27. Brighton TA, Evans PA, Castaldi CN, Chesterman CN, Chong BH. Prospective evaluation of the clinical usefulness of an antigen-specific Assay (MAIPA) in idiopathic thrombocytopenic purpura and other immune cytopenias. Blood. 1996;88:194–201.
28. Psaila B, Bussel JB. Fc receptors in immune thrombocytopenias: a target for immunomodulation? J Clin Invest. 2008;118:2677–81.
29. Cooper N, Bussel J. The pathogenesis of immune thrombocytopaenic purpura. Br J Haematol. 2006;133: 364–74.
30. Breunis WB, van Mirre E, Bruin M, Geissler J, de Boer M, Peters M, Roos D, de Haas M, Koene HR, Kuijpers TW. Copy number variation of the activating FcGR2C gene predisposes to idiopathic thrombocytopenic purpura. Blood. 2008;111:1029–38.

31. Cooper N, Heddle NM, Haas M, Reid ME, Lesser ML, Fleit ME, Woloski BMR, Bussel JB. Intravenous immunoglobulin and intravenous anti RhD achieve acute platelet increases by different mechanisms: modulation of cytokine and platelet responses to IV anti-D by FcgRIIa and FcgRIIa polymorphisms. Br J Haematol. 2004;124:511–8.
32. Olson B, Anderson PO, Jernas M, Jacobson S, Carlson B, Carlson LMS, Wadenvik H. T-cell-mediated cytotoxicity toward platelets in chronic idiopathic thrombocytopenic purpura. Nat Med. 2003;9:1123–4.
33. Semple JW, Freedman J. Increased antiplatelet T helper lymphocyte reactivity in patients with immune thrombocytopenia. Blood. 1991;78:2619–25.
34. Semple JW, Milev Y, Cosgrave D, Mody M, Hornstein A, Blanchette V, Freedman J. Differences in serum cytokine levels in acute and chronic ITP: relationship to platelet phenotype and antiplatelet T-cell reactivity. Blood. 1996;87:4245–54.
35. Chow L, Aslam R, Speck E, Kim M, Criland N, Webster ML, Chen P, Sanib K, Ni H, Lazarus AH, Garvey B, Freedman J, Semple JW. A murine model of severe immune thrombocytopenia is induced by antibody and CD8+ T cell mediated responses that are differentially sensitive to therapy. Blood. 2010;115(6):1247–53.
36. Stasi R, Cooper N, Poeta G, Stipa E, Evangelista ML, Abruzzese E, Amadori S. Analysis of regulatory T-cell changes in patients with idiopathic thrombocytopenic purpura receiving B-cell depleting therapy with rituximab. Blood. 2008;112:1147–50.
37. Yu J, Heck S, Patel V, Levan J, Yu Y, Bussel J, Yazdanbakhsh N. Defective circulating CD25 regulatory T cells in patients with chronic ITP. Blood. 2008;112:1325–8.
38. Solanila A, Pasquet JM, Viallard JF, Contin C, Grosset C, Dechanet-Merville J. Platelet associated CD 154 in idiopathic thrombocytopenic purpura. Blood. 2005;105:215–8.
39. Gernsheimer T, Stratton J, Ballem PJ, Sluchter SJ. Mechanisms of response to treatment in ITP. N Engl J Med. 1989;320:974–8.
40. Mc Millan R, Wang L, Tomer A, Nichola J, Pistillo J. Suppression of in vitro megakaryocyte production by antiplatelet antibodies from adult patients with chronic ITP. Blood. 2004;103:1364–9.
41. Houwerzijl EJ, Blom NR, Want JJL, Esselink MT, Koornstra JJ, Smit JW, Louwes H, Vellenga E, Wolf JTM. Ultrastructural study shows morphologic features of apoptosis and para-apoptosis in megakaryocytes from patients with idiopathic thrombocytopenic purpura. Blood. 2004;103:500–6.
42. Houwerzijl EJ, Blom NR, Want JJL, Esselink MT, Koornstra JJ, Smit JW, Louwes H, Vellenga E, Wolf JTM. Increased peripheral platelet destruction and caspase -3 independent programmed cell death of bone marrow megakaryocytes in myelodysplastic patients. Blood. 2005;105:3472–9.
43. Stasi R, Sarpatwari A, Segal JB, Osborn J, Evangelista ML, Cooper N, Provan D, Newland A, Amadori S, Bussel JB. Effects of eradication of helicobacter pylori infection in patients with immune thrombocytopenic purpura: a systematic review. Blood. 2009;113:1231–40.
44. Ali R, Ozkalemkac F, Ozcelik T, Ozkocaman V, Ozan U, Kimya T, Koksal N, Bulbul-Baskan E, Develioglu O, Tufekci M, Tunali A. Idiopathic thrombocytopenic purpura in pregnancy: a single institutional experience with maternal and neonatal outcomes. Ann Hematol. 2003;82:348–52.
45. George JN, Woolf SH, Raskob GE, Wasser JS, Aledort LM, Balem PJ, Blanchette VS, Bussel JB, Cines DB, Kelton JG, Lichtin AE, Mc Millan R, Okerbloom JA, Regan DH, Warrier I. Idiopathic thrombocytopenic purpura: a practice guideline developed by methods for the American Society of Hematology. Blood. 1996;88:3–40.
46. Boehlen F, Hohlfeld P, Extermann P, De Moerloose P. Maternal antiplatelet antibodies in predicting risk of neonatal thrombocytopenia. Obstet Gynecol. 1999;93:169–73.
47. Samuels P, Bussel JB, Braitman LE, Tomaski A, Druzin ML, Mennuti MT, Cines DB. Estimation of the risk of thrombocytopenia in the offspring of pregnant women with presumed immune thrombocytopenic purpura. N Engl J Med. 1990;323:229–35.
48. Beilin Y, Zahn J, Comerford M. Safe epidural analgesia in thirty parturients with platelet counts between 69,000 and 98,000 mm^{-3}. Anesth Analg. 1997;85:385–8.
49. Neunert C, Lim W, Crowther M, Cohen A, Solberg L, Crowther MA. The American Society of Hematology 2011 evidence-based practice guideline for immune thrombocytopenia. Blood. 2011;117:4190–207.
50. Cooper N. Intravenous immunoglobulin and intravenous anti RhD therapy in the management of idiopathic thrombocytopenic purpura. Hematol Oncol Clin North Am. 2009;23:1317–27.
51. Marti-Carvajal AJ, Pena-Marti GE, Comunian-Carrasco G. Medical treatments for idiopathic thrombocytopenic purpura during pregnancy. Cochrane Libr. 2009;4:1–25.
52. Fujimura K, Harada Y, Fujimoto T, Ikeda Y, Kuramoto A, Akatsua J, Kazuo D, Mitsuhiro O, Mizoguchi H. Nationwide study of Idiopathic Thrombocytopenic Purpura in pregnant women and clinical influence on neonates. Int J Hematol. 2002;75:426–33.
53. Clark AL, Gall SA. Clinical uses of intravenous immunoglobulin in pregnancy. Am J Obstet Gynecol. 1997;176:241–53.
54. Cook RL, Miller RC, Katz VL, Cefalo RC. Immune thrombocytopenic purpura in pregnancy: a reappraisal of management. Obstet Gynecol. 1991;78:578–83.
55. Siragam V, Crow AR, Brinc D, Song S, Freedman J, Lazarus AH. Intravenous immunoglobulin ameliorates ITP activating Fc gamma receptors on dendritic cells. Nat Med. 2006;12:688–92.
56. Bussel J. Intravenous immune serum globulin in immune thrombocytopenia: clinical results and biochemical evaluation. Vox Sang. 1985;49 Suppl 1:44–50.

57. Cromwell C, Tarantino M, Aledort LM. Safety of anti-D during pregnancy. Am J Hematol. 2009;84: 261–2.
58. Michel M, Novoa MV, Bussel JB. Intravenous anti-D as a treatment for immune thrombocytopenic purpura (ITP) during pregnancy. Br J Haematol. 2003;123: 142–6.
59. Sulkenik-Halevy R, Ellis HH, Fejgin MD. Management of immune thrombocytopenic purpura in pregnancy. Obstet Gynecol Surv. 2008;63:182–8.
60. Sieunarine K, Shapiro S, Obaidi MJ, Girling J. Intravenous anti-D immunoglobulin in the treatment of resistant immune thrombocytopenic purpura in pregnancy. BJOG. 2007;114:505–7.
61. Song S, Crow AR, Siragam V, Freedman J, Lazarus AH. Monoclonal antibodies that mimic the action of anti-D in the amelioration of murine ITP act by a mechanism distinct from that of IVIG. Blood. 2005;105:1546–8.
62. Crow AR, Lazarus AH. Role of Fcgamma receptors in the pathogenesis and treatment of ITP. J Pediatr Hematol Oncol. 2003;25(S1):S14–8.
63. Newland A, Provan D, Myint S. Preventing severe infection after splenectomy. BMJ. 2005;331(7514): 417–8.
64. Stasi R, Poeta G, Stipa E, Evangelista ML, Trawinska M, Cooper N, Amadori S. Response to B-cell depleting therapy with rituximab reverts the abnormalities of T-cell subsets in patients with idiopathic thrombocytopenic purpura. Blood. 2007;110:2924–30.
65. Klink DT, van Elburg RM, Schreurs MWJ, van Well GTJ. Rituximab administration in third trimester of pregnancy suppresses neonatal B-cell development. Clin Dev Immunol. 2008;51:1–6.
66. Cooper N, Arnold DM. The effect of rituximab on humoral and cell mediated immunity and infection in the treatment of autoimmune diseases. Br J Haematol. 2010;149(1):3–13.
67. Provan D, Moss AJ, Newland AC, Bussel JB. Efficacy of mycophenolate mofetil as single-agent therapy for refractory immune thrombocytopenic purpura. Am J Hematol. 2006;81(1):19–25.
68. Kotb R, Pinganaud C, Trichet C, et al. Efficacy of mycophenolate mofetil in adult refractory autoimmune cytopenias: a single center preliminary study. Eur J Haematol. 2005;75(1):60–4.
69. Kaushansky K. Thrombopoietin: the primary regulator of megakaryocyte and platelet production. Thromb Haemost. 1995;74(1):521–5.
70. Bussel JB, Kuter DJ, George JN, et al. AMG 531, a thrombopoiesis-stimulating protein, for chronic ITP. N Engl J Med. 2006;355(16):1672–81.
71. Kuter DJ. New thrombopoietic growth factors. Blood. 2007;109(11):4607–16.
72. Bussel JB, Cheng G, Saleh MN, et al. Eltrombopag for the treatment of chronic idiopathic thrombocytopenic purpura. N Engl J Med. 2007;357(22): 2237–47.
73. Kuter DJ, Bussel JB, Lyons RM, et al. Efficacy of romiplostim in patients with chronic immune thrombocytopenic purpura: a double-blind randomised controlled trial. Lancet. 2008;371(9610):395–403.
74. Nplate (Romiplostim). Amgen. Summary of product characteristics last updated on the eMC: 15/01/2014. Available from: https://www.medicines.org.uk/
75. Revolade (Eltrombopag). GlaxoSmithKlein. Summary of product characteristics last updated on the eMC: 19/05/2014. Available from: https://www.medicines.org.uk/
76. Alkaabi JK, Alkindi S, Riyami NA, Zia F, Balla LM, Balla SM. Successful treatment of severe thrombocytopenia with romiplostim in a pregnant patient with systemic lupus erythematosus. Lupus. 2012;21(14): 1571–4.
77. Bussel JB, Sola-Visner M. Current approaches to the evaluation and management of the fetus and neonate with immune thrombocytopenia. Semin Perinatol. 2009;33:35–42.
78. Veneri D, Franchini M, Raffaeli R, Musola M, Memmo A, Franchi M, Pizzolo G. Idiopathic thrombocytopenic purpura in pregnancy: analysis of 43 consecutive cases followed at a single Italian institution. Ann Hematol. 2006;85:552–4.
79. Won YW, Moon W, Yun YS, Oh HS, Choi JH, Lee YY, Kim IS, Choi IY, Ahn MJ. Clinical aspects of pregnancy and delivery in patients with chronic idiopathic thrombocytopenic purpura (ITP). Korean J Intern Med. 2005;20:129–34.

Thrombocytopenia in Pregnancy: Fetal and Neonatal Alloimmune Thrombocytopenia

16

Sukrutha Veerareddy and Pranav P. Pandya

Abstract

Fetal/neonatal alloimmune thrombocytopenia (FNAIT) results from the formation by the mother of antibodies that are directed against a fetal platelet alloantigen inherited from its father. The maternal alloantibodies cross the placenta and destroy the baby's platelets, and the resulting fetal thrombocytopenia may cause bleeding, particularly into the brain, before or shortly after birth. Approximately 10–20 % of affected fetuses have intracranial hemorrhages, one quarter to one half of which occur in utero. There are considerable controversies regarding the optimal management of FNAIT-affected pregnancies. There is no clear approach to the antenatal management of first affected pregnancies, and several questions remain around the approaches to the management of second and subsequent affected pregnancies. Currently, antenatal management of FNAIT consists of weekly maternal intravenous immunoglobulin (IVIg) infusions, with or without oral steroid therapy – the optimal steroid dosages and protocols remain to be defined. Some centers continue to offer serial intrauterine platelet transfusions as first-line therapy, but the multiple cordocenteses required to administer the platelets carry substantial risk of fetal demise. Potential techniques for antenatal screening of first pregnancies are being developed. Postnatal screening does not prevent neonatal morbidity and mortality.

Keywords

Fetal/neonatal alloimmune thrombocytopenia • FNAIT • Platelets • Maternal intravenous immunoglobulin infusions • Serial intrauterine platelet transfusions

S. Veerareddy, BSc, MBBS, MRCOG, PhD
Women's Health Services,
Queen Elizabeth Hospital, Lewisham
and Greenwich NHS Trust, Stadium Road,
London SE18 4QH, UK
e-mail: sukrutha.veerareddy@nhs.net

P.P. Pandya, BSc, MBBS, MD, FRCOG (✉)
Fetal Medicine Unit, University College
London Hospitals NHS Foundation Trust,
1 Elizabeth Garrett Anderson Wing,
25 Grafton Way, London WC1E 6DB, UK
e-mail: pranav.pandya@uclh.nhs.uk

H. Cohen, P. O'Brien (eds.), *Disorders of Thrombosis and Hemostasis in Pregnancy: A Guide to Management*, DOI 10.1007/978-3-319-15120-5_16, © Springer-Verlag London 2015

16.1 Introduction

Fetal and neonatal alloimmune thrombocytopenia (FNAIT) occurs when the mother produces antibodies against a platelet alloantigen that the fetus has inherited from its father [1, 2] These maternal alloantibodies cross the placenta and destroy the baby's platelets, which may result in internal bleeding, in particular into the fetal brain [3–5]. As a result, babies may die in utero or have long-lasting disability. FNAIT is usually diagnosed following the birth of a thrombocytopenic baby, or less commonly, it may be suspected following the antenatal detection of a fetal intracranial hemorrhage (ICH).

16.2 Nature and Incidence of Fetal Neonatal Autoimmune Thrombocytopenia (FNAIT)

Platelet-specific alloantigens or human platelet alloantigens (HPAs) are expressed predominantly on platelets. If the fetus has inherited a HPA type from its father that is incompatible with the HPA type of its mother, antibodies against that specific HPA type may be produced by the mother [6–9]. These IgG antibodies can easily cross the placenta as early as the 14th week of gestation, prompting the fetal reticuloendothelial system to remove antibody-coated platelets from the fetal circulation [6, 10, 11]. This can cause fetal thrombocytopenia, the severity of which depends on several variables, such as (a) the concentration and subclass of maternal IgG alloantibodies; (b) the density of the target antigens on the fetal platelets; (c) the activity of phagocytes in the fetal reticuloendothelial system; and (d) the ability of the fetal bone marrow to compensate for the accelerated destruction of antibody-sensitized platelets [4]. Transfer of antibodies increases as gestation progresses, until a maximum level is attained in the late third trimester [12]. The first case of FNAIT within a family is usually detected at or shortly after birth. The newborn usually presents with skin bleeding or, in a small percentage of cases, is found to have a low platelet count. However, in severe cases, ICH may occur in utero during the antenatal period or during labor, or shortly after birth.

The incidence of FNAIT in Caucasian populations is between 1 in 1,000 and 1 in 1,500 live births [7, 13–16]. The incidence of severe thrombocytopenia ($<50 \times 10^9$/L) is 1 in 1,695 live births [17]. However, the true incidence is likely to be higher; in one study [17] only 37 % of cases with severe FNAIT were detected.

In the Caucasian population, 98 % of people are HPA-1a positive; consequently, 2 % of pregnant women are HPA-1a negative (HPA1bb). These women are most likely to carry a HPA-1a-positive fetus and are therefore at risk of being immunized. Interestingly, only 6–12 % of HPA1bb pregnant women develop anti-HPA-1a antibodies [15]. This is because the mother's immunogenetic background plays a major role [7, 18, 19]. Several studies have shown that anti-HPA-1a sensitization occurs only if the mother is HLA type DR52a, and anti-HPA-5b sensitization occurs only with HLA type DRw6 [17, 18, 20–22].

In Caucasians, antibodies to HPA-1a are the major cause of FNAIT (75 %), followed by HPA-5b (15 %) and HPA-3a (5 %), whereas in the Japanese population most cases involve antibodies to HPA-4b (Table 16.1) [12, 23–36]. The diagnosis of FNAIT is made by identifying maternal HPA antibodies and documenting parental incompatibility for the HPA allele in question.

16.3 Differences Between NAIT and Rhesus D Hemolytic Disease of the Fetus and Newborn

Unlike in hemolytic disease of the fetus and newborn (HDFN) caused by maternal sensitization to fetal Rhesus D (RhD) inherited from the father (the red cell equivalent of FNAIT), FNAIT often occurs in the first pregnancy. However, there is currently no consensus regarding the utility of screening in previously unaffected women for antiplatelet antibodies and thus identifying women whose babies could be affected by FNAIT early in gestation (discussed in Sect. 16.11). Active antenatal manage-

Table 16.1 HPA antibodies involved in FNAIT in Caucasians and their prevalences: literature review

Author and year	HPA-1a (%)	HPA-1b (%)	HPA-3a (%)	HPA-5a (%)	HPA-5b (%)	HPA-15 (%)	HPA-1a & HPA-5b (%)	Other (%)
Reznikoff-Etievant (1988) [23]	90							
Mueller-Eckhardt et al. (1989) [24]	90				8			2
Kornfeld et al. (1996) [25]	90				10			
Letsky and Greaves (1996) [26]	80–90				5–15			
Khouzami et al. (1996) [27]	75							
Kanhai et al. (1996) [28]	79		5	11				
Uhrynowska et al. (1997) [29]	91	4			4			
Spencer and Burrows (2001) [12]	78		4		4			
Davoren et al. (2002) [30]	94		3		3			
Davoren et al. (2004) [31]	79	4	2	1	9		2	
Rayment et al. (2003) [32]	85				10	5		
Mandelbaum et al. (2005) [33]						2		
Ertel et al. (2005) [34]						1		
Kroll et al. (2005) [35]	75		2		18		2	
Porcelijn et al. (2006) [36]	73	1	5	1	15			

Table 16.2 Differences between RhD HDFN and FNAIT

	Rh	FNAIT
Incidence	1/100	1/1,000
First child affected	No	Yes
Routine screening in place	Yes	No
Testing readily available	Yes	No
Prophylaxis available	Yes	No
Severe clinical phenotype	Hydrops	Intracranial hemorrhage
Management of next pregnancy	Red cell transfusions in utero	IVIg ± prednisolone ± platelet transfusions

ment of this disease is confined to those women who have had a previously affected fetus [7]. There are important differences between RhD isoimmunization and FNAIT (Table 16.2).

16.4 Diagnosis

The diagnosis of FNAIT is based on clinical and serological findings. The typical picture is of a neonate presenting with purpura within minutes to hours after birth, born to a healthy mother with no history of a bleeding disorder, after an uneventful pregnancy with a normal maternal platelet count [37–40]. The first step in the diagnosis of FNAIT is confirmation of neonatal thrombocytopenia, followed by exclusion of the most frequent causes of neonatal thrombocytopenia such as infection, disseminated intravascular coagulation, and maternal immune thrombocytopenia (ITP) [11, 39]. The platelet count is low at birth and tends to fall further during the first 24–48 h of life. Laboratory diagnosis involves the detection of maternal circulating alloantibodies against a HPA type shared by neonatal and paternal platelets. This is accomplished using the monoclonal antibody-specific immobilization of platelet antigen (MAIPA) test [41], the platelet immunofluorescence test, or a novel antigen-specific particle assay [11, 26, 42–46]. The diagnosis of FNAIT is unequivocal when a parental incompatibility with corresponding maternal alloantibody is present [4, 10, 39, 47].

Recognition of FNAIT and appropriate therapy are important both for the affected neonate and for the management of subsequent pregnancies [48]. Indications for testing for FNAIT prenatally include any fetus with ICH, selected cases of ventriculomegaly (e.g., moderate to severe unilateral), neonates with thrombocytopenia of unclear etiology, neonatal ICH with significant thrombocytopenia, and familial transient neonatal thrombocytopenia [49–52]. A number of FNAIT cases (10 %) have been reported in which no HPA antibody could be detected [53–56]. The diagnosis is then based on maternal-fetal or maternal-paternal HPA incompatibility and exclusion of other causes of thrombocytopenia [54, 57, 58]. In some cases, antibodies may become detectable in the weeks or months after delivery or during/after a subsequent pregnancy [39, 40, 59, 60]. In unconfirmed FNAIT cases, antibodies detected before 20 weeks in a subsequent pregnancy require confirmation by a later specimen, because early transient antibodies may exist and do not seem to be of clinical significance [60]. Some studies have demonstrated significant correlation between high anti-HPA-1a antibody titers (>1:32) and a fetal platelet count below 50×10^9/L [21, 59, 60], whereas others have not [17, 36, 61]. This discrepancy may be due to differences in the size of the series, parity of the women, timing of blood sampling, or the method of antibody titration [61].

HPA typing of mother, father and fetus/neonate is important, not only for the diagnosis of FNAIT but also for provision of HPA-matched blood components to neonates with FNAIT, for genetic counseling and for estimation of the recurrence risk [62]. Conventional serological immuno-phenotyping for HPA is limited by the lack of certain rare but well-characterized typing antisera, such as anti-HPA-1b and anti-HPA-4b [62]. Even when non-paternity has been ruled out, it is not always possible to demonstrate parental incompatibility of platelet-specific alloantigens in the presence of corresponding maternal alloantibodies, especially if the mother is sensitized to a rare paternal antigen, making the diagnosis more difficult [63]. If there is a strong suspicion of FNAIT, testing the maternal serum against the paternal platelets (using a blood sample from the father or the fetus/neonate) may confirm incompatibility.

16.5 Fetal/Neonatal Risks

FNAIT may affect the fetus as early as the beginning of the second trimester and usually remits spontaneously within 1–3 weeks after delivery, depending on the rate of removal of maternal platelet antibodies from the neonatal circulation. Thrombocytopenia can be severe and can cause antenatal ICH in around 10–30 % of severe cases. ICH is associated with death in 10 % and neurological sequelae in a further 10–20 % [6, 11, 39, 50]. Chaoying et al. [64] found that FNAIT is the most important cause of ICH and poor outcome in neonates.

Around 25–50 % of cases of FNAIT-related ICH occur in utero. The majority occur between 30 and 35 weeks of gestation [7, 50], but ICH have also been reported at earlier gestations. The international No IntraCranial Haemorrhage (NOICH) registry, an observational cohort study, characterised pregnancies between 2001 and 2010 where the fetus or neonate was diagnosed with fetal and neonatal alloimmune thrombocytopenia (FNAIT) and suffered from intracranial haemorrhage (ICH), with special focus on time of bleeding onset. Of 592 FNAIT cases in the registry, 43 confirmed cases of ICH due to FNAIT were included in the study. The majority of bleeding episodes (23/43; 54 %) occurred before 28 weeks of gestation and often affected the first born child (27/43; 63 %). One-third (35 %) of the children died within 4 days after delivery. Twenty-three (53 %) children survived with severe neurological disabilities and only 5 (12 %) were alive and well at time of discharge. Antenatal treatment was not given in most (91 %) cases of fetal/neonatal ICH. The authors concluded that ICH caused by FNAIT often occurs during second trimester and the clinical outcome is poor. In order to prevent ICH caused by FNAIT, at-risk pregnancies must be identified and prevention and/ or interventions should start early in the second trimester [65]. Without treatment, there is a risk of ICH as long as severe thrombocytopenia persists [23]. Thrombocytopenia is most severe in the presence of HPA-1a incompatibility, which accounts for most cases of in utero ICH.

Although high levels of maternal anti-HPA-1a may correlate with the severity of thrombocytopenia [21, 66], in up to 30 % of cases no antibody is found [67]. In some cases, antibody detection can be improved by varying assay conditions [68, 69]. Severe thrombocytopenia or ICH in HPA-1a-alloimmunized pregnancies cannot be predicted with sufficient sensitivity and specificity for clinical application from maternal anti-HPA-1a potency, bioactivity or isotype [32, 70, 71]. The maternal antibody level therefore has limited use in prediction of the severity of fetal/neonatal thrombocytopenia.

Neonatal thrombocytopenia due to FNAIT usually becomes progressively more severe and occurs earlier in subsequent pregnancies [10, 38, 44]. Following severe neonatal thrombocytopenia ($<50 \times 10^9$/L), a cerebral ultrasound or nuclear magnetic resonance (MRI) scan is advised to detect clinically silent ICH [7, 11]. A few cases of ICH resulting from incompatibility for HPA-3a, HPA-4b, HPA-5b, or HPA-9b alloantigens have been reported [72, 73].

16.6 Antenatal Management and Outcomes

The goal of antenatal management is to prevent severe thrombocytopenia and thus ICH which may result in death, either in utero or after birth, or long-lasting disability. A balance must be found between the inherent risks of the condition itself and the risks of diagnostic testing and therapy. The antenatal treatment of FNAIT has evolved over the past 25 years, largely based on published case series, detailing outcomes with differing regimens. They include: (a) fetal blood sampling (FBS) and serial intrauterine platelet transfusions (IUT) [54, 74]; (b) weekly intravenous immunoglobulin (IVIg) infusions; and (c) immunosuppression with corticosteroids [5, 57, 75]. Over the last 15 years, there has been a gradual change from invasive management to a less invasive management protocol to a completely non-invasive approach. However, controversy still exists over the optimal antenatal management strategy.

16.6.1 Diagnostic Fetal Blood Sampling and Intrauterine Platelet Transfusions

Fetal blood sampling (FBS) involves the insertion of a needle into the umbilical or intrahepatic vein to sample fetal blood in order to ascertain the fetal platelet count. The procedure is usually complemented by the transfusion of a specially selected, very concentrated platelet suspension that is both HPA and ABO and RhD blood group compatible, to reduce the risk of bleeding associated with individual procedures [74, 76, 77]. With reports of a fetal loss rate of around 6 % per pregnancy [78], serial (weekly) intrauterine platelet transfusions (IUPT) are reserved for the management of affected fetuses that do not respond to medical management alone. An important unresolved issue in the management of at-risk pregnancies is how to safely minimize or eliminate FBS [66, 79]. FBS, with its associated risks of bleeding, boosting antibody levels, fetal bradycardia requiring emergency (preterm) Cesarean section, and fetal loss, may not be necessary before medical therapy for FNAIT is instituted, but may be required subsequently to determine the fetal response to treatment and IUPT in selected cases [56, 80–82].

16.6.2 Intravenous Immunoglobulin

After anecdotal observation by Bussel et al. [50] that antenatal maternal treatment with high-dose IVIg seemed to prevent ICH in high-risk pregnancies, IVIg became increasingly popular in the treatment of FNAIT [83]. It is often given to the mother on a weekly basis, using various regimens, until delivery. After birth, the neonatal platelet count and the absence of ICH provide measures of IVIg efficacy.

The mechanism of action of IVIg in FNAIT is still unclear. Four possible explanations are cited in the literature. First, in the maternal circulation IVIg will dilute the anti-HPA antibodies, resulting in a lower proportion of anti-HPA antibodies within the IgG transferred to the fetus via the Fc-receptors in the placenta. Secondly, in the placenta, IVIg may block the placenta receptor (Fc-R) and reduce the placental transmission of maternal antibodies, including anti-HPA antibodies. Thirdly, in the fetus, IVIg can block the Fc-receptors on the macrophages and thereby prevent the destruction of antibody-covered cells [66]. A fourth possible mechanism could be that IVIg may enhance the expression of inhibitory receptors on splenic macrophages [84] and, as a result, suppress maternal antibody production and reduce placental transfer of the antibodies [85]. So far, evidence for only the first mechanism exists.

Short-term mild side effects that have been associated with IVIg therapy include headache, febrile reactions, nausea, malaise and myalgia, but these are more common with rapid infusion and can be minimized by slowing the infusion rate. Several rare but serious side-effects such as aseptic meningitis, acute renal failure, thrombosis, transmission of blood-borne diseases, and reactions including severe headache and fever, and anaphylaxis, have also been reported.

The long-term side effects of IVIg for mother and child are still unclear, but it is generally considered safe. A possible increase of IgE in children after maternal IVIg administration compared to the normal population has been suggested. However, no clinically apparent adverse effects in early childhood could be demonstrated [66]. Since IVIg is known for its immunomodulating characteristics, there is always a possibility of long-time side-effects for the mother and child. Furthermore, weekly IVIg administration is expensive.

Weekly maternal IVIg is the most commonly used therapy today. Following IVIg infusion, the IgG level falls by 30 % after 24 h and by 50 % after 72 h [64]. Maternal administration of IVIg has been reported to increase the fetal platelet count and/or prevent ICH in 55–85 % of FNAIT cases [38, 86–88]. IVIg treatment seems to reduce the risk of ICH even if the fetal platelet count is not altered [79, 89]; the mechanism of this latter effect is unclear. There is conflicting evidence on the efficacy of IVIg in preventing ICH, with most reports documenting favorable results [53, 86, 88] while others report failure of IVIg to prevent ICH [48, 75, 90]. However, in the latter reports, the IVIg dose used was only 1.0 g/kg/week.

The study by Bussel et al. [86] suggested a substantial elevation in fetal platelet count following treatment with IVIg 1.0 g/kg/week; the reported response rate in the literature varies from 30 to 85 %. Results from a randomized placebo-controlled trial [86] suggest no beneficial effect of adding dexamethasone to the administered IVIg. The dose of IVIg of 1.0 g/kg/week has been commonly used ever since the first publication by Bussel et al. in 1988 [57]. However, the optimal treatment dose regimen of IVIg has not been formally evaluated. In treating chronic ITP, the standard dose is 400 mg/kg daily for 5 days, although 1 g/kg/day for 2 days may be more effective. Placental antibody transfer does not appear to be further increased despite high IgG concentrations in the mother resulting from IVIg treatment. This suggests a limitation of the placental Fc receptor [66].

High levels of maternal anti-HPA 1a have been reported to be strongly associated with severe thrombocytopenia in the neonate [21, 66]. This has prompted the suggestion that in cases of low maternal titers of anti-HPA antibodies, a lower dose of IVIg may be sufficient to reduce transmission of pathogenic HPA antibodies leading to thrombocytopenia. Van den Akker et al. conducted a randomized international multicenter trial to compare the effectiveness of a low dose of IVIg (0.5 g/kg/week) with the commonly used dose (1.0 g/kg/week). Survival was 100 % and none of the neonates had an ICH. However, unfortunately this trial ended prematurely because of inadequate patient recruitment [91]. This study might be regarded as a successful pilot study, and the use of 0.5 g/kg/week IVIg in pregnant women with FNAIT and a previous child without ICH is still an option. However, this should be restricted to patients that participate in a formal prospective study. Van den Akker et al. also recommend non-invasive treatment without recourse to invasive strategies, which is both safe and effective in the antenatal management of FNAIT [56].

16.6.3 Corticosteroids

The administration of steroids as the sole treatment for FNAIT is controversial, as their efficacy is variable and chronic steroid therapy has been associated with adverse effects [57]. In a selection of studies corticosteroids have been administered as a means of supporting the action of IVIg. A study in which very high-risk patients (initial fetal platelet count $<20\times10^9$/L or a sibling with perinatal ICH) received weekly IVIg infusions along with daily corticosteroid therapy showed that the combination was more effective than IVIg alone in eliciting a satisfactory fetal platelet response (82 % vs. 18 %) [49, 79]. Both IVIg alone and IVIg combined with any corticosteroids resulted in an improved clinical outcome in treated FNAIT fetuses compared to their untreated siblings [92]. At present, prednisone seems to be the corticosteroid of choice for treatment of FNAIT [49, 79].

Dexamethasone is now avoided as it may cross the fetal blood-brain barrier. In addition, at higher doses it has been associated with oligohydramnios [57] and, at lower doses, a lack of efficacy [86]. Although mothers may experience side-effects of systemic corticosteroids, clinical experience suggests no abnormalities in children of mothers treated with usual doses of prednisone throughout pregnancy.

In summary, IVIg is the mainstay of the antenatal management of FNAIT. It is recommended that treatment is started 4–6 weeks before the estimated gestational age at which the ICH occurred or severe thrombocytopenia was detected in the previous affected fetus. If this information about the previous pregnancy is unavailable or if the previous sibling did not suffer ICH, IVIg therapy can be instituted at 26–28 weeks' gestation because intrauterine ICH has generally been reported after 30 weeks [73, 89].

The role of concomitant steroids alongside IVIg needs further clarification. Bussel et al. [93] treated women with a history of previous early ICH at various gestations. Treatment comprised initial IVIg 1 or 2 g/kg/week infusion at 12 weeks, with the addition of prednisone later only if the fetal platelet count fell below 30×10^9/L in non-responders to IVIg therapy alone. Clinical outcomes in this study were favorable. Similarly, Berkowitz et al. [79] have proposed that 1 g/kg/week of IVI alone is clearly insufficient in siblings of fetuses with a previous ICH in utero. If the initial fetal platelet count is $<20\times10^9$/L at 20 weeks of gestation, IVIg alone 1 g/kg/week has a substantially lesser effect, and a lower response rate, than IVIg and prednisone combined [49, 79]. Furthermore, they claim that prednisone in low doses is almost as good as 1 g/kg/week of IVIg in the least affected fetuses (those with a sibling without an ICH and with a pre-treatment fetal platelet count of $<20\times10^9$/L) [79].

Since there are substantial risks associated with FBS [80–82] and non-invasive treatment is effective, therapy for FNAIT can be instituted without invasive procedures [38, 89, 94].

A Cochrane review in 2010 [95] concluded that there are insufficient data from randomized controlled trials to determine the optimal antenatal management of FNAIT and that future trials should consider the dose of IVIg, the timing of initial treatment, monitoring of response to treatment, laboratory measures to define pregnancies with a high risk of ICH, management of non-responders, and long-term follow-up of children.

16.6.4 Implications for Practice

1. IVIg can be used as first-line treatment for standard-risk FNAIT, where there was no peripartum ICH in an affected sibling and the pre-treatment fetal platelet count (if performed) is $>20\times10^9$/L. However, the optimal dose of IVIg has not been established and further guidance based on the results of the NOICH 2 study is awaited.
2. IVIg in combination with prednisone may be more effective in raising the fetal platelet count than IVIg alone in high-risk pregnancies, where the pre-treatment fetal platelet count $<20\times10^9$/L or the affected sibling sustained a peripartum ICH. The optimal timing of administration and the dose of prednisone and IVIg are unclear, but studies have demonstrated efficacy when treatment was initiated at 20–26 weeks.

16.7 Suggested Antenatal Management of a Subsequent Affected Fetus

Following the affected pregnancy, the father should be tested for the presence of the relevant HPA. The risk of recurrence in subsequent pregnancies is virtually 100 % if the father is homozygous for the responsible HPA and 50 % if he is heterozygous. In the latter case, it is possible to determine the fetal platelet type by 16 weeks of gestation via PCR amplification of DNA obtained from amniocytes (obtained at amniocentesis). If the fetus is found to be negative for the HPA allele, no further testing is indicated [12, 96, 97]. Pre-implantation diagnosis (PGD) can be considered [98]. Non-invasive prenatal diagnosis (NIPD) using cell-free fetal DNA obtained from maternal plasma and serum is now a clinical reality, particularly in the management of RhD hemolytic disease, and many investigators are evaluating NIPD in FNAIT that may in the future form part of national antenatal screening programs.

The severity of FNAIT usually increases with each pregnancy. Attempts have been made to predict a fetus at risk from severe thrombocytopenia by the use of serial antibody titers in order to determine which fetus needs treatment. As stated above (Sect. 16.5), the antibody titer measurements are not a reliable predictor of the severity of FNAIT and are thus of limited use in the clinical management of FNAIT. The clinical history of an affected sibling is currently the best indicator of risk in a current pregnancy [37, 38, 99]. The recurrence rate of ICH in the subsequent pregnancies of women with FNAIT was 72 % (when the previous pregnancy was without fetal death) and 79 % (when the previous pregnancy included a fetal death). Conversely, the risk of ICH in those with a history of FNAIT but without ICH was estimated at 7 % [99].

It is presumed that, in fetuses with early severe fetal thrombocytopenia, ICH will be seen in a second pregnancy even though this did not occur in the first sibling. In a study by Bussel and Kaplan [47], 50 % of 98 affected fetuses already had a platelet count of $<20\times10^9$/L by 25 weeks' gestation, indicating early severity. Forty percent had a lower fetal platelet count at that time than their previously affected siblings had at birth, indicating increasing severity in subsequent pregnancies. These authors concluded that when FNAIT occurs at an early gestation, it is severe; and it is more severe in fetuses with an older affected sibling that had an antenatal ICH. This suggests that fetuses may require different management strategies depending on the history of their previous sibling. There has been a trend and a strong recommendation to utilize non-invasive strategies (IVIg) in the management of FNAIT at high risk of in utero or postnatal ICH [100, 101].

For platelet antigen incompatibilities other than HPA-1a, much less data exist regarding antenatal management and clinical course. Incompatibility of HPA-3a, while infrequent, is as severe as that of HPA-1a [102], while incompatibilities of HPA-5b and HPA-9b are less severe [103]. HPA-4 incompatibility also seems to be severe [104], and most rare antigens are identified because of a severe case of neonatal FNAIT.

16.8 Timing and Mode of Birth

The delivery plan should be based on the patient's risk category, the response to treatment, and the most recent fetal platelet count, if pertinent [105]. The appropriate gestational age for delivery has not been established. The risk of prematurity and the costs of neonatal intensive care unit admission should be weighed against the risk of continued exposure of the fetus to the harmful antibodies and the cost of IVIg therapy. Different units recommend delivery between 35 weeks and term. Vaginal delivery is reasonable if the fetal platelet count exceeds 50×10^9/L [87]. With platelet counts below 50×10^9/L, IUPT has been performed before vaginal delivery for protection against bleeding at the time of delivery, with its associated risks. There is no evidence that vaginal delivery of a fetus with a platelet count below 50×10^9/L increases the risk of ICH. In a Dutch study of 32 pregnancies complicated by FNAIT in which the thrombocytopenic sibling did not have an ICH, vaginal delivery was not associated with neonatal intracranial bleeding, even though the platelet count was $<50\times10^9$/L in 4 neonates [106]. Cesarean delivery alone is not considered effective in preventing antenatal or perinatal hemorrhage [11, 107]. Instrumental vaginal delivery, ventouse, fetal scalp electrode and fetal scalp blood sampling should be avoided. The neonatologist on duty during delivery should be informed in advance, as should a consultant in hematology/transfusion medicine, and the blood transfusion laboratory should also be asked in advance to obtain HPA compatible platelets.

16.9 Treatment of the Neonate

Treatment of the neonate is dictated by its condition. If there are no signs of bleeding and the thrombocytopenia is mild or moderate, no therapy is necessary. In cases of neonatal bleeding or a platelet count below 30×10^9/L, therapy is needed and must be rapid and effective. First-line therapy is prompt transfusion of (ideally) HPA-compatible platelets that will not be destroyed by maternal antibodies in the neonate's circulation. Blood centers should be able to supply HPA-1a and 5b negative platelets. If these are not available, an amendment to the British Committee in Standards for Haematology (BCSH) guidelines recommends using platelets that are not selected for HPA status [60]. Treatment of neonatal FNAIT with IVIg and/or steroids is advised when severe thrombocytopenia and/or hemorrhage persist despite transfusion of HPA-compatible platelets. Platelet transfusion thresholds of 20–30 $\times10^9$/L and 50×10^9/L are recommended for neonates, depending on the clinical situation [60]. The effectiveness of IVIg in the neonate has not been shown in some studies [108]. The therapeutic effect on the platelet count, however, is delayed for 24–48 h, during which time the neonate remains at risk of ICH.

16.10 Preconception Counseling

Pregnant women are at risk of FNAIT if they have a history of a previous neonate with FNAIT or are known to have circulating alloantibodies [4]. Before a subsequent pregnancy, these women should be referred to a tertiary center that specializes in the treatment of FNAIT. The risks of ICH in a subsequent pregnancy and the diagnosis and treatment strategies that might be of benefit should be discussed, as addressed above. If the previously affected child had an ICH, there is a 70–80 % chance that the next affected child will have an ICH. However, if the pregnancy complicated by FNAIT did not involve ICH, the risk of ICH in a subsequent pregnancy is less than 10 % [38, 99, 109]. Counseling is most effective after HPA typing of the father. If the father is homozygous for the HPA allele, the risk of recurrence of FNAIT is 100 %, whereas the risk of recurrence is 50 % if the father is heterozygous.

16.11 Screening for FNAIT in the First Pregnancy

The implementation of an antenatal screening program for FNAIT depends on cost-effectiveness and is currently under debate. Several studies provided calculations and reached the conclusion that screening is likely to be cost-effective [38, 55, 110–112], although this was not a universal view [113]. Antenatal screening for FNAIT might identify alloimmunized women during their first pregnancy, allowing antenatal intervention to prevent ICH. Even if no antenatal intervention was undertaken, delivery could be planned so that compatible platelets would be available [7].

The major determinants of the costs are the initial HPA typing, antibody detection in those at risk, and costs of interventions. Although these costs are considerable, even for the most expensive strategy (e.g. offering IVIg to all immunized women), they are easily outweighed by the savings made in preventing most cases of life-long severe neurological morbidity.

Three large studies of antenatal screening for HPA-1a incompatibility have been performed [15, 17, 114]. Two, from East Anglia [114] and Scotland [17] in the UK, were performed in approximately 25,000 cases each. The largest study in Norway included more than 100,000 pregnancies [15]. Another study from Norway concluded that, without a screening programme, the detection rate of NAIT in Norway is only 14 % of expected [115]. Key findings from these studies suggest that the incidence of FNAIT in the neonate was approximately 1:5,000 but, on antenatal screening, a higher incidence of 1:1,000 using HPA-1a incompatibility only was noted. A systematic review suggests that screening for HPA-1a alloimmunization detects around 2 cases in 1,000 pregnancies and that severe FNAIT occurs in around 40 per 1,000,000 pregnancies. Despite several antenatal interventions, severe ICH occurred in 3–4 children per 1,000,000 pregnancies screened. Furthermore, the review highlighted that the incidence of ICH in non-screened populations is likely to be higher. Screening of all pregnancies together with effective antenatal treatment such as IVIg may reduce the mortality and morbidity associated with FNAIT without known risks for the mother or child [14, 82, 83, 116]. These data indicate that large-scale screening studies including comparison of intervention strategies are warranted [117, 118].

Conclusions

The most serious complication of FNAIT is ICH, which occurs in 10–30 % of severe cases, causing death (10 %) and neurological sequelae (10–20 %). In the majority of cases, fetal thrombocytopenia is more severe and occurs successively earlier in subsequent pregnancies [50]. There is a 70–80 % risk of antenatal ICH in a subsequent pregnancy complicated by FNAIT if a previous child had ICH [38, 90]. Most cases of in utero ICH involve HPA-1a incompatibility with severe thrombocytopenia, although a few cases have resulted from incompatibility for HPA-3a, HPA-4b, HPA-5b, or HPA-9b alloantigens.

Antenatal management of FNAIT includes weekly maternal IVIg infusions which are very effective. Concomitant usage of steroids alongside IVIg has been suggested to show favorable results in high-risk fetuses that have not responded to IVIg alone [49, 94, 109, 119]. Treatment should start 4–6 weeks before the estimated gestational age at which ICH or severe thrombocytopenia occurred in the previous pregnancy, or at approximately 28 weeks' gestation [73, 89].

FBS with its significant associated risks may not be necessary before therapy for FNAIT is instituted, but may become necessary to determine the fetal response to treatment [56]. Spontaneous vaginal delivery is preferred in FNAIT cases, while avoiding procedures that might increase the risk of fetal hemorrhage (such as fetal scalp electrode, fetal scalp blood sampling, forceps or ventouse assistance) [106]. Cesarean section may be performed in selected high-risk fetuses.

At present, there is no approved method of antenatal screening to detect the first affected pregnancy [59, 114, 120]. Postnatal screening, although simple, cannot prevent neonatal morbidity and mortality [55].

The aim of current research must be to develop reliable predictors of disease severity in affected infants and to increase the effectiveness of non-invasive treatment strategies for FNAIT. Prospective trials are necessary to evaluate different treatment strategies and to acquire additional data on optimal prevention programs.

16.12 Case Studies

Case Study 1

A 36 year old primigravida delivered a baby girl vaginally at 41 weeks' gestation. The Apgar scores were 8 at 1 min and 9 at 5 min. The 1-h assessment was normal except for bruising on the scalp. By 6 h of age, however, the infant was feeding poorly and was hypothermic, with decreased tone, irritability, and hyper-responsiveness to stimulation; her anterior and posterior fontanelles were full. Bruising was noted over the entire scalp, with petechiae covering the entire chest, abdomen, and upper and lower limbs.

A full blood count showed severe thrombocytopenia (platelets 16×10^9/L). A coagulation screen (prothrombin time (PT), activated partial thromboplastin time (APTT) and fibrinogen) was normal. The CT scan showed a very large acute subdural hematoma on the right side of the cerebellum, with midline shift to the left. The compressed cerebellum caused obstruction of the cisterns and increased the size of the temporal horns of the lateral ventricles, resulting in increased intracranial pressure (ICP). A repeat platelet count was 6×10^9/L. The infant was transferred to a neonatal intensive care unit and emergency surgery was undertaken to evacuate the subdural hematoma. After surgery, the ICP dropped, and the ventricular size was normal on repeat CT scan.

In the meantime, the mother, who had a normal platelet count, was tested for antibodies. Her platelet count was normal, but her screen was positive for anti-HPA-1 antibodies, consistent with a diagnosis of neonatal alloimmune thrombocytopenia (NAIT) (confirmation of the diagnosis would require maternal-fetal or maternal-paternal HPA incompatibility and exclusion of other causes of thrombocytopenia). During the first 36 h of life, the infant was transfused with random donor platelets, red blood cells, FFP, and cryoprecipitate. The platelet count improved and by day 5 was 228×10^9/L, increasing to 346×10^9/L by discharge on Day 7 of life. The infant was eating well and gaining weight by discharge. The platelet count remained stable at 2 weeks and 1 month of age. At 1-year follow-up, the infant was thriving and developmentally appropriate [121].

Case Studies 2 & 3

Maternal immunization against low-frequency, platelet (PLT)-specific antigens is being recognized with increasing frequency as a cause of NAIT. These two cases of severe NAIT were caused by maternal immunization against previously unrecognized, low-frequency antigens created by amino acid substitutions in GPIIb/IIIa (αIIb/β3 integrin). They highlight that a search should be conducted for novel paternal antigens in cases of apparent NAIT not explained on the basis of maternal-fetal incompatibility for known human platelet antigens.

Case Study 2 (HPA-22bw, Sey)

A 31 year old mother had a spontaneous vaginal birth of a female infant. The baby had scattered petechial hemorrhages at birth associated with severe thrombocytopenia (platelets 13×10^9/L), with the remainder of the blood count normal. A random-donor platelet transfusion and intravenous immunoglobulin (IVIg) 1.0 g/kg body weight were administered, after which the platelet count increased to 80×10^9/L. During the next 11 days, the baby received two additional platelet transfusions and two IVIg infusions. After each transfusion, the platelet count increased to the range of 50×10^9/L to 80×10^9/L, but subsequently declined. On Day 9, the platelet count had fallen to 22×10^9/L and bloody stools were observed. A platelet transfusion and IVIg were again administered. The platelets rose to 65×10^9/L and increased steadily thereafter. The child was discharged on Day 15 with a normal platelet count.

Case Study 3 (HPA-23bw, Hug)

The second child, a boy, was born to a 22-year-old woman by spontaneous vaginal delivery.

He developed widespread petechial and subconjunctival hemorrhages soon after birth and was found to have a platelet count of 13×10^9/L. Other hematological findings were unremarkable except for a weakly positive direct antiglobulin test thought to be a consequence of maternal-fetal incompatibility for blood group B. At 1 day of age, the baby's petechial hemorrhages were resolving and its platelet count was 27×10^9/L. IVIg, 1 g/kg body weight, was administered. The platelet counts were 38×10^9/L the next day and 102×10^9/L 2 days later. The baby was discharged on day 5 [122].

Key Learning Points

- All cases of FNAIT should be managed by maternal-fetal medicine specialists in tertiary referral centers, with appropriate liaison with specialists in neonatology and hematology/transfusion medicine.
- If the previously affected sibling had an ICH, the next affected fetus is highly likely to have early, severe thrombocytopenia and in utero ICH, in the absence of effective treatment.
- Effective non-invasive antenatal treatment (IVIg) exists for cases recognized as a result of a previously affected sibling.
- Invasive treatment (intrauterine platelet transfusions) appears to be required only in non-responders.

References

1. Moulinier J. Alloimmunisation maternelle antiplaquettaire duzo. In: Proceedings of the 6th congress of the European society of haematology. Paris: European Society of Hematology; 1953. p. 817–20.
2. Shulman NR, Marder VJ, et al. Platelet and leukocyte isoantigens and their antibodies: serologic physiologic and clinical studies. Prog Hematol. 1964;4:222–304.
3. Burrows RF, Kelton JG. Fetal thrombocytopenia and its relation to maternal thrombocytopenia. N Engl J Med. 1993;329:1463–6.
4. Blanchette VS, Johnson J, Rand M. The management of alloimmune neonatal thrombocytopenia. Baillieres Best Pract Res Clin Haematol. 2000;13: 365–90.
5. Kaplan C, Murphy MF. Feto-maternal alloimmune thrombocytopenia: antenatal therapy with IvIgG and steroids – more questions than answers. European Working Group on FMAIT. Br J Haematol. 1998; 100(1):62–5.
6. Kaplan C, Forestier F, Daffos F. Management of fetal and neonatal alloimmune thrombocytopenia. Transfus Med Rev. 1996;10:233–40.
7. Murphy MF, Williamson LM. Antenatal screening for fetomaternal alloimmune thrombocytopenia: an evaluation using the criteria of the UK National Screening Committee. Br J Haematol. 2000;111:726–32.
8. Proulx C, Filion M, Goldman M. Analysis of immunoglobulin class, IgG subclass and titre of HPA-1a antibodies in alloimmunized mothers giving birth to babies with or without neonatal alloimmune thrombocytopenia. Br J Haematol. 1994;87:813–7.
9. Rothenberger S. Neonatal alloimmune thrombocytopenia. Ther Apher. 2002;6:32–5.
10. Kaplan C. Platelet alloimmunity: the fetal/neonatal alloimmune thrombocytopenia. Vox Sang. 2002;83 Suppl 1:289–91.
11. Murphy MF, Manley R, Roberts D. Neonatal alloimmune thrombocytopenia. Haematologica. 1999;84: 110–4.
12. Spencer JA, Burrows RF. Feto-maternal alloimmune thrombocytopenia: a literature review and statistical analysis. Aust N Z J Obstet Gynaecol. 2001;41:45–55.
13. Blanchette VS, Chen L, de Friedberg ZS. Alloimmunisation to the PlA1 platelet antigen: results of a prospective study. Br J Haematol. 1990;74:209–15.
14. Kamphuis MM, Paridaans N, Porcelijn L, De Haas M, van der Schoot CE, Brand A, Bonsel GJ, Oepkes D. Screening in pregnancy for fetal or neonatal alloimmune thrombocytopenia: systematic review. BJOG. 2010;117(11):1335–43.
15. Kjeldsen-Kragh J, Killie MK, Tomter G, Golebiowska E, Randen I, Hauge R. A screening and intervention program aimed to reduce mortality and serious morbidity associated with severe neo-natal alloimmune thrombocytopenia. Blood. 2007;110:833.
16. Mueller-Eckhardt C, Mueller-Eckhardt G, Willen-Ohff H, Horz A, Kuenzlen E, O'Neill GJ. Immunogenicity of and immune response to the human platelet antigen Zwa is strongly associated with HLAB8 and DR3. Tissue Antigens. 1985;26:71–6.
17. Turner ML, Bessos H, Fagge T. Prospective epidemiologic study of the outcome and cost-effectiveness of antenatal screening to detect neonatal alloimmune thrombocytopenia due to anti-HPA-1a. Transfusion. 2005;45:1945–56.
18. Decary F, L'Abbe D, Tremblay L. The immune response to the HPA-1a antigen: association with HLA-DRw52a. Transfus Med. 1991;1:55–62.
19. Mueller-Eckhardt C, Santoso S, Kiefel V. Platelet alloantigens molecular, genetic, and clinical aspects. Vox Sang. 1994;67S3:89–93.
20. Doughty HA, Murphy MF, Metcalfe P. Antenatal screening for fetal alloimmune thrombocytopenia: the results of a pilot study. Br J Haematol. 1995;90:321–5.
21. Jaegtvik S, Husebekk A, Aune B. Neonatal alloimmune thrombocytopenia due to anti-HPA-1a antibodies; the level of maternal antibodies predicts the severity of thrombocytopenia in the newborn. Br J Obstet Gynaecol. 2000;107:691–4.
22. Valentin N, Vergracht A, Bignon JD. HLA-DRw52a is involved in alloimmunization against PL-A1 antigen. Hum Immunol. 1990;27:73–9.
23. Reznikoff-Etievant MF. Management of alloimmune neonatal and antenatal thrombocytopenia. Vox Sang. 1988;55:193–201.
24. Mueller-Eckhardt C, Grubert A, Weisheit M. 348 cases of suspected neonatal alloimmune thrombocytopenia. Lancet. 1989;1:363–6.
25. Kornfeld I, Wilson RD, Ballem P. Antenatal invasive and noninvasive management of alloimmune thrombocytopenia. Fetal Diagn Ther. 1996;11:210–7.
26. Letsky EA, Greaves M. Guidelines on the investigation and management of thrombocytopenia in pregnancy and neonatal alloimmune thrombocytopenia. Br J Haematol. 1996;95:21–6.
27. Khouzami AN, Kickler TS, Callan NA. Devastating sequelae of alloimmune thrombocytopenia: an entity that deserves more attention. J Matern Fetal Med. 1996;5:137–41.
28. Kanhai HHH, Porcelijn L, van Zoeren D. Antenatal care in pregnancies at risk of alloimmune thrombocytopenia: report of 19 cases in 16 families. Eur J Obstet Gynecol Reprod Biol. 1996;68:67–73.
29. Uhrynowska M, Maslanka K, Zupanska B. Neonatal thrombocytopenia: incidence, serological and clinical observations. Am J Perinatol. 1997;14:415–8.
30. Davoren A, McParland P, Barnes CA. Neonatal alloimmune thrombocytopenia in the Irish population: a discrepancy between observed and expected cases. J Clin Pathol. 2002;55:289–92.
31. Davoren A, Curtis BR, Aster RH. Human platelet antigen-specific alloantibodies implicated in 1162 cases of neonatal alloimmune thrombocytopenia. Immunohematology. 2004;44:1220–5.

32. Rayment R, Birchall J, Yarranton H, Hewertson J, Allen D, Murphy MF. Neonatal alloimmune thrombocytopenia. BMJ. 2003;327:331–2.
33. Mandelbaum M, Koren D, Eichelberger B. Frequencies of maternal platelet alloantibodies and autoantibodies in suspected fetal/neonatal alloimmune thrombocytopenia, with emphasis on human platelet antigen-15 alloimmunization. Vox Sang. 2005;89:39–43.
34. Ertel K, Al-Tawil M, Santoso S. Relevance of the HPA-15 (Gov) polymorphism on CD109 in alloimmune thrombocytopenic syndromes. Transfusion. 2005;45:366–73.
35. Kroll H, Yates J, Santoso S. Immunization against a low-frequency human platelet alloantigen in fetal alloimmune thrombocytopenia is not a single event: characterization by the combined use of reference DNA and novel allele-specific cell lines expressing recombinant antigens. Transfusion. 2005;45:353–8.
36. Porcelijn L, Huiskes E, Overbeeke M. Rare anti HPA-5a NAIT cases. Vox Sang. 2006;91S2:Abstract 55.
37. Ahya R, Turner ML, Urbaniak SJ. Fetomaternal alloimmune thrombocytopenia. Transfus Apher Sci. 2001;25:139–45.
38. Birchall J, Murphy MF, Kaplan C. European collaborative study of the antenatal management of feto-maternal alloimmune thrombocytopenia. Br J Haematol. 2003;122:275–88.
39. Kaplan C, Morel-Kopp MC, Clemenceau S. Fetal and neonatal alloimmune thrombocytopenia: current trends in diagnosis and therapy. Transfus Med. 1992; 2:265–71.
40. Taaning E. HLA antibodies and fetomaternal alloimmune thrombocytopenia: myth or meaningful? Transfus Med Rev. 2000;14:275–80.
41. Kiefel V. The MAIPA assay and its applications in immunohaematology. Transfus Med. 1992;2:181–8.
42. Bertrand G, Jallu V, Gouet M. Quantification of human platelet antigen-1a antibodies with monoclonal antibody immobilization of platelet antigens procedure. Transfusion. 2005;45:1319–23.
43. Goldman M, Trudel E, Richard L. Report on the eleventh international society of blood transfusion platelet genotyping and serology workshop. Vox Sang. 2003;85:149–55.
44. Kaplan C. Alloimmune thrombocytopenia of the fetus and the newborn. Blood Rev. 2002;16:69–72.
45. Killie MK, Kjeldsen-Kragh J, Skogen B. Maternal anti-HPA1a antibody level as predictive value in neo-natal alloimmune thrombocytopenic purpura (NAITP). Blood. 2004;104:Abstract 2072.
46. Meyer O, Agaylan A, Borchert H. A simple and practical assay for the antigen-specific detection of platelet antibodies. Transfusion. 2006;46:1226–31.
47. Bussel JB, Kaplan C. The fetal and neonatal consequences of maternal alloimmune thrombocytopenia. Baillieres Clin Haematol. 2007;11:391–408.
48. Sainio S, Teramo K, Kekomaki R. Prenatal treatment of severe fetomaternal alloimmune thrombocytopenia. Transfus Med. 1999;9:321–30.
49. Berkowitz RL, Kolb A, Mcfarland JG. Parallel randomized trials of risk-based therapy for fetal alloimmune thrombocytopenia. Obstet Gynecol. 2006;107:91–6.
50. Bussel JB, Skupski DW, Mcfarland JG. Fetal alloimmune thrombocytopenia: consensus and controversy. J Matern Fetal Med. 1996;5:281–92.
51. Kuhn MJ, Couch SM, Binstadt DH. Prenatal recognition of central nervous system complications of alloimmune thrombocytopenia. Comput Med Imaging Graph. 1992;16:137–42.
52. Stanworth SJ, Hackett G, Williamson LM. Feto-maternal alloimmune thrombocytopenia presenting antenatally as hydrops fetalis. Prenat Diagn. 2001; 21:418–24.
53. Bussel JB. Immune thrombocytopenia in pregnancy: autoimmune and allo-immune. J Reprod Immunol. 1997;37:35–61.
54. Kaplan C, Daffos F, Forestier F. Management of alloimmune thrombocytopenia: antenatal diagnosis and in utero transfusion of maternal platelets. Blood. 1988;72:340–3.
55. Murphy MF, Williamson LM, Urbaniak SJ. Antenatal screening for fetomaternal alloimmune thrombocytopenia: should we be doing it? Vox Sang. 2002;83 Suppl 1:409–16.
56. Van den Akker ES, Oepkes D, Lopriore E, Brand A, Kanhai HH. Noninvasive antenatal management of fetal and neonatal alloimmune thrombocytopenia: safe and effective. BJOG. 2007;114(4):469–73.
57. Bussel JB, Berkowitz RL, McFarland JG. Antenatal treatment of neonatal alloimmune thrombocytopenia. N Engl J Med. 1988;319:1374–8.
58. Ohto H, Yamaguchi T, Takeuchi C. Anti-HPA-5b-induced neonatal alloimmune thrombocytopenia: antibody titre as predictor. Br J Haematol. 2000;110:223–7.
59. Killie MK, Husebekk A, Kjeldsen-Kragh J. Significance of antibody quantification. Vox Sang. 2006;91:15. Abstract 51.
60. BCSH guidelines, Gibson BES, Bolton-Maggs PHB, Pamphilon D, et al. Transfusion guidelines for neonates and older children. Br J Haematol. 2004;124:433–53;2005 amendment to these guidelines: www.bcshguidelines.com.
61. Bessos H, Turner M, Urbaniak SJ. Is there a relationship between anti-HPA-1a concentration and severity of neonatal alloimmune thrombocytopenia? Immunohematology. 2005;21:102–8.
62. Lyou JY, Chen YJ, Hu HY. PCR with sequence-specific primer-based simultaneous genotyping of human platelet antigen-1 to -13w. Transfusion. 2002; 42:1089–95.
63. Peterson JA, Balthazor SM, Curtis BR. Maternal alloimmunization against the rare platelet-specific antigen HPA-9b (Max-a) is an important cause of neonatal alloimmune thrombocytopenia. Transfusion. 2005;45:1487–95.
64. Chaoying M, Junwu G, Chituwo BM. Intraventricular haemorrhage and its prognosis, prevention and treatment in term infants. J Trop Pediatr. 1999;45: 237–9.

65. Tiller H, Kamphuis MM, Flodmark O, Papadogiannakis N, David AL, Sainio S, Koskinen S, Javela K, Wikman AT, Kekomaki R, Kanhai HH, Oepkes D, Husebekk A, Westgren M. Fetal intracranial haemorrhages caused by fetal and neonatal alloimmune thrombocytopenia: an observational cohort study of 43 cases from an international multicentre registry. BMJ Open. 2013;3(3). pii:e002490. doi:10.1136/bmjopen-2012-002490.
66. Radder CM, Kanhai HH, Brand A. On the mechanism of high dose maternal intravenous immunoglobulin (IVIG) in alloimmune thrombocytopenia. In: Management of fetal alloimmune thrombocytopenia. Amsterdam: Print Partners Ipskamp; 2004. p. 69–81.
67. Kaplan C, Daffos F, Forestier F, Morel MC, Chesnel N, Tchernia G. Cur- rent trends in neonatal alloimmune thrombocytopenia: diagnosis and therapy. In: Kaplan-Gouet C, Schlegel N, Salmon C, McGregor J, editors. Platelet immunology: fundamental and clinical aspects. Paris: Colloque INSERM/John Libbey Eurotext; 1991. p. 267–78.
68. Prouix C, Filion M, Goldman M, Bradley A, Devine D, Decary F, Chartrand P. Analysis of immunoglobulin class, IgG subclass and titre of HPA-1a antibodies in alloimmunised mothers giving birth to babies with or without neonatal alloimmune thrombocytopenia. Br J Haematol. 1994;87:813–7.
69. Marzusch K, Fischer Dietl J, Wiest E, Volklein K, Schnaid M. Difficulties in the antenatal assessment of neonatal alloimmune thrombocytopenia. Acta Obstet Gynecol Scand. 1993;72:583–5.
70. Bertrand G, Martageix C, Jallu V. Predictive value of sequential maternal anti-HPA-1a antibody concentrations for the severity of fetal alloimmune thrombocytopenia. J Thromb Haemost. 2006;4:628–37.
71. Ghevaert C, Campbell K, Stafford P, Metcalfe P, Casbard A, Smith GA, Allen D, Ranasinghe E, Williamson LM, Ouwehand WH. HPA-1a antibody potency and bioactivity do not predict severity of feto-maternal alloimmune thrombocytopenia. Transfusion. 2007;7:1296–305.
72. Ino H, Torigoe K, Numata O. A case of neonatal alloimmune thrombocytopenic purpura by anti-HPA-4b with intracranial hemorrhage. J Jpn Pediatr Soc. 2000;104:682–5.
73. Radder CM, Kanhai HH, de Beaufort AJ. Evaluation of gradual conversion to a less invasive therapeutic strategy for pregnant women with alloimmune thrombocytopenia in the fetus for prevention of intracranial hemorrhage. Ned Tijdschr Geneeskd. 2000;144:2015–8.
74. Murphy MF, Pullon HWH, Metcalfe P, Chapman JF, Jenkins E, Waters AH. Management of fetal alloimmune thrombocytopenia by weekly in utero platelet transfusions. Vox Sang. 1990;58:45–9.
75. Murphy MF, Waters AH, Doughty HA, Hambley H, Mibashan RS, Nicolaides K. Antenatal management of fetal alloimmune thrombocytopenia. Transfus Med. 1994;4:281–92.
76. Paidas MJ, Berkowitz RL, Lynch L, Lockwood CJ, Lapinski R, McFarland JG. Alloimmune thrombocytopenia: fetal and neonatal losses related to cordocentesis. Am J Obstet Gynecol. 1995;172:475–9.
77. Simsek S, Christiaens GCLM, Kanhai HHH. Human platelet antigen-1 (Zw) typing of fetuses by analysis of polymerase chain reaction-amplified genomic DNA from amniocytes. Transfus Med. 1994;4: 15–9.
78. Overton TG, Duncan KR, Jolly M, Letsky E, Fisk NM. Serial aggressive platelet transfusion for fetal alloimmune thrombocytopenia: platelet dynamics and peri-natal outcome. Am J Obstet Gynecol. 2002;186(4):826–31.
79. Berkowitz RL, Lesser ML, McFarland JG, Wissert M, Primiani A, Hung C. Antepartum treatment without early cordocentesis for standard-risk alloimmune thrombocytopenia: a randomised controlled trial. Obstet Gynecol. 2007;110(2 Pt 1):249–55.
80. Nicolini U, Kochenour NK, Greco P, Letsky EA, Johnson RD, Contreras M. Consequences of fetomaternal haemorrhage after intrauterine transfusion. BMJ. 1988;297:1379–81.
81. Radder CM, Roelen DL, Van de Meer-Prins EM, Claas FHJ, Kanhai HHH, Brand A. The immunologic profile of infants born after maternal immunoglobulin treatment and intrauterine platelet transfusions for fetal/neonatal alloimmune thrombocytopenia. Am J Obstet Gynecol. 2004;191:815–20.
82. Radder CM, de Haan MJJ, Brand A, Stoelhorst GMSJ, Veen S, Kanhai HHH. Follow up of children after antenatal treatment for alloimmune thrombocytopenia. Early Hum Dev. 2004;80:65–76.
83. Zimmermann R, Huch A. In utero therapy with immunoglobulin for alloimmune thrombocytopenia. Lancet. 1992;340:1034–5.
84. Samuelsson A, Towers TL, Ravetch JV. Anti-inflammatory activity of IVIG mediated through the inhibitory Fc receptor. Science. 2001;291:484–6.
85. Clark AL, Gall SA. Clinical uses of intravenous immunoglobulin in pregnancy. Am J Obstet Gynecol. 1998;176:241–53.
86. Bussel JB, Berkowitz RL, Lynch L, Lesser ML, Paidas MJ, Huang CL. Antenatal management of alloimmune thrombocytopenia with intravenous gamma-globulin: a randomized trial of the addition of low dose steroid to intravenous gamma-globulin. Am J Obstet Gynecol. 1996;174(5):1414–23.
87. Gaddipati S, Berkowitz RL, Lembet AA. Initial fetal platelet counts predict the response to intravenous gammaglobulin therapy in fetuses that are affected by PLA1 incompatibility. Am J Obstet Gynecol. 2001;185:976–80.
88. Lynch L, Bussel JB, McFarland JG, Chitkara U, Berkowitz RL. Antenatal treatment of alloimmune thrombocytopenia. Obstet Gynecol. 1992;80:67–71.
89. Radder CM, Brand A, Kanhai HH. A less invasive treatment strategy to prevent intracranial hemorrhage in fetal and neonatal alloimmune thrombocytopenia. Am J Obstet Gynecol. 2001;185:683–8.

90. Kroll H, Kiefel V, Giers G, Bald R, Hoch J, Hanfland P. Maternal intravenous immunoglobulin treatment does not prevent intracranial haemorrhage in fetal alloimmune thrombocytopenia. Transfus Med. 1994;4(4):293–6.
91. Van den Akker ESA, Westgren M, Husbekk A, Kanhai HHH, Oepkes D. Fetal or neonatal alloimmune thrombocytopenia: a new randomized con-trolled trial and international multicenter data collection [abstract]. J Obstet Gynaecol. 2006;26 Suppl 1:S63.
92. Ward MJ, Pauliny J, Lipper EG, Bussel JB. Long-term effects of fetal and neonatal alloimmune thrombocytopenia and its antenatal treatment on the medical and developmental outcomes of affected children. Am J Perinatol. 2006;23(8):487–92.
93. Bussel JB, Berkowitz RL, Hung C, Kolb EA, Wissert M, Primiani A, Tsaur FW, Macfarland JG. Intracranial hemorrhage in alloimmune thrombocytopenia: stratified management to prevent recurrence in the subsequent affected fetus. Am J Obstet Gynecol. 2010;203(2):135.e1–14.
94. Paternoster DM, Cester M, Memmo A. The management of feto-maternal alloimmune thrombocytopenia: report of three cases. J Matern Fetal Neonatal Med. 2006;19:517–20.
95. Rayment R, Brunskill SJ, Soothill PW, Roberts DJ, Bussel JB, Murphy MF. Antenatal interventions for fetomaternal alloimmune thrombocytopenia. Cochrane Database Syst Rev. 2011;(5):CD004226. doi:10.1002/14651858.CD004226.pub3.
96. Bennett PR, Warwick R, Vaughan J. Prenatal determination of human platelet antigen type using DNA amplification following amniocentesis. Br J Obstet Gynaecol. 1994;101:246–9.
97. Sainio S, Jarvenpaa AL, Renlund M. Thrombocytopenia in term infants: a population-based study. Obstet Gynecol. 2000;95:441–6.
98. Bennett PR, Vaughan J, Handyside A. Potential for pre-implantation determination of human platelet antigen type using DNA amplification: a strategy for prevention of allo-immune thrombocytopenia. Fetal Diagn Ther. 1994;9:229–32.
99. Radder CM, Brand A, Kanhai HHH. Will it ever be possible to balance the risk of intracranial haemorrhage in fetal or neonatal alloimmune thrombocytopenia against the risk of treatment strategies to prevent it? Vox Sang. 2003;84:318–25.
100. Deruelle P, Wibaut B, Manessier L, Subtil D, Vaast P, Puech F, Valat AS. Is a non-invasive management allowed for maternofetal alloimmune thrombocytopenia? Experience over a 10-year period. Gynecol Obstet Fertil. 2007;35(3):199–204.
101. Kanhai HH, van den Akker ES, Walther FJ, Brand A. Intravenous immunoglobulins without initial and follow-up cordocentesis in alloimmune fetal and neonatal thrombocytopenia at high risk for intracranial hemorrhage. Fetal Diagn Ther. 2006;21(1):55–60.
102. Glade-Bender J, McFarland JG, Kaplan C, Porcelijn L, Bussel JB. Anti-HPA-3A induces severe neonatal alloimmune thrombocytopenia. J Pediatr. 2001;138:862–7.
103. Kaplan C, Morel-Kopp MC, Kroll H, Kiefel V, Sohlege N, Chesnel N, Mueller-Eckhardt C. HPA-5b (Br(a)) neonatal alloimmune thrombocytopenia: clinical and immunological analysis of 39 cases. Br J Haematol. 1991;78:425–9.
104. Friedman JM, Aster RH. Neonatal alloimmune thrombocytopenic purpura and congenital porencephaly in two siblings associated with a "new" maternal antiplatelet antibody. Blood. 1985;65:1412–5.
105. Gyamfi C, Eddleman KA. Alloimmune thrombocytopenia. Clin Obstet Gynecol. 2005;48:897–909.
106. Van den Akker E, Oepkes D, Brand A, Kanhai HH. Vaginal delivery for fetuses at risk of alloimmune thrombocytopenia? BJOG. 2006;113(7):781–3.
107. Sia CG, Amigo NC, Harper RG. Failure of cesarean section to prevent intracranial hemorrhage in siblings with isoimmune neonatal thrombocytopenia. Am J Obstet Gynecol. 1985;153:79–81.
108. te Pas AB, Lopriore E, van den Akker ES, Oepkes D, Kanhai HH, Brand A, Walther FJ. Postnatal management of fetal and neonatal alloimmune thrombocytopenia: the role of matched platelet transfusion and IVIG. Eur J Pediatr. 2007;166(10):1057–63.
109. Berkowitz R, Bussel JB, Hung C, Wissert M. A randomised prospective treatment trial for patients with "standard risk" alloimmune thrombocytopenia (AIT). Am J Obstet Gynecol. 2006;195 Suppl 1:S23.
110. Gafni A, Blanchette VS. Screening for alloimmune thrombocytopenia: an economic perspective. Curr Stud Hematol Blood Transfus. 1988;54:140–7.
111. Killie MK, Kjeldsen-Kragh J, Husebekk A, Skogen B, Olsen JA, Kristiansen IS. Cost-effectiveness of ante-natal screening for neonatal alloimmune thrombocytopenia. BJOG. 2007;114:588–95.
112. Kjedsen-Kragh J, Husebekk A, Kjaer Killie M, Skogen B. Is it time to include screening for neonatal alloimmune thrombocytopenia in the general antenatal health program? Transfus Apher Sci. 2008;38:183–8.
113. Durand-Zaleski I, Schlegel N, Blum-Boisgard C, Uzan S, Dreyfus M, Kaplan C. Screening primiparous women and newborns for fetal/neonatal alloimmune thrombocytopenia: a prospective comparison of effectiveness and costs. Am J Perinatol. 1996;13:423–31.
114. Williamson LM, Hackett G, Rennie J. The natural history of fetomaternal alloimmunization to the platelet-specific antigen hpa-1a (pi-a1, zw-a) as determined by antenatal screening. Blood. 1998;92:2280–7.
115. Tiller H, Killie MK, Skogen B, Øian P, Husebekk A. Neonatal alloimmune thrombocytopenia in Norway: poor detection rate with nonscreening versus a general screening programme. BJOG. 2009; 116(4):594–8.
116. Kaplan C. Alloimmune thrombocytopenia of the fetus and neonate: prospective antenatal screening. Third European symposium on platelet and granulocyte immunobiology, Cambridge; 26–29 June 1994.
117. Husebekk A, Killie MK, Kjeldsen-Kragh J. General overview over screening programs. Vox Sang. 2006;91:15. Abstract 49.

118. Husebekk A, Killie MK, Kjeldsen-Kragh J, Skogen B. Is it time to implement HPA-1 screening in pregnancy? Curr Opin Hematol. 2009;16(6):497–502.
119. Berkowitz RL, Bussel JB, Mc Farland JG. Alloimmune thrombocytopenia: state of the art. Am J Obstet Gynecol. 2006;195:907–13.
120. Murphy MF, Bussel JB. Advances in the management of alloimmune thrombocytopenia. Br J Haematol. 2007;136:366–78.
121. Beachy J. Neonatal alloimmune thrombocytopenia: a case study (Lab Values). Neonatal Netw J Neonatal Nurs. 2011;30(6):407.
122. Peterson JA, Pechauer SM, Gitter ML, Kanack A, Curtis BR, Reese J, et al. New platelet glycoprotein polymorphisms causing maternal immunization and neonatal alloimmune thrombocytopenia. Transfusion. 2012;52(5):1117–24.

Thrombotic Microangiopathies in Pregnancy

17

Marie Scully and Patrick O'Brien

Abstract

Thrombotic microangiopathies (TMAs) describe a collection of disorders with similar presenting features but different underlying pathogenesis and often differing therapies. TMAs are defined by the presence of thrombocytopenia, hemolytic anemia and fragmented red blood cells on a blood film, which is due to shearing of red blood cells caused by the presence of microthrombi. TMAs can present during or unrelated to pregnancy, and in pregnancy it can be difficult in the acute situation to confirm the underlying diagnosis. This chapter focuses on the diagnosis, pathophysiology and management of TMAs that are primarily precipitated by pregnancy.

Keywords

Thrombotic microangiopathies • Pre-eclampsia • HELLP syndrome • Thrombotic thrombocytopenic purpura • Haemolytic uremic syndrome • Systemic lupus erythematosus • Antiphospholipid syndrome • Acute fatty liver of pregnancy

M. Scully, MB ChB, BSc (Hons), MD, MRCP, FRCPath (✉)
Thrombotic Microangiopathy, Department of Haematology, University College London Hospitals NHS Foundation Trust, Whitfield St., London W1T 4EU, UK
e-mail: scully@ucl.ac.uk

P. O'Brien, MBBCh, FRCOG, FICOG, FFSRH
Institute for Women's Health, University College London Hospitals NHS Foundation Trust, 250 Euston Road, London NW1, UK
e-mail: patobrien64@yahoo.co.uk

17.1 Introduction

Thrombotic microangiopathies (TMAs) describe a collection of disorders with similar presenting features but different underlying pathogenesis and often differing therapies. TMAs are defined by the presence of thrombocytopenia, hemolytic anemia and fragmented red blood cells on a blood film, which is due to shearing of red blood cells caused by the presence of microthrombi. TMAs can present during or unrelated to pregnancy, and in pregnancy it can be difficult in the acute situation

H. Cohen, P. O'Brien (eds.), *Disorders of Thrombosis and Hemostasis in Pregnancy: A Guide to Management*, DOI 10.1007/978-3-319-15120-5_17, © Springer-Verlag London 2015

to confirm the underlying diagnosis. The features of TMA can occur in disseminated intravascular coagulation (DIC), but in this chapter we will focus on the diagnosis, pathophysiology and management of those conditions that are primarily precipitated by pregnancy and, unlike DIC, typically associated with a normal coagulation screen. Included in the differential diagnosis are pre-eclampsia (PET) or eclampsia, HELLP (hemolysis, elevated liver enzymes, low platelets) syndrome, thrombotic thrombocytopenic purpura (TTP), hemolytic uremic syndrome (HUS), systemic lupus erythematosus (SLE), antiphospholipid syndrome (APS) and acute fatty liver of pregnancy (AFLP) (Table 17.1).

17.2 Moderate to Severe Thrombocytopenia Presenting During Pregnancy

Thrombocytopenia is defined as a platelet count <150 × 10⁹/L and results from increased destruction/consumption or decreased production. Thrombocytopenia can affect 10 % of pregnancies. However, a platelet count of under 100 × 10⁹/L, as defined by an international working group [1], is encountered in 1 % of pregnant women. The challenge is to determine the underlying pathophysiology. The most common is gestational thrombocytopenia, occurring in 75 % of all cases, in which the platelet count is rarely below 70 × 10⁹/L. It is characterised by a normal platelet count at the antenatal booking visit, is most apparent in the third trimester and returns to normal within 12 weeks postpartum. Gestational thrombocytopenia is thought to result from the hemodilutional effect of pregnancy and placental platelet destruction [2].

Idiopathic thrombocytopenic purpura (ITP) occurs in 5 % of pregnancies and is a result of peripheral platelet destruction [3]. Occasionally maternal treatment (oral steroids or IV immunoglobulin) and precautions during delivery (avoidance of fetal scalp blood sampling, fetal scalp electrode, ventouse delivery or difficult forceps delivery) may be required, but rarely does it have an affect on the fetus prior to labor and delivery. PET and HELLP account for 21 % of all cases of thrombocytopenia and the platelet count usually returns to normal within 3–5 days after delivery.

17.3 Acute Renal Injury in Pregnancy

Serum creatinine normally falls as pregnancy proceeds because of hemodilution, hyperfiltration and reduced oncotic pressures. Seventy-five percent of cases of renal impairment in pregnancy occur in the third trimester and postpartum. The leading cause of acute kidney injury in pregnancy is the hypertensive disorders of pregnancy; other causes include sepsis, hemorrhage, intrauterine fetal death (IUFD), AFLP and TMAs. For most of these differential diagnoses, pregnancy plays a primary role. However, in the case of TMAs, pregnancy is the trigger for a condition primarily associated with an underlying genetic risk. Acute renal injury may range from increased creatinine levels to dialysis dependence, and can be associated with significant feto-maternal morbidity and mortality.

17.4 Pre-eclampsia

17.4.1 Clinical Features

The definition of PET specifies *de novo* hypertension (i.e. blood pressure >140/90 mmHg) and proteinuria (>0.3 g/24 h) occurring after 20 weeks of gestation [4]. This definition encompasses the triad of hypertension, proteinuria and edema, but this is essentially a multisystem disorder that affects 5–10 % of pregnancies. PET is the second most common cause of thrombocytopenia in the second half of pregnancy and accounts for approximately 20 % of all cases. Platelet counts <50 × 10⁹/L occur in less than 5 % of women with PET and, in the presence of intravascular hemolysis, other TMAs such as TTP must be excluded. Indeed, consideration should be given to checking ADAMTS 13 activity and giving treatment for TTP, if appropriate. Liver involvement in PET is the most common

Table 17.1 A summary of the characteristics of thrombotic microangiopathies

	Primary features	Pathophysiology	Complications	Treatment
DIC	Abnormal coagulation (increased PT, APTT, reduced fibrinogen and platelets)	Underlying precipitant, e.g. placental abruption, sepsis	Excessive bleeding or thrombosis	Treat the underlying cause and support with blood components/ products as required
PET	Hypertension (>140/90 mmHg), proteinuria (>0.3 g/24 h), edema	Dysfunctional spiral artery development and release of trophoblast derived factors, e.g. increased VEGF-1 (s-Flt-1) and sEng; reduced VEGF and PIGF	Thrombocytopenia, HELLP syndrome; renal impairment; eclampsia (convulsions); stroke; placental abruption; IUGR and preterm delivery	Symptomatic control of hypertension. If severe, delivery. Antiplatelets +/– LMWH for prevention in high risk women
HELLP	Upper abdominal pain and tenderness, nausea, vomiting, malaise, headache, rarely jaundice	Result of endothelial cell injury. Bilirubin is typically not raised, transferases are increased from only marginally to 20-fold. The degree of thrombocytopenia defines type (I, II or III)	DIC, placental abruption, acute renal failure, pulmonary edema, hepatic failure (occasionally requiring liver transplantation), hepatic rupture	Symptomatic control of seizures, hypertension and thrombocytopenia. If severe, delivery. PEX may be required. Steroids may improve thrombocytopenia
TTP	Primarily neurological and cardiac features acutely, but features in pregnancy may be non-specific	ADAMTS 13 deficiency. Either congenital TTP (with no antibody present, and confirmed by mutational analysis) or antibody mediated disease (with proven Anti-ADAMTS 13 antibodies)	IUGR, IUFD, PET, renal impairment	PEX required for acute presentation. Subsequent pregnancies require therapy throughout. Acquired TTP requires associated immunosuppressive therapy
HUS	Renal impairment or failure	Complement dysfunction	Dialysis, ESRF, hypertension	PEX, eculizumab
SLE	Thrombocytopenia, hemolytic anemia, pancytopenia, nephritis	ANA, dsDNA	Hypertension, preterm delivery, IUGR	Immunosuppression, symptomatic
APLS	Recurrent miscarriages or IUFD	LA, ACLA result in abnormal placentation	IUGR, IUFD, preterm delivery	LDA, LMWH, PEX
AFLP	Non-specific features, RUQ pain, GI hemorrhage, coagulation abnormalities/DIC, acute renal failure, pancreatitis, hypoglycemia, liver failure, encephalopathy	Fetal deficiency of LCHAD, a mitochondrial enzyme	Within hours of birth, the fetus presents with non-ketotic hypoglycemia, which can quickly progress to coma and death	Treat hypoglycemia. Genetic screening

All these conditions present with features of thrombocytopenia and hemolytic anemia

DIC disseminated intravascular coagulation, *PT* prothrombin time, *APTT* activated partial thromboplastin time, *PET* pre-eclampsia, *VEGF* vascular endothelial growth factor, *sFlt-1* soluble fms-like tyrosine kinase 1, *sEng* soluble endoglin, *PlGF* placental growth factor, *HELLP* hemolysis, elevated liver enzymes and low platelets, *IUGR* intrauterine fetal growth restriction, *LMWH* low molecular weight heparin, *PEX* plasma exchange, *TTP* thrombotic thrombocytopenic purpura, *ADAMTS*-13 a disintegrin and metalloproteinase with a thrombospondin type 1 motif, member 13 – also known as von Willebrand factor-cleaving protease (vWFCP), *IUFD* intrauterine fetal death, *HUS* hemolytic uremic syndrome, *ESRF* end-stage renal failure, *SLE* systemic lupus erythematosis, *ANA* anti-nuclear antibodies, *dsDNA* double stranded deoxyribonucleic acid, *APLS* antiphospholipid syndrome, *LA* lupus anticoagulant, *ACLA* anticardiolipin antibodies, *LDA* low dose aspirin, *AFLP* acute fatty liver of pregnancy, *RUQ* right upper quadrant, *GI* gastrointestinal, *LCHAD* long chain 3-hydroxyacyl-CoA dehydrogenase cause of hepatic tenderness and liver dysfunction in pregnancy. It is one of the indicators that should prompt consideration of delivery because of the high perinatal morbidity and mortality and the increased risk of eclampsia (seizures), hepatic rupture and necrosis. In 2–12 % of cases of eclampsia, the condition is complicated by HELLP syndrome. Other potential complications include renal impairment, stroke, placental abruption and abnormalities of the coagulation system. As with all the TMA's, adverse affects on the placenta can result in fetal growth restriction and premature birth (usually as a result of medical intervention).

17.4.2 Serum Markers for Predicting Pre-eclampsia

The placenta is central to the pathogenesis of PET, and the only curative treatment is delivery and removal of the placenta, with symptoms usually improving within days. Failure of trophoblastic invasion of the maternal spiral arteries results in inadequate vascular remodelling. This in turn results in placental ischemia and infarction, which can be confirmed histologically. Uteroplacental ischemia is associated with the release of soluble factors that lead to widespread maternal endothelial dysfunction that manifest as the clinical features of PET. It is the disturbed balance between placenta derived anti-angiogenic factors and proangiogenic factors that are thought to contribute to the pathogenesis of PET [5, 6]. Placental ischemia can also cause IUGR, and PET and IUGR often present together. Therefore, early diagnosis and timely delivery are imperative for perinatal survival.

17.4.2.1 Placental Growth Factor (PIGF) and Soluble Fms-Like Tyrosine Kinase-1 (sFlt-1)

Fms-like tyrosine kinase-1 (Flt-1, soluble Flt (sFlt-1) and their ligands PIGF and vascular endothelial growth factor A (VEGF-A) are expressed by trophoblasts and their expression is altered in PET compared to normotensive controls. In PET, PIGF levels are reduced; serum concentrations of sFlt-1 and soluble endoglin (sEng) are increased, and the increase appears to correlate with disease severity. In a rodent model, overexpressing sFlt can trigger PET [7]. Furthermore, in other disease states, such as cancer, anti-VEGF therapy was associated with the development of hypertension and proteinuria [8].

In normal pregnancy, serum PIGF levels decrease and sFlt-1 levels increase in the third trimester. In PET, these changes are seen earlier in pregnancy and can be used to predict the disease 5 weeks before the onset of clinical symptoms. PIGF levels were lower before 12 weeks' gestation in women who subsequently developed PET later in pregnancy [9, 10]. It has also been shown that women who have had a pregnancy affected by PET are at increased risk of cardiovascular disease (stroke, ischemic heart disease) later in life (see Sect. 17.4.7).

17.4.2.2 Placental Protein 13

The levels of placental protein 13 (PP13) are decreased in women who develop pre-eclampsia. The utility of a combination of uterine artery Doppler pulsatility index (PI) and maternal serum PP-13 measured in the first trimester (between 11 and 13 weeks) for the prediction of PET has been investigated [11]. PP-13 levels were lower and pulsatility indices higher in women that subsequently developed PET. This study had a high detection rate (90 %) for a false positive rate of 6 %.

17.4.2.3 Soluble Endoglin (sEng)

Endoglin is a co-receptor for transforming growth factors β1 and β3, expressed on trophoblasts. Its levels are increased in PET [12] and in pregnant rats this has been associated with increased vascular permeability and hypertension. When both sFlt-1 and sEng levels were elevated, symptoms were markedly worse, and associated with the development of HELLP syndrome. In a longitudinal analysis, the rise in sEng concentrations occurred earlier and was more marked in pregnancies in women that subsequently developed PET [13].

17.4.3 Management of Pre-eclampsia

The three main aspects of therapy are the management of hypertension (both systolic and diastolic), prevention and treatment of eclampsia, and careful fluid balance management. Delivery is the ultimate cure and particularly in women near term delivery may be appropriate, especially if there is associated HELLP syndrome. However, if anti-hypertensive treatment is required, one option is nifedipine, which is associated with reduced maternal hypotension. However, it should be avoided in women with known coronary heart disease or diabetes (for more than 15 years) or who are older than 45 years because of the risk of sudden cardiac death. Labetalol is less effective, but has a preferred side-effect profile compared to hydralazine. In severe PET, magnesium sulphate ($MgSO_4$) should be used to reduce the risk of seizures. In general, timing of delivery depends on the maternal condition, fetal wellbeing (which can be assessed by umbilical artery Doppler), the gestational age and the neonatal care facilities available. Steroids for fetal lung maturation should be considered for pregnancies less than 36 weeks' gestation.

Blood component support may be required, particularly in women with a coagulopathy. Platelets are not usually administered, but may be indicated if platelet counts are $<50 \times 10^9/L$ and particularly if the platelet count is dropping precipitously [14].

17.4.4 Antiplatelet Agents for the Prevention of Pre-eclampsia

Placental ischemia and infarction in PET is thought to be a result of platelet aggregation and activation of the coagulation system and platelets. Initial trials suggested that antiplatelet therapy might prevent PET [4, 15, 16]. The PARIS (perinatal antiplatelet review of International studies) collaboration undertook a systematic review and meta-analysis to assess the use of antiplatelet agents for the primary prevention of PET and to explore women most likely to benefit from such treatment [17]. There was a 10 % reduction in the relative risk of both PET ($p=0.004$) and preterm delivery before 34 weeks ($p=0.011$). However, there was no difference in antepartum haemorrhage (APH), postpartum haemorrhage (PPH) or placental abruption compared to controls. There was a 7 % reduction in the RR of preterm birth before 37 weeks ($p=0.003$). The conclusion was that antiplatelet agents are associated with a reduction in the relative risk of PET, preterm birth before 34 weeks and serious adverse pregnancy outcomes. The PREDO (Prediction and Prevention of Pre-eclampsia) group which included 152 women with risk factors for PET and abnormal uterine artery Dopplers, showed that low dose aspirin (LDA) did not prevent PET unless started before 16 weeks' gestation [18].

17.4.5 Future Therapeutic Targets

Over 50 proteins synthesised by the placenta have been investigated, and an understanding of their identities and role is being elucidated by genetic techniques including mRNA expression [19]. sFlt-1 ligands such as VEGF or PIGF have been shown in animal studies to improve PET [20]. More recently, it has been shown that low molecular weight heparin (LMWH) increases levels of both circulating and urinary sFlt-1; and that heparin bound sFlt-1 has decreased affinity to negatively charged surfaces when compared to sFlt-1 alone. It is speculated that upon heparin treatment, sFlt-1 bound to heparan sulfate proteoglycans of the extracellular matrix are mobilized into the circulation [21]. Furthermore, in a meta-analysis of randomized controlled trials comparing prophylactic LMWH with no therapy, there was a significant relative risk reduction in adverse pregnancy outcomes (18.7 % vs 42.9 % in treated and non-treatment groups, respectively). These adverse outcomes include PET, severe PET, small for gestational age (<10 % percentile), preterm delivery <37 weeks and preterm delivery <34 weeks. Therefore, LMWH may be a useful therapy for placenta mediated pregnancy complications but further trials are required [22]. Statins can upregulate pro-angiogenic factors and also improve PET in animal models [23].

17.4.6 Outcome of Subsequent Pregnancy After First Pregnancy with Early Onset PET

Presentation with PET is generally near term, and much more common in nulliparous women. However, 10 % of women who develop PET will present before 34 weeks. Earlier presentations are associated with worse outcomes for both mother and fetus. Recurrence rates in subsequent pregnancies are variably quoted between 15 and 65 % [24]. Treatment in subsequent pregnancies with LMWH and LDA has been reported to improve outcomes [25]; LMWH is thought to have a dual role as an anti-inflammatory and anti-thrombotic agent. Furthermore, women with a history of chronic hypertension also had an improved outcome with this therapy. More recently, using LDA alone before 16 weeks' gestation reduced the risk of PET and severe PET in high-risk women [17, 18].

17.4.7 Long-Term Effects of Pre-eclampsia

Later in life, women with a history of PET have an increased risk of cerebrovascular complications such as hypertension, ischemic heart disease and stroke, that is thought to stem from endothelial dysfunction [26, 27]. This risk appears to be greater in women who have preterm PET or PET complicated by IUGR [28]. There is an increased risk of peripartum cardiomyopathy and it has been suggested that the babies are at increased long-term risk of pulmonary hypertension. There is also a suggestion of an increased relative risk of end stage renal failure, although the absolute risk remains low [26]. What remains unclear is whether the long-term cardiovascular risks associated with PET are due to damage caused by the pre-eclamptic process, or whether women who develop PET have a pre-existing cardiovascular phenotype that predispose them to both PET and later cardiovascular disease.

17.5 Thrombotic Thrombocytopenic Purpura

17.5.1 Clinical and Laboratory Features

TTP is an acute life-threatening disorder associated with thrombocytopenia, microangiopathic hemolytic anemia and symptoms related to microvascular thrombosis. Clinically, in addition to a low platelet count ($<150\times10^9$/L, but typically $<50\times10^9$/L), patients are anemic secondary to hemolysis, with acute consumption of folate. Corresponding blood film changes include polychromasia, anemia, reduced platelets and fragmented red blood cells. Bilirubin is often raised but the direct antiglobulin test is negative and the clotting screen is normal. Lactate dehydrogenase (LDH) is increased, often to a greater extent than the degree of hemolysis, due to associated tissue ischemia [29].

17.5.2 Pathophysiology

von Willebrand factor (vWF), a plasma glycoprotein synthesized by megakaryocytes and endothelial cells, normally circulates as multimers of 500–20,000 kDa. Ultra-large vWF multimers (ULvWFM), >20,000 kDa, not normally detected in plasma, have been detected in patients with chronic relapsing TTP [30]. The deficiency of vWF-cleaving protease in patients with TTP has been identified as a disintegrin and metalloprotease with thrombospondin type 1 motif, member 13' or ADAMTS 13 [31, 32]. This enzyme is required to break down ULVWF multimers, and failure to do so, due to an inherited deficiency of ADAMTS 13 (in congenital TTP) or an acquired reduction (due to antibodies to ADAMTS 13), leads to platelet adhesion and aggregation on ULvWF multimers, which results in microvascular thrombosis. Hence, platelet transfusions are contraindicated in TTP, as infusions potentiate the effects of platelet aggregation on ULvWF multimers.

As a precipitating cause of acute TTP, pregnancy accounts for only a small proportion of all cases in women [33, 34]. TTP is more common in women than in men (3:2) and 45 % of all cases occur in women of childbearing age. There is also the risk of relapse of TTP during subsequent pregnancies once women have been diagnosed. Other pregnancy related thrombotic microangiopathies, such as PET/HELLP (hemolysis, elevated liver enzymes, low platelets) and hemolytic-uremic syndrome (HUS) may further complicate the diagnosis of TTP but may also be part of the TTP syndrome.

17.5.3 Hemostatic Changes of Normal Pregnancy: Factor VIII, von Willebrand Factor (vWF) and ADAMTS 13

Normal pregnancy is associated with marked prothrombotic changes in hemostasis that are hormonally mediated and protect against severe hemorrhage at the time of birth, but result in a hypercoagulable state. Factor VIII and vWF increase in parallel in the first half of pregnancy; thereafter, the increase in vWF is greater throughout the remainder of pregnancy, returning to normal levels over the 6 postpartum weeks. Reciprocal changes of vWF and ADAMTS 13 have been documented. Therefore, with the increased vWF in pregnancy, ADAMTS 13 would be expected to decrease.

A review of ADAMTS 13 in normal women with no history of TTP documented a reduction in ADAMTS 13 activity in the 2nd and 3rd trimesters of pregnancy [35]. Another study in healthy women confirmed a reduction in ADAMTS 13 activity after the first trimester (weeks 12–16) up until the end of the postnatal period, when levels normalised to pre-pregnancy levels. Interestingly, this group found that ADAMTS 13 activity was lower in non-pregnant nulliparous women (mean 65 %) compared to parous women (mean 83 %). In pregnancy and postpartum, mean ADAMTS 13 activity was slightly, but non-significantly, lower in primigravidae than in multigravidae (68 % vs 74 %). ADAMTS 13 was unaffected by platelet count, but was significantly higher in smokers than in non-smokers during pregnancy (mean 79 % vs 70 %, respectively). There was a significant inverse correlation between vWF: Ag levels and ADAMTS 13 activity [36]. The cause of the decrease in ADAMTS 13 during pregnancy may be twofold. Firstly, enzyme levels decrease with excess substrate, namely vWF. Secondly, a hormonal influence, possibly estrogen, may reduce ADAMTS13 levels.

17.5.4 Women Presenting with Acute TTP During Pregnancy

Women presenting with TTP during pregnancy appear to fall into two groups; those with congenital TTP and those with acquired, antibody mediated TTP. Congenital TTP may first present during pregnancy; indeed, it is more likely that presentation in pregnancy will be congenital TTP [37, 38] and these women will relapse in subsequent pregnancies. Diagnosis of congenital TTP is confirmed in patients with ADAMTS 13 activity <5 %, no evidence of an inhibitor and confirmation by mutational analysis of the ADAMTS 13 gene, revealing a homozygous or compound heterozygous abnormality.

17.5.5 Risks in Pregnancy in Women with Previous Acquired Idiopathic (Non-pregnancy Associated) TTP

A particular concern in women who have had acute TTP unrelated to pregnancy is the risk of relapse during pregnancy. This occurs in 30–50 % of cases and the risk of fetal loss is significant. In those patients in whom ADAMTS 13 was tested, normal levels pre-pregnancy or at the onset of pregnancy were associated with a lower likelihood of relapse. Another important feature is the associated complications in TTP, such as pre-eclampsia and HELLP. Thrombotic microangiopathies during pregnancy may be clinically indistinguishable from one another and very difficult to treat. Because the reduction in ADAMTS 13 levels occurs from the onset of the second trimester, it had originally been proposed that this was the time of increased presentation of acute TTP. However, it now appears that the time of greatest risk is in the 3rd trimester or postpartum.

17.5.6 Management of TTP in Pregnancy

The primary decision is whether delivery will be associated with remission of the TMA (as it is in PET and HELLP) or whether plasma exchange (PEX) should be instigated, if recovery following delivery is unlikely and there is a risk of multi-organ dysfunction or death. A further complicating issue is the possible development of

HELLP/PET following delivery, which may occur in 20–30 % of cases. If TTP develops in the first trimester, PEX may allow continuation of pregnancy with delivery of a live infant. However, in contrast to PET and HELLP, delivery does not necessarily induce remission of TTP [39–41]. Later in pregnancy, differentiation from other pregnancy associated TMAs can be very difficult, but is important. Delivery is the definitive treatment of choice for pregnancy associated TMAs and, with recovery after delivery, TTP can be excluded. If there is progression of symptoms despite delivery, PEX is the most appropriate option.

A prospective study of TTP cases from the United Kingdom TTP Registry with clinical and laboratory data from the largest cohort of pregnancy-associated TTP [42] describes management through pregnancy, averting fetal loss and maternal complications. The study included 35 women who presented with a first TTP episode during pregnancy: 23/47 pregnancies with their first congenital TTP (cTTP) episode and 12/47 with acute acquired TTP in pregnancy. The conclusions from this study are that careful diagnosis, monitoring, and treatment in congenital and acquired TTP have assisted in excellent pregnancy outcomes [42].

With the availability of ADAMTS 13 activity measurement and detection of inhibitors to ADAMTS 13 or more specifically IgG antibodies, these markers may be helpful to distinguish TTP from other pregnancy associated TMAs. Specifically, if ADAMTS 13 activity is under 5 % and/or there are anti-ADAMTS 13 IgG autoantibodies, it is diagnostic of TTP. In HELLP, ADAMTS 13 activity is reduced (median 31 %, range 12–43 %) but with no inhibitor/antibodies to ADAMTS 13 and higher VWF levels [43]. Women presenting with thrombocytopenia, microangiopathic haemolytic anaemia (MAHA), neurological features (such as stroke/TIA, seizures, encephalopathy) or renal impairment, should be treated with PEX until the diagnosis of TTP is excluded.

Steroids may be useful in TTP and HELLP, but for differing reasons. They have been empirically used in TTP because of the underlying autoimmune basis of the disorder. In HELLP, steroids may accelerate platelet recovery and predelivery, dexa-/betametasone will aid fetal lung maturity.

In women with congenital TTP, the risk of relapse in subsequent pregnancy is such that elective plasma therapy, to provide ADAMTS 13 supplementation, throughout pregnancy and the post-partum period, is warranted. Plasma infusions may be satisfactory; however, in order to deliver sufficient volumes, PEX may be required. The precise optimal frequency of plasma replacement is unknown; the half-life of ADAMTS 13 is 2–3 days [44] and plasma therapy every 2 weeks appears satisfactory. However, this often needs to be increased to weekly from the 2nd trimester, and the appropriate frequency can be determined by monitoring platelet counts and LDH.

In women with acquired TTP, it is not as easy to predict which patients are likely to relapse and the literature is sparse in this area. A previous history of TTP and ADAMTS 13 activity at the onset of pregnancy may be helpful in differentiating patients most likely to relapse in subsequent pregnancies. A normal ADAMTS 13 at the onset of pregnancy appears to predict women at reduced risk of subsequent relapse [45]. However, low ADAMTS 13 activity (<5 %) prior to pregnancy should prompt consideration of elective therapy to prevent relapse. In contrast, women with normal ADAMTS 13 activity at the onset of pregnancy who maintain normal routine laboratory parameters, ADAMTS 13 activity and antibody/inhibitor levels throughout pregnancy, do not usually require intervention for TTP. A reduction in ADAMTS 13 activity (<10 %) may be the catalyst to instigate elective therapy to prevent microvascular thrombosis during pregnancy.

Adjunctive therapy during pregnancy has not been addressed in the literature; specifically, LDA and/or prophylactic LMWH administration. LDA throughout pregnancy should be considered, and women with a documented thrombophilia or a past history of venous thromboembolism associated with TTP, may require prophylactic LMWH. The aim is to optimize implantation and preserve placental function, as abnormalities of the uteroplacental circulation resulting in placental insufficiency are established in the first trimester [46]. LDA/LMWH may be beneficial in other thrombophilia disorders during pregnancy due to the effects of placental abnormalities secondary to infarction. However, this therapy has not been formally evaluated in pregnancy associated TTP. There are no data on the microvascular effects of 'subacute' TTP prior to presentation with thrombocytopenia. Therefore, women with a previous pregnancy loss due to TTP or low ADAMTS 13 activity at the onset of pregnancy can be assumed to be at increased risk of further episodes in subsequent pregnancies. Women who have a past history of TTP may have an increased risk of complications, such as pre-eclampsia, which could in part be attributable to placental infarction due to thrombotic occlusion of the decidual arterioles. Supportive measures may help to reduce such complications in those at risk. Red cell transfusion should be administered according to clinical need especially if there is cardiac involvement. Due to the risk of precipitating further thrombotic events, platelet transfusions are contraindicated unless there is life- threatening haemorrhage [29].

In summary, women with congenital TTP require therapy with plasma, either as infusions or PEX to provide ADAMTS 13 supplementation, throughout pregnancy and the post-partum period. In women with acquired TTP and previous acute TTP, the baseline ADAMTS 13 activity and inhibitor/antibody status may be useful in the identification of those most likely to relapse. Monitoring of enzyme activity in those with normal pregnancy levels may be useful, but in women with low (<5 %) ADAMTS 13 activity and/or raised IgG antibody levels, who appear to be at increased risk of relapse during pregnancy, elective PEX may be useful. Adjunctive therapy with LDA in all women +/− prophylactic LMWH should be added to help prevent complications related to placental thrombosis. Close liaison with an obstetrician with a special interest in feto-maternal medicine is required in mothers with TTP. Pre-conceptual counselling is advised for subsequent pregnancies and women of child bearing age should be counselled about potential risks of pregnancy and COCP.

17.6 Liver Disease in Pregnancy

Clinically relevant changes in liver function are seen in only 3–5 % of all pregnancies and in the majority pregnancy is the primary precipitant. In the first trimester, hyperemesis gravidarum is the main cause; in the 2nd and 3rd trimesters, the primary culprit is intrahepatic cholestasis of pregnancy.

17.6.1 Intrahepatic Cholestasis of Pregnancy

17.6.1.1 Clinical and Laboratory Features

The first feature of intrahepatic cholestasis of pregnancy (ICP) is usually pruritus (10–25 % of patients), followed by jaundice and a 10–20-fold increase in aminotransferases (bilirubin is not usually raised to the same extent). The diagnosis is confirmed by measuring bile acid levels. The ultimate treatment is delivery, but management in the interim (in order to gain fetal maturity) is with ursodeoxycholic acid (UDCA), which can both improve symptoms of itching and reduce levels of bile acids and aminotransferases. Steroids have not been shown to be useful in managing ICP (although may be used to improve fetal maturity when preterm delivery because of the ICP is anticipated. Raised bile acid levels may be associated with placental insufficiency. The condition resolves with delivery, but recurrence is seen in approximately 50 % of cases in future pregnancies or with the use of the combined oral contraceptive pill. Underlying abnormalities of progesterone are thought to be the pathological defect [47].

17.6.2 Acute Fatty Liver of Pregnancy

17.6.2.1 Clinical Features

AFLP is a rare disorder the incidence of which is estimated at 1 in 13,000 births, but it is an acute life-threatening illness associated with significant maternal and perinatal mortality [48]. It presents primarily in the third trimester, usually affecting women in their first pregnancy, but recurrence in subsequent pregnancies has been reported.

Clinically, the presentation is non specific, with headache, fatigue, nausea, vomiting (70 %) and right upper quadrant or epigastric pain (50 %). There may be gastrointestinal hemorrhage, coagulation abnormalities, acute renal failure, infection, pancreatitis and hypoglycemia early in the presentation. Usually there is progression to liver failure and hepatic encephalopathy. Improvement occurs 1–4 weeks post-partum.

17.6.2.2 Diagnosis

The diagnosis is usually clinical but, if there is uncertainty, may be confirmed by liver biopsy. Histologically, in the liver there is characteristic microvesicular steatosis and, with Oil Red O staining, cytoplasmic vesiculation as a result of microvesicular fat. However, it is often not possible to undertake a liver biopsy if coagulation is affected because of the increased risk of hemorrhage.

Laboratory testing reveals a raised white cell count and thrombocytopenia, with evidence of DIC (with prolonged prothrombin time (PT), activated partial thromboplastin time (APPT) and reduced fibrinogen). Urea, creatinine and uric acid levels are raised, as are ammonia levels, and there is hypoglycemia. Serum aminotransferases are raised and alkaline phosphatase is three to four times higher than normal. The primary differential diagnoses are acute fulminant hepatitis and severe HELLP syndrome, although these conditions are less likely to feature hypoglycemia or a prolonged PT.

17.6.2.3 Pathophysiology

The pathophysiology of AFLP is interesting. This condition results from mitochondrial dysfunction, associated with a deficiency of the enzyme long chain 3-hydroxyacyl-CoA dehydrogenase (LCHAD) in the fetus. This enzyme is important in mitochondrial fatty acid β-oxidation [49]. β-oxidation of fatty acids is a major source of energy for skeletal muscle and the heart. The liver oxidizes fatty acids under conditions of prolonged fasting, during illness and at periods of increased muscular activity. Mitochondrial β-oxidation of fatty acids is a complex process. LCHAD is part of an enzyme complex, the mitochondrial trifunctional protein (MTP), which is associated with the inner mitochondrial membrane [49, 50]. Defects in the MTP complex are recessively inherited and are due to an isolated LCHAD deficiency, specifically associated with a G1548C mutation. A few hours after birth, the newborn presents with non-ketotic hypoglycemia and hepatic encephalopathy, progressing to coma or death, if untreated.

It is suggested that there is an association between fetal MTP defects and AFLP. In one study, in all pregnancies with a fetus affected by LCHAD deficiency, the mother had AFLP or HELLP in each pregnancy. In pregnancies in which the fetus was not LCHAD deficient, the pregnancy progressed normally with no liver dysfunction. In a study which prospectively screened mothers who developed AFLP (27 pregnancies) or HELLP (81 pregnancies), 5 fetuses had MTP mutations in the AFLP group, but none in the HELLP group [51].

The precise mechanism by which an LCHAD deficient fetus causes AFLP in a heterozygote mother remains unclear, but several possible explanations are hypothesized. The heterozygote mother for an MTP defect has reduced capacity to oxidise long chain fatty acids. The maternal stress of pregnancy associated with altered metabolism, increased lipolysis and decreased β-oxidation, is combined with the accumulation in the maternal circulation of the hepatotoxic LCHAD produced by the fetus or placenta. Whatever the mechanism, approximately one in five women who develop AFLP may carry an LCHAD-deficient fetus. Screening of newborn infants at birth for this disorder of fatty acid oxidation can be lifesaving and allows for genetic counselling in subsequent pregnancies.

17.7 Hemolysis, Elevated Liver Enzymes and Low Platelets Syndrome

17.7.1 Clinical Features and Diagnosis

HELLP syndrome is a microangiopathy related to endothelial cell injury, fibrin deposition, platelet activation and consumption, and areas of hepatic hemorrhage and necrosis. The underlying precipitating cause is unknown, but it occurs only in pregnancy, with an incidence between 0.17 and 0.85% of all live births. Maternal mortality is 3–4 % with fetal mortality approximately 25 %. Diagnostically, there is considerable overlap with other TMA's, in particular PET. HELLP typically presents in the 2nd and 3rd trimesters, although a quarter of all cases occur postpartum [52]. Presenting symptoms include upper abdominal pain and tenderness, nausea, vomiting, malaise, headache, and rarely jaundice.

There are no pathognomonic clinical or laboratory features of HELLP syndrome. Bilirubin is not usually raised and aminotransferases can be increased only marginally or up to 20-fold. HELLP syndrome may be classified according to the degree of thrombocytopenia: HELLP 1 ($<50\times10^9$/L), HELLP 2 (between 50 and 100×10^9/L) and HELLP 3 (between 100 and 150×10^9/L) [53].

Serious maternal complications include DIC, placental abruption, acute renal failure, pulmonary edema and hepatic failure, occasionally requiring liver transplantation [54]. Hepatic rupture is a rare, acute, life-threatening complication. However, in patients with HELLP-associated acute kidney injury, renal biopsy rarely finds typical features of TMA (only 15 %). The most common lesions in these patients are glomerular endotheliosis, similar to the lesions seen in acute tubular necrosis.

17.7.2 Diagnostic Markers of HELLP Syndrome

The liver is the organ primarily affected in HELLP syndrome. Pregnancy is a hypermetabolic condition and protein production is mainly hepatic; compared to those with normal pregnancy, women with HELLP syndrome have increased serum amyloid A (SAA). However, further work is needed to determine if this is truly a predictive marker for the development of HELLP or if it is merely a surrogate of liver impairment. Other hypotheses for the causation of HELLP syndrome are activation of complement factors, which stimulate monocytes to produce sFlt-1, thus inhibiting placental trophoblast differentiation and invasion. This is thought to be involved directly in abnormal placental development.

Complement dysregulation associated with a genetic predisposition has been identified in HELLP syndrome patients. Of 11 patients with HELLP syndrome and relatively significant renal involvement, four had complement gene mutations and three had stigmata of complement activation (low C3 and factor B serum levels) without documented complement gene mutations.

17.7.3 Management of HELLP Syndrome

Stabilisation of hypertension and other manifestations of HELLP, such as seizures or DIC, are necessary. Fetal monitoring is important as the condition may compromise fetal wellbeing. The primary treatment is delivery of the baby. After 34 weeks of gestation, in women with severe or progressive disease, delivery should be expedited. Induction of labor and vaginal delivery is sometimes possible, but up to 50 % result in Cesarean section. Evidence does not support a role for steroids in the routine treatment of HELLP syndrome other than to improve fetal lung maturity. In the majority of patients, following delivery, normalisation of platelet count and resolution of HELLP occurs by day 5. However, in those cases with persistent thrombocytopenia, hemolysis, organ failure or life-threatening complications, plasma exchange has been used, but this is anecdotal and not based on clinical trial evidence.

In subsequent pregnancies, there is an increased risk of uteroplacental pathology, including PET, recurrent HELLP syndrome, IUGR, prematurity and placental abruption. One review included 341 patients followed up 2–14 years after an initial episode of HELLP syndrome, who had 152 subsequent pregnancies. A control group of 139 normotensive women had 192 subsequent pregnancies. Complications included preeclampsia (19 %), preterm delivery (21 %), IUGR (12 %), placental abruption (2 %), perinatal death (4 %), and HELLP syndrome

(3 %). 6.2 % had chronic hypertension and 13 women with pre-existing chronic hypertension had 20 subsequent pregnancies. These women had a higher rate of PET (75 %), preterm delivery (80 %), IUGR (45 %), placental abruption (20 %), and perinatal death (40 %), but a low rate of recurrent HELLP syndrome (5 %) [55].

17.7.4 PEX and HELLP Syndrome

HELLP syndrome is usually self-limiting, recovering quickly after delivery, but rarely it can be complicated by multi-organ failure and require intensive care support. The use of PEX in HELLP is reported only in single case reports or small case series, and its value is debated. With an increasing association of HELLP with complement dysregulation, the rationale for the use of PEX becomes more cogent; it is proposed that PEX may be beneficial in patients in whom HELLP persists for 48–72 h.

17.7.5 Steroids and HELLP Syndrome

In a placebo controlled trial of 31 pregnant women with HELLP syndrome presenting before 30 weeks of gestation, with platelet counts $<100 \times 10^9$/L, 100 mg of intravenous prednisolone daily was compared to no treatment. The prednisolone group had a significantly lower risk of another HELLP exacerbation after the initial crisis, and had a faster platelet count recovery. Prednisolone was chosen as the most suitable steroid as it has low transplacental passage. The beneficial action of the steroid was considered to be an anti-inflammatory effect, which may stabilise activated endothelium and inhibit platelet aggregation. However, the time from the first dose of steroid to delivery did not differ between the groups. In summary, the steroid group had a faster time to platelet recovery and improved liver function, and a reduction in exacerbation of HELLP, but did not result in prolongation of pregnancy. There were four perinatal deaths in the prednisolone group compared to none in the placebo group. Long-term follow-up (to 24 months) of the infants showed no difference between the groups [56].

Previously, observational studies had found relatively positive outcomes of dexamethasone therapy in HELLP syndrome, which has been the main steroid used in this disorder. A prospective double blind placebo controlled trial recruited 132 women with HELLP syndrome class 1 and 2, and they were given 20 mg daily dexamethasone versus placebo until delivery and continued 3 days postpartum. There were no differences between the groups in hospital stay, platelet recovery time, liver function tests, maternal complications or the need for blood products. Other studies that have suggested a benefit for steroids are smaller series, with no placebo control groups, and usually including only patients with severe disease, although definition may be variable. However, in a subgroup analysis of class 1 HELLP (platelet count $<50 \times 10^9$/L), there was a shorter average platelet count recovery time and reduced hospital in-patient stay [57].

A Cochrane Database systematic review of 11 trials (550 women) compared corticosteroids with placebo or no treatment. There was no difference in the risk of maternal death, maternal death or severe maternal morbidity, or perinatal/infant death. The only clear effect of treatment on individual outcomes was improved platelet count, with the effect strongest in women who commenced treatment antenatally, and in women receiving dexamethasone compared with those receiving betamethasone. The authors concluded that there was no clear evidence of any effect of corticosteroids on substantive clinical outcomes to support the routine use of steroids for the management of HELLP. They suggested that the use of corticosteroids may be justified in clinical situations in which an increased rate of recovery in platelet count is considered clinically worthwhile [58].

17.7.6 Platelet Transfusions and HELLP Syndrome

A randomised trial of women with class 1 HELLP syndrome who received either dexamethasone alone (n = 26) or dexamethasone plus platelet transfusions (n=20) found that liver function tests were significantly worse in the steroid plus platelets group. Platelet count normalised significantly faster in the dexamethasone alone group and the postpartum stay was longer in the dexamethasone plus platelets group. The group that received platelets had an increased incidence of wound dehiscence, wound infection and pulmonary edema. The use of intrapartum platelet transfusions when the platelet count was $<40\times10^9$/L did not reduce the incidence of hemorrhagic complications [59].

17.8 Hemolytic Uremic Syndrome

17.8.1 Clinical Features and Pathogenesis

HUS includes verotoxin associated HUS, secondary HUS (due to pregnancy) and atypical HUS [60]. The predominant clinical feature in this TMA is renal impairment or failure, although rarely there is cardiac or neurological involvement. Most cases are caused by complement dysregulation involving the alternative pathway, with inactivating mutations of the three main genes, for Factor H, Factor I or MCP (membrane cofactor protein). Less commonly, there are gain-of-function mutations affecting C3 or Factor B. Rarely, HUS is caused by acquired autoantibodies to Factor H. Mutations in these genes can be identified in only around 50 % of aHUS cases; in these cases, disease is associated with environmental triggers, of which pregnancy is one recognised cause. aHUS has a poorer prognosis, with an overall mortality of 25 % in the acute phase and 50 % requiring chronic renal replacement. Based on retrospective data, the greatest risk of pregnancy-associated aHUS is with CFH and C3 mutations; the risk is less with CFI and MCP mutations. Pregnancy associated aHUS accounts for 20 % of all aHUS cases, with increased rates of fetal loss and maternal PET; however, 75 % of pregnancy associated cases occur postpartum. Furthermore, genetic analysis of the PROMISSE cohort suggests that there is evidence supporting a role of complement in patients with SLE/APLS and those with antibody negative PET, in which abnormalities of CFI and MCP have been identified in 18 % and 8.5 % of the cohorts, respectively [61].

17.8.2 Management of Pregnancy Associated HUS

PEX is the mainstay of therapy of HUS, the aim being to reduce complement activation. However, PEX response may not be optimal, particularly in, for example, CFH and C3 mutations; despite improvements in the platelet count, renal function may not respond as quickly. In this scenario, the use of eculizumab may be considered. Eculizumab is a humanized IgG monoclonal therapy that is a potent inhibitor of C5 cleavage. It thus inhibits the generation of C5a, that is a potent anaphylatoxin, and C3b, that prevents activation of the membrane attack complex (MAC). Its use should be considered early in disease presentation; the dose is 900 mg weekly for 4 weeks and 1,200 mg every 2 weeks thereafter. Meningococcal prophylaxis and prophylactic penicillin V are required, and patients should be warned of the potential risk of meningococcal infection [62–64].

Mutational screening of family members is not currently undertaken because of low penetrance and unpredictability. However, relatives of an index case should be monitored for HELLP during pregnancy, by checking urine dipstick analysis for protein/blood, blood pressure and serum creatinine and protein-creatinine ratio.

17.9 Exacerbation of Systemic Lupus Erythematosus

SLE is a multisystem, autoimmune disease, the active phase of which may be associated with thrombocytopenia, hemolytic anemia, pancytopenia and an increase in double stranded DNA. Serum complement levels may be normal or decreased. An acute exacerbation occurs during pregnancy in 25–30 % of women with SLE; alternatively, SLE may present for the first time during pregnancy or in the postpartum period. An acute episode of lupus nephritis, associated with hypertension and proteinuria, may be difficult to differentiate from HELLP or pre-eclampsia.

Associated antiphospholipid antibodies (aPL) may be present in 30–49 % of women with lupus [65, 66]; if present, they increase the risk of thrombotic events, tissue ischemia and TMA. Thrombocytopenia is present in 40–50 % and hemolytic anemia in around a quarter of cases. Neurological symptoms may result from cerebral vasculitis or vaso-occlusive disease [67].

Maternal and perinatal morbidity and mortality are specifically associated with lupus nephritis, central nervous system disease and aPL. aPL positivity in particular is associated with higher miscarriage rates, intrauterine fetal death (IUFD; 4–10 %), intrauterine growth restriction (IUGR) and preterm delivery (38–54 %), due to vascular thrombosis, placental infarction and hemorrhage. Maternal complications include high rates of early onset PET and complications related to thromboembolism and microangiopathy.

17.10 Plasma Exchange and Pregnancy Outcomes in Antiphospholipid Syndrome

The live birth rate in APS was previously between 10 and 59 %, but has increased to over 70 % with the use of heparins, LDA, prednisolone and intravenous immunoglobulin (IVIg) [68–75]. However, pregnancy-associated complications are common, including PET, IUGR, and preterm birth [46]. Several case reports document the successful use of PEX in APS [76, 77] as well as other TMAs. El Haieg et al. (2007) investigated the effect of plasmapheresis with low dose prednisone (10 mg daily) on obstetric and neonatal outcomes among unsuccessfully treated pregnant high-risk women with APS, defined by a poor obstetric history, positive lupus anticoagulant (LA) and levels of anticardiolipin antibodies (aCL) over 40 GPL units/mL (with APS diagnosis as per international consensus criteria [78]). When apheresis was performed initially three times a week, reducing once aCL levels fell below 15 GPL units/mL and LA was no longer detectable, there were no maternal complications with severe PET, abruption or thrombotic events. All women delivered after 32 weeks, with a 100 % live birth rate and no perinatal deaths. Mild pre-eclampsia occurred in 5.5 % of women, with preterm deliveries in 22 % and intrauterine growth restriction in 11 % [79]. The authors suggested that plasmapheresis may be used to treat pregnant women with documented APS when first lines (aspirin and/or heparin) fail to prevent pregnancy loss. Previous studies have confirmed the significant benefit of heparin and aspirin, but there has often been variability in the laboratory methodology used to diagnose APS. A reduction or disappearance of aCL may correlate with improved fetal prognosis in patients with APS.

Abnormal placentation is thought to be a result of direct damage to trophoblasts by aPL, resulting in decidual vasculopathy, thrombi in the intervillous spaces and impaired maternal spiral arterial blood flow. The antibodies inhibit phospholipid binding proteins on endothelial surfaces, platelets or gestational tissue. A reduction in obstetric complications and normalization of uterine artery blood flow suggests that early removal of aPL with PEX ameliorates aPL effects on the trophoblast and improves placentation. aPL binding to trophoblasts activates complement, leading to activation of inflammatory cells and injury to the fetal-maternal unit. This effect has been verified in mouse models of APS, suggesting that pregnancy complications are initiated by inflammation rather than thrombosis [80]. It has been suggested that heparin prevents obstetric complications caused by aPL because it blocks complement activation rather than through its antithrombotic properties [34]. This supports the use of heparin/LMWH as a first-line treatment in pregnancy. In a subgroup of patients with poor obstetric outcome and high positive aPL, PEX may be an alternative therapy, although this has not been evaluated in a larger trial setting.

17.10.1 Catastrophic Antiphospholipid Syndrome

Catastrophic APS (CAPS) occurs in less than 1 % of patients with positive aPL. This condition is associated with acute TMA affecting the small vessels of multiple organs, typically the kidneys, and cardiorespiratory and central nervous systems. Maternal mortality is almost 50 %. The management is based on anecdotal and case reports, and includes therapeutic dose anticoagulation, IVIg, PEX, and immunosuppressive therapy, including high-dose corticosteroids, cyclophosphamide, rituximab and eculizumab [81–86].

17.11 Disseminated Intravascular Coagulation

DIC must not be forgotten in pregnancy as a cause of thrombocytopenia with an abnormal clotting screen, with hypofibrinogenaemia characteristic. Usually, there is an underlying precipitating cause that must be treated, to remove the driver for DIC, and DIC can be a complication of a severe case of any of the TMAs discussed above. Treatment of DIC requires supportive treatment with blood components to correct the haemostatic derangement: platelet transfusions aimed at maintaining the platelet count above 50×10^9/L; and fresh frozen plasma and cryoprecipitate, which may be given, depending on the degree of abnormality of the coagulation parameters [87].

Conclusions

In conclusion, the TMAs often prove to be a challenging group of disorders, and require careful and repeated review of clinical and laboratory features. They are either inherent to, or precipitated by, pregnancy, and usually improve following delivery. As our understanding of the underlying pathophysiology has increased, more specific therapies have become available for some of these conditions.

17.12 Case Study

A 33 year old presented with acute TTP associated with bruising, symptomatic anemia and fetal loss at 25 weeks gestation in her first pregnancy. She received three single-volume plasma exchanges (PEX) with FFP and four separate infusions of FFP, 15 mg/kg. She remained in clinical remission despite documented ADAMTS-13 activity less than 5 %. A year later she had a miscarriage at 8 weeks gestation. During her third pregnancy, fortnightly PEX was commenced from 12 weeks gestation given her history of a pregnancy associated TTP episode, fetal loss and persistently low ADAMTS-13 activity (<5 %). Increased red cell fragmentation on her blood film was noted at 28 weeks. The remaining blood parameters were normal, but PEX was continued weekly. She was induced at 35 weeks because of further red cell fragmentation associated with an elevated LDH (526 IU/L; normalrange, < 480 IU/L), a decrease in the platelet count (113×10^9/L), proteinuria and hypertension. She had an uncomplicated vaginal delivery of a live male infant. Cord blood platelet count was 63×10^9/L, with a reticulocytosis (2.8 %), raised LDH (1,023 IU/L), bilirubin of 105 μmol/L, a negative direct antiglobulin test and both mother and infant blood groups were A-positive. The neonatal blood film was normal. Both maternal and neonatal blood counts were in the normal range on discharge 2 days later. ADAMTS-13 assays were performed on cord blood and repeated on venous samples 6 weeks later. The neonatal cord ADAMTS-13 activity was slightly low at 63 % (normal range, 80–120 %) and at 6 weeks was normal at 90 %. The father's ADAMTS-13 activity was 99 % [41].

Key Learning Points

- Thrombotic microangiopathies describe a collection of disorders with similar presenting features but different underlying pathogenesis and often differing therapies.
- Delivery is the ultimate cure for pre-eclampsia. However, in contrast to pre-eclampsia and HELLP syndrome,

delivery does not necessarily induce remission of TTP.

- If ADAMTS 13 activity is under 5 % and/or there are anti-ADAMTS 13 IgG autoantibodies, it is diagnostic of TTP. Women presenting with thrombocytopenia, microangiopathic haemolytic anaemia (MAHA), neurological features (such as stroke/TIA, seizures, encephalopathy) or renal impairment, should be treated with plasma exchange until the diagnosis of TTP is excluded.
- Women with congenital TTP require therapy with plasma, either as infusions or plasma exchange, to provide ADAMTS 13 supplementation, throughout pregnancy and the post-partum period.
- In women with acquired TTP and previous acute TTP, the baseline ADAMTS 13 activity and inhibitor/antibody status may be useful in the identification of those most likely to relapse. Monitoring of enzyme activity in those with normal pregnancy levels may be useful, but in women with low (<5 %) ADAMTS 13 activity and/or raised IgG antibody levels, who appear to be at increased risk of relapse during pregnancy, elective plasma exchange may be useful.
- In women with acute TTP or previous acute TTP, adjunctive therapy with LDA +/− prophylactic LMWH should be added to help prevent complications related to placental thrombosis.
- Red cell transfusion should be administered according to clinical need especially if there is cardiac involvement. Due to the risk of precipitating further thrombotic events, platelet transfusions are contraindicated unless there is life-threatening hemorrhage.
- Women who have had a pregnancy affected by pre-eclampsia are at increased risk of cardiovascular disease (stroke, ischemic heart disease) later in life.

References

1. Provan D, Stasi R, Newland AC, et al. International consensus report on the investigation and management of primary immune thrombocytopenia. Blood. 2010;115:168–86.
2. Gernsheimer T, James AH, Stasi R. How I treat thrombocytopenia in pregnancy. Blood. 2013;121:38–47.
3. Cines DB, Blanchette VS. Immune thrombocytopenic purpura. N Engl J Med. 2002;346:995–1008.
4. Sibai B, Dekker G, Kupferminc M. Pre-eclampsia. Lancet. 2005;365:785–99.
5. Naljayan MV, Karumanchi SA. New developments in the pathogenesis of preeclampsia. Adv Chronic Kidney Dis. 2013;20:265–70.
6. Staff AC, Benton SJ, von Dadelszen DP, et al. Redefining preeclampsia using placenta-derived biomarkers. Hypertension. 2013;61:932–42.
7. Maynard SE, Venkatesha S, Thadhani R, Karumanchi SA. Soluble Fms-like tyrosine kinase 1 and endothelial dysfunction in the pathogenesis of preeclampsia. Pediatr Res. 2005;57:1R–7.
8. Yang JC, Haworth L, Sherry RM, et al. A randomized trial of bevacizumab, an anti-vascular endothelial growth factor antibody, for metastatic renal cancer. N Engl J Med. 2003;349:427–34.
9. Chen CW, Jaffe IZ, Karumanchi SA. Pre-eclampsia and cardiovascular disease. Cardiovasc Res. 2014; 101(4):579–86.
10. Smith GC, Pell JP, Walsh D. Pregnancy complications and maternal risk of ischaemic heart disease: a retrospective cohort study of 129,290 births. Lancet. 2001;357:2002–6.
11. Nicolaides KH, Bindra R, Turan OM, et al. A novel approach to first-trimester screening for early pre-eclampsia combining serum PP-13 and Doppler ultrasound. Ultrasound Obstet Gynecol. 2006;27:13–7.
12. Venkatesha S, Toporsian M, Lam C, et al. Soluble endoglin contributes to the pathogenesis of preeclampsia. Nat Med. 2006;12:642–9.
13. Levine RJ, Lam C, Qian C, et al. Soluble endoglin and other circulating antiangiogenic factors in preeclampsia. N Engl J Med. 2006;355:992–1005.
14. Steegers EA, von Dadelszen P, Duvekot JJ, Pijnenborg R. Pre-eclampsia. Lancet. 2010;376:631–44.
15. CLASP (Collaborative Low-dose Aspirin Study in Pregnancy) Collaborative Group. CLASP: a randomised trial of low-dose aspirin for the prevention and treatment of pre-eclampsia among 9364 pregnant women. Lancet. 1994;343:619–29.
16. Golding J. A randomised trial of low dose aspirin for primiparae in pregnancy. The Jamaica Low Dose Aspirin Study Group. Br J Obstet Gynaecol. 1998; 105:293–9.
17. Askie LM, Duley L, Henderson-Smart DJ, Stewart LA. Antiplatelet agents for prevention of pre-eclampsia: a meta-analysis of individual patient data. Lancet. 2007;369:1791–8.

18. Villa PM, Kajantie E, Raikkonen K, et al. Aspirin in the prevention of pre-eclampsia in high-risk women: a randomised placebo-controlled PREDO Trial and a meta-analysis of randomised trials. BJOG. 2013; 120:64–74.
19. Kleinrouweler CE, van Uitert M, Moerland PD, et al. Differentially expressed genes in the pre-eclamptic placenta: a systematic review and meta-analysis. PLoS One. 2013;8:e68991.
20. Gilbert JS, Verzwyvelt J, Colson D, et al. Recombinant vascular endothelial growth factor 121 infusion lowers blood pressure and improves renal function in rats with placentalischemia-induced hypertension. Hypertension. 2010;55:380–5.
21. Hagmann H, Bossung V, Belaidi AA, et al. Low-Molecular Weight Heparin Increases Circulating sFlt-1 Levels and Enhances Urinary Elimination. PLoS One. 2014;9:e85258.
22. Rodger MA, Carrier M, Le GG, et al. Meta-analysis of low-molecular-weight heparin to prevent recurrent placenta-mediated pregnancy complications. Blood. 2014;123:822–8.
23. Kumasawa K, Ikawa M, Kidoya H, et al. Pravastatin induces placental growth factor (PGF) and ameliorates preeclampsia in a mouse model. Proc Natl Acad Sci U S A. 2011;108:1451–5.
24. Witlin AG, Saade GR, Mattar F, Sibai BM. Predictors of neonatal outcome in women with severe preeclampsia or eclampsia between 24 and 33 weeks' gestation. Am J Obstet Gynecol. 2000;182:607–11.
25. Sergio F, Maria CD, Gabriella F, et al. Prophylaxis of recurrent preeclampsia: low-molecular-weight heparin plus low-dose aspirin versus low-dose aspirin alone. Hypertens Pregnancy. 2006;25:115–27.
26. Funai EF, Friedlander Y, Paltiel O, et al. Long-term mortality after preeclampsia. Epidemiology. 2005;16: 206–15.
27. Brown MC, Best KE, Pearce MS, Waugh J, Robson SC. Bell R Cardiovascular disease risk in women with pre-eclampsia: systematic review and meta-analysis. Eur J Epidemiol. 2013;28(1):1–19.
28. Ray JG, Vermeulen MJ, Schull MJ, Redelmeier DA. Cardiovascular health after maternal placental syndromes (CHAMPS): population-based retrospective cohort study. Lancet. 2005;366:1797–803.
29. Scully M, Hunt BJ, Benjamin S, et al. Guidelines on the diagnosis and management of thrombotic thrombocytopenic purpura and other thrombotic microangiopathies. Br J Haematol. 2012;158:323–35.
30. Moake JL, Rudy CK, Troll JH, et al. Unusually large plasma factor VIII: von Willebrand factor multimers in chronic relapsing thrombotic thrombocytopenic purpura. N Engl J Med. 1982;307:1432–5.
31. Fujikawa K, Suzuki H, McMullen B, Chung D. Purification of human von Willebrand factor-cleaving protease and its identification as a new member of the metalloproteinase family. Blood. 2001;98: 1662–6.
32. Levy GG, Nichols WC, Lian EC, et al. Mutations in a member of the ADAMTS gene family cause thrombotic thrombocytopenic purpura. Nature. 2001;413: 488–94.
33. Bell WR, Braine HG, Ness PM, Kickler TS. Improved survival in thrombotic thrombocytopenic purpura-hemolytic uremic syndrome. Clinical experience in 108 patients. N Engl J Med. 1991;325:398–403.
34. Scully M, Yarranton H, Liesner R, et al. Regional UK TTP registry: correlation with laboratory ADAMTS 13 analysis and clinical features. Br J Haematol. 2008;142:819–26.
35. Mannucci PM, Canciani MT, Forza I, et al. Changes in health and disease of the metalloprotease that cleaves von Willebrand factor. Blood. 2001;98: 2730–5.
36. Sanchez-Luceros A, Farias CE, Amaral MM, et al. von Willebrand factor-cleaving protease (ADAMTS13) activity in normal non-pregnant women, pregnant and post-delivery women. Thromb Haemost. 2004;92:1320–6.
37. Fujimura Y, Matsumoto M, Kokame K, et al. Pregnancy-induced thrombocytopenia and TTP, and the risk of fetal death, in Upshaw-Schulman syndrome: a series of 15 pregnancies in 9 genotyped patients. Br J Haematol. 2009;144(5):742–54.
38. Moatti-Cohen M, Garrec C, Wolf M, et al. Unexpected frequency of Upshaw-Schulman syndrome in pregnancy-onset thrombotic thrombocytopenic purpura. Blood. 2012;119:5888–97.
39. Ambrose A, Welham RT, Cefalo RC. Thrombotic thrombocytopenic purpura in early pregnancy. Obstet Gynecol. 1985;66:267–72.
40. Rozdzinski E, Hertenstein B, Schmeiser T, et al. Thrombotic thrombocytopenic purpura in early pregnancy with maternal and fetal survival. Ann Hematol. 1992;64:245–8.
41. Scully M, Starke R, Lee R, Mackie I, Machin S, Cohen H. Successful management of pregnancy in women with a history of thrombotic thrombocytopaenic purpura. Blood Coagul Fibrinolysis. 2006;17: 459–63.
42. Scully M, Thomas M, Underwood M, Watson H, Langley K, Camilleri RS, et al.; Collaborators of the UK TTP Registry. Thrombotic thrombocytopenic purpura and pregnancy: presentation, management, and subsequent pregnancy outcomes. Blood. 2014; 124(2):211–9.
43. Lattuada A, Rossi E, Calzarossa C, Candolfi R, Mannucci PM. Mild to moderate reduction of a von Willebrand factor cleaving protease (ADAMTS-13) in pregnant women with HELLP microangiopathic syndrome. Haematologica. 2003;88:1029–34.
44. Furlan M, Robles R, Morselli B, Sandoz P, Lammle B. Recovery and half-life of von Willebrand factor-cleaving protease after plasma therapy in patients with thrombotic thrombocytopenic purpura. Thromb Haemost. 1999;81:8–13.

45. Ducloy-Bouthors AS, Caron C, Subtil D, et al. Thrombotic thrombocytopenic purpura: medical and biological monitoring of six pregnancies. Eur J Obstet Gynecol Reprod Biol. 2003;111:146–52.
46. Gris JC, Mercier E, Quere I, et al. Low-molecular-weight heparin versus low-dose aspirin in women with one fetal loss and a constitutional thrombophilic disorder. Blood. 2004;103:3695–9.
47. Dann AT, Kenyon AP, Seed PT, et al. Glutathione S-transferase and liver function in intrahepatic cholestasis of pregnancy and pruritus gravidarum. Hepatology. 2004;40:1406–14.
48. Riely CA. Acute fatty liver of pregnancy. Semin Liver Dis. 1987;7:47–54.
49. Uchida Y, Izai K, Orii T, Hashimoto T. Novel fatty acid beta-oxidation enzymes in rat liver mitochondria. II. Purification and properties of enoyl-coenzyme A (CoA) hydratase/3-hydroxyacyl-CoA dehydrogenase/3-ketoacyl-CoA thiolase trifunctional protein. J Biol Chem. 1992;267:1034–41.
50. Jackson S, Kler RS, Bartlett K, et al. Combined enzyme defect of mitochondrial fatty acid oxidation. J Clin Invest. 1992;90:1219–25.
51. Yang Z, Yamada J, Zhao Y, Strauss AW, Ibdah JA. Prospective screening for pediatric mitochondrial trifunctional protein defects in pregnancies complicated by liver disease. JAMA. 2002;288:2163–6.
52. Rath W, Faridi A, Dudenhausen JW. HELLP syndrome. J Perinat Med. 2000;28:249–60.
53. Martin Jr JN, Blake PG, Perry Jr KG, et al. The natural history of HELLP syndrome: patterns of disease progression and regression. Am J Obstet Gynecol. 1991;164:1500–9.
54. Barton JR, Sibai BM. Diagnosis and management of hemolysis, elevated liver enzymes, and low platelets syndrome. Clin Perinatol. 2004;31:807–33.
55. Sibai BM, Ramadan MK, Chari RS, Friedman SA. Pregnancies complicated by HELLP syndrome (hemolysis, elevated liver enzymes, and low platelets): subsequent pregnancy outcome and long-term prognosis. Am J Obstet Gynecol. 1995;172:125–9.
56. Runnard Heimel PJ, Huisjes AJ, Franx A, et al. A randomised placebo-controlled trial of prolonged prednisolone administration to patients with HELLP syndrome remote from term. Eur J Obstet Gynecol Reprod Biol. 2006;128:187–93.
57. Fonseca JE, Mendez F, Catano C, Arias F. Dexamethasone treatment does not improve the outcome of women with HELLP syndrome: a double-blind, placebo-controlled, randomized clinical trial. Am J Obstet Gynecol. 2005;193:1591–8.
58. Woudstra DM, Chandra S, Hofmeyr GJ, Dowswell T. Corticosteroids for HELLP (hemolysis, elevated liver enzymes, low platelets) syndrome in pregnancy. Cochrane Database Syst Rev. 2010;(9):CD008148.
59. Roberts WE, Perry Jr KG, Woods JB, et al. The intrapartum platelet count in patients with HELLP (hemolysis, elevated liver enzymes, and low platelets) syndrome: is it predictive of later hemorrhagic complications? Am J Obstet Gynecol. 1994;171:799–804.
60. Hofer J, Giner T, Józsi M. Complement factor h-antibody-associated hemolytic uremic syndrome: pathogenesis, clinical presentation, and treatment. Semin Thromb Hemost. 2014;40(4):r431–43.
61. Salmon JE, Heuser C, Triebwasser M, Liszewski MK, Kavanagh D, Roumenina L, et al. Mutations in complement regulatory proteins predispose to preeclampsia: a genetic analysis of the PROMISSE cohort. PLoS Med. 2011;8(3):e1001013. doi:10.1371/journal.pmed.1001013.
62. Fremeaux-Bacchi V, Fakhouri F, Roumenina L, Dragon-Durey MA, Loirat C. Atypical hemolytic-uremic syndrome related to abnormalities within the complement system. Rev Med Interne. 2011;32:232–40.
63. Fang CJ, Richards A, Liszewski MK, Kavanagh D, Atkinson JP. Advances in understanding of pathogenesis of aHUS and HELLP. Br J Haematol. 2008;143: 336–48.
64. Cortes-Hernandez J, Ordi-Ros J, Paredes F, et al. Clinical predictors of fetal and maternal outcome in systemic lupus erythematosus: a prospective study of 103 pregnancies. Rheumatology (Oxford). 2002;41: 643–50.
65. Tincani A, Bompane D, Danieli E, Doria A. Pregnancy, lupus and antiphospholipid syndrome (Hughes syndrome). Lupus. 2006;15:156–60.
66. Levine JS, Branch DW, Rauch J. The antiphospholipid syndrome. N Engl J Med. 2002;346:752–63.
67. Chakravarty EF, Colon I, Langen ES, et al. Factors that predict prematurity and preeclampsia in pregnancies that are complicated by systemic lupus erythematosus. Am J Obstet Gynecol. 2005;192:1897–904.
68. Mak A, Cheung MW, Cheak AA, Ho RC. Combination of heparin and aspirin is superior to aspirin alone in enhancing live births in patients with recurrent pregnancy loss and positive anti-phospholipid antibodies: a meta-analysis of randomized controlled trials and meta-regression. Rheumatology (Oxford). 2010;49(2):281–8.
69. Rai R, Cohen H, Dave M, Regan L. Randomised controlled trial of aspirin and aspirin plus heparin in pregnant women with recurrent miscarriage associated with phospholipid antibodies (or antiphospholipid antibodies). BMJ. 1997;314(7076):253–7.
70. Goel N, Tuli A, Choudhry R. The role of aspirin versus aspirin and heparin in cases of recurrent abortions with raised anticardiolipin antibodies. Med Sci Monit. 2006;12:CR132–6.
71. Farquharson RG, Quenby S, Greaves M. Antiphospholipid syndrome in pregnancy: a randomized, controlled trial of treatment. Obstet Gynecol. 2002;100:408–13.
72. Bramham K, Thomas M, Nelson-Piercy C, Khamashta M, Hunt BJ. First-trimester low-dose prednisolone in refractory antiphospholipid antibody-related pregnancy loss. Blood. 2011;117(25):6948–51.
73. Branch DW, Peaceman AM, Druzin M, et al. A multicenter, placebo-controlled pilot study of intravenous immune globulin treatment of antiphospholipid syn-

drome during pregnancy. The Pregnancy Loss Study Group. Am J Obstet Gynecol. 2000;182:122–7.
74. Rosove MH, Tabsh K, Wasserstrum N, et al. Heparin therapy for pregnant women with lupus anticoagulant or anticardiolipin antibodies. Obstet Gynecol. 1990;75:630–4.
75. Silveira LH, Hubble CL, Jara LJ, et al. Prevention of anticardiolipin antibody-related pregnancy losses with prednisone and aspirin. Am J Med. 1992;93:403–11.
76. Szodoray P, Hajas A, Toth L, Szakall S, Nakken B, Soltesz P, Bodolay E. The beneficial effect of plasmapheresis in mixed connective tissue disease with coexisting antiphospholipid syndrome. Lupus. 2014;23(10):1079–84.
77. Tsagalis G, Psimenou E, Nakopoulou L, Laggouranis A. Effective treatment of antiphospholipid syndrome with plasmapheresis and rituximab. Hippokratia. 2010;14(3):215–6.
78. Miyakis S, Lockshin MD, Atsumi T, Branch DW, Brey RL, Cervera R, Derksen RH, De Groot PG, Koike T, Meroni PL, et al. International consensus statement on an update of the classification criteria for definite antiphospholipid syndrome (APS). J Thromb Haemost. 2006;4:295–306.
79. El Haieg DO, Zanati MF, El Foual FM. Plasmapheresis and pregnancy outcome in patients with antiphospholipid syndrome. Int J Gynaecol Obstet. 2007;99:236–41.
80. Salmon JE, Girardi G, Lockshin MD. The antiphospholipid syndrome as a disorder initiated by inflammation: implications for the therapy of pregnant patients. Nat Clin Pract Rheumatol. 2007;3:140–7.
81. Cervera R, Serrano R, Pons-Estel GJ, Ceberio-Hualde L, Shoenfeld Y, de Ramón E, et al.; on behalf of the Euro-Phospholipid Project Group (European Forum on Antiphospholipid Antibodies). Morbidity and mortality in the antiphospholipid syndrome during a 10-year period: a multicentre prospective study of 1000 patients. Ann Rheum Dis. 2014. doi:10.1136/annrheumdis-2013-204838 [Epub ahead of print].
82. Bucciarelli S, Erkan D, Espinosa G, Cervera R. Catastrophic antiphospholipid syndrome: treatment, prognosis, and the risk of relapse. Clin Rev Allergy Immunol. 2009;36(2–3):80–4.
83. Berman H, Rodríguez-Pintó I, Cervera R, Morel N, Costedoat-Chalumeau N, Erkan D, et al.; Catastrophic Antiphospholipid Syndrome (CAPS) Registry Project Group (European Forum on Antiphospholipid Antibodies). Rituximab use in the catastrophic antiphospholipid syndrome: descriptive analysis of the CAPS registry patients receiving rituximab. Autoimmun Rev. 2013;12(11):1085–90.
84. Mar N, Kosowicz R, Hook K. Recurrent thrombosis prevention with intravenous immunoglobulin and hydroxychloroquine during pregnancy in a patient with history of catastrophic antiphospholipid syndrome and pregnancy loss. J Thromb Thrombolysis. 2014;38(2):196–200.
85. Espinosa G, Berman H, Cervera R. Management of refractory cases of catastrophic antiphospholipid syndrome. Autoimmun Rev. 2011;10(11):664–8.
86. Shapira I, Andrade D, Allen SL, Salmon JE. Brief report: induction of sustained remission in recurrent catastrophic antiphospholipid syndrome via inhibition of terminal complement with eculizumab. Arthritis Rheum. 2012;64:2719–23.
87. Wheeler AP, Bernard GR. Treating patients with severe sepsis. N Engl J Med. 1999;340:207–14.

18 The Management and Outcome of Pregnancy in Patients with Myeloproliferative Neoplasms

Susan E. Robinson and Claire N. Harrison

Abstract

The myeloproliferative neoplasms are rare blood cancers that are characterised by increased risks of thrombosis, haemorrhage and also risk of transformation to acute myeloid leukaemia. These conditions are common in older adults but they do occur in children and young adults, and as a consequence fertility and management of pregnancy is an issue for patients with these conditions. In this chapter we briefly review the pathogenesis of MPN before describing what is known about pregnancy outcomes for these patients and presenting an algorithm for pregnancy management.

Keywords

Myeloproliferative neoplasms • Essential thrombocythemia • Polycythemia vera • Primary myelofibrosis • JAK2V617F mutation

18.1 Introduction

The myeloproliferative disorders are clonal, generally indolent stem cell malignancies that are characterized by clinical features of thrombosis, hemorrhage, and transformation to myelofibrosis or acute myeloid leukemia. The World Health Organization classification of hemato-oncology [1] has renamed these conditions myeloproliferative neoplasms (MPN), and currently this category includes the following disorders: essential thrombocythemia (ET), polycythemia vera (PV), primary myelofibrosis (PMF), MPN unclassified, MPN syndromes overlapping with myelodysplasia, mast cell disorders, chronic neutrophilic leukemia, and hypereosinophilic syndrome. These are all rare myeloid malignancies, and in this chapter we focus on the management of pregnancy in the commoner MPNs – ET, PV, and PMF.

MPN are rare (e.g., the incidence of ET is 1–1.5/100,000 per annum) and are usually diagnosed in patients who are in their sixth or seventh decade. However, for ET in particular, there is another peak in women of reproductive age,

S.E. Robinson, MB ChB, MRCP, FRCPath, MDRes
C.N. Harrison, MB ChB, DM, FRCP, FRCPath (✉)
Department of Haematology,
Guy's Hospital, Guy's and St. Thomas'
NHS Foundation Trust, London, UK
e-mail: claire.harrison@gstt.nhs.uk

H. Cohen, P. O'Brien (eds.), *Disorders of Thrombosis and Hemostasis in Pregnancy: A Guide to Management*, DOI 10.1007/978-3-319-15120-5_18, © Springer-Verlag London 2015

and 15 % of patients with PV are aged less than 40 years at the time of diagnosis. These diseases are therefore encountered in patients with reproductive potential and may indeed be first diagnosed in pregnancy. Furthermore, pregnancy in these conditions may be complicated, and current data suggest that a proportion of patients with MPN will require disease-specific intervention in pregnancy, without which they risk significant complications for themselves and their pregnancy.

18.2 Pathogenesis of MPN

Our understanding of the molecular pathogenesis of MPN was revolutionized in 2005 when four groups simultaneously reported the discovery of a point mutation in exon 14 of Janus kinase 2 (JAK2V617F) [2–5]. Here, a bulky phenylalanine is substituted by valine, which causes constitutive activation of JAK2. Both wild-type and mutant JAK2 are bound to the intracytoplasmic tail of many common hemopoietic cytokine receptors including those for erythropoietin, thrombopoietin, and granulocyte colony-stimulating factor. When the ligand binds to one of these cognate receptors, phosphorylation of JAK2 and the receptor itself occurs, leading to signaling via JAK-STAT, MAPK, and PI3K pathways. This process occurs independent of ligand receptor interaction in the presence of JAK2V617F. Strikingly, the JAK2V617F mutation is highly prevalent in these patients, affecting 95 % of patients with PV (most of the remaining PV patients have a mutation in exon 12 of JAK2 [6]) and 50 % of patients with ET or PMF. In patients with ET or PMF, a proportion have one of several mutations of the transmembrane domain of the thrombopoietin receptor cMPL which also causes constitutive activation of the receptors [7]. All these mutations produce the phenotype of MPN in a mouse transplantation model. The clinical and molecular features of PV, ET, and PMF are shown in Fig. 18.1.

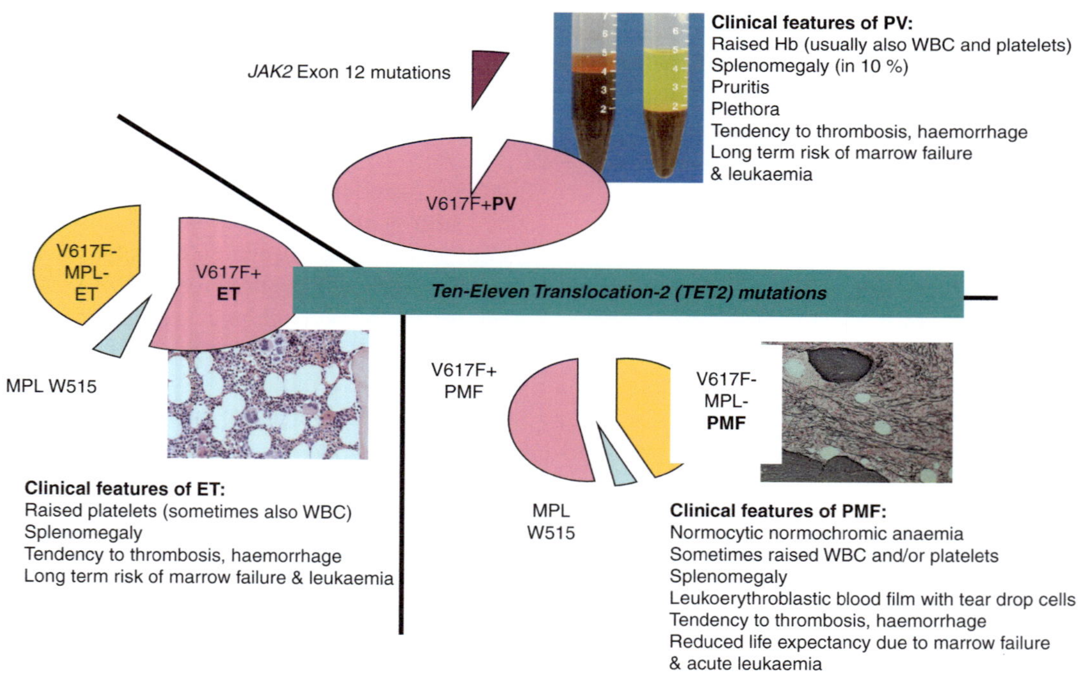

Fig. 18.1 Summary of clinical and molecular features in MPN

18.3 Diagnosis and Natural History of MPN

18.3.1 Diagnosis

The discovery of the JAK2V617F mutation has also had a major impact on the diagnostic process for these patients. In the past, these diagnoses were made by exclusion and frequently involved multiple tests to exclude other potential disorders such as an underlying malignancy in patients with isolated thrombocytosis. The current diagnostic criteria for MPN are shown in Table 18.1. It is apparent that any patients with sustained elevation of hemoglobin (i.e., a hematocrit or packed cell volume (PCV) of more than 0.51 for men and 0.48 for women), elevated platelet count (in excess of 450×10^9/L), and splenomegaly should be investigated. These disorders should also be suspected in patients presenting with thrombosis in an unusual site; for example, 60 % of patients with no clear cause for a splanchnic vein thrombosis have been reported to have a JAK2V617F-positive MPN [8]. In the context of pregnancy, it is important to consider a diagnosis of MPN in a patient with adverse pregnancy outcome, even if the blood count is normal; this is because the dilutional effect of the expanded plasma volume during the second and third trimesters may cause blood counts to completely normalize in these conditions.

18.3.2 Natural History

The patient with MPN has an enhanced risk of thrombotic complications. This increased risk is thought to be due to platelet-platelet and platelet-

Table 18.1 Diagnostic algorithm for MPNs

Careful clinical assessment to evaluate for secondary cause and additional risk factors	
Screen for V617F JAK2 ± CMPLW515L/K	
Positive V617F JAK2	**Negative V617F JAK2**
PV: if V617F JAK2 *and all of*:	PV: *if 1 + 2 and either one A or two B criteria*:
1. PCV >0.51 in Males and >0.48 in Females or raised red cell mass	1. PCV >0.60 in Males and >0.56 Females or raised red cell mass
2. No secondary cause of high PCV	2. No secondary cause of high PCV and normal erythropoietin
3. Normal/low serum erythropoietin	A Palpable splenomegaly A Presence of acquired cytogenetic abnormality B Neutrophilia (>10 × 10^9/L; or >12.5 × 10^9/L in smokers B Splenomegaly on imaging B Endogenous erythroid colonies or low erythropoietin B Thrombocytosis (plts >400 × 10^9/L)
ET: *if V617F JAK2 and all of*: Platelet count > upper limit normal range No other myeloid disease (includes PV, MDS, MF)	ET: *if all of*: Platelet count >600 × 10^9/L No other myeloid disease (includes CML, PV, MDS, MF) No reactive cause and normal iron status
MF: *if V617F JAK2* and: Reticulin > grade three-fourths or presence of collagen	MF: *if all of*: Reticulin > grade three-fourths or presence of collagen Absence of V617F JAK2 and BCR/ABL
And any two of: Palpable splenomegaly Unexplained anemia Teardrop red cells Leucoerythroblastic film Systemic symptoms (night sweats, >10 % weight loss, bone pain) Biopsy proven extramedullary hematopoiesis	*And any two of*: Palpable splenomegaly Unexplained anemia Teardrop red cells Leucoerythroblastic film Systemic symptoms (night sweats, >10 % weight loss, bone pain) Biopsy proven extramedullary hematopoiesis

leukocyte interaction, possibly directly related to the pathological activation of JAK2, although other as yet unclear factors are likely to contribute, for example, perturbation of the bone marrow microenvironment. Yet, not all patients will suffer from this complication, and thus risk assessment has been developed to tailor treatment strategies appropriately. It is well recognized that the risk of thrombosis latent to MPN is increased by age and history of a prior thrombotic event [9]. Interestingly, there is poor correlation between the degree of elevation of blood counts and thrombosis. However, patients with a platelet count in excess of $1{,}500 \times 10^9$/L are considered as a high-risk group because of their predisposition to hemorrhage (see below). Many clinicians would also include patients currently receiving antihypertensives and hypoglycemic agents as high-risk candidates. Hemorrhage, usually characterized by mucocutaneous bleeding, is less common and may be due to a reduction in the number of high molecular weight von Willebrand factor multimers, which are thought to bind to the megakaryocyte and platelet membranes. This causes an acquired von Willebrand disease (vWD), but the presence of these laboratory features may not necessarily indicate risk of future clinically significant acquired vWD. These and other factors should be considered to assess risk in the context of the current or indeed planned pregnancy; this is discussed in further detail below.

18.4 The Potential for Genetic Susceptibility to MPN

Patients diagnosed with MPN in their youth pose particular management problems over and above those faced by older patients. These include the potential for enhanced risk of long-term treatment toxicity, as well as management of fertility and pregnancy, including consideration of potential heritability of the disease. An inherited tendency to develop MPN was previously assumed to be uncommon. However, during the 1990s, studies of large kindreds with an apparent predisposition to an MPN phenotype (i.e., thrombocytosis) allowed the identification of mutations in 5′ untranslated [10] region of the thrombopoietin (TPO) gene and in cMpl, the cognate receptor for TPO [11]. Interest in a potential genetic predisposition to MPN was rekindled following the discovery of the JAK2V617F mutation in 2005, as previously described. However, this mutation has not been reported in constitutional DNA, and families have been reported in which members affected with MPN are discordant for the JAK2V617F mutation. In addition, epidemiological studies indicate that inherited factors may predispose to the development of many MPNs. The largest study assessed the risk of MPN in 24,577 first-degree relatives of 11,039 MPN patients in Sweden. The results suggest that these relatives have a significantly increased risk of developing an MPN. For example, a first-degree relative of a subject with PV has a relative risk (RR) of 5.7 (95 % confidence interval 3.5–9.1); for ET, the RR is 7.4 (3.7–14.8). For all of these cases, there was no evidence of anticipation of the age at presentation [12]. In Spring 2009, three papers appeared in the same edition of the journal Nature Genetics describing a common haplotype (single-nucleotide polymorphism) designated 46/1 conferring susceptibility to JAK2V617F-positive MPNs [13–15]. The exact mechanism of this predisposition remains uncertain, but one hypothesis suggests the "fertile ground" idea, that is, that the presence of 46/1 increases the probability of the V617F mutation occurring downstream. Despite this evidence of genetic susceptibility, routine testing of the offspring of MPN patients would not at present be recommended.

18.5 Management of MPN

Patients with MPN are generally treated according to an assessment of their risk of thrombotic or hemorrhagic potential (Fig. 18.2). Agents such as low-dose aspirin (LDA), hydroxycarbamide, anagrelide, or interferon alpha are used to reduce the risk of thrombotic events; patients with PV may require venesection and aspirin, either alone or in addition to the cytoreductive agents listed.

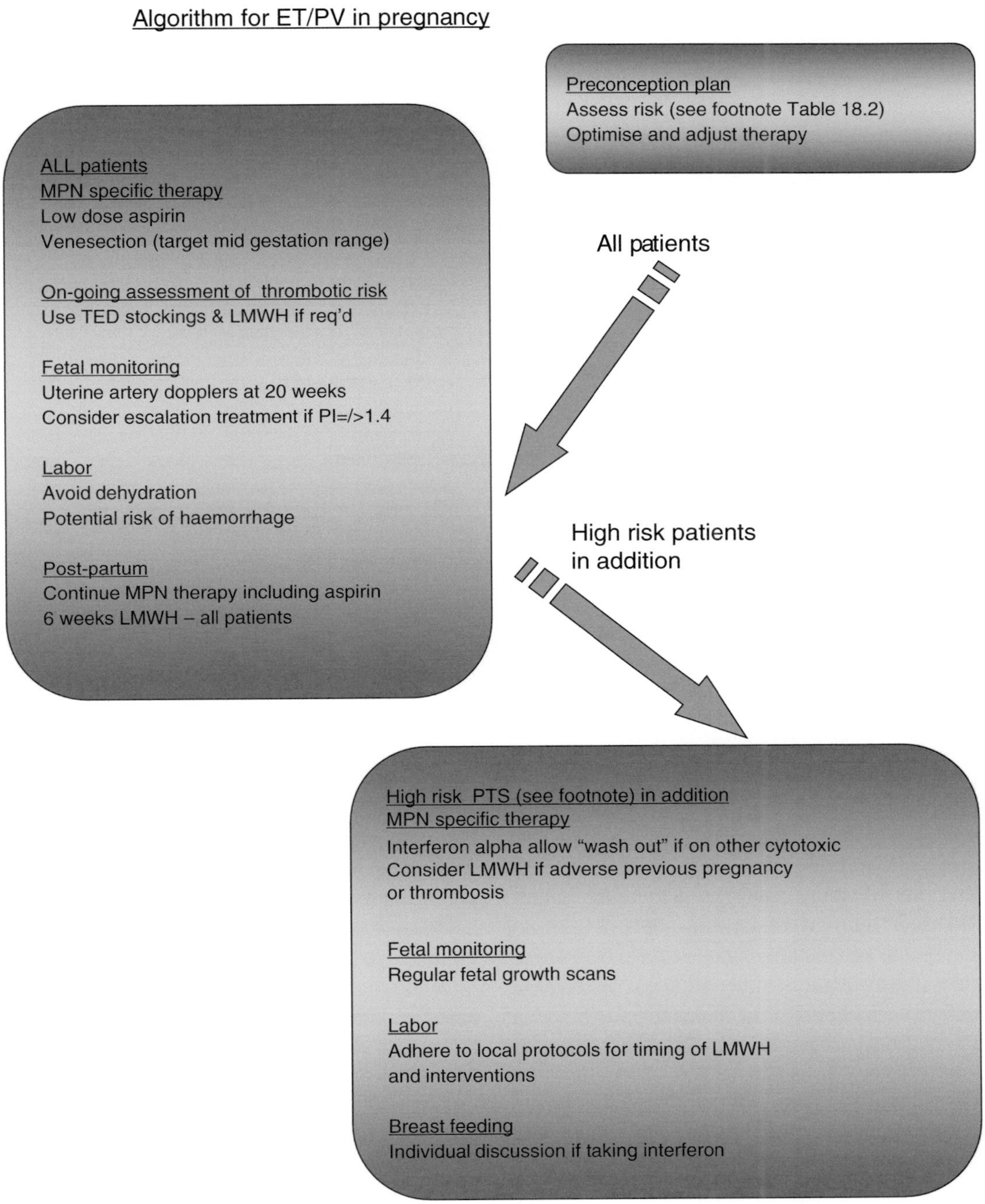

Fig. 18.2 Algorithm for MPN management in pregnancy

LDA and low molecular weight heparin (LMWH) are variably used in pregnancy, which is clearly a time of transient increased thrombotic risk. However, of the cytoreductive agents, only interferon alpha would generally be recommended for the management of high-risk patients in pregnancy. Hydroxycarbamide and anagrelide both have potential to harm the fetus [16] and should ideally be stopped prior to conception (see below); for male patients wishing to father a child, both anagrelide and interferon are appropriate, but hydroxycarbamide should be stopped for 3 months prior to trying to conceive and substituted with another agent where appropriate. There is increasing interest in the utility of a pegylated interferon as a better-tolerated agent with the potential to induce complete remission at a clinical and molecular level in a cohort of patients [17]. However, the safety of this agent in pregnancy has yet to be established. JAK2 inhibitors are currently the subject of clinical trials, largely in patients with PMF, and are not yet licensed or considered standard of care. Only a very small proportion of patients with MPN will undergo bone marrow transplantation when the severity of their disease merits this high-risk approach; the management of fertility and pregnancy in this cohort of patients is beyond the scope of this text.

The development of long-term complications of ET and PV, such as transformation to acute leukemia and the more aggressive disorder myelofibrosis, appears to be dependent upon time. These complications are an inherent tendency of these conditions, possibly related to genetic instability that has been described in association with the JAK2V617F mutation. Leukemic transformation may also be related to the use of drugs such as alkylating agents. However, current therapeutic options are not thought to significantly increase the risk of leukemic transformation although there is ongoing debate with regard to the leukemogenic potential of hydroxycarbamide [9]. Whether treatment strategies can influence the risk of myelofibrotic transformation is currently the subject of debate. Pregnancy does not affect the risk of either leukemic or myelofibrotic transformation.

Table 18.2 Risk factors for complications in pregnancy

Risk factors
Marked sustained rise in platelet count rising to above $1,500 \times 109$/L[a]
Previous venous or arterial thrombosis in mother (whether pregnant or not)
Previous hemorrhage attributed to ET (whether pregnant or not)
Development of persistent notching of uterine artery Dopplers
Previous pregnancy complication that may have been caused by ET, for example:
Unexplained recurrent first trimester loss (three unexplained first trimester losses)
Intrauterine growth restriction (birthweight <5th centile for gestation)
Intrauterine death or stillbirth (with no obvious other cause, evidence of placental dysfunction, and growth restricted fetus)
Severe preeclampsia (necessitating preterm delivery <34 weeks) or development of any such complication in the index pregnancy
Placental abruption
Significant ante- or postpartum hemorrhage (requiring red cell transfusion)

[a]These would represent indications for interferon only rather than interferon plus low molecular weight heparin

18.6 Pregnancy Outcomes

ET is the commonest MPN in women of childbearing age, and a significant number of pregnancies have been described in the literature, but these data do not enable confident management guidelines to be drawn up. A number of factors have variably been used to identify high-risk pregnancies in patients with MPN, and these are shown in Table 18.2. Analysis of pregnancy outcomes in women with ET suggests that the presence of JAK2V617F may increase the risk of pregnancy loss [18]. However, the strength of this association is not sufficient to recommend adjusting management strategy on this basis. It should be noted that thrombophilia screening, unless in specific situations (e.g., a strong personal or family history of thrombotic events), does not contribute to risk assessment for pregnancy in MPNs. The current literature for pregnancy outcome in MPN is relatively sparse, and it is important to recognize that it is likely to be subject to reporting bias; the details are summarized as follows:

ET: As ET has a second peak in incidence in women of reproductive age, the medical literature for these patients is much more abundant than for the other MPNs. A meta-analysis reported data from 461 pregnancies in women with ET whose median age was 29 years and platelet count at the outset of pregnancy $1,000 \times 109$/L, declining to 599×10^9/L in the second trimester. The live birth rate ranged from 50 to 70 %; first trimester loss affected 25–40 % and late pregnancy loss 10 %; the rate of placental abruption was 3.6 % and intrauterine growth restriction (IUGR) 4.5 % [19]. Maternal morbidity is rare in ET, but stroke has been reported [20].

PV: The reported outcomes of 18 pregnancies combined with a literature review of an additional 20 cases is available in the literature; outcomes were concordant with those for ET [21]. First trimester loss was most prevalent, occurring in 21 % and late pregnancy loss in 18 %; IUGR was reported in 15 % and preterm delivery in 13 %, associated with three neonatal deaths. The overall successful pregnancy rate was 50 %. Maternal morbidity was significant including one maternal death due to thrombosis and disseminated intravascular coagulation. It should be noted, however, that the literature review included cases reported in the 1960s, at which time treatment had not yet been standardized.

PMF: A report of four pregnancies in PMF combined with four historical cases suggests a 50 % risk of fetal loss but no evidence of maternal complications [22].

The literature in this area, particularly that relating to PV and PMF, is too small to permit conclusions about the current risks and makes a strong case for international collaboration to document pregnancy outcomes.

18.7 Therapeutic Strategies for Pregnancy in MPN

Therapeutic strategies for MPN in pregnancy are influenced by the patients' disease status and prior obstetric history. For this reason, it is useful to discuss pregnancy with young MPN patients. It is of course integral to consenting patients for cytoreductive agents that the implications of unplanned pregnancy while taking these agents are discussed. The majority of patients can and should be managed in local obstetric units under the combined care of obstetric and hematology teams. However, detailed discussion of pregnancy would ideally be provided in the form of preconception counseling when a formal risk assessment and management strategy can be developed. The key components of such a meeting would include:

- Risk assessment for pregnancy
- Discussion of therapeutic options
- Need for additional monitoring during pregnancy
- A comprehensive delivery and postpartum plan
- Discussion about breast-feeding
- Options to optimize disease control if fertility is an issue
- Informed multidisciplinary care and education

18.7.1 Fertility Treatment and Contraception

There is currently insufficient evidence to either support or refute an association between estrogen-based hormone treatment and thrombosis risk in ET and no evidence with regard to PV or PMF. A retrospective review of thrombotic events in a total of 305 women with ET followed for a median of 133 months suggested that combined oral contraceptive pill use might be associated with an increased risk of deep venous thrombosis, but other estrogen-based hormone therapies may be safe in ET [23]. Therefore, the use of combined oral contraceptives is discouraged for women for MPN. There are no data with regard to ovarian stimulation therapy in MPN. However, ovarian hyperstimulation increases the risk of thrombosis, so each case should be assessed individually and offered thromboprophylaxis when appropriate. This would include, for example, patients with previous arterial or venous thrombotic events.

18.7.2 Standard Pregnancy Management

Low-dose aspirin is safe in pregnancy and seems advantageous in ET [24] and probably PV [21]. We would therefore recommend that, in the absence of a clear contraindication, all patients should receive LDA (75 mg once daily) throughout pregnancy. For patients with PV, venesection can be continued to maintain the hematocrit within a target range which will alter through the course of pregnancy due to the expansion of the plasma volume relative to the red cell mass. Venesection may be associated with a risk of syncope, particularly for patients in the third trimester; this is due to reduced venous return, and formal intravenous fluid replacement may be required in this context.

18.7.3 High-Risk Pregnancies

A pregnancy is likely to be at high risk of maternal or fetal complications if one or more of a number of factors are either present at the outset or develop during the pregnancy (see Table 18.2). In addition to the standard measures described above, cytoreductive therapy and LMWH should be considered for patients with any such factors present at the outset or developing during pregnancy.

If cytoreductive treatment is deemed necessary (see Table 18.2), interferon alpha is the drug of choice, for there have been no reports of teratogenic effects with this agent in animals or adverse effects in the small numbers of reported human pregnancies exposed to this drug, with the exception of one possibly related case of neonatal lupus [25]. However, interferon alpha may impair fertility [26] so may be better avoided in women who have difficulty in conceiving. A few pregnancies have been reported in patients treated with hydroxycarbamide [16, 27], most without fetal complications. However, hydroxycarbamide is probably contraindicated around the time of conception (this also applies to male patients) and during pregnancy due to the risk of teratogenicity. Anagrelide is not recommended because there are insufficient data regarding its use in pregnancy and the molecule is small enough to cross the placenta. Thus, hydroxycarbamide and/or anagrelide should ideally be gradually withdrawn 3–6 months prior to planned conception and substituted by interferon alpha if necessary. The dose of interferon alpha should be titrated against the blood count with a target platelet count of 400×10^9/L and hematocrit within the gestation appropriate normal range.

LMWH is safe in pregnancy; heparin-induced thrombocytopenia has not been described with LMWH in pregnancy, and the risk of osteopenia is extremely low [28]. It has been used anecdotally in women with MPN and previous thrombosis and/or fetal morbidity, when an empirical dose of LMWH (e.g., enoxaparin 40 mg o.d.) has been used throughout pregnancy. This dose may be altered at extremes of body weight (e.g., <50 kg or >90 kg) [29]. If the patient has had a previous venous thromboembolism, thromboprophylaxis is indicated during pregnancy, with unmonitored intermediate dose LMWH being widely used (e.g., for venous thromboprophylaxis, enoxaparin 40 mg o.d. initially, increasing to 40 mg twice daily from 16 weeks' gestation and dropping to 40 mg o.d. for 6 weeks postpartum). Patients with previous or current arterial or recurrent thrombosis may require higher doses of LMWH and should be discussed on an individual basis with a hematologist. At 20 weeks uterine artery dopplers and anomaly scan are performed. A mean pulsatility index greater than or equal to 1.40 is a predictor of potential placental dysfunction. Some consider this an additional indication for LMWH or escalation of LMWH dose, although its benefit is uncertain when started at this late gestation.

18.7.4 Thromboprophylaxis

The Royal College of Obstetricians and Gynaecologists' (RCOG) guideline [29] for thromboprophylaxis in pregnancy recommends continual reassessment of the venous thrombotic risk during pregnancy and that all women with previous VTE should be encouraged to wear graded elastic compression stockings (GECS) throughout pregnancy and for 6–12 weeks after delivery. The use of GECS is also recommended for pregnant women traveling by air [30], while patients with two additional risk factors (one of which would be ET) should receive one prophylactic dose of LMWH prior to the flight.

18.7.5 Fetal Assessment

Standard care includes ultrasound scans at 12 and 20 weeks, with assessment of uterine artery Doppler at 20 weeks. A mean pulsatility index greater than or equal to 1.40 is a predictor of potential placental dysfunction and should prompt consideration of escalating therapy. These options include the addition, or increasing the dose, of either LMWH or interferon alpha. Regular growth scans should also be performed throughout the remainder of the pregnancy.

18.7.6 Intrapartum

It is important to discuss the implications of the use of thromboprophylaxis with the obstetrician and obstetric anesthetist and plan for eventualities including instrumental delivery, Cesarean section, and epidural or spinal anesthesia. Local guidelines with regard to interruption of LMWH should be adhered to during labor, and dehydration should be avoided (see Chap. 3).

18.7.7 Postpartum

In the puerperium, we recommend thromboprophylaxis with 6 weeks of prophylactic dose LMWH for all mothers with MPN, in addition to ongoing management of their MPN. It is important to note that changes due to increased plasma volume and the well-described tendency for the platelet count to fall during the third trimester will reverse during the puerperium, and this is a time when thrombotic events have been described [20].

18.7.8 Breastfeeding

Breastfeeding is safe with LMWH and warfarin but is traditionally contraindicated with the cytoreductive agents. However, the recommendation to avoid breastfeeding during maternal interferon-alpha therapy is based on reports that this agent is variably excreted in breast milk and may be active orally [31, 32]. In essence, this represents an absence of evidence of safety, rather than any evidence of harm to the neonate. The substantial benefits of breastfeeding are well documented and include a reduced risk of infection and gastroenteritis. Any decision about breastfeeding should therefore be made on an individual basis, after discussion of the possible risks and benefits.

Conclusions

The current literature suggests that pregnancy in women with MPN is associated with increased morbidity and mortality to both mother and child. The retrospective nature of reports, case study reporting bias, and lack of standardized management historically limits interpretation regarding the current epidemiology and outcome of these pregnancies. This is particularly true in the light of the recent revival of interest in MPNs and their modern-day management.

A prospective UK-based survey of pregnancy in women with MPN is being run in association with the UK Obstetric Surveillance System (UKOSS). This will enable an up-to-date review of the epidemiology and outcome of pregnancy in women with this diagnosis and an assessment of variation in current practice. This survey should provide more robust evidence on which to base management of these pregnancies.

As outlined in this chapter, all women with MPN should have a detailed plan of management for pregnancy, which should encompass preconception planning, individual risk assessment, and a treatment strategy agreed in a multidisciplinary setting.

18.8 Case Studies

Case Study 1

A pregnant 26-year-old woman, diagnosed with PV following investigation of menorrhagia and epistaxis 4 years previously, attends clinic 9 weeks pregnant.

- No prior obstetric history;
- Current management is low dose aspirin and venesection;

- Full Blood Count: Hemoglobin 150 g/L, PCV 0.49, platelets 567×10^9/L.

What would you advise?

The history of menorrhagia +/− epistaxis may be attributed to MPD in this case and, if so, the woman would meet the criteria to consider interferon in this pregnancy, but this is a relatively soft indication alone.

With no history of thrombotic events or pregnancy complications, antenatal LMWH prophylaxis is not considered to be indicated, although it is prudent to give this for 6 weeks postpartum. Aspirin should be continued throughout pregnancy. The current PCV is outside the appropriate range for the first trimester and venesection should be considered if tolerated.

Case Study 2

- A 32-year-old woman;
- Diagnosed with PMF 3 years ago following a hepatic vein thrombosis; attends clinic to discuss treatment options regarding future pregnancies. She has one healthy daughter of 5 years delivered by Cesarean section following a trial of labour which failed to progress;
- Medication: aspirin, warfarin & hydroxyurea;
- Full Blood Count: Hemoglobin 110 g/L, PCV 0.35, Platelets 147×10^9/l, White Cell Count 7.6×10^9/L.

What would you advise?

In the pre-conception planning, a management plan regarding anticoagulation, cytoreductive therapy, and a plan for specialist review of concomitant liver disease status is required.

The aspirin should be continued throughout pregnancy. Pregnancy testing should be performed in the fortnight following a possible conception in order to stop the warfarin as early as possible and commence LMWH, before 6 weeks of gestation to avoid warfarin –related teratogenicity. In view of the history of a hepatic vein thrombosis, a high prophylactic dose of LMWH should be used and switched back to warfarin postpartum.

Three months prior to conception the hydroxyurea needs to be stopped and interferon commenced. Optimization of any concomitant liver pathology and portal hypertension secondary to the previous hepatic vein thrombosis is important. The management and follow up during pregnancy including delivery planning according to concomitant pathology should be within a multidisciplinary setting, with specialist obstetric, haematology, hepatology and anesthetic input.

Key Learning Points

- A proportion of patients with MPN will require disease-specific intervention in pregnancy, without which they risk significant complications for themselves and their pregnancy.
- A Preconception meeting to risk assess regarding future pregnancy, discuss therapeutic options and additional monitoring during pregnancy, is beneficial.
- Low dose aspirin is safe in pregnancy. In the absence of a clear contraindication, all patients should receive aspirin 75 mg once daily throughout pregnancy.
- In pregnancies considered to be 'high risk', additional therapy including low molecular weight heparin and interferon should be considered.
- Uterine artery dopplers should be performed to screen for placental dysfunction at 20 weeks followed by serial growth scans.
- Consider postpartum thromboprophylaxis in all women with MPN.

References

1. Swerdlow SH. WHO classification of tumours of haematopoietic and lymphoid tissues, IARC WHO classification of tumours, vol. 2. 2nd ed. Geneva: World Health Organization; 2008.
2. Baxter EJ, Scott LM, Campbell PJ, East C, Fourouclas N, Swanton S, et al.; Cancer Genome Project. Acquired mutation of the tyrosine kinase JAK2 in human myeloproliferative disorders. Lancet. 2005;365(9464):1054–61.
3. James C, Ugo V, Le Couédic JP, Staerk J, Delhommeau F, Lacout C, et al. A unique clonal JAK2 mutation leading to constitutive signalling causes polycythaemia vera. Nature. 2005;434(7037):1144–8.

4. Kralovics R, Passamonti F, Buser AS, Teo SS, Tiedt R, Passweg JR, et al. A gain-of-function mutation of JAK2 in myeloproliferative disorders. N Engl J Med. 2005;352(17):1779–90.
5. Levine RL, Wadleigh M, Cools J, Ebert BL, Wernig G, Huntly BJ, et al. Activating mutation in the tyrosine kinase JAK2 in polycythemia vera, essential thrombocythemia, and myeloid metaplasia with myelofibrosis. Cancer Cell. 2005;7(4):387–97.
6. Scott LM, Tong W, Levine RL, Scott MA, Beer PA, Stratton MR, et al. JAK2 exon 12 mutations in polycythemia vera and idiopathic erythrocytosis. N Engl J Med. 2007;356(5):459–68.
7. Pikman Y, Lee BH, Mercher T, McDowell E, Ebert BL, Gozo M, et al. MPLW515L is a novel somatic activating mutation in myelofibrosis with myeloid metaplasia. PLoS Med. 2006;3(7):e270.
8. Patel RK, Lea NC, Heneghan MA, Westwood NB, Milojkovic D, Thanigaikumar M, et al. Prevalence of the activating JAK2 tyrosine kinase mutation V617F in the Budd-Chiari syndrome. Gastroenterology. 2006;130(7):2031–8.
9. Harrison CN. Essential thrombocythaemia: challenges and evidence-based management. Br J Haematol. 2005;130(2):153–65.
10. Wiestner A, Schlemper RJ, van der Maas AP, Skoda RC. An activating splice donor mutation in the thrombopoietin gene causes hereditary thrombocythaemia. Nat Genet. 1998;18(1):49–52.
11. Ding J, Komatsu H, Wakita A, Kato-Uranishi M, Ito M, Satoh A, et al. Familial essential thrombocythemia associated with a dominant-positive activating mutation of the c-MPL gene, which encodes for the receptor for thrombopoietin. Blood. 2004;103(11):4198–200.
12. Landgren O, Goldin LR, Kristinsson SY, Helgadottir EA, Samuelsson J, Bjorkholm M. Increased risks of polycythemia vera, essential thrombocythemia, and myelofibrosis among 24,577 first-degree relatives of 11,039 patients with myeloproliferative neoplasms in Sweden. Blood. 2008;112(6):2199–204.
13. Jones AV, Chase A, Silver RT, Oscier D, Zoi K, Wang YL, et al. JAK2 haplotype is a major risk factor for the development of myeloproliferative neoplasms. Nat Genet. 2009;41(4):446–9.
14. Kilpivaara O, Mukherjee S, Schram AM, Wadleigh M, Mullally A, Ebert BL, et al. A germline JAK2 SNP is associated with predisposition to the development of JAK2 (V617F)-positive myeloproliferative neoplasms. Nat Genet. 2009;41(4):455–9.
15. Olcaydu D, Harutyunyan A, Jager R, Berg T, Gisslinger B, Pabinger I, et al. A common JAK2 haplotype confers susceptibility to myeloproliferative neoplasms. Nat Genet. 2009;41(4):450–4.
16. Harrison C. Pregnancy and its management in the Philadelphia negative myeloproliferative diseases. Br J Haematol. 2005;129(3):293–306.
17. Kiladjian JJ, Cassinat B, Chevret S, Turlure P, Cambier N, Roussel M, et al. Pegylated interferon-alfa-2a induces complete hematologic and molecular responses with low toxicity in polycythemia vera. Blood. 2008;112(8):3065–72.
18. Passamonti F, Randi ML, Rumi E, Pungolino E, Elena C, Pietra D, et al. Increased risk of pregnancy complications in patients with essential thrombocythemia carrying the JAK2 (617 V >F) mutation. Blood. 2007;110(2):485–9.
19. Barbui T, Finazzi G. Myeloproliferative disease in pregnancy and other management issues. Hematology Am Soc Hematol Educ Program. 2006;109:246–52.
20. Willoughby SJ, Fairhead S, Woodcock BE, Pearson TC. Postpartum thrombosis in primary thrombocythaemia. Eur J Haematol. 1997;59(2):121–3.
21. Robinson S, Bewley S, Hunt BJ, Radia DH, Harrison CN. The management and outcome of 18 pregnancies in women with polycythemia vera. Haematologica. 2005;90(11):1477–83.
22. Tulpule S, Bewley S, Robinson SE, Radia D, Nelson-Piercy C, Harrison CN. The management and outcome of four pregnancies in women with idiopathic myelofibrosis. Br J Haematol. 2008;142(3):480–2.
23. Gangat N, Wolanskyj AP, Schwager SM, Mesa RA, Tefferi A. Estrogen-based hormone therapy and thrombosis risk in women with essential thrombocythemia. Cancer. 2006;106(11):2406–11.
24. Gangat N, Wolanskyj AP, Schwager S, Tefferi A. Predictors of pregnancy outcome in essential thrombocythemia: a single institution study of 63 pregnancies. Eur J Haematol. 2009;82(5):350–3.
25. Fritz M, Vats K, Goyal RK. Neonatal lupus and IUGR following alpha-interferon therapy during pregnancy. J Perinatol. 2005;25(8):552–4.
26. Griesshammer M, Bergmann L, Pearson T. Fertility, pregnancy and the management of myeloproliferative disorders. Baillieres Clin Haematol. 1998;11(4):859–74.
27. Liebelt EL, Balk SJ, Faber W, Fisher JW, Hughes CL, Lanzkron SM, et al. NTP-CERHR expert panel report on the reproductive and developmental toxicity of hydroxyurea. Birth Defects Res B Dev Reprod Toxicol. 2007;80(4):259–366.
28. Greer IA, Nelson-Piercy C. Low-molecular-weight heparins for thromboprophylaxis and treatment of venous thromboembolism in pregnancy: a systematic review of safety and efficacy. Blood. 2005;106(2):401–7.
29. Royal College of Obstetricians and Gynaecologists. Thrombosis and embolism during pregnancy and the puerperium, reducing the risk (Green-top guideline no. 37). 2009. https://www.rcog.org.uk/guidelines.
30. Royal College of Obstetricians and Gynaecologists. Air travel and pregnancy. Scientific Advisory Committee Opinion Paper 1. London: RCOG Press; 2008. https://www.rcog.org.uk/guidelines.
31. Bayley D, Temple C, Clay V, Steward A, Lowther N. The transmucosal absorption of recombinant human interferon-alpha B/D hybrid in the rat and rabbit. J Pharm Pharmacol. 1995;47(9):721–4.
32. Kumar AR, Hale TW, Mock RE. Transfer of interferon alfa into human breast milk. J Hum Lact. 2000;16(3):226–8.

19

Paroxysmal Nocturnal Hemoglobinuria in Pregnancy

Deepa Jayakody Arachchillage and Peter Hillmen

Abstract

Paroxysmal nocturnal hemoglobinuria (PNH) is a rare disease of hematopoietic stem cells characterized by hemolytic anemia, bone marrow failure, and thromboembolism. Pregnancy in women with PNH is associated with an increased risk of complications for the mother with high maternal morbidity and mortality rates, mainly due to either thrombosis or complications of bone marrow failure. These maternal complications are associated with fetal morbidity including fetal loss. Eculizumab appears safe to use in this setting and is likely to prevent many of the complications usually observed. This chapter addresses the pathogenesis of PNH and the management of pregnancy in women with this disorder.

Keywords

Paroxysmal nocturnal hemoglobinuria (PNH) • Complement • Hemolytic anemia • Pregnancy • Eculizumab • Thrombosis

19.1 Introduction

Paroxysmal nocturnal hemoglobinuria (PNH) is a rare disease of hematopoietic stem cells caused by a somatic mutation in the X-linked phosphatidylinositol glycan complementation class A (*PIGA*) gene. PNH is characterized by hemolytic anemia, bone marrow failure, and thromboembolism [1]. PNH was first described as a distinct clinical entity in 1882 [2], and the term "paroxysmal nocturnal hemoglobinuria" introduced by Enneking in 1925 [3]. In 1937, Thomas Ham found that PNH erythrocytes hemolysed when incubated with normal, acidified serum. This pivotal discovery resulted in the first diagnostic test for PNH, the acidified serum or Ham test [4]. Red cell lysis in acidified serum appeared to be complement dependent, since red cell lysis was abolished by heat inactivation. However, it wasn't until 1954,

D.J. Arachchillage, MBBS, MRCP, FRCPath
Department of Haematology, University College London Hospitals NHS Foundation Trust, 250 Euston Road, London NW1 2PG, UK
e-mail: d.arachchillage@ucl.ac.uk

P. Hillmen, MB ChB, PhD, FRCP, FRCPath (✉)
Department of Haematology, St James's University Hospital NHS Trust, Beckett Street, Leeds LS9 7TF, UK
e-mail: peter.hillmen@nhs.net

H. Cohen, P. O'Brien (eds.), *Disorders of Thrombosis and Hemostasis in Pregnancy: A Guide to Management*, DOI 10.1007/978-3-319-15120-5_19,

with the discovery of the alternative pathway of complement activation, that increased complement sensitivity was substantively proven as the cause the hemolysis of PNH red cells. In the 1980s, it was discovered that PNH cells display a global deficiency in a group of proteins attached to the cell surface via a glycosylphosphatidylinositol (GPI) anchor that the PNH cells cannot synthesize due to the mutation in the *PIGA* gene.

The prevalence of PNH is estimated at 15.9 cases per million of the general population [5]. Patients with PNH can present at any age but the median age of first diagnosis is in the early to mid-30s, which includes women of childbearing age. Males and females are equally affected [6]. The median survival in PNH is 10–15 years, with thromboembolism being the leading cause of death [2, 7]. Other causes of death include complications of bone marrow failure, renal failure, myelodysplastic syndrome and leukemia [8]. In PNH, thrombosis may occur at any site. In addition to lower limb deep venous thrombosis (DVT) and pulmonary embolism (PE), common sites include the intra-abdominal and cerebral veins, for reasons still unknown, making thrombosis a leading cause of morbidity as well as mortality. Arterial thromboses are also increased in patients with PNH, frequently involving the cerebral and coronary arteries [9, 10].

Until recently, bone marrow transplantation was the only effective treatment for PNH. However, the development of eculizumab an anti-complement antibody targeting the C5 complement component, has revolutionized the approach to the management of PNH [11]. Pregnancy in women with PNH is associated with an increased risk of complications for the mother, with high maternal morbidity and mortality rates, mainly due to either thrombosis or complications of associated bone marrow failure. These maternal complications are associated with fetal morbidity including fetal loss. Therefore, pregnancy has generally been discouraged in the past [12–14]. However, accumulating evidence supports the safe and effective use of eculizumab in pregnancy, with successful pregnancy outcomes [15, 16].

19.2 Pathogenesis of PNH

The *PIGA* gene mutation that characterises PNH impairs the membrane expression of a number of glycosylphosphatidylinositol-anchored complement regulatory proteins (GPI-AP), including the complement regulators CD55 and CD59 on affected blood cells [17–19]. The role of CD55, or decay accelerating factor (DAF), is a 68,000 Dalton (Da) molecular weight glycoprotein whose role is to accelerate the rate of destruction of membrane bound C3 convertase [20]. CD59, or membrane inhibitor of reactive lysis (MIRL), a 19,000 Da molecular weight glycoprotein, is the main regulator of terminal complement. It does this by directly interacting with the membrane attack complex (MAC) to prevent lytic pore formation by blocking the aggregation of C9 [21, 22]. Reduction or complete absence of CD55 and CD59 causes inappropriate and uncontrolled activation of the complement pathway, leading to intravascular hemolysis. Figure 19.1 summarises the pathophysiology of PNH in line with available evidence and current understanding of the disease. Intravascular hemolysis causes anemia and release of free hemoglobin, leading to subsequent depletion of nitric oxide (NO). Depletion of NO causes vaso-occlusion and platelet activation, leading to dysphagia, fatigue, abdominal pain, bloating, chest pain, erectile dysfunction, pulmonary hypertension and other end organ damage [23, 24].

19.3 Pregnancy and PNH

Pregnancy and childbirth pose particular clinical challenges in women with PNH. Information about the management of PNH during pregnancy is limited to case reports and small studies [15, 25–27]. Pregnancy in PNH patients is associated with high rates of maternal and fetal morbidity and mortality, and there is further increased risk during the post-partum period [14, 27, 28]. Maternal mortality has been reported to be as high at 12–21 % [14, 27], although this is probably an overestimate due to over-reporting of eventful cases. However, there is also a significant risk of

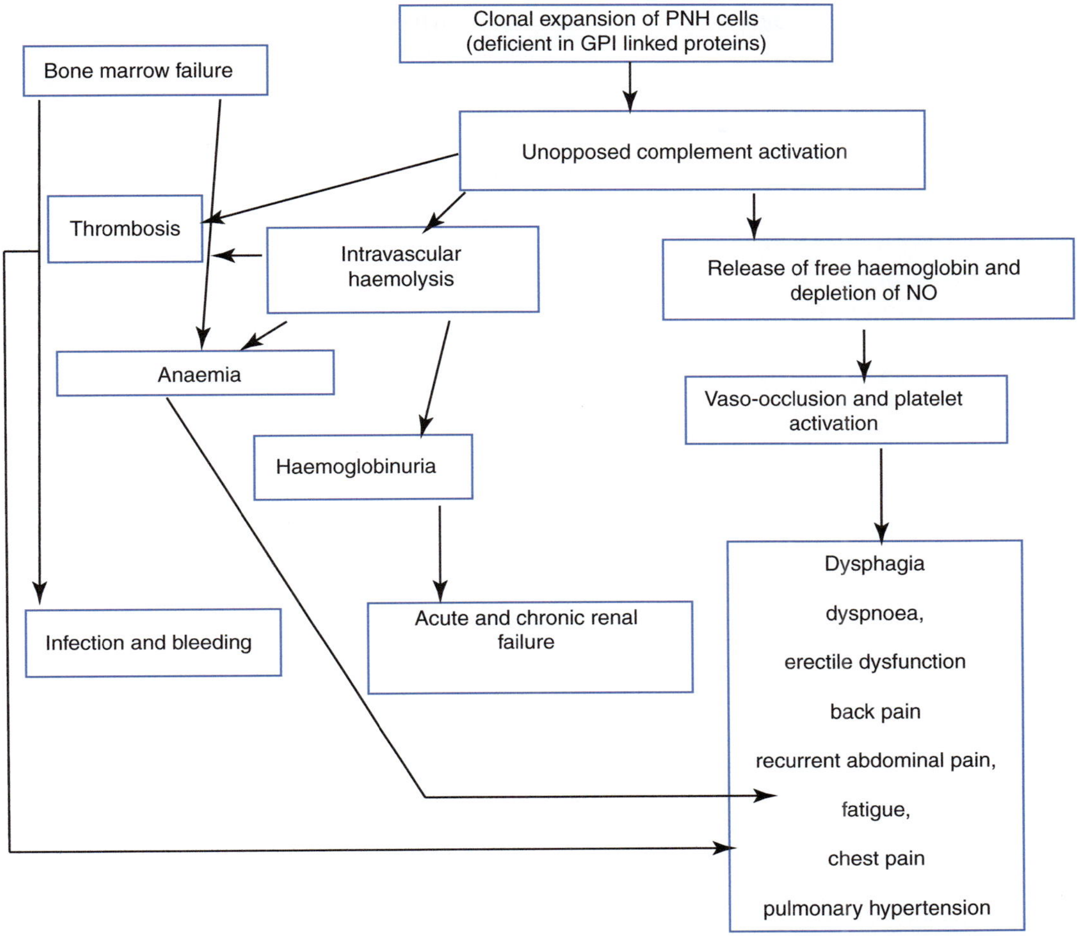

Fig. 19.1 Pathophysiology of PNH

complications such as stroke, which, although not always fatal, can lead to permanent deterioration in health. The main causes of death have been thromboembolism, more often in unusual sites such as hepatic and cerebral veins, and infections. The perinatal mortality rate has been reported to be 7–9 %, with prematurity the main risk to the baby [14, 27]. Stillbirth and miscarriage is also common and over 45 % of pregnancies in women with PNH result in either spontaneous miscarriages or early termination [12]. It has been reported that only half of the pregnancies progress to term. Major maternal complications requiring hospitalization and/or admission to an intensive care unit can occur in 16 % of women, with the highest incidence during the post-partum period [14]. Women with PNH may present for the first time during pregnancy. A retrospective review demonstrated that the diagnosis of PNH in women was made during pregnancy in 25 % of cases [27]. As for most other rare diseases, the primary step in the successful management of PNH is to consider the diagnosis as it can be mistaken for other conditions in pregnancy. PNH should be considered as a diagnosis in pregnant women presenting with unexplained anemia and/or thrombocytopenia with intravascular hemolysis as well as thrombosis in unusual sites [29, 30]. Worsening anemia due to increased intravascular hemolysis and thrombocytopenia are often more severe during pregnancy than in the non-pregnant state, resulting in an increased red cell transfusion requirement throughout pregnancy [14, 27, 28, 31]. The platelet count is often less than 50×10^9/L [27], which makes the antithrombotic management of thrombosis more challenging during pregnancy.

19.3.1 Thrombosis During Pregnancy and the Postpartum Period

Normal pregnancy is accompanied by increased concentrations of fibrinogen, FVII, FVIII, FX, and von Willebrand factor, particularly marked in the third trimester [32–35]. The active form of protein S is decreased during pregnancy, secondary to increased levels of its binding protein, the complement component C4b [32, 36]. Plasminogen activator inhibitor type 1 (PAI-1) levels are also increased [37]. All of these changes contribute to the hypercoagulable state seen in pregnancy and in women with PNH contribute to the further increased risk of thrombosis. Venous thromboembolism (VTE), comprising DVT and PE, is a leading cause of morbidity and mortality during pregnancy in the western world. The risk of pregnancy associated VTE has been estimated from 0.5 to 2 per 1,000 pregnancies [38–40]. The risk of developing DVT and PE in pregnancy is five to tenfold higher than in non-pregnant women of child-bearing age [41]. The incidence of postpartum VTE is more common than antepartum and 20 times more likely following Cesarean section than vaginal birth [38]. VTE accounts for 0.79 deaths per 100,000 pregnancies [42]. Compared to VTE, arterial thrombosis is far less common in pregnancy, with the reported incidence of stroke and myocardial infarction being 0.18 and 0.1 per 1,000 births, respectively [43].

In PNH, there is an increased risk of both venous and arterial thromboembolism, with the incidence of VTE in patients with PNH around 40 % [2]. VTE is the main cause of mortality in PNH, accounting for 40–67 % of PNH-related deaths whose cause is known [44]. As in the non-pregnant state, as well as lower limb DVT and PE, the hepatic and cerebral veins are the sites most commonly affected with thrombosis in PNH [2, 45]. The mechanism of thrombosis in PNH is not fully understood and multiple mechanisms have been proposed [46], including endothelial damage caused by the free hemoglobin released from intravascular hemolysis, platelet activation and microparticle formation [47]. It has been shown that there is increased procoagulant and fibrinolytic activity in patients with PNH, suggesting increased fibrin generation [48]. Several defects have been observed in the fibrinolytic system, including a deficiency of urokinase-type plasminogen activator receptor on PNH granulocytes, and increased plasma levels of soluble urokinase-type plasminogen activator receptors [49]. Furthermore, it has been shown that patients with a large PNH clone have a greater risk of developing thrombosis, suggesting a direct relationship between the PNH clone size and risk of thrombosis [44, 50]. Thrombosis may occur despite anticoagulation, and in one reported case a pregnant woman developed Budd–Chiari syndrome whilst on therapeutic dose anticoagulation, as well as bone marrow failure [51]. Another case report (Case Study 1 below) describes a woman with PNH who appears to have developed sagittal sinus thrombosis despite prophylactic dose low molecular weight heparin (LMWH) [30].

19.3.2 Renal Disease

Although renal failure itself is not a common problem during pregnancy in women with PNH, it contributes to 8–18 % of PNH related deaths [52]. Renal damage in PNH is associated with chronic hemosiderosis and/or microvascular thrombosis, renal vein thrombosis and recurrent urinary tract infections [53, 54]. Evidence of renal damage (on renal biopsy, by using imaging techniques or at post-mortem examination) can be seen in almost all PNH patients [52, 55–60]. Repeated exposure to cell-free hemoglobin release from intravascular hemolysis causes hemosiderin accumulation in renal tubules, tubulo-interstitial inflammation and renal damage [58].

Free hemoglobin scavenges NO leading to its depletion. NO is of critical importance in the regulation of vascular tone with the greatest effect on the afferent renal arterioles [61]. Impairment of renal blood flow because of alteration of vascular tone due to lack of NO can have a direct effect on the glomerular filtration rate and renal plasma flow [61–64]. During pregnancy, there is a risk of renal vein thrombosis leading to acute renal failure and increased hemolysis, which in turn leads to release of more free hemoglobin. Hemoglobinuria is associated with recurrent urinary tract infections, predominantly in women with PNH [54], with a further increased risk during pregnancy. Good hydration and careful monitoring of blood pressure, in addition to other management strategies, is critical during pregnancy and will be discussed later in the chapter.

19.3.3 Bone Marrow Failure and Increased Hemolysis During Pregnancy

Physiological hematological changes in pregnancy include dilutional anemia, relative neutropenia and gestational thrombocytopenia [65]. In addition, iron deficiency anemia is common during pregnancy and folate deficiency can also occur. It may sometimes be difficult to distinguish the manifestations of PNH from those of normal pregnancy and from other pathological conditions which can occur during pregnancy such as HELLP syndrome (Hemolysis, Elevated Liver enzymes and Low Platelets), preeclampsia, gestational thrombocytopenia and immune thrombocytopenia [66]. HELLP syndrome, in particular, is often difficult to distinguish from a PNH crisis during pregnancy as both conditions share common features. Normally, HELLP syndrome develops in the third trimester of pregnancy and clinical features can include right upper quadrant or epigastric abdominal pain and tenderness, nausea, and vomiting. Laboratory abnormalities include thrombocytopenia $<100\times10^9$/L, low haptoglobin, elevated lactate dehydrogenase (LDH) and indirect (unconjugated) bilirubin [67]. These laboratory findings are almost always present in PNH too, and patients with PNH commonly experience abdominal pain, which can also be due to PNH-related hepatic vein thrombosis. HELLP syndrome is typically associated with microangiopathic changes (i.e. red cell fragmentation in association with thrombocytopenia) on the blood film that are not usually seen in PNH. Although hypertension is not a feature of PNH, it may accompany a PNH crisis or can occur due to renal damage, which is common in patients with PNH. Furthermore, a woman with PNH can present with preeclampsia/HELLP syndrome during pregnancy [27]. The severity of hemolysis increases during pregnancy especially in later pregnancy. Women with PNH have been noted to experience hemoglobinuria prior to their next dose of eculizumab even if they had well controlled hemolysis on the standard fortnightly doses of eculizumab for years prior to becoming pregnant [15].

Both anemia and thrombocytopenia are common in women with PNH during pregnancy, and in the pre-eculizumab era often necessitated red cell and platelet transfusion [25, 27]. A series of 27 pregnancies in 22 women with PNH from France reported that the majority (95 %) developed at least minor complications, mainly cytopenias, during pregnancy, requiring transfusion in more than half, while two women developed aplastic anemia (AA) during pregnancy [25]. In this case series, it was observed that in one of the cases with AA, spontaneous improvement of hematological parameters occurred after delivery with only persistent asymptomatic hemolysis. In a review of 20 published reports describing the outcome of 33 pregnant women with PNH [27], there were 73 and 27 % event rates for anemia and thrombocytopenia, respectively. The hemoglobin levels were typically below 80 g/L and, of those who developed anemia, 83 % required red cell transfusion, often more than once. Platelet counts were typically less than 50×10^9/L and some women developed major bleeding events, whilst one of these women developed a major VTE episode with a platelet count of 10×10^9/L. In this report the authors were unable to assess the rate of pancytopenia.

19.4 Diagnosis of PNH

PNH may be diagnosed during or outside of pregnancy. A comprehensive clinical history is critical and PNH should be suspected and investigated in patients presenting with any of the following: hemoglobinuria; direct antiglobulin test (DAT) negative hemolytic anemia; thrombosis in unusual sites such as Budd-Chiari syndrome, other intra-abdominal sites (e.g. mesenteric or portal veins), cerebral veins, dermal veins; aplastic anemia (such patients should be screened for PNH at diagnosis and annually even in the absence of evidence of intravascular hemolysis), refractory anemia/myelodysplastic syndrome (MDS); and episodic dysphagia or abdominal pain with evidence of intravascular hemolysis [68].

Laboratory investigations for PNH include:

- Full blood count (FBC), reticulocytes and blood film, particularly to check for red cell fragmentation
- LDH, total bilirubin, direct bilirubin, haptoglobin, serum B12 and folate levels, urinary hemosiderin, serum iron studies (iron concentration, total iron binding capacity, transferrin saturation index, and ferritin concentration, with C-reactive protein estimation as ferritin is an acute phase reactant)
- Direct antiglobulin test (DAT); blood group and red cell alloantibody screen
- Flow-cytometric analysis of GPI-anchored proteins
- Bone-marrow diagnostics including cytology, cytogenetics and histology, in patients with significant cytopenia of such an extent that PNH is suspected in the context of another hematological disease (especially aplastic anemia or MDS).

Flow cytometric analysis using antibodies directed against GPI-AP is the most sensitive and informative assay available for diagnosis of PNH [68–70]. For initial studies, quantitation of at least 2 GPI-APs is recommended to exclude the possibility that the clinical process is a consequence of an inherited, isolated deficiency of a single GPI-AP [71, 72]. For patients with established, stable disease, annual analysis of peripheral blood GPI-AP expression is recommended; however, a change in clinical parameters (worsening or more frequent hemolysis, or a thromboembolic event) warrants immediate re-evaluation [68]. The flow cytometric analysis can both determine the percentage of cells that are abnormal and identify discrete populations with different degrees of deficiency (particularly on red cells; Fig. 19.2). Red cells with complete deficiency of GPI-APs are called PNH III, those with subtotal deficiency (usually around 10 % of normal expression) PNH II, and those with normal expression PNH I (Fig. 19.2). In order to obtain accurate information about the percentage of GPI-AP–deficient erythrocytes, flow cytometric analysis should be performed prior to red cell transfusion; in a transfused patient, the analysis should be deferred for at least 4 weeks or longer if clinically safe to do so. This is because the flow cytometric histogram will be affected by the normal (transfused) red cells by increasing the proportion of red cells expressing CD55 and CD59, although it is unlikely to obscure the diagnosis of PNH. Analysis of expression of GPI-AP on granulocytes provides additional clinically useful information such as aiding the decision to start prophylactic anticoagulation as the size of the PNH clone has a direct relationship to the risk of thrombosis, as mentioned previously. The current recommendation is to commence prophylactic anticoagulation if the PNH granulocytes clone is >50 % [50]. Unlike GPI-AP–deficient red cells, the life span of PNH granulocytes is normal [73, 74], hence the proportion of abnormal granulocytes more accurately reflects the PNH clone size and is unaffected by red cell transfusion [68] (Fig. 19.3).

19.5 Management of PNH During Pregnancy

The management of women with PNH during pregnancy and postpartum is challenging and should be undertaken in a multidisciplinary high risk clinic setting, with specialist hematological and obstetric input. It is important to refer these patients to a tertiary centre with experience in managing patients with PNH for further advice and management. Women with PNH should receive pre-pregnancy counselling, preferably at an early stage of management. The patient's age, overall health, previous history of thrombosis, degree of hemolysis and bone marrow failure, particularly thrombocytopenia, the size of the PNH clone, other co-existing medical conditions and the degree of personal support should all be taken into account [68]. The management of patients with hemolytic or thrombotic PNH (generally those with a PNH granulocyte clone of over 50 %) is described below and in Table 19.1. Patients with predominantly aplastic anemia and those with small PNH clones should be monitored closely but do not necessarily require anticoagulation and/or eculizumab. An individualised management plan should be established and documented for each patient.

19.5.1 Supportive Therapy and Anticoagulation

Close monitoring of the pregnancy, both clinical and laboratory, with regular ultrasound scans to monitor the fetus is important. Both anemia and thrombocytopenia frequently worsen during pregnancy. Red cell and platelet transfusion should be administered as clinically required. In the case of significant bleeding during pregnancy or at delivery, fresh frozen plasma (FFP) should be used with great caution, as it contains a large amount of complement, which markedly increases the risk of thrombosis and intravascu-

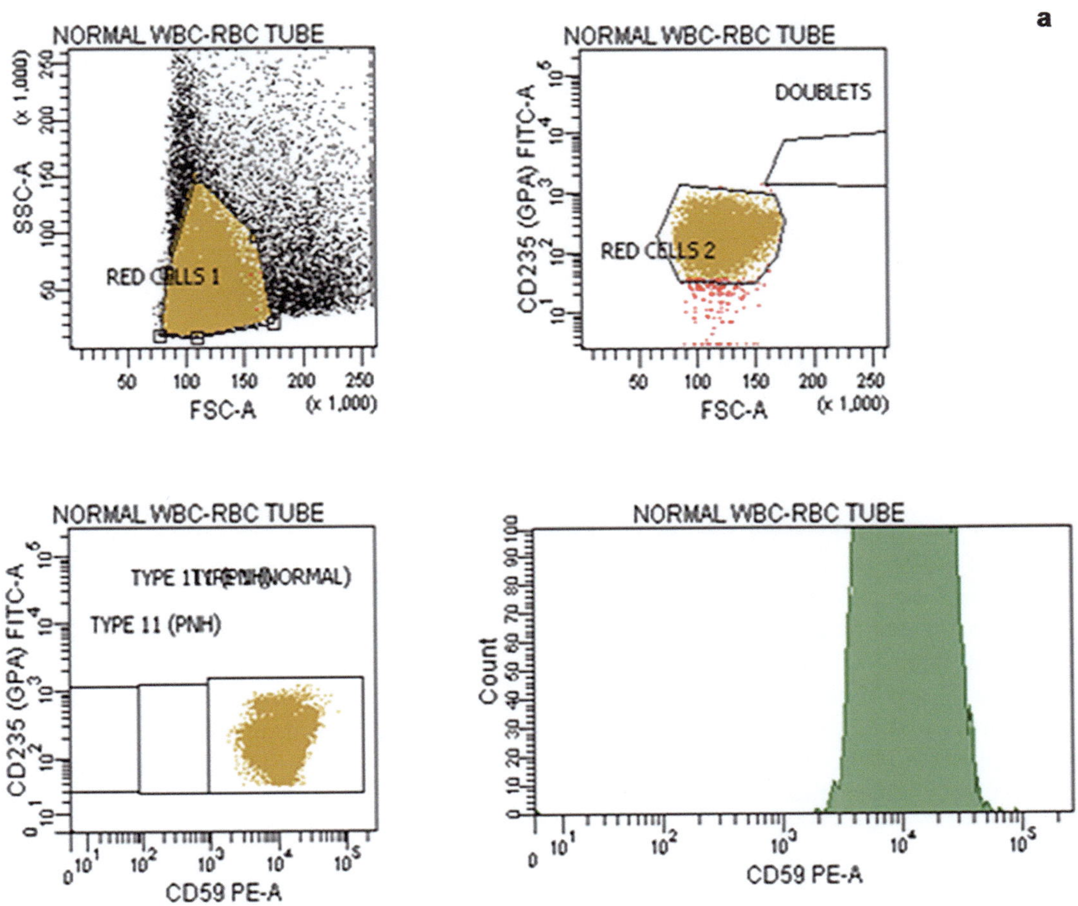

Fig. 19.2 Flow cytometric analysis of red cells in a normal individual (**a**) and in a patient with PNH (**b**) using anti-CD59. A normal individual's histogram analysis of CD59 expression shows a single population of cells positive for CD59. In a patient with PNH, the histogram demonstrates that, in addition to a major population of CD59 positive normal red cells, there are two populations of red cells deficient in CD59. These are PNH red cells

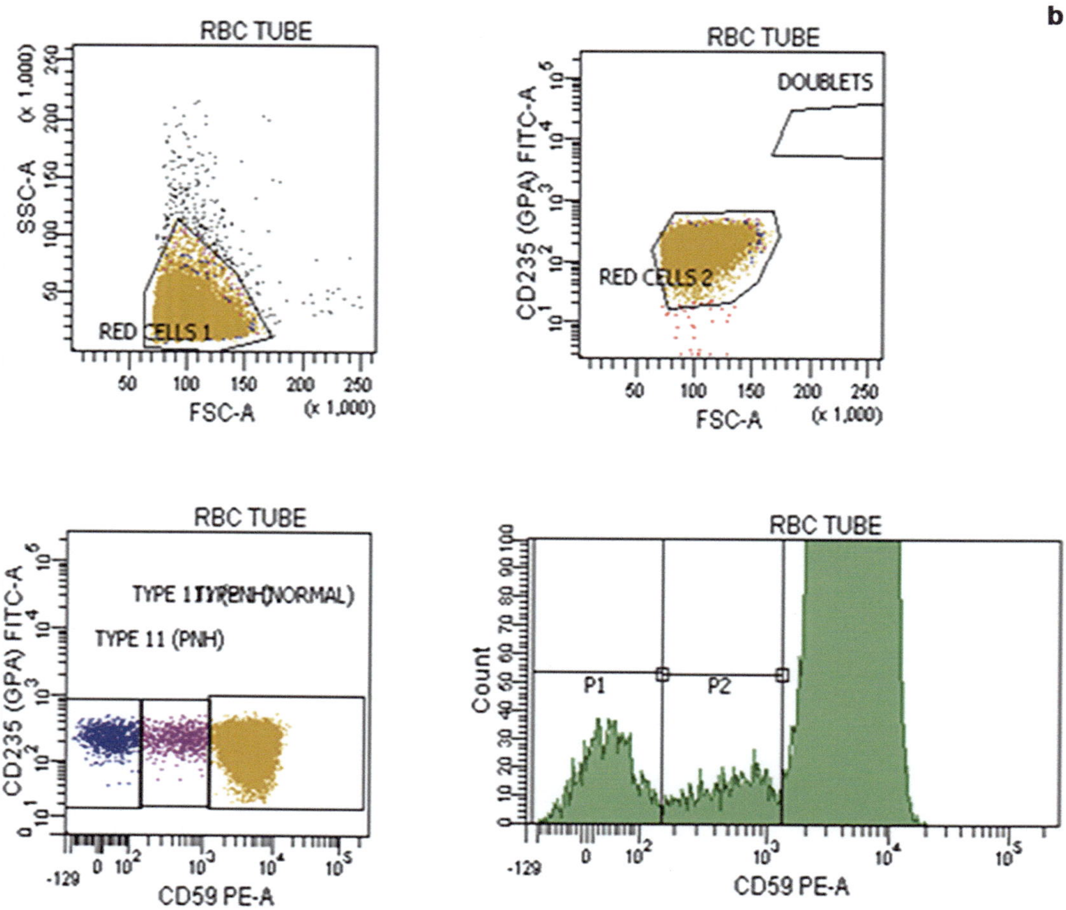

Fig. 19.2 (continued)

lar hemolysis [66]. If its use is essential, FFP must be covered with eculizumab [66]. Prothrombin complex concentrate may be considered but should be used with caution due to the risk of thrombosis [15]. Iron and folic acid supplements should be given to all women with PNH throughout pregnancy. Although the role of prophylactic anticoagulation during pregnancy has not been studied systematically, given the high risk of thrombosis during pregnancy, which carries significant risk of morbidity and mortality, the current approach is to start anticoagulation with therapeutic dose LMWH as soon as the pregnancy is confirmed and continue throughout pregnancy and for at least 6 weeks post-partum [68]. It is important that women who are already on anticoagulation for previous thrombosis with warfarin or other vitamin K antagonists (VKA) should be switched to split therapeutic dose LMWH (i.e. 12 hourly) as soon as pregnancy is confirmed, and before 6 weeks' gestation, due to the risk of teratogenicity in the first trimester. Regular monitoring of the blood count as well as the reticulocyte count and LDH is required to assess the degree of intravascular hemolysis, and liver function and renal function tests should be undertaken. Close monitoring of the platelet count should be undertaken, and prophylactic platelet transfusion should be administered if required to avoid bleeding, particularly with concurrent use of anticoagulation. Anti-Xa levels are useful to monitor the anticoagulant intensity of LMWH. The lower anti-Xa peak levels achieved with split dose LMWH minimise the risk of bleeding should the platelet count fall.

19.5.2 Use of Eculizumab During Pregnancy

Eculizumab [75], a humanized monoclonal antibody, inhibits the terminal complement cascade by binding uniquely to human complement protein C5, thereby inhibiting the formation of pro-inflammatory, prothrombotic C5a and C5b, with subsequent inhibition of assembly of the membrane attack complex [11, 76, 77] (Fig. 19.4). Following a series of multinational clinical trials demonstrating the efficacy and safety of eculizumab in patients with PNH [11, 44, 78, 79], it was approved for use in PNH by the United States Food and Drug Administration (FDA) in March 2007 and by the European Medicines Agency (EMA) in June 2007. Eculizumab is well tolerated, leads to a rapid and clinically significant reduction in intravascular hemolysis, thus providing substantial clinical benefit [77] and improvement in patients' quality of life [11]. Eculizumab is given initially as 600 mg once weekly by intravenous infusion (IVI) for 4 weeks followed by 900 mg 1 week later, and thereafter

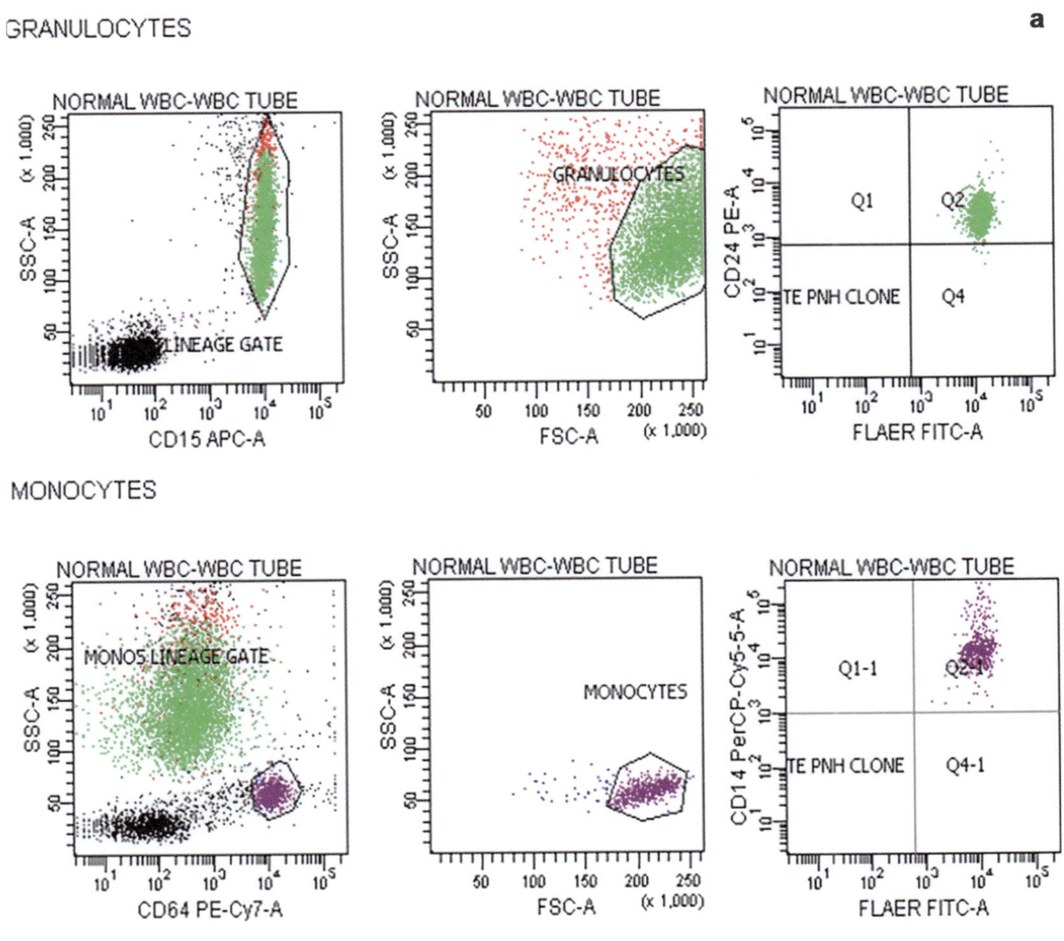

Fig. 19.3 Flow cytometric analysis of granulocytes in a normal individual (**a**) and in a patient with PNH (**b**) using anti-CD15 and anti-CD64. In the patient with PNH there are two populations of cells that are outside the normal CD15 and CD64 gated area. These are PNH granulocytes

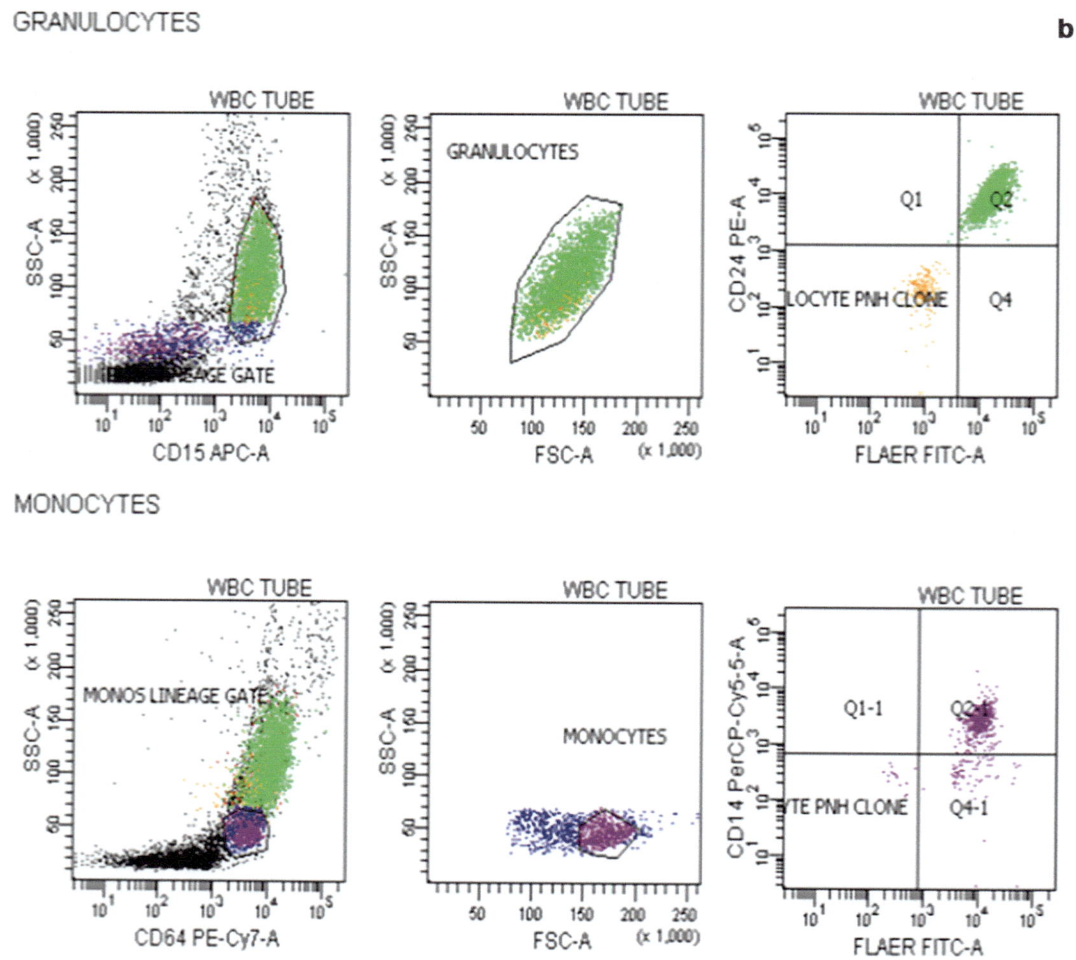

Fig. 19.3 (continued)

900 mg every 14 days [11, 78]. However, under certain circumstances a dose adjustment will be necessary because of the occurrence of breakthrough hemolysis during pregnancy (e.g. maintenance therapy with 900 mg weekly rather than fortnightly). As terminal complement deficiency is associated with an increased risk of infections with encapsulated organisms [80], mainly Neisseria meningitides, all patients must be must be given meningococcal vaccine. The risk of meningococcal infection following vaccination is low and it has been reported as an infection rate of 0.42 per 100 patient-years [77]. The current practice in the UK is to administer tetravalent meningococcal vaccine on the day the patient starts eculizumab (given the potential for complement activation and complications with vaccination) and to cover the first 2 weeks of therapy with an effective dose of ciprofloxacin followed by penicillin V 500 mg bd indefinitely. In the last 4 years since the UK policy was changed there have been no episodes of meningococcal infection in over 150 patients treated.

The observation that eculizumab was effective and well tolerated in red cell transfusion-dependent patients with PNH were demonstrated to be also applicable to a broader PNH patient population, which included those with minimal transfusion requirements or with thrombocytopenia, in the phase 3 open-label non-placebo-controlled

Table 19.1 The management of pregnancy in patients with haemolytic and/or thrombotic PNH

The management of women with PNH during pregnancy requires close monitoring and specialist hematological and obstetric input
An individualised management plan should be established and documented for each patient
Eculizumab should be administered during and immediately after pregnancy, with the dose increased should there be breakthrough haemolysis during pregnancy
Split therapeutic dose low molecular weight heparin (LMWH) should be commenced as soon as pregnancy is confirmed, and continued throughout pregnancy and for at least 6 weeks postpartum
Red cell and platelet transfusions should be administered as required
Delivery should be planned in advance and undertaken in a hospital with expertise in obstetric high risk patients and specialist haematological input
Normal vaginal delivery is recommended unless there is an obstetric reason for instrumental delivery or cesarean section
Anticoagulation should be restarted as soon as is feasible post-delivery, in order to minimise the additional risk of thrombosis during this period of high risk due to excessive complement activation resulting from tissue injury
In the case of significant bleeding during pregnancy or at delivery, fresh frozen plasma (FFP) should be used with great caution, as it contains a large amount of complement, which markedly increases the risk of thrombosis and intravascular hemolysis. If its use is essential, FFP must be covered with eculizumab. Prothrombin complex concentrate may be considered but should be used with caution due to the risk of thrombosis

SHEPHERD (Safety and Efficacy of the Terminal Complement Inhibitor Eculizumab in Patients with Paroxysmal Nocturnal Hemoglobinuria) study. This international multicenter study included 97 patients from 33 sites. Treatment with eculizumab resulted in an 87 % reduction in hemolysis. It also led to an improvement in anemia despite a 52 % reduction in transfusions, with 49 (51 %) of patients not requiring transfusion for the study period of 52 weeks. The improvements in hemolysis, fatigue, and transfusion requirements with eculizumab were independent of baseline levels of hemolysis and degree of thrombocytopenia. Quality of life measures were also broadly improved with eculizumab treatment [81]. The long-term safety and efficacy of eculizumab was investigated in 195 patients over 66 months, and found to have a substantial impact on the symptoms and complications of PNH and result in a significant improvement in patient survival [77].

With regard to its use in pregnancy, eculizumab is categorised as a class C drug (i.e. potential benefits may warrant its use in pregnancy, despite the potential risks). The Summary of Product Characteristics (SPC) indicates that as human IgG are known to cross the human placental barrier, eculizumab may potentially cause terminal complement inhibition in the fetal circulation and should be given to a pregnant woman only if clearly needed [75]. However, based on published case reports of 9 patients [15, 16, 26] and unpublished data on the use of eculizumab during pregnancy, it appears to be safe for the treatment of pregnant patients with PNH and likely to prevent many of the usual complications. Moreover, eculizumab does not appear to cross the placenta or to be excreted in breast milk, and no maternal morbidity attributable to PNH has been observed [15]. Out of 9 cases treated with eculizumab at some point during pregnancy, 8 had normal healthy babies with one pregnancy electively terminated [26]. In a case series describing 7 pregnancies, only 2 patients had eculizumab throughout the whole pregnancy including the post-partum period. The eculizumab dose requirement was higher during the latter part of pregnancy than prior to pregnancy, as there was breakthrough hemolysis prior to the next dose of eculizumab [15]. Therefore, it appears that eculizumab is probably safe in pregnancy but, as these observations are based on a small number of patients, more evidence are needed to determine the safety and efficacy profile for eculizumab in pregnancy. Nevertheless, taking the risk and benefit ratio into account, eculizumab is currently recommended during pregnancy; in the UK, women with hemolytic PNH not requiring eculizumab pre-pregnancy are routinely offered it during pregnancy and in the immediate post-partum period. Further information regarding PNH in the UK is available at http://www.specialisedservices.nhs.uk/library/36/Service_Specification_and_Standards___Paroxysmal_Nocturnal_Hemoglobinuria_Service_1.pdf. Information on its safety and efficacy during pregnancy continues to accumulate.

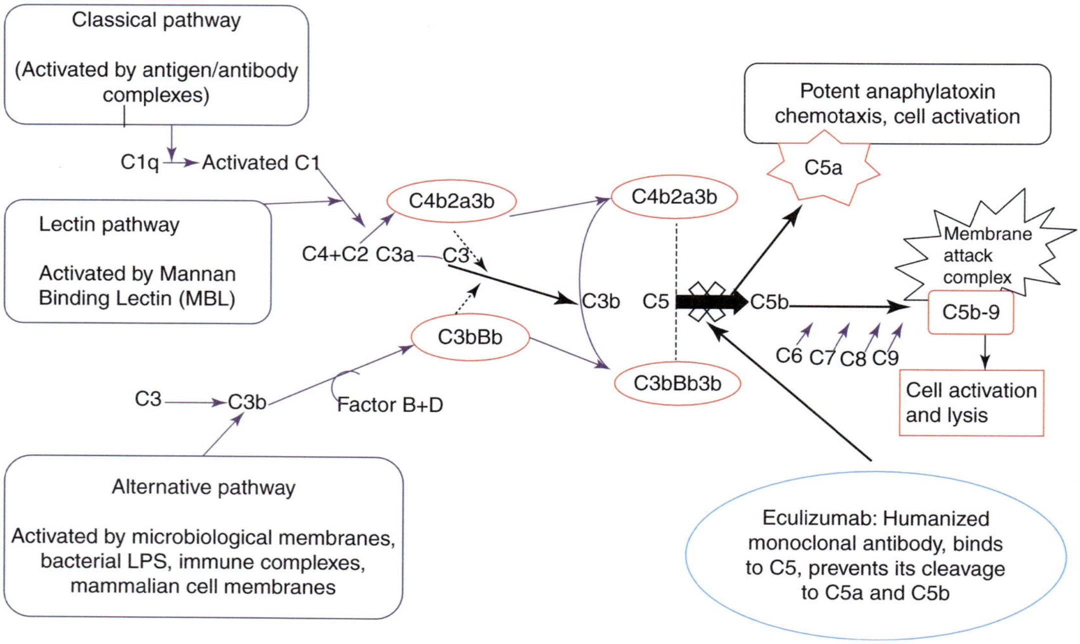

Fig. 19.4 Eculizumab a humanized monoclonal antibody, inhibits the terminal complement cascade by binding uniquely to human complement protein C5, thereby inhibiting the formation of pro-inflammatory, prothrombotic C5a, and C5b, with subsequent inhibition of assembly of the membrane attack complex

19.5.3 Management of Delivery and the Postpartum Period

Aiming for a normal vaginal delivery is recommended; Cesarean section or instrumental delivery should only be for obstetric reasons. Considering the risk of bleeding during delivery, anticoagulation should be withheld for a short period after birth. For patients on therapeutic anticoagulation, delivery should be along the lines detailed in Chap. 5. Anticoagulation should be restarted as soon as is feasible post-delivery, in order to minimise the additional risk of thrombosis during this period of high risk due to excessive complement activation resulting from tissue injury. As stated above, FFP should generally be avoided and, if essential for major bleeding, then its use must be covered with eculizumab. Prothrombin complex concentrate may be considered but should be used with caution due to the risk of thrombosis [15]. Therapeutic dose LMWH should be continued for at least 6 weeks postpartum. In women on long-term warfarin or another VKA, LMWH can be switched back to warfarin (or another VKA) postpartum.

19.6 Case Studies

Case Study 1 [30]

A 29-year-old woman, diagnosed with PNH 5 years previously, was reviewed at 9 weeks' gestation in her first pregnancy. At this stage, she had moderate hemolytic anemia and had been commenced on oral iron supplementation and low dose aspirin. She had no history of thrombosis and had not required transfusion prior to pregnancy. During pregnancy, she required transfusion of a total of 7 units of red cells to maintain her Hb at around 100 g/L. At 33 weeks' gestation, she developed frontal headache and was started on prophylactic dose LMWH. Two weeks later, she was admitted to hospital with persistent headache. She improved following treatment with intravenous analgesia. Cerebral magnetic resonance imaging (MRI) showed no abnormalities and she was discharged from hospital. Her headache worsened and at 37 weeks' gestation she was readmitted. Computerised tomography (CT) of the brain showed a sagittal sinus thrombosis. Treatment dose unfractionated heparin (UFH) was commenced by intravenous infusion (IVI). Delivery was performed by Cesarean section. Her daughter (birth weight 2.3 kg), was well with no complications. The puerperium was uneventful and her anticoagulation was switched back to warfarin.

Case Study 2

A 23-year-old woman was diagnosed with PNH in the postpartum period following her first pregnancy. She developed hepatic and cerebral vein thrombosis 6 weeks following her second delivery and was started on warfarin anticoagulation. Eculizumab was commenced. Prior to starting eculizumab, she required regular red cell transfusion, every 4–8 weeks, to maintain her Hb around 100 g/L, but further red cell transfusion was not required following commencement of eculizumab. She became pregnant for the third time whilst on eculizumab. Warfarin was stopped and split treatment dose LMWH was commenced (dalteparin 7,500 units 12 hourly, appropriate for her antenatal booking weight of 70 kg), with regular anti-Xa monitoring and dose adjustment to maintain the peak anti-Xa above 0.5 IU/mL. She continued fortnightly eculizumab 900 mg by IVI, together with oral folic acid 5 mg daily, ferrous sulphate 200 mg daily and calcium and vitamin D supplementation. Her blood count, reticulocytes, LDH level, and liver function and renal function tests were monitored regularly throughout pregnancy. Her hemoglobin remained around 100 g/L and platelet count above 100×10^9/L throughout pregnancy. At 35 weeks' gestation, her hemoglobin was 115 g/L, reticulocytes 4.62×10^9/L, platelets 109×10^9/L, haptoglobin <0.1 mg/dL, LDH 467 IU/L and anti Xa level therapeutic at 0.5 units/mL. She had an uncomplicated vaginal delivery following induction of labour at 38 weeks' gestation. Her son (birth weight 3.2 kg), was well with no complications. Post-delivery, she was maintained on treatment dose LMWH, with warfarin introduced on day 4 postpartum, until the International Normalised Ratio (INR) was within the target therapeutic range (2.0–3.0) 1 week following delivery.

Key Learning Points

- Paroxysmal nocturnal hemoglobinuria (PNH) is a rare disease of hematopoietic stem cells characterized by hemolytic anemia, bone marrow failure and thromboembolism.
- Pregnancy in women with PNH is associated with an increased risk of complications for the mother, with high maternal morbidity and mortality rates, mainly due to either thrombosis or complications of bone marrow failure.
- The primary step in successful management of PNH is to consider the diagnosis, as this disorder can be mistaken for other conditions in pregnancy. PNH should be suspected and investigated in patients presenting with some or all of the following: hemoglobinuria; direct antiglobulin test (DAT) negative hemolytic anemia; thrombosis in unusual sites such as Budd-Chiari syndrome, other intra-abdominal sites (e.g. mesenteric or portal veins), cerebral veins, dermal veins; aplastic anemia, refractory anemia/myelodysplastic syndrome (MDS); and episodic dysphagia or abdominal pain with evidence of intravascular hemolysis.
- The management of women with PNH during pregnancy and postpartum is challenging and should be undertaken in a multidisciplinary high risk clinic setting, with specialist hematological and obstetric input.
- Split therapeutic dose LMWH should be commenced as soon as pregnancy is confirmed, and continued throughout pregnancy and for at least 6 weeks postpartum.
- Women who are already on therapeutic anticoagulation for previous thrombosis

with warfarin or other vitamin K antagonists should be switched to LMWH as soon as pregnancy is confirmed, and before 6 weeks' gestation, in view of the risk of teratogenicity in the first trimester.

- The use of eculizumab during pregnancy appears to be safe and it is likely to prevent many of the complications usually observed in PNH.

References

1. Hillmen P, Richards SJ. Implications of recent insights into the pathophysiology of paroxysmal nocturnal haemoglobinuria. Br J Haematol. 2000;108(3):470–9.
2. Hillmen P, Lewis SM, Bessler M, Luzzatto L, Dacie JV. Natural history of paroxysmal nocturnal hemoglobinuria. N Engl J Med. 1995;333(19):1253–8.
3. Enneking J. Eine neue form intermittierender haemoglobinurie (Haemoglobinuria paroxysmalis nocturia). Klin Wochenschr. 1928;7:2045.
4. Ham TH, Dingle JH. Studies on destruction of red blood cells. II. Chronic hemolytic anemia with paroxysmal nocturnal hemoglobinuria: certain immunological aspects of the hemolytic mechanism with special reference to serum complement. J Clin Invest. 1939;18(6):657–72.
5. Jarva H, Meri S. Paroxysmal nocturnal haemoglobinuria: the disease and a hypothesis for a new treatment. Scand J Immunol. 1999;49(2):119–25.
6. de Latour RP, Mary JY, Salanoubat C, Terriou L, Etienne G, Mohty M, et al.; French Association of Hematology; French Association of Young Hematologists. Paroxysmal nocturnal hemoglobinuria: natural history of disease subcategories. Blood. 2008;112(8):3099–106.
7. Ware RE, Hall SE, Rosse WF. Paroxysmal nocturnal hemoglobinuria with onset in childhood and adolescence. N Engl J Med. 1991;325(14):991–6.
8. Brodsky RA. How I, treat paroxysmal nocturnal hemoglobinuria. Blood. 2009;113(26):6522–7.
9. von Stuckrad-Barre S, Berkefeld J, Steckel D, Sitzer M. Cerebral arterial thrombosis in paroxysmal nocturnal hemoglobinuria. J Neurol. 2003;250(6):756–7.
10. Hill A, Kelly RJ, Kulasekararaj AG, Gandhi SA, Mitchell LD, Elebute M, et al. Eculizumab in paroxysmal nocturnal hemoglobinuria (PNH): a report of all 153 patients treated in the UK. Abstract Presented at the 54th Annual Meeting of the American Society of Hematology (ASH), Atlanta, GA, December 10, 2012: abstract 3472. Blood. 2012;120(21):3472.
11. Hillmen P, Young NS, Schubert J, Brodsky RA, Socié G, Muus P, et al. The complement inhibitor eculizumab in paroxysmal nocturnal hemoglobinuria. N Engl J Med. 2006;355(12):1233–43.
12. Bais J, Pel M, von dem Borne A, van der Lelie H. Pregnancy and paroxysmal nocturnal hemoglobinuria. Eur J Obstet Gynecol Reprod Biol. 1994;53(3):211–4.
13. Bjørge L, Ernst P, Haram KO. Paroxysmal nocturnal hemoglobinuria in pregnancy. Acta Obstet Gynecol Scand. 2003;82(12):1067–71.
14. Fieni S, Bonfanti L, Gramellini D, Benassi L, Delsignore R. Clinical management of paroxysmal nocturnal hemoglobinuria in pregnancy: a case report and updated review. Obstet Gynecol Surv. 2006;61(9):593–601.
15. Kelly R, Arnold L, Richards S, Hill A, Bomken C, Hanley J, et al. The management of pregnancy in paroxysmal nocturnal haemoglobinuria on long term eculizumab. Br J Haematol. 2010;149(3):446–50.
16. Marasca R, Coluccio V, Santachiara R, Leonardi G, Torelli G, Notaro R, Luzzatto L. Pregnancy in PNH: another eculizumab baby. Br J Haematol. 2010;150(6):707–8.
17. Bessler M, Mason PJ, Hillmen P, Miyata T, Yamada N, Takeda J, et al. Paroxysmal nocturnal haemoglobinuria (PNH) is caused by somatic mutations in the PIG-A gene. EMBO J. 1994;13(1):110–7.
18. Miyata T, Takeda J, Iida Y, Yamada N, Inoue N, Takahashi M, et al. The cloning of PIG-A, a component in the early step of GPI-anchor biosynthesis. Science. 1993;259(5099):1318–20.
19. Takeda J, Miyata T, Kawagoe K, Iida Y, Endo Y, Fujita T, et al. Deficiency of the GPI anchor caused by a somatic mutation of the PIG-A gene in paroxysmal nocturnal hemoglobinuria. Cell. 1993;73(4):703–11.
20. Medof ME, Kinoshita T, Nussenzweig V. Inhibition of complement activation on the surface of cells after incorporation of decay-accelerating factor (DAF) into their membranes. J Exp Med. 1984;160(5):1558–78.
21. Meri S, Morgan BP, Davies A, Daniels RH, Olavesen MG, Waldmann H, Lachmann PJ. Human protectin (CD59), an 18,000-20,000 MW complement lysis restricting factor, inhibits C5b-8 catalysed insertion of C9 into lipid bilayers. Immunology. 1990;71(1):1–9.
22. Rollins SA, Sims PJ. The complement-inhibitory activity of CD59 resides in its capacity to block incorporation of C9 into membrane C5b-9. J Immunol. 1990;144(9):3478–83.
23. Hill A, Rother RP, Wang X, Morris Jr SM, Quinn-Senger K, Kelly R, et al. Effect of eculizumab on haemolysis-associated nitric oxide depletion, dyspnoea, and measures of pulmonary hypertension in patients with paroxysmal nocturnal haemoglobinuria. Br J Haematol. 2010;149(3):414–25.
24. Rother RP, Bell L, Hillmen P, Gladwin MT. The clinical sequelae of intravascular hemolysis and extracellular plasma hemoglobin: a novel mechanism of human disease. JAMA. 2005;293(13):1653–62.
25. de Guibert S, Peffault de Latour R, Varoqueaux N, Labussière H, Rio B, Jaulmes D, et al. Paroxysmal nocturnal hemoglobinuria and pregnancy before the eculizumab era: the French experience. Haematologica. 2011;96(9):1276–83.

26. Morita Y, Nishimura J, Shimada T, Tanaka H, Serizawa K, Taniguchi Y, et al. Successful anticoagulant therapy for two pregnant PNH patients, and prospects for the eculizumab era. Int J Hematol. 2013; 97(4):491–7.
27. Ray JG, Burows RF, Ginsberg JS, Burrows EA. Paroxysmal nocturnal hemoglobinuria and the risk of venous thrombosis: review and recommendations for management of the pregnant and nonpregnant patient. Haemostasis. 2000;30(3):103–17.
28. Tichelli A, Socié G, Marsh J, Barge R, Frickhofen N, McCann S, et al.; European Group for Blood and Marrow Transplantation Severe Aplastic Anaemia Working Party. Outcome of pregnancy and disease course among women with aplastic anemia treated with immunosuppression. Ann Intern Med. 2002;137(3):164–72.
29. Higgins SP, McMahon LP, Brennecke SP. Paroxysmal nocturnal haemoglobinuria in pregnancy–not to be confused with pre-eclampsia or HELLP syndrome. Case report and literature review. J Obstet Gynaecol. 2004;24:83–5.
30. Melo A, Gorgal-Carvalho R, Amaral J, Marques MC, Andrade J, et al. Clinical management of paroxysmal nocturnal haemoglobinuria in pregnancy: three case reports. Blood Transfus. 2011;9:99–103.
31. Spencer JA. Paroxysmal nocturnal haemoglobinuria in pregnancy: case report. Br J Obstet Gynaecol. 1980;87:246–8.
32. Bremme KA. Haemostatic changes in pregnancy. Best Pract Res Clin Haematol. 2003;16:153–68.
33. Sanchez-Luceros A, Meschengieser SS, Marchese C, Votta R, Casais P, et al. Factor VIII and von Willebrand factor changes during normal pregnancy and puerperium. Blood Coagul Fibrinolysis. 2003;14:647–51.
34. Stirling Y, Woolf L, North WR, Seghatchian MJ, Meade TW. Haemostasis in normal pregnancy. Thromb Haemost. 1984;52:176–82.
35. Wickstrom K, Edelstam G, Lowbeer CH, Hansson LO, Siegbahn A. Reference intervals for plasma levels of fibronectin, von Willebrand factor, free protein S and antithrombin during third-trimester pregnancy. Scand J Clin Lab Invest. 2004;64:31–40.
36. Bremme K, Ostlund E, Almqvist I, Heinonen K, Blomback M. Enhanced thrombin generation and fibrinolytic activity in normal pregnancy and the puerperium. Obstet Gynecol. 1992;80:132–7.
37. Sie P, Caron C, Azam J, Goudemand J, Grandjean H, Boneu B, Fournie A. Reassessment of von Willebrand factor (VWF), VWF propeptide, factor VIII:C and plasminogen activator inhibitors 1 and 2 during normal pregnancy. Br J Haematol. 2003;121:897–903.
38. Gherman RB, Goodwin TM, Leung B, Byrne JD, Hethumumi R, Montoro M. Incidence, clinical characteristics, and timing of objectively diagnosed venous thromboembolism during pregnancy. Obstet Gynecol. 1999;94:730–4.
39. James AH, Jamison MG, Brancazio LR, Myers ER. Venous thromboembolism during pregnancy and the postpartum period: incidence, risk factors, and mortality. Am J Obstet Gynecol. 2006;194:1311–5.
40. Vora S, Ghosh K, Shetty S, Salvi V, Satoskar P. Deep venous thrombosis in the antenatal period in a large cohort of pregnancies from western India. Thromb J. 2007;5:9.
41. Pomp ER, Lenselink AM, Rosendaal FR, Doggen CJ. Pregnancy, the postpartum period and prothrombotic defects: risk of venous thrombosis in the MEGA study. J Thromb Haemost. 2008;6:632–7.
42. Cantwell R, Clutton-Brock T, Cooper G, Dawson A, Drife J, et al. Saving Mothers' Lives: Reviewing maternal deaths to make motherhood safer: 2006–2008. The Eighth Report of the Confidential Enquiries into Maternal Deaths in the United Kingdom. BJOG. 2011;118 Suppl 1:1–203.
43. Walker ID. Venous and arterial thrombosis during pregnancy: epidemiology. Semin Vasc Med. 2003;3: 25–32.
44. Hillmen P, Muus P, Duhrsen U, Risitano AM, Schubert J, et al. Effect of the complement inhibitor eculizumab on thromboembolism in patients with paroxysmal nocturnal hemoglobinuria. Blood. 2007;110:4123–8.
45. de Latour RP, Mary JY, Salanoubat C, Terriou L, Etienne G, et al. Paroxysmal nocturnal hemoglobinuria: natural history of disease subcategories. Blood. 2008;112:3099–106.
46. Hill A, Kelly RJ, Hillmen P. Thrombosis in paroxysmal nocturnal hemoglobinuria. Blood. 2013;121:4985–96.
47. Van Bijnen ST, Van Heerde WL, Muus P. Mechanisms and clinical implications of thrombosis in paroxysmal nocturnal hemoglobinuria. J Thromb Haemost. 2012;10:1–10.
48. Grunewald M, Siegemund A, Grunewald A, Schmid A, Koksch M, et al. Plasmatic coagulation and fibrinolytic system alterations in PNH: relation to clone size. Blood Coagul Fibrinolysis. 2003;14:685–95.
49. Gao W, Wang Z, Bai X, Li Y, Ruan C. Diagnostic significance of measurement of the receptor for urokinase-type plasminogen activator on granulocytes and in plasma from patients with paroxysmal nocturnal hemoglobinuria. Int J Hematol. 2002;75:434–9.
50. Hall C, Richards S, Hillmen P. Primary prophylaxis with warfarin prevents thrombosis in paroxysmal nocturnal hemoglobinuria (PNH). Blood. 2003;102:3587–91.
51. Bjorge L, Ernst P, Haram KO. Paroxysmal nocturnal hemoglobinuria in pregnancy. Acta Obstet Gynecol Scand. 2003;82:1067–71.
52. Nishimura J, Kanakura Y, Ware RE, Shichishima T, Nakakuma H, et al. Clinical course and flow cytometric analysis of paroxysmal nocturnal hemoglobinuria in the United States and Japan. Medicine (Baltimore). 2004;83:193–207.
53. Hillmen P, Elebute M, Kelly R, Urbano-Ispizua A, Hill A, et al. Long-term effect of the complement inhibitor eculizumab on kidney function in patients with paroxysmal nocturnal hemoglobinuria. Am J Hematol. 2010;85:553–9.
54. Bessler M, Hiken J. The pathophysiology of disease in patients with paroxysmal nocturnal hemoglobinuria. Hematology Am Soc Hematol Educ Program. 2008;1:104–10.

55. Jose MD, Lynn KL. Acute renal failure in a patient with paroxysmal nocturnal hemoglobinuria. Clin Nephrol. 2001;56:172–4.
56. Mathieu D, Rahmouni A, Villeneuve P, Anglade MC, Rochant H, Vasile N. Impact of magnetic resonance imaging on the diagnosis of abdominal complications of paroxysmal nocturnal hemoglobinuria. Blood. 1995;85:3283–8.
57. Mulopulos GP, Turner DA, Schwartz MM, Murakami ME, Clark JW. MRI of the kidneys in paroxysmal nocturnal hemoglobinuria. AJR Am J Roentgenol. 1986;146:51–2.
58. Nath KA, Vercellotti GM, Grande JP, Miyoshi H, Paya CV, et al. Heme protein-induced chronic renal inflammation: suppressive effect of induced heme oxygenase-1. Kidney Int. 2001;59:106–17.
59. Rimola J, Martin J, Puig J, Darnell A, Massuet A. The kidney in paroxysmal nocturnal haemoglobinuria: MRI findings. Br J Radiol. 2004;77:953–6.
60. Suzukawa K, Ninomiya H, Mitsuhashi S, Anno I, Nagasawa T, Abe T. Demonstration of the deposition of hemosiderin in the kidneys of patients with paroxysmal nocturnal hemoglobinuria by magnetic resonance imaging. Intern Med. 1993;32:686–90.
61. Schlaich MP, Schmitt D, Ott C, Schmidt BM, Schmieder RE. Basal nitric oxide synthase activity is a major determinant of glomerular haemodynamics in humans. J Hypertens. 2008;26:110–6.
62. Delles C, Klingbeil AU, Schneider MP, Handrock R, Schaufele T, Schmieder RE. The role of nitric oxide in the regulation of glomerular haemodynamics in humans. Nephrol Dial Transplant. 2004;19:1392–7.
63. Gabbai FB. Effects of nitric oxide synthase blockers on renal function. Nephrol Dial Transplant. 2001;16 Suppl 1:10–3.
64. Schneider R, Raff U, Vornberger N, Schmidt M, Freund R, et al. L-Arginine counteracts nitric oxide deficiency and improves the recovery phase of ischemic acute renal failure in rats. Kidney Int. 2003;64: 216–25.
65. Peck TM, Arias F. Hematologic changes associated with pregnancy. Clin Obstet Gynecol. 1979;22:785–98.
66. Danilov AV, Brodsky RA, Craigo S, Smith H, Miller KB. Managing a pregnant patient with paroxysmal nocturnal hemoglobinuria in the era of eculizumab. Leuk Res. 2010;34:566–71.
67. Sibai BM. Evaluation and management of severe preeclampsia before 34 weeks' gestation. Am J Obstet Gynecol. 2011;205:191–8.
68. Parker C, Omine M, Richards S, Nishimura J, Bessler M, et al. Diagnosis and management of paroxysmal nocturnal hemoglobinuria. Blood. 2005;106:3699–709.
69. Richards SJ, Rawstron AC, Hillmen P. Application of flow cytometry to the diagnosis of paroxysmal nocturnal hemoglobinuria. Cytometry. 2000;42:223–33.
70. Schubert J, Alvarado M, Uciechowski P, Zielinska-Skowronek M, Freund M, et al. Diagnosis of paroxysmal nocturnal haemoglobinuria using immunophenotyping of peripheral blood cells. Br J Haematol. 1991;79:487–92.
71. Daniels G. Cromer-related antigens–blood group determinants on decay-accelerating factor. Vox Sang. 1989;56:205–11.
72. Yamashina M, Ueda E, Kinoshita T, Takami T, Ojima A, et al. Inherited complete deficiency of 20-kilodalton homologous restriction factor (CD59) as a cause of paroxysmal nocturnal hemoglobinuria. N Engl J Med. 1990;323:1184–9.
73. Brubaker LH, Essig LJ, Mengel CE. Neutrophil life span in paroxysmal nocturnal hemoglobinuria. Blood. 1977;50:657–62.
74. Rosse WF. The life-span of complement-sensitive and -insensitive red cells in paroxysmal nocturnal hemoglobinuria. Blood. 1971;37:556–62.
75. Soliris. Summary of product characteristics (SPC), Alexion Pharma UK. Available from http://www.medicines.org.uk/emc/medicine/19966/SPC/soliris/. Last updated on the eMC: 26 Mar 2014.
76. Brodsky RA. Advances in the diagnosis and therapy of paroxysmal nocturnal hemoglobinuria. Blood Rev. 2008;22:65–74.
77. Hillmen P, Muus P, Roth A, Elebute MO, Risitano AM, et al. Long-term safety and efficacy of sustained eculizumab treatment in patients with paroxysmal nocturnal haemoglobinuria. Br J Haematol. 2013;162:62–73.
78. Hillmen P, Hall C, Marsh JC, Elebute M, Bombara MP, et al. Effect of eculizumab on hemolysis and transfusion requirements in patients with paroxysmal nocturnal hemoglobinuria. N Engl J Med. 2004;350:552–9.
79. Hillmen P. The role of complement inhibition in PNH. Hematology Am Soc Hematol Educ Program. 2008;1:116–23.
80. Morgan BP, Walport MJ. Complement deficiency and disease. Immunol Today. 1991;12:301–6.
81. Brodsky RA, Young NS, Antonioli E, Risitano AM, Schrezenmeier H, et al. Multicenter phase 3 study of the complement inhibitor eculizumab for the treatment of patients with paroxysmal nocturnal hemoglobinuria. Blood. 2008;111:1840–7.

Hemoglobinopathies in Pregnancy

20

Joanna Howard, Susan M. Tuck, Asma A. Eissa, and John Porter

Abstract
Pregnancies in women with both sickle and thalassemia disorders are seen increasingly worldwide, but outside a small number of specialist centers, most obstetricians and hematologists will see only a few affected pregnancies. Prospective trials addressing the challenges of managing these disorders in pregnancy remain limited so that current management often differs between centers. Both sickle and thalassemia disorders share increased thromboembolic and infection risks, but other complications differ. The UK and international data on maternal and fetal morbidity and mortality in pregnancies complicated by maternal sickle cell disease and thalassaemia disorders are described here in order to assist both obstetricians and haematologists in arriving at informed decisions.

Keywords
Sickle cell • Alpha thalassaemia • Beta thalassaemia

John Porter is supported by the National Institute of Health Research, University College London Hospitals, Biomedical Research Institute.

J. Howard, MBBS, MRCP, FRCPath (✉)
Department of Haematology, Guy's Hospital, Guy's and St Thomas' NHS Foundation Trust, Great Maze Pond, London SE1 9RT, UK
e-mail: jo.howard@gstt.nhs.uk

S.M. Tuck, MB ChB, MD, MRCGP, FRCOG
Department of Obstetrics and Gynaecology, The Royal Free Hospital, Royal Free London NHS Foundation Trust, Pond Street, London NW3 2QG, UK

A.A. Eissa, MBBS, MRCOG, MD
Department of Obstetrics and Gynaecology, The Royal Free Hospital, Royal Free London NHS Foundation Trust, Pond Street, London NW3 2QG, UK
e-mail: asma.eissa@nhs.net

J. Porter, MB ChB, MA, MD, FRCP, FRCPath
Department of Haematology, University College London Hospitals NHS Foundation Trust, 72 Huntley St., London NW1 2PJ, UK
e-mail: j.porter@ucl.ac.uk

H. Cohen, P. O'Brien (eds.), *Disorders of Thrombosis and Hemostasis in Pregnancy: A Guide to Management*, DOI 10.1007/978-3-319-15120-5_20, © Springer-Verlag London 2015

20.1 Introduction

Pregnancies in women with both sickle and thalassemia disorders are increasing in numbers, but outside a small number of specialist centers, most obstetricians and hematologists will see only a few episodes. Prospective trials addressing the challenges of managing these disorders in pregnancy remain limited so that current management often differs between centers. Both sickle and thalassemia disorders share increased thromboembolic and infection risks, but other complications differ. For example, in sickle syndromes, the risk of exacerbating the underlying condition with vasoocclusive crisis and sickle chest syndrome needs to be considered, whereas in thalassemia syndromes, the risks of exacerbating iron-mediated complications such as cardiomyopathy or diabetes need careful consideration. Women with hemoglobinopathy traits have few complications in pregnancy, other than the difficulty of distinguishing concurrent iron deficiency and the increased incidence of urinary tract infections in women with sickle cell trait. The UK and international data on maternal and fetal morbidity and mortality in pregnancies complicated by maternal sickle cell disease and thalassaemia disorders are described here in order to assist both obstetricians and haematologists in arriving at informed decisions.

20.2 Sickle Cell Disease

20.2.1 Key Issues

Sickle cell disease (SCD) is one of the most common inherited conditions worldwide, and in the UK, there are over 12,000 affected individuals with over 300 affected babies born each year. The term SCD refers to both homozygous sickle cell disease (HbSS) and compound heterozygotes with a clinically significant phenotype, such as those with HbSC, HbS-beta thalassemia, HbSD, and HbSO-Arab. SCD is associated with lifelong hemolytic anemia, intermittent episodes of severe pain from vasoocclusion and tissue ischemia, and chronic complications including stroke, pulmonary hypertension, renal disease, and retinal damage. Previously, SCD was associated with early mortality, but the majority of children born in the UK now survive to adulthood [1] with median survival to at least to the sixth decade [2]. Increased birth rates with SCD and improved survival have led to increasing numbers of women of childbearing age with SCD.

Pregnancy with SCD is associated with increased maternal and fetal morbidity and mortality, although these can be improved with comprehensive multidisciplinary care. Even if the clinical phenotype is mild before pregnancy, affected women should be treated as high risk and offered antenatal, intrapartum, and postnatal care by a team with appropriate experience. Multidisciplinary care by a team which includes a hematologist, is essential. Prophylactic blood transfusion throughout pregnancy is not necessary for all women, but should be discussed in the multidisciplinary setting, and is advisable in higher-risk situations. Women with SCD often face practical difficulties in receiving appropriate advice on safe and effective contraception, which would enable their pregnancies to be planned. Such advice would allow women to aim for pregnancy when their SCD and related health issues were in an optimal state which would be associated with improved outcomes.

20.2.2 Maternal Mortality Data

The Confidential Enquiries into Maternal Deaths in England and Wales show small numbers of maternal deaths in most triennia. Between 1973 and 1981 there were eight deaths [3, 4]. If one estimates 30 sickle cell disease pregnancies per year in the UK, this would equate to a mortality rate of 3 %. This is 200 times higher than the contemporaneous overall maternal UK mortality rate of 15 per 100,000 births. However, an almost contemporaneous survey of 125 pregnancies in women with SCD in the UK from 1975 to 1981 which only surveyed centers with ten or more adult SCD patients [5] included no maternal deaths. The Confidential Enquiries looking at the 16 years between 1982 and 1996 show four maternal deaths due to SCD, despite an increase in numbers of pregnancies in women with SCD over this time. The most recent Confidential Enquiries reports indicate similar rates of maternal mortality, with three deaths in the 2000–2002 triennium (two with HbSS and one with HbSC), two deaths in the 2003–2005 triennium (one with HbSS and one with HbSC) and one death in the 2006–2008 triennium (in a woman with HbSC) [6, 7] despite increasing numbers of pregnancies in women with SCD. However, contemporaneous series from three centers in London, with well-established specialist services, reported no maternal deaths in series of 25, 62, and 71 pregnancies, respectively, between 2000 and 2007 [8–10]. Taken together, these data raise concern that there is an increased risk of maternal mortality in hospitals without regular experience of patients with SCD. Indeed, this is a general concern raised in the National Confidential Enquiry into Deaths in sickle cell disease in the United Kingdom covering the years 2005 and 2006 [11].

The UK data are echoed in the published international data. Mortality rates from the 1980s and 1990s vary from 0.4 % (2 deaths in 445 pregnancies) in the US cooperative study of 19 hospitals [12] to 9.2 % (7 deaths in 76 pregnancies) in a 1980–1988 series from a hospital in Ile-Ife, Nigeria [13]. Figures from Benin (in West Africa), Lagos (Nigeria), Guadeloupe (in the French Antilles), and Bahrain fall between these extremes [14–17]. The women with SCD in the Benin study were provided with information and education about SCD and were advised on nutrition, malarial prevention, and early detection of bacterial infections. While maternal mortality was 1.8 %, it was not markedly higher than the 1.2 % maternal mortality in their maternity unit [17]. Some of the more recent data have shown improvement in maternal mortality. The USA's Nationwide Inpatient Sample for 2000–2003, which included nearly 18,000 pregnant women with SCD, found a mortality rate of 72 per 100,000 deliveries (0.07 %), which is sixfold higher than their rate of 12.7 per 100,000 deliveries in women without SCD [18]. In Saudi Arabia, one maternal death (0.4 %) was reported in a series of 255 pregnancies between 2000 and 2007 although this may reflect the more benign natural history of the prevailing mutation in that country [19]. Figures from Bahrain [20] reported four maternal deaths in 351 pregnancies between 1998 and 2002 (1.1 % maternal mortality). Evidence from the Jamaican cohort study showed 2 deaths in 94 pregnancies in women with HbSS (a mortality rate of 2.1 %) [21] but no maternal deaths in 95 pregnancies in women with HbSC [22].

20.2.3 Perinatal Mortality Data

Perinatal mortality data (i.e., stillbirths and deaths in the first week after live birth) show a similar variability, although the absolute numbers are not so much higher than the prevailing rates in the general population. In the UK, the perinatal mortality rate (PMR) in the 1975–1981 series was 48 per 1,000 births (four times the national PMR) [23] and in the 1991–1993 series was 60 per 1,000 (six times the contemporary national rate) [24]. International data show similar outcomes, with perinatal mortality varying from 44 per 1,000 in Guadeloupe [16] to 78.2 per 1,000 deliveries in Saudi Arabia [19] and 134–187 per 1,000 in Nigeria [14, 17]. Several reports support the impression that outcomes can be better in hospitals where there is expertise with the condition, with one perinatal loss in the three UK series, among a total of 158 pregnancies [8–10].

20.2.4 Maternal Morbidity

Maternal morbidity is also increased in SCD pregnancies. The US Nationwide Inpatient Sample showed increased antenatal hospital admissions in women with SCD [25], partly as a result of increased painful crises, and other studies have shown a rate of antenatal painful crisis, which occur most commonly in the third trimester, varying from 20 to 56 % [10, 12, 20, 21, 26, 27]. Painful crises also occurred postnatally in 7.7 % of SCD pregnancies [26], and were also seen in women with HbSC [22].

Infection is also more common, especially urinary tract infections (seen in 16–23 % of pregnancies)[10, 26–28]. Pulmonary complications have an incidence of 11–17 % [10, 26–28] and include the acute chest syndrome. This is a serious potentially life-threatening complication of

SCD, caused by sequestration of sickle cells in the pulmonary vasculature, and characterized by signs and symptoms of chest consolidation with decreased oxygen saturation and new infiltrates on chest X-ray.

Patients with SCD show laboratory evidence of hypercoagulability, with increased thrombin generation, tissue factor [29], and expression of procoagulants on sickle cells and microparticles [30], as well as decreased markers of fibrinolysis. However, linking these prothrombotic changes to an increased risk of venous thromboembolism (VTE) in a given individual is not usually possible unless independent additional prothrombotic risk factors are identified or there is a previous history of VTE, which has been reported at increased frequency in some SCD pregnancies in some studies, but not in others. These differences are probably due in part to the small size of studies and because the differential diagnosis of pulmonary embolism (PE) and pneumonia or acute chest syndrome can be difficult without modern imaging techniques. Therefore, data may not be accurate in older studies or in centers without imaging techniques that allow differentiation between chest syndrome and VTE. VTE is 40 % more common in black Americans than white controls, and this can be a confounding factor in the interpretation of incidence data [31]. The Nationwide Inpatient Sample in the USA, which is the largest reported series and analyzed the inpatient admissions in nearly 18,000 pregnant women with SCD, showed a significant increase in deep venous thrombosis (DVT) and cerebral vein thrombosis, but a nonsignificant increase in PE [18]. Deaths due to VTE are well described, however, and are often associated with prolonged immobilization or admission for painful crisis [15].

An increased incidence of preeclampsia and pregnancy-induced hypertension has been reported in some studies [5, 12, 19] but not in others [14, 20, 21], but a significant increase was seen in large US inpatient data surveys, implying that severe hypertension, requiring hospital admission, was more common in women with SCD [18, 25]. This link may be related to the endothelial damage resulting from the altered shape and increased rigidity of sickled red blood cells.

20.2.5 Fetal and Neonatal Morbidity

These are nonspecific and are as would be expected from a suboptimal intrauterine environment. They include intrauterine fetal growth restriction (IUGR), (in 10–44 %), increased preterm delivery (in 16–33 %), and fetal distress during labor [8–10, 12, 14, 20, 21, 24, 25].

20.2.6 Pre-pregnancy Care

A survey of 149 sexually active women with SCD in north London [24] indicated that 64 % of pregnancies had been unplanned, suggesting a lack of practical help with optimal planning and effective contraception. Only 28 % had a correct under-standing of the relevant genetics of their condition, although 60 % had heard of the concept of prenatal testing of fetuses. This information should ideally be clarified before pregnancy, so that the relevant options can be considered without the pressure of time. Partner screening should be encouraged preconceptually, and if the partner is a hemoglobinopathy carrier, the couple should be counseled accordingly about the availability of prenatal diagnosis and of preimplantation genetic screening (if in vitro fertilization is used). Preconceptual advice to the woman should include screening for hepatitis B and C, HIV, and rubella, and pneumococcal and hepatitis vaccination should be administered if not already done. Screening investigations such as protein-creatinine ratio, echocardiography, and ophthalmology screening should be performed if not done in the recent past. A specific assessment of any additional thrombotic conditions should be made, so that appropriate prophylaxis during pregnancy can be planned.

Medications should be reviewed, and the woman should be advised to take folic acid supplements 5 mg daily and penicillin prophylaxis (because of functional hyposplenism) [32]. Any other medication should be reviewed in the context of possible teratogenicity and stopped or changed to alternatives, as appropriate. Hydroxycarbamide (hydroxyurea) is used to decrease the incidence of painful crisis and acute chest syndrome, but it is teratogenic in animals, and current UK advice is that women should stop taking hydroxycarbamide for 3 months before they conceive. There are anecdotal reports of women who have received hydroxycarbamide in pregnancy without adverse effects; therefore, if a woman conceives while taking it, they should not automatically be advised to consider termination of the pregnancy, but detailed anomaly scans are indicated. Some women may be taking iron chelators, which are essential treatment to reduce the organ damage which would result from excessive iron deposition derived from multiple blood transfusions, and these should be stopped prior to pregnancy or as soon as pregnancy is diagnosed, because of possible teratogenicity [33–35]. Vitamin C, which is usually given with desferrioxamine to enhance efficacy, should also be stopped when the chelators are stopped. Some women will be taking ACE inhibitors or angiotensin receptor blockers for the treatment of proteinuria, and these should be stopped pre-conceptually. There may also be general health issues that need to be addressed before pregnancy, such as advising on smoking cessation, alcohol intake, or blood pressure control. Women should be made aware of local arrangements for pregnancy care and whom to inform when they become pregnant.

20.2.7 Pregnancy Care

The level of care and attention in pregnancy and the puerperium should be the same for women with all types of SCD including those with infrequent complications prior to their pregnancy, as it is not possible to predict which individuals will have complications during pregnancy. Care should be provided by a multi-disciplinary team including obstetricians and midwives, haematologists and obstetric anaesthetists who are all experienced in the care of high-risk pregnancies. It is also helpful to have access to a health psychology team as there are often psychosocial issues involved with coming to terms with chronic health problems and motherhood [36]. There should be a clearly coordinated plan of care, with effective communication between all those involved, including a clear system for enabling the patient to seek emergency help without delay. This needs to continue into the puerperium, when the patient is still at risk of sickle cell crises and other serious complications.

Women should be encouraged to come to hospital promptly if they experience pain which does not rapidly settle with simple analgesia at home. Treatment should include rapid assessment and analgesia with opiates, if required, which can be given orally, by intermittent subcutaneous injection or via a patient-controlled analgesia device. Pethidine should be avoided, because it is less effective, its metabolites have longer-lasting depressant effects and it is associated with an increased risk of seizures. Nonsteroidal anti-inflammatory drugs should be avoided from 28 weeks gestation because they can cause premature closure of the ductus arteriosus in the fetus. Further supportive care should include hydration, infection screening, and early recourse to antibiotics for any infection, which may have been the trigger for the crisis. This particularly includes urinary and chest infections, endometritis in the puerperium, and malaria in those who have undertaken recent foreign travel. Oxygen saturations on air should be measured and oxygen therapy given if saturations are less than 97 %. Oxygen saturations which fall to below 94 % or 3 % below baseline may indicate pulmonary complications such as PE, or acute chest syndrome, and the patient should have an immediate medical review. Treatment with oxygen or other respiratory support may be indicated and in addition, intravenous antibiotics, thromboprophylaxis, or exchange transfusion may be required. There should be a low threshold for transfer to a high dependency unit or intensive care unit.

Planned antenatal care should be tailored to the individual patient and should include a review at least at 2- to 4-week intervals throughout pregnancy. The hemoglobin concentration, hematocrit, platelet count, bilirubin, transaminase, and lactate dehydrogenase levels should be checked at least every 4 weeks. Blood pressure checks and urine checks for infection, hematuria, and proteinuria should be made at least every 4 weeks.

Fetal growth should be monitored at least 4 weekly from 24 weeks with serial ultrasound scans.

A thromboprophylactic plan should be made both antenatally and postpartum, which, as a minimum, should include daily injections of low molecular weight heparin while an inpatient and for at least 7 days postpartum. Additional risk factors (e.g., age, obesity, operative delivery) should be considered using the recommendations in the RCOG guidelines [37]. The timing and mode of delivery should depend on the individual pregnancy, along standard obstetric lines. Vigilance and care should be sustained into the postnatal period, when there is also an increased incidence of painful crises and thromboembolic events.

20.2.8 The Use of Blood Transfusion

During pregnancy, blood transfusions can be given either on an "as required basis" for the treatment of acute complications or on a prophylactic basis. Two Cochrane Database Systematic Reviews [38] concluded that there is "not enough evidence to draw conclusions" on the extent to which prophylactic blood transfusions help pregnancy outcomes. Both a randomized controlled trial [39] and retrospective studies [26, 40] have shown that prophylactic transfusion decreased maternal painful crises but did not show other measurable differences in fetal or maternal outcome. However, the randomized study was small, and the number of units ultimately transfused during pregnancy in those randomized to "no blood transfusion" did not differ significantly from those randomized to "transfusion" because many in the "no transfusion" arm received emergency blood transfusion for vasoocclusive crises. Many centers still advise prophylactic top-up or exchange transfusion for SCD during pregnancy, particularly for high-risk cases or where potential organizational delays in providing timely emergency transfusions would increase the maternal and fetal risks. There are significant risks of transfusion, that include alloimmunization, delayed hemolytic transfusion reactions [26, 41], hemolytic disease of the newborn, and infection transmission. Iron overload from repeated transfusions in SCD rarely deposits in organs other than the liver [42], but if patients receive prophylactic top-up transfusions in several pregnancies, iron loading of the liver may require treatment in the longer term. The need for prophylactic transfusion throughout pregnancy should therefore be discussed in the multidisciplinary clinic and considered if the woman has a poor obstetric or previous sickle history, if there are the increased demands of a twin pregnancy or if the woman has stopped hydroxycarbamide in order to conceive. Most clinicians will have a greater readiness to give blood transfusions during the third trimester of pregnancy.

Ad hoc top-up blood transfusions for correction of anemia are indicated where the hematocrit has dropped below 0.26 and/or significantly below the patient's normal steady-state values. An emergency exchange transfusion, either by the manual or automated route, is indicated when a patient presents with an acute chest syndrome or a stroke and should be considered when persistent or recurrent acute pain develops. Once a patient has required a blood transfusion during pregnancy, prophylactic transfusions should be continued to maintain the hematocrit and suppress the HbS level. There is no clear guidance on target HbS level, but many centres will use a target of below 30 or 50 %, depending on indication. The resulting hematocrit needs to be a compromise between sufficient red blood cells to provide adequate oxygen delivery, without increasing the viscosity of the blood to a level which may precipitate vasoocclusion. To reduce alloimmunization (the formation of antibodies to red cell antigens), patients with SCD should have an extended red cell phenotype performed at presentation, and all transfusions should be matched for C, E, and Kell antigens [43]. If red cell antibodies are already present, extended red cell matching may be required.

20.2.9 Contraception in SCD

As many as two-thirds of pregnancies are unplanned, with the attendant lost opportunity to optimize the health of the woman and the potential outcome of her pregnancy [24]. Barrier methods of contraception are safe and effective. There is limited evidence about the efficacy and safety of hormonal contraception. A Cochrane review [44] identified only one randomized controlled trial which included 25 women with HbSS studied over a 2-year period in a single-blind crossover design of depot medroxyprogesterone acetate. A reduction in acute sickling and hemolysis was found in those receiving the active injections [45]. A further study randomly assigned women to intramuscular depo-medroxyprogesterone (DMPA) or Microgynon (combined oral contraceptive pill) and showed a decrease of painful episodes in both groups, more in the DMPA group [46]. Thus, progestogen-containing contraceptives appear to be safe and effective, and there is a suggestion that they may decrease painful episodes. Women who take oral contraceptive pills may have "pill failures" when treatment is interrupted by an emergency admission to hospital. Also, the efficacy of the contraceptive pill may be compromised by the use of broad-spectrum antibiotics, which are frequently prescribed. Clinicians are often reluctant to advise use of the intrauterine contraceptive device, because of the potential complications of menorrhagia, exacerbating anemia and infection, provoking acute sickling crises. Both these concerns would, in principle, be avoided by use of the progestogen-releasing intrauterine system (Mirena). Some clinicians have concerns about using the combined oral contraceptive pill in women with SCD because of the risk of venous thromboembolism, but there is no evidence to confirm this.

SCD is listed by the British National Formulary and by manufacturers' literature as a contraindication to the prescription of combined oral contraceptive pills. The UK Medical Eligibility Criteria (UKMEC) which is based on the World Health Organization criteria to classify contraceptive use classifies the combined oral contraceptive pill and the copper intrauterine device as category 2, which means the advantages outweigh the disadvantages. However, other methods of contraception, including the progestogen-only pill, Depo-Provera, and the levonorgestrel intrauterine system (Mirena), and emergency contraception are rated as category 1, implying there is no restriction on their use. The level 2 methods should therefore be used as second line.

The outcome of this paucity of guidance is that the majority of women with SCD receive either confused advice or none at all. A survey of 149 sexually active women with SCD in north London in 1993 [24] found that 36 % had been specifically advised to avoid pregnancy. Concerns of the significant mortality risks both for the mother and the baby, as well as a consideration of the generally reduced ability of the woman to care for her child subsequently, are perhaps less likely to prevail nowadays.

20.3 Sickle Cell Trait

20.3.1 Genetic Counseling

Genetic counseling for women with sickle cell trait (HbAS) should be provided as part of the United Kingdom national antenatal hemoglobinopathy screening program, introduced in 2001. Ideally, the woman's carrier status should be identified as part of general pre-pregnancy health advice prior to planning pregnancy. Failing that, in high-prevalence areas, all women are offered hemoglobinopathy screening at the time of booking for antenatal care. In low-prevalence areas (with fewer than 1.5 per 10,000 pregnancies with sickle cell disease fetuses/babies per year), initial screening is undertaken by ascertaining ethnicity using a standardized family origin questionnaire, followed by laboratory testing, when relevant. Currently 1 in 35 pregnant women in the UK are identified by the national screening program as carrying a hemoglobinopathy.

If the screening of a woman by full blood count and Hb electrophoresis suggests she is a carrier of a sickle hemoglobin (or of thalassemia or another significant haemoglobin variant, see below), her partner's hemoglobinopathy carrier status should be ascertained as a matter of urgency. If he also carries a significant hemoglobinopathy, the expected inheritance pattern is that of an autosomal recessive condition, and genetic counseling should be given in a timely manner at an expert center that is able to provide full and balanced relevant information of the risks for the child. The possibilities of fetal testing by chorionic villus sampling (from 11 weeks of pregnancy) or amniocentesis or fetal blood sampling later in pregnancy should be explained, together with their potential complications and the possibility of selective termination of the pregnancy if the fetus is found to be affected. As in all such counseling, it is important to give the couple full and up-to-date information on the potential health issues and care for the expected child, all of which is available through the NHS Sickle Cell and Thalassaemia Screening Programme (www.screening.nhs.uk/sickleandthal).

20.3.2 Other Pregnancy Complications

Few additional complication rates in sickle trait compared with other women of the same ethnic and obstetric backgrounds have been reported, the main issue of significance being a susceptibility to urinary tract infections. Studies in the USA and in the UK found recurrent urinary tract infections in 6 % of women during pregnancy, with 16 % showing microscopic hematuria [5, 47]. The latter finding is a reflection of microinfarcts from localized sickling in the peculiarly challenging renal microenvironment, which may be sufficient to provoke sickling of red blood cells, even when only half the hemoglobin they contain is Hb S.

20.3.3 Thromboembolism

A case–control study suggests an increased incidence of VTE [48] with a statistically significant increase in pulmonary embolism, compared with similar individuals without sickle hemoglobin, and a non-significant increase in DVT. A further study looking at hormonal contraception found a non-statistically significant increase in VTE in the sickle trait group [49]. Published studies however have not included pregnant women, who already have an increased likelihood of VTE by virtue of the changes related to pregnancy itself. Whether this is sufficient justification for specific thromboprophylaxis with heparin preparations is debatable, but this and other standard risk reduction precautions should be considered if any further complications were to be added to the pregnancy or delivery.

20.4 β-Thalassemia Major (TM)

Pregnancy in TM was rarely seen before the 1970s, before iron chelation became available, because hypogonadotropic hypogonadism (HH) rendered patients infertile (see below) and, in any case, most died before the age of 20. There has however been a gradual increase in experience of managing pregnancies in the last two decades. Chelation therapy was introduced in the early 1970s, and despite there being only about 800 patients with TM in the UK, early experience in the management of TM was described [50]. However, the probability of most doctors in the United Kingdom encountering a pregnant woman with TM is very small, as there are only an estimated 800 patients with TM in the UK. Many of the challenges of fertility and management of pregnancy are peculiar to TM. The input of a specialist center in the planning and management of pregnancy in this condition is therefore essential.

20.4.1 Pregnancy Outcomes in TM

Prior to the 1980s, experience with pregnancy in true TM was not described, but as cohorts of patients who had been treated with DFO entered reproductive age, occasional cases of spontaneous pregnancy were reported [51–54]. Later, the deliberate induction of ovulation with successful pregnancies in patients with hypogonadotropic hypogonadism (HH) also began to be reported [51, 55]. The first successful twin pregnancy following in vitro fertilization and tubal embryo transfer was described in 1994 [56]. There are now several relatively large series of pregnancies in women with TM described in the literature.

In a series of 29 pregnancies in 22 women cared for at the Royal Free Hospital, London, between 1989 and 2005 (Tuck S, 2005, personal communication), 13 followed ovulation induction therapy. Four women had preexisting diabetes. Five had hepatitis C and one had hepatitis B before pregnancy. Five women had significant cardiomyopathy prior to pregnancy, two of whom died during the postnatal period. Of the 29 pregnancies, two resulted in miscarriage and three had termination procedures. There were 26 live births, including two sets of twins (both following gonadotrophin stimulation of ovulation). Only four of the pregnancies were delivered before 37 weeks' gestation, and the birth weights of the 21 term babies ranged from 2,050 to 4,100 g, with a mean of 3,240 g. The rate of delivery by Cesarean section was high, involving 18 of the 24 relevant pregnancies, and in 14 cases this was because of fetomaternal cephalopelvic disproportion.

In a review of 14 pregnancies in 11 TM patients over the last 15 years at UCLH [57], there were two sets of twins and one set of triplets. One patient developed a thromboembolic episode and two had preeclampsia. The mean serum ferritin concentration increased from a pre-pregnancy value of 2,000 to 5,000 mg/L postdelivery. Although no significant cardiac complications and no mortality were encountered, the incidence of preterm labor and growth restriction was threefold higher than in the background population. None of the fetuses had congenital malformations. The mean fetal birth weight was 2.5 kg. Breast-feeding was encouraged in all cases. In high-risk cases, planned Cesarean was recommended and this was performed in 73 % of cases. In the remaining pregnancies, planned induction of labor was undertaken before full term. In high-risk cardiac cases (as currently assessed by myocardial T2*, left ventricular ejection fraction (LVEF) by MRI, and by serial echocardiography), labour was preceded by the use of DFO at low continuous doses. DFO was also recommenced in the immediate postpartum period and, in high-risk cases, from the third trimester of pregnancy. No case of maternal mortality was seen, but at least one woman showed increased cardiac iron deposition during pregnancy (see case discussion) having had normal cardiac iron immediately before becoming pregnant. Rapid myocardial iron loading in a pregnant TM woman was also reported in another case [58].

In an Italian series of 58 pregnancies in 46 TM women, conception was achieved after gonadotrophin-induced ovulation in 33 of these women. Ninety-one percent of the pregnancies resulted in successful delivery of 45 singleton live-born neonates, five sets of twins, and one set of triplets. When considering only the singleton pregnancies, the proportion of babies with intrauterine growth restriction did not differ from that reported in the general Italian population [59]. Although chelation was continued in the first few weeks of pregnancy in some unplanned cases, chelation was not given in the later stages of pregnancy. Overall, left ventricular ejection fraction did not change significantly during the pregnancies, although significant increases in left ventricular end diastolic dimension were seen, which returned to pre-pregnancy levels following delivery. Longitudinal myocardial T2* data were not available except in two patients, but values fell from 16.9 to 8.4 ms in one of these, where myocardial T2* measurement was undertaken. In this series, there were five spontaneous miscarriages, one termination of pregnancy, and a high prevalence of preterm births [59].

Thus, despite some differences in obstetric management between centers, there are some consistent themes. Overall there is a good fetal outcome, although there is some evidence of increased premature labor. It is clear that cardiac risks from iron overload are not trivial and risks can be decreased by selecting patients with the lowest cardiac risk and by the use of intensive chelation pre-pregnancy, where appropriate. Where this is not possible, the maternal risks may be decreased by the use of Cesarean section and the avoidance of prolonged labor. Some centers have also used DFO in the latter weeks of pregnancy, without adverse fetal effects.

20.4.2 Fertility and Other Endocrine Complications in TM

Individuals with TM major are dependent on regular and frequent (at least monthly) blood transfusions. As each unit of blood contains about 200 mg of iron, which cannot be physiologically excreted, repeated transfusion results in the accumulation of iron in the liver and subsequently in endocrine tissues such as the anterior pituitary, the islet cells of the pancreas, the thyroid and parathyroids, and the heart, if the iron burden is not well managed with adequate chelation therapy. Ovarian function, however, is usually well preserved. Hypogonadotropic hypogonadism (HH), from iron deposition in the anterior pituitary, is one of the earliest manifestations of insufficient control of iron overload, leading to poor growth and sexual development, often with primary amenorrhea or early secondary amenorrhea [60, 61]. Once HH has developed, there is no evidence that it can be reversed with intensive chelation therapy. However, with optimal chelation therapy during childhood and adolescence, HH can usually be prevented in many cases and its frequency is falling. For example in 1996, a study of 97 individuals in London found 66 % of young adult thalassemics with HH, 20 % with diabetes, and 10 % with hypothyroidism [62]. A slightly later study in over 1,000 patients in Italy found hypogonadism in 55 % of patients over 12 years old [63]. Progressive birth cohorts treated from an early age with desferrioxamine (DFO) show a falling incidence of HH; at the age of 20, 65 % of patients born between 1970 and 1974 had evidence of hypogonadism, but this fell to 14 % in the 1980–1984 birth cohort [64].

Because ovarian function is usually well preserved, the effects of HH on fertility in TM women can be circumvented by induction of ovulation with gonadotrophins [65] and successful pregnancy is often achievable. The success rate in pregnancies following induction of ovulation is surprisingly high. For example, in 11 women with TM managed at University College London Hospitals (UCLH), over the last 15 years and who had HH but functionally intact ovaries, 14 healthy newborn infants were delivered [57]. Worldwide over 350 successful pregnancies have been reported with this approach.

It is important that the management of infertility includes comprehensive pre-pregnancy counseling of the couple and should include evaluation of the partner according to standard criteria as well as assessment for his hemoglobinopathy carrier status. If the partner of a patient with TM is heterozygous for beta-thalassemia, there is a 1 in 2 chance of the baby having TM. If such a couple proceeds with ovulation induction and wishes to have prenatal diagnosis, the acceptability to the couple of a 1 in 2 chance of an affected pregnancy needs to be discussed in advance. At UCLH, we have encountered two couples where both had TM but wished to conceive. The use of donor gametes, preferably using donor sperm, is an option in such circumstances, as sperm is relatively easily available from sperm banks, whereas the use of donor eggs is technically more complicated with unpredictable success rates [57]. In TM patients with severe organ damage or where both partners have TM, adoption should be considered. Preimplantation testing is also theoretically possible if in vitro fertilization techniques are used to achieve pregnancy [66], provided the couple are prepared to accept the lower overall chances of pregnancy compared with the combination of natural conception and the use of antenatal diagnostic procedures.

20.4.3 Pre-pregnancy Assessment in TM

Most but not all patients will require induction of ovulation, allowing a planned approach to the management of pregnancy [57, 67, 68]. Previous long-term treatment with iron chelation therapies such as desferrioxamine (DFO), deferasirox (DFX), and deferiprone (DFP) usually prevents the extrahepatic effects of iron overload, if used appropriately and regularly. While these therapies are offered to all patients treated in the UK, adherence is not always ideal, and they may not be available to patients treated elsewhere. The main cause of early mortality in poorly chelated patients with TM has been due to cardiac toxicity. Important decisions concerning the maternal risk with respect to cardiomyopathy during pregnancy and labor will therefore need to be made, as healthy cardiac function is essential for the increased demands of pregnancy. Indeed there have been several reported maternal deaths from cardiac failure in pregnancy (see below). A detailed assessment of cardiac function is therefore essential before a planned pregnancy. This should involve a myocardial T2*, assessment of LVEF, a detailed assessment of any history of previous heart failure and/or arrhythmias and review by a cardiologist with expertise in this area. If the myocardial T2* shows evidence of cardiac iron overload, especially in the presence of decreased left ventricular function, a course of intensive chelation therapy will be necessary before considering pregnancy. This may take over a year to achieve, so long-term planning of pregnancies is an important aspect of overall management. This decision is not always straightforward however: the development of cardiac iron overload as a result of withholding chelation during the entirety of pregnancy has been seen at UCLH (see Case study 2). In the same clinic, patients with evidence of moderate cardiac iron loading but with well-preserved cardiac function have been successfully managed using small doses of DFO in the final trimester (see below).

A detailed assessment for other comorbidities is required, including glucose tolerance, and bone densitometry [34, 35]. Hypothyroidism and diabetes are recognized complications of hemosiderosis in adults with transfusion-dependent thalassemias. Treatment should be optimized before pregnancy, in the same way as in the general population, with the same issues being relevant, including the risks of fetal anomalies and miscarriage, if not closely controlled. Given their lifelong dependence on transfusions with donated blood, hepatitis B, hepatitis C, and HIV status should be checked before pregnancy, although the risk of transmission from the UK blood supply is extremely low. Appropriate antiviral treatment should be given before conception if required, both for the benefit of the woman herself and in order to reduce the risk of transmission to the fetus, but this may take months or years to complete. The risk of transmission of hepatitis C and HIV to the baby is relatively low if managed appropriately.

Osteoporosis is a significant problem, affecting about 40 % of adult patients, caused by a combination of endocrine, genetic factors, and direct effects of the dysfunctional bone marrow on the skeleton. During pregnancy, a degree of bone loss is seen physiologically, and as TM patients often start from a low baseline of bone density, this can be a particular problem. Many TM patients now routinely receive bisphosphonates to improve bone density, and a careful plan of stopping these several months before conception is required, due to the long biological half-life of these agents and their potential adverse effects on fetal skeletal development. Stopping these agents can add to bone loss during pregnancy. Prolonged heparin anticoagulation during pregnancy, which is necessary in some women, (see below) may exacerbate bone loss in this patient group. Other supportive measures, such as weight-bearing exercise and appropriate calcium and vitamin D supplements, can, however, be continued. Patients should therefore be advised of the risks of worsening osteopenia before embarking on induction of ovulation. Ideally, a TM woman who wishes to become pregnant at a future date should have the opportunity of discussing how to maximize bone mass several years before a planned pregnancy. Efforts should be made to minimize activities which may increase the risk of spinal fractures, such as heavy lifting.

The presence of atypical red cell antibodies should be reviewed prior to pregnancy and assessed for the risk of haemolytic disease of the fetus and newborn (HDFN). The likelihood of new alloantibodies forming during pregnancy in someone who has received lifetime transfusions is small.

20.4.4 Care of Thalassemia Major During Pregnancy

20.4.4.1 Transfusion

The dilutional effects of the physiological anaemia in pregnancy are also seen in TM, and blood transfusions may be needed at more frequent intervals than before pregnancy, in order to maintain the same mean hemoglobin and to minimize major fluctuations in the hemoglobin concentration and cardiac workload, particularly in the later stages of pregnancy. In the Italian study [59], blood consumption increased significantly, from 132 to 157 mL of red cells per kg per year during pregnancy.

Although there is some variation in transfusion practice worldwide, usually the aim should be to maintain the hemoglobin concentration above 100 g/L for TM patients. Reported policy from an Italian study was to transfuse only if the hemoglobin concentration fell below 100 g/L [59]. It has been argued that the relatively high rate of intrauterine growth restriction (IUGR) of 22 % in this study suggests that a more aggressive transfusion policy may be needed [69, 70]. If IUGR is present despite maintaining the hemoglobin concentration above 100 g/L, other fetoplacental and maternal factors should be considered (bearing in mind that 30 % of IUGR in the general population have no identifiable underlying cause).

20.4.4.2 Cardiac Risk and Chelation Therapy in TM Pregnancy

The physiological effects of pregnancy with an increased blood volume, hemodilution, increased stroke volume, heart rate, and cardiac output may precipitate heart failure in patients with preexisting LV dysfunction or with evidence of myocardial siderosis. Progressive changes in many body systems during pregnancy result in increased basal oxygen consumption and increased susceptibility to oxidative stress that peaks by the second trimester of pregnancy [71], but is also likely to increase during prolonged labor. Added to this risk is the common practice of withholding chelation therapy during pregnancy because of potential teratogenic risks. Indeed, some pregnancies have been terminated because of concern about DFO toxicity [35, 72, 73]. Thus, although patients with normal resting cardiac performance and adequate pregestational chelation therapy usually proceed through pregnancy and delivery without complications, a woman with marginally impaired cardiac performance or with myocardial hemosiderosis may be at risk of developing heart failure. There have been at least four case reports of fatal heart failure during pregnancy in the literature [35, 69, 70]. In another report of three cases, end-systolic diameters, fractional shortening, and ejection fraction were within the normal range before pregnancy, but worsened during gestation, and one patient developed incipient congestive heart failure [74]. Key aspects of avoiding such complications are careful pre-pregnancy counseling and full cardiovascular assessment, aimed at avoiding pregnancy in high-risk patients. In an Italian study, patients with impaired LV function were not given induction of ovulation or were advised not to become pregnant until intensive chelation therapy had been undertaken [59].

If a patient with preexisting myocardial siderosis or LV dysfunction becomes pregnant, the risk and benefits of chelation therapy, particularly with DFO, need to be carefully considered. When a woman with TM is actively trying for pregnancy or receiving fertility treatment, her iron chelation therapy is usually discontinued, because of possible teratogenic risks from chelation therapy, in line with the manufacturers' recommendations. This approach has not been universally adopted, however. In the Origa study [59], chelation therapy [deferoxamine (n=31), deferiprone (n=2), and deferasirox (n=2)] was being taken at the time of conception and was continued for the following 2–10 weeks in the spontaneous pregnancies and in ten pregnancies achieved by ovarian stimulation with no adverse fetal effects. In patients with a history of high myocardial iron load, the withholding of chelation therapy for repeated cycles of ovulation induction may pose an unacceptable risk. In such cases, some patients at UCLH have continued DFO (but not other chelators) until pregnancy has been confirmed. No fetal abnormalities have been seen. Furthermore, in the latter part of pregnancy, where teratogenic effects are theoretically less than in the first trimester, the potential benefits of DFO in high-risk cases may need to be considered. The potential teratogenic effects of DFP are well recognized [75], but with DFO, the risks may not be as great as hitherto considered. Firstly, DFO, by nature of its positive charge, its relative hydrophilic properties, and its larger molecular weight than orally absorbed chelators, transits biomembranes more slowly [76], and this would also be expected with placental transfer [33]. Although teratogenic effects and skeletal anomalies were noted in animal studies with DFO, it can be difficult to extrapolate the degree of placental transfer to humans. Furthermore, over three decades, there have been over 40 pregnancies reported in iron-overloaded subjects given DFO at various stages of pregnancy without apparent teratogenic effects [77–84]. There have also been reports of DFO use throughout the second and third trimesters of pregnancy without adverse fetal effects [70, 82]. At UCLH [57], it has been recent practice to give low doses of DFO (1 g/day) in the later stages of pregnancy to patients with a high risk of heart disease, based on either a previous history of LV dysfunction or with evidence of myocardial iron deposition, either immediately before pregnancy or of progressive myocardial iron accumulation during pregnancy. Such patients are admitted for early induction of labor or Cesarean section, to avoid spontaneous (i.e. unplanned) labor, and DFO is given in the days immediately preceding induction of labor.

20.4.4.3 Thrombosis Risk in TM Pregnancy

Thalassemic patients have a chronic hypercoagulable state, with an increased incidence of thromboembolic episodes (TE). In a survey of Italian thalassemic centers, 32 TE episodes were identified in a total of 735 subjects [85], but this series also included thalassemia intermedia (TI) patients. As will be seen below, thromboembolism is generally two to four times greater in TI than TM [85–87]. Sites of TE risks included the central nervous system (with a clinical picture of headache, seizures, and hemiparesis), pulmonary, mesenteric, and portal sites [85, 87]. Deep venous thrombosis, intracardiac thrombosis, and laboratory signs of disseminated intravascular coagulation (DIC) have also been observed during pregnancy in two patients [85].

The mechanisms for the increased thrombotic tendency include the presence of abnormal red cells that express phosphatidylserine on their cell surface [29] and that shed prothrombotic microvesicles [30]. A wide variety of laboratory changes are seen including increased urinary excretion of thromboxane A2 metabolites, enhanced expression of P-selectin in intact thalassemic platelets, elevated plasma levels of thrombin-antithrombin complexes, elevated levels of endothelial adhesion protein (ICAM-1, ELAM-1, VCAM-1, von Willebrand factor, and thrombomodulin) [78], and low plasma levels of the natural anticoagulants, protein C and protein S, and heparin cofactor II [88, 89].

Many TM and TI patients will have undergone splenectomy and this further increases the risk of thrombosis [87] and the number of PS-expressing red-cell-derived microparticles [30]. VTE appears more common in patients with associated organ dysfunction [85] such as diabetes, cardiopulmonary abnormalities, hypothyroidism, and liver function anomalies. These risks may be combined with the known effects of pregnancy such as increased levels of clotting factors II, VII, VIII, and X, increased fibrin formation, decreased fibrinolysis, decreased free-protein S levels, and acquired resistance to activated protein C. Many of these effects can be partially abrogated by hyper-transfusion, which will suppress endogenous red cell production, and hence thromboses are less likely in TM than TI syndromes. It is therefore not surprising that the incidence of VTE is less common in TM than in TI, occurring in to 3.95 and 9.61 % of patients, respectively [85]. Thus, unless there is a history of VTE or additional risk factors such as antiphospholipid syndrome, routine thromboprophylaxis has not generally been used in TM pregnancies. In splenectomized patients, low-dose aspirin has been suggested, as its use does not seem to be associated with risk to the central and regional circulation of the fetus [90]. The risks of VTE postpartum are increased, and it is routine practice at UCLH to recommend subcutaneous low molecular weight heparin prophylaxis postdelivery for 6 weeks.

20.4.4.4 Endocrine Issues During TM Pregnancy

The care of diabetes and hypothyroidism is along the same principles as in all women with these conditions, recognizing that endocrine disorders are more common in TM and may manifest themselves for the first time during pregnancy. Tight glycemic control requires multidisciplinary care, and additional ultrasound scans are needed to check for fetal anomalies and to monitor the fetal growth pattern. Delivery at between 38 and 39 weeks' gestation is likely to be advised, to reduce the risk of sudden intrauterine fetal death in late pregnancy with maternal diabetes. The mother should be checked in each trimester for possible retinal and renal complications of her diabetes. For those with hypothyroidism, their dose of thyroxine replacement therapy usually needs to be increased during pregnancy, because of the physiological increase in carrier proteins, but this can be easily monitored by measurements of serum TSH and free thyroxine at intervals of approximately 6–8 weeks, as appropriate for the individual patient.

20.4.4.5 Infection Risk in TM Pregnancy

In TM patients who have undergone splenectomy, there is an increased risk of bacterial infections, particularly streptococcal infections. Pneumococcal vaccination is advised, and a booster dose should be given prior to planned pregnancy if required. Splenectomized patients are commonly maintained on prophylactic penicillin V, which should be continued prior to and during pregnancy, with an ongoing awareness of the patient's susceptibility to infections. Patients with severe iron overload are also at increased risk of infection with organisms such as Klebsiella and Yersinia *enterocolitica.*

20.4.4.6 Optimal Timing and Method of Delivery

A series of 58 pregnancies showed a high prevalence of preterm births (33 %) [59]. Therefore, if the mother is being managed in a specialist thalassemia center at a significant geographical distance from her home, a planned antenatal admission for induction of labor or Cesarean section may be appropriate. If a TM mother is significantly iron overloaded, the risks of prolonged labor with attendant acidosis and the risk of liberating toxic iron pools should also be taken into account. In a series from Italy, with all the women cared for in the centers at Cagliari, Genoa, and Brindisi, 67 % of women in Turin gave birth by Cesarean section [59]. In series from Greece, all were delivered by elective Cesarean section [72, 73, 91]. The fact that most patients with transfusion-dependent thalassemia are themselves of shorter than average stature means that they often require Cesarean delivery because of cephalopelvic disproportion. However, elective Cesarean section is not a universal approach, and in the absence of the confounding influences of maternal diabetes, fetal growth restriction, or high maternal cardiac risk, pregnancy often proceeds normally, allowing plans for timing and mode of delivery to be made along relatively standard obstetric principles.

20.4.4.7 Postnatal Care and Complications in TM

Because of the increased thrombotic risks described above, it is usual practice to recommend low molecular weight heparin prophylaxis in the postpartum period and in splenectomized women to continue low-dose aspirin [59]. The longer-term risks of being without chelation therapy for 9 months have not been studied systematically, but there is some evidence of significant consequences. In one study, endocrine complications developed during the 6 months following delivery, with two women developing diabetes [35]. In the same study, two developed new significant cardiomyopathy, and five women developed secondary amenorrhea. It is therefore recommended to reinstitute chelation therapy as soon as practical postnatally. If the mother wishes to breast-feed, DFO is the chelator of choice, as it is not absorbed by the oral route. In a twin pregnancy where DFO was given to the mother postnatally, normal iron levels were observed in breast milk, and no clinical or hematological abnormalities due to DFO therapy could be shown in the breast-fed newborns [92]. At UCLH,

DFO has been given to some mothers while breast-feeding, and although low levels of DFO were found in the breast milk, no clinical or hematological abnormalities due to DFO have been observed in the babies.

20.5 Thalassemia Intermedia (TI)

20.5.1 Overview of Management Issues

Unlike TM, patients with TI do not usually receive regular transfusion therapy. The frequency of transfusion is highly variable between TI patients and also within individual patients during their lifetime, with a tendency to increasing transfusion requirements with advancing age. The lack of regular transfusion in TI has three major consequences relevant to pregnancy: firstly, iron overload will have previously advanced more slowly than in TM so that cardiomyopathy and other risks from iron overload are less common. Hypogonadotropic hypogonadism is therefore less common or occurs later than in TM. Thus, pregnancy can usually occur without the need for induction of ovulation. The second consequence is that previous exposure to red cell alloantigens is less in TI than in TM, so the formation of new red cell alloantibodies, if transfusion is given during pregnancy, is more likely. Thirdly, because a higher proportion of red cells are endogenous in TI and express PS on their cell surface, there is an increased risk of thrombin generation. VTE is two to three times more common in TI than TM. Rarer issues that have occasionally arisen in TI pregnancy include worsening extramedullary hematopoiesis [93] and spinal cord compression [94].

20.5.2 Pregnancy Outcome and Management of Anemia

Pregnancy outcome in TI has been described in 44 women, with 83 pregnancies from Lebanon and Italy [95]. Spontaneous miscarriages occurred in 21 % of pregnancies, with two intrauterine fetal deaths, at 26 weeks' and 36 weeks' gestation. In pregnancies progressing beyond 20 weeks' gestation, preterm delivery and IUGR were noted in 32 and 24 %, respectively. Transfusion was given in 80 % of women during pregnancy, with 27 % receiving transfusion for the first time. Two women developed severe alloimmune hemolytic anemia, one of whom progressed to cardiac failure at 35 weeks' gestation and was delivered by Cesarean section. Thrombotic events during pregnancy were seen in 7 % of patients.

Several patient series from Asia have described pregnancy outcomes in HbE-beta thalassemia (E-β Thal), a clinical syndrome that ranges in phenotype from TI to TM. In a series of 80 pregnancies from Thailand [96], outcomes were examined retrospectively in 80 patients with E-β Thal (29 %) or HbH (65 %). (Hemoglobin H disease is a form of alpha thalassemia, in which three of the four genes responsible for the production of the alpha-globin chains for hemoglobin are defective). In general, a less aggressive transfusion policy was given in E-β Thal than is typically recommended in Europe to TM patients in pregnancy. Overall, fetal growth restriction was seen in 27 %, with preterm births in 21 % and low birth weight (<2,500 g) in 44 %. The mean gestational age at delivery was 37 weeks (range 27–42). Thirty-three percent had delivery by Cesarean section, and the remainder had successful vaginal deliveries. Baseline hemoglobin (Hb) levels and the mean birth weight of babies born to women with E-β Thal were significantly lower than in those with HbH disease. This suggests that the lower Hb level in E-β Thal may have contributed to the less desirable obstetric outcomes. This conclusion is supported by a retrospective case control cohort study from Thailand in 54 E-β Thal women with singleton pregnancies that has relevance to transfusion policy in TI phenotypes [97]. Although maternal outcomes were similar in both groups, gestational age at birth and birth weight were significantly lower in the E-β Thal women, and the Cesarean section rate was higher (relative risk 2.1). The incidences of fetal growth restriction, preterm birth, and low birth weight were also significantly higher, with relative risks of 2.8, 2.7, and 5.6, respectively. The influence of transfusion policy on these outcomes is of potential importance. The patient population consisted mainly of people with milder forms E-β Thal, and 35 % of patients had not received blood transfusions before pregnancy. The mean Hb levels during pregnancy were significantly lower in the E-β Thal than in the control group (81 g/L vs. 128 g/L). However, most women received 1–5 transfusions during pregnancy (mean 2.4 transfusions), based on an intention to keep the patients' hemoglobin higher than 70 g/L. This transfusion policy differs from studies of TM populations in Europe where there has typically been an intention to maintain Hb >100 g/L [34]. There is some evidence that anemia <100 g/L is an independent risk factor for low birth weight and preterm delivery in non-thalassemic women [98]. However, in the clinical management of TI (or E-β Thal), the potential risk of low birth weight and preterm delivery has to be balanced against the risk of alloimmunization in otherwise infrequently transfused patients.

20.5.3 Management of Thrombotic Risk

The greater inherent risks of TI compared with TM are well recognized, with VTE being two to four times more frequent [85, 87]. Thrombotic risks in TI in descending order of frequency include DVT, PE, superficial thrombophlebitis, portal vein thrombosis, and stroke [87]. Venous thrombotic events are proportionately greater in TI compared with TM, whereas arterial events are more common in TM. Splenectomy is a clear risk factor for thrombosis in TI [87, 99], as is a high nucleated red cell count (>300 × 10^9 L), a platelet count >500 × 109/L, evidence of pulmonary hypertension (PHT), or being transfusion naïve [87, 99]. The median time to thrombosis following splenectomy is 8 years in Middle Eastern and Italian TI populations [87]. The prothrombotic mechanisms for thalassemia syndromes have been outlined above, but transfusion appears to have a protective influence. Transfused patients have lower numbers of thrombogenic red cells and microparticles [30], and transfusion also corrects deficiency of natural anticoagulants in TI [88]. The practical implication of these findings for pregnant TI patients with identifiable risk factors, such as a previous history of thrombosis, splenectomy, high platelet and nucleated red blood cell counts, or in whom laboratory investigations demonstrate thrombophilia risk, is that prophylactic measures need to be considered. Options are anticoagulation [100] and/or hypertransfusion. Anticoagulation alone may not protect against thrombosis in high-risk cases [101], and at UCLH, cases of intractable ongoing VTE in TI have been corrected by hypertransfusion, when anticoagulation therapy alone has failed, one of these cases occurring during pregnancy. Although transfusion may decrease the risk of VTE, as well as low birth weight deliveries, these potential advantages need to be balanced against the risk of alloimmunization [95, 102]. With the current level of evidence, clinical decisions about whether to institute transfusion and/or anticoagulation in TI pregnancies need to be made on a case-by-case basis.

20.6 α- and β-Thalassemia Traits

Antenatal counseling is a key part of the management of thalassemia traits. The identification of at-risk couples before pregnancy and/or early in pregnancy and the provision of appropriate expert counseling in a timely manner are critical but beyond the scope of this chapter.

Once genetic counseling is completed, the presence of β-thalassemia trait or α-thalassemia trait usually has little impact on the care of pregnancy. The effects of thalassaemia traits have been reported in a large study of over 2,000 thalassemia trait patients and healthy controls [103], in healthy women the Hb fell by about 7 % from the end of the first trimester associated with the increase in plasma volume, and the fall in haemoglobin in β-thalassemia trait was marginally greater at 10 %. In healthy women, the Hb fell from a mean of 126 g/L in the first trimester to 117 g/L in the second trimester, whereas in women with β-thalassemia trait this fell from 108 to 96 g/L [103]. This means that some women with β-thalassemia trait will develop Hb values <100 g/L during pregnancy without any other factors contributing to anemia. However, if values fall below 90 g/L, some additional cause for anemia should be considered such as concomitant iron or folate deficiency. For alpha-thalassemia traits, similar or slightly smaller decrements in Hb values during pregnancy have been reported. Interestingly, patients with alpha-thalassemia traits seem to have the same incidence of iron deficiency as the normal pregnant patients, whereas in those with β trait, it was four times less common [103]. Iron supplements do not improve the erythropoietic response unless there is coexisting iron deficiency, which is best confirmed by measurement of serum ferritin levels. With maternal thalassemia traits, no abnormality of placental function as assessed by serum estriol concentration or fetal growth was found, and no increase in maternal or fetal morbidity was documented.

20.7 Case Studies

Case Study 1

Case 1 has homozygous sickle cell disease (hemoglobin SS). She is of Jamaican origin and was aged 24 when she delivered her first child and 31 when she delivered her second child. A year before her first pregnancy, she had a total hip replacement on the right side, having become increasingly disabled because of avascular necrosis of the femoral head. This is a common chronic complication of sickle cell disease. She was in hospital with multiple severe painful episodes during her first pregnancy and spent most of the third trimester in hospital. Because of this, she was delivered by elective Cesarean section at 36 weeks and had a healthy girl, birth weight 2.931 kg. Four weeks after delivery, she had a deep vein thrombosis in her left leg. In her second pregnancy, she was given low molecular weight heparin prophylaxis from 24 weeks' gestation. She had mild bone pains throughout, but no crisis severe enough to require hospital admission. She had a normal delivery, after spontaneous onset of labor at 38 weeks, with a healthy girl, birth weight 2.928 kg. Since then, she has a progestogen-releasing intrauterine system in place for contraception and is not planning any further pregnancies.

Case Study 2

A 39-year-old woman with thalassemia major became pregnant following induction of ovulation. In her past history, she started transfusion when aged 2 years and desferrioxamine at the age of 14. She had primary amenorrhea, secondary hypothyroidism, secondary hypoparathyroidism, osteopenia, and had hepatitis C at the age of 21, but remained HCV-RNA negative. She currently had good compliance with desferrioxamine 2.5 g five times per week, a serum ferritin of 1,734 mg/L, and this had been consistently <2,500 mg/L for the previous 3 years. Immediately prior to induction of ovulation, the myocardial T2* was 19.9 ms, the LVEF was 82 %, and liver iron was 5 mg/g dw by MRI. DFO was stopped at the commencement of ovulation induction, and she became pregnant in the first cycle of therapy. At 12 weeks, the ferritin was 3,591 mg/L, LVEF 73 %, and the myocardial T2* 22 ms. She was admitted for induction of labor at 39 weeks and given low-dose DFO infusion during labor. Due to poor progression of cervical dilatation, Cesarean section was performed, and a healthy baby was born. Thromboprophylaxis with LMW heparin was given postdelivery. Because of the high ferritin and borderline myocardial T2* pre-pregnancy, subcutaneous DFO was given after delivery at standard doses. The baby was breast-fed and measurement of DFO in breast milk showed a very low concentration (0.18 mM). Four months postdelivery, the serum ferritin had fallen to 2,789 mg/L, but the myocardial T2* was now 11.8 ms. She continued subcutaneous DFO at standard doses, and at 7 months' postdelivery, the ferritin was 2,623 mg/L and the myocardial T2* had improved to 17.9 ms. Twelve months after delivery, the myocardial T2* was 31 ms and ferritin 2,124 mg/L.

Key Learning Points

- Pregnancy in women with sickle cell disease continues to show high rates of maternal and fetal mortality and morbidity.
- Outcomes can be improved by providing care in centers with specialist expertise.
- Routine prophylactic blood transfusion may not be required in pregnant women with sickle cell disease, but has a role in selected cases.
- Ad hoc transfusions may be required during pregnancy for women experiencing complications.
- Women with TM can sometimes develop rapid myocardial iron loading during pregnancy when chelation is not used.
- If the patient has a history of myocardial iron loading, close monitoring is recommended (possibly including myocardial T2* in late pregnancy).
- If the LVEF falls or myocardial T2* falls, there is a case for giving low-dose DFO in the latter weeks of pregnancy even though chelation therapy is not officially sanctioned in drug licensing.

References

1. Telfer P, Coen P, Chakravorty S, Wilkey O, Evans J, Newell H, Smalling B, Amos R, Stephens A, Rogers D, Kirkham F. Clinical outcomes in children with sickle cell disease living in England: a neonatal cohort in East London. Haematologica. 2007;92:905–12.
2. Wierenga KJ, Serjeant BE, Serjeant GR. Cerebrovascular complications and parvovirus infection in homozygous sickle cell disease. J Pediatr. 2001;139:438–42.
3. DHSS D.o.H.S.S. Report on confidential enquiries into maternal deaths in England and Wales, 1991–93. London: Her Majesty's Stationery Office; 1994.
4. DHSS D.o.H.S.S. Reports on confidential enquiries into maternal deaths in England and Wales, 1967–69, 1970–72, 1973–75, 1976–78, 1979–81. London: Her Majesty's Stationery Office; 1976, 1979, 1982.
5. Tuck SM, Studd JW, White JM. Pregnancy in sickle cell disease in the UK. Br J Obstet Gynaecol. 1983;90:112–7.
6. Lewis GE. The confidential enquiry into maternal and child health, 2000–02, 2003–05. Reports on confidential enquiries into maternal deaths in the United Kingdom. London: CEMACH; 2004, 2007.
7. Lewis GE. Confidential enquiry into maternal and child health. Saving mothers' lives: reviewing maternal deaths to make motherhood safer, 2006–08. The eighth report of the confidential enquiries into maternal deaths in the United Kingdom. London: CEMACH; 2011. www.cmace.org.uk/Publications/CEMACHPublications/Maternal-and-Perinatal-Health.aspx
8. Chase AR, Sohal M, Howard J, Laher R, McCarthy A, Layton DM, Oteng-Ntim E. Pregnancy outcomes in sickle cell disease: retrospective cohort study of two tertiary referral centres in the UK. Obstet Med. 2010;3:110–2.
9. Sohal M, Davies J, Howard J, Vogt K, McCarthy A, Layton D. Pregnancy in sickle cell disease (SCD): experience in a single tertiary centre. Br J Haematol. 2008;141:111.
10. Yu CK, Stasiowska E, Stephens A, Awogbade M, Davies A. Outcome of pregnancy in sickle cell disease patients attending a combined obstetric and haematology clinic. J Obstet Gynaecol. 2009;29:512–6.
11. Lucas SB, et al. A report of the National Confidential Enquiry into Patient Outcome and Death (NCEPOD): a sickle crisis? 2008. http://www.ncepod.org.uk/2008report1/Downloads/Sickle_report.pdf.
12. Smith J, Espeland M, Bellevue R, Bonds D, Brown A, Koshy M. Pregnancy in sickle cell disease: experience of the cooperative study of sickle cell disease. Obstet Gynecol. 1996;87:199–204.
13. Dare F, Makinde O, Faasuba O. The obstetric performance of sickle cell disease patients and homozygous haemoglobin C patients in Ile-Ife, Nigeria. Int J Gynaecol Obstet. 1992;37(3):163–8.
14. Afolabi BB, Iwuala NC, Iwuala IC, Ogedengbe OK. Morbidity and mortality in sickle cell pregnancies in Lagos, Nigeria: a case control study. J Obstet Gynaecol. 2009;29:104–6.
15. El-Shafei AM, Dhaliwal JK, Sandhu AK. Pregnancy in sickle cell disease in Bahrain. Br J Obstet Gynaecol. 1992;99:101–4.
16. Leborgne-Samuel Y, Janky E, Venditelli F, Salin J, Daijardin JB, Couchy B, Etienne-Julan M, Berchel C. Sickle cell anemia and pregnancy: review of 68 cases in Guadeloupe. J Gynecol Obstet Biol Reprod (Paris). 2000;29:86–93.
17. Rahimy MC, Gangbo A, Adjou R, Deguenon C, Goussanou S, Alihonou E. Effect of active prenatal management on pregnancy outcome in sickle cell disease in an African setting. Blood. 2000;96:1685–9.
18. Villers MS, Jamison MG, De Castro LM, James AH. Morbidity associated with sickle cell disease in pregnancy. Am J Obstet Gynecol. 2008;199(125):e121–5.

19. Al Jama FE, Gasem T, Burshaid S, Rahman J, Al Suleiman SA, Rahman MS. Pregnancy outcome in patients with homozygous sickle cell disease in a university hospital, Eastern Saudi Arabia. Arch Gynecol Obstet. 2009;280:793–7.
20. Rajab KE, Issa AA, Mohammed AM, Ajami AA. Sickle cell disease and pregnancy in Bahrain. Int J Gynaecol Obstet. 2006;93:171–5.
21. Serjeant GR, Loy LL, Crowther M, Hambleton IR, Thame M. Outcome of pregnancy in homozygous sickle cell disease. Obstet Gynecol. 2004;103:1278–85.
22. Serjeant GR, Hambleton I, Thame M. Fecundity and pregnancy outcome in a cohort with sickle cell-haemoglobin C disease followed from birth. BJOG. 2005;112:1308–14.
23. Tuck SM, Studd J. Sickle haemoglobin and pregnancy. Br Med J (Clin Res Ed). 1983;287:1143–4.
24. Howard RJ, Lillis C, Tuck SM. Contraceptives, counselling, and pregnancy in women with sickle cell disease. BMJ. 1993;306:1735–7.
25. Chakravarty EF, Khanna D, Chung L. Pregnancy outcomes in systemic sclerosis, primary pulmonary hypertension, and sickle cell disease. Obstet Gynecol. 2008;111:927–34.
26. Howard RJ, Tuck S, Pearson T. Pregnancy in sickle cell disease in the UK: results of a multicentre survey of the effect of prophylactic blood transfusion on maternal and fetal outcome. Br J Obstet Gynaecol. 1995;102:947–51.
27. Powars DR, Sandhu M, Niland-Weiss J, Johnson C, Bruce S, Manning PR. Pregnancy in sickle cell disease. Obstet Gynecol. 1986;67:217–28.
28. Al-Suleiman S, Rahman M, Rahman J, Al-Najashi S. Sickle cell disease and pregnancy in Saudi Arabia. J Obstet Gynaecol. 1991;11:331–5.
29. Cappellini MD. Coagulation in the pathophysiology of hemolytic anemias. Hematology Am Soc Hematol Educ Program. 2007;2007:74–8.
30. Westerman M, Pizzey A, Hirschman J, Cerino M, Weil-Weiner Y, Ramotar P, Eze A, Lawrie A, Purdy G, Mackie I, Porter J. Microvesicles in haemoglobinopathies offer insights into mechanisms of hypercoagulability, haemolysis and the effects of therapy. Br J Haematol. 2008;142:126–35.
31. Heit JA, Beckman MG, Bockenstedt PL, Grant AM, Key NS, Kulkarni R, Manco-Johnson MJ, Moll S, Ortel TL, Philipp CS. Comparison of characteristics from White- and Black-Americans with venous thromboembolism: a cross-sectional study. Am J Hematol. 2010;85:467–71.
32. UK-Standards. Standards for the clinical care of adults with sickle cell disease in the UK. Sickle Cell Society publication. 2008. www.sicklecellsociety.
33. Curry SC, Bond GR, Raschke R, Tellez D, Wiggins D. An ovine model of maternal iron poisoning in pregnancy. Ann Emerg Med. 1990;19:632–8.
34. Jensen CE, Tuck SM, Wonke B. Fertility in ß thalassaemia major: a report of 16 pregnancies, preconceptual evaluation and a review of the literature. Br J Obstet Gynaecol. 1995;102:625–9.
35. Tuck SM, Jensen CE, Wonke B, Yardumian A. Pregnancy management and outcomes in women with thalassaemia major. J Pediatr Endocrinol Metab. 1998;11 Suppl 3:923–8.
36. Thomas VJ, Rawle H, Howard J, Abedian M, Westerdale N, Oteng-Ntim E, Musumadi L. Psychological help for pregnant women with sickle cell disease. Prim Health Care. 2009;19: 26–9.
37. Royal College of Obstetricians and Gynaecologists. Thrombosis and embolism during pregnancy and the puerperium, Reducing the risk (Green-top guideline no. 37). 2009. https://www.rcog.org.uk/guidelines.
38. Mahomed K. Prophylactic versus selective blood transfusion in sickle cell disease pregnancies. Cochrane Database Syst Rev. 2000 and 2006;(2):CD000040, and update in (3):CD000040.
39. Koshy M, Burd L, Wallace D, Moawad A, Baron J. Prophylactic red-cell transfusions in pregnant patients with sickle cell disease. A randomized cooperative study. N Engl J Med. 1988;319:1447–52.
40. Ngo C, Kayem G, Habibi A, Benachi A, Goffinet F, Galacteros F, Haddad B. Pregnancy in sickle cell disease: maternal and fetal outcomes in a population receiving prophylactic partial exchange transfusions. Eur J Obstet Gynecol Reprod Biol. 2010;152:138–42.
41. Tuck SM, James CE, Brewster EM. Prophylactic blood transfusion in maternal sickle cell syndromes. Br J Obstet Gynaecol. 1987;94:121–5.
42. Walter PB, Harmatz P, Vichinsky E. Iron metabolism and iron chelation in sickle cell disease. Acta Haematol. 2009;122:174–83.
43. Vichinsky EP. Current issues with blood transfusions in sickle cell disease. Semin Hematol. 2001;38:14–22.
44. Manchikanti A, Grimes DA, Lopez LM, Schulz KF. Steroid hormones for contraception in women with sickle cell disease. Cochrane Database Syst Rev. 2007;(2):CD006261.
45. De Ceulaer K, Gruber C, Hayes R, Serjeant GR. Medroxyprogesterone acetate and homozygous sickle-cell disease. Lancet. 1982;2:229–31.
46. de Abood M, de Castillo Z, Guerrero F, Espino M, Austin KL. Effect of Depo-Provera or microgynon on the painful crises of sickle cell anemia patients. Contraception. 1997;56:313–6.
47. Blank AM, Freedman WL. Sickle cell trait and pregnancy. Clin Obstet Gynecol. 1969;12(1):123–33.
48. Austin H, Key NS, Benson JM, Lally C, Dowling NF, Whitsett C, Hooper WC. Sickle cell trait and the risk of venous thromboembolism among blacks. Blood. 2007;110:908–12.
49. Austin H, Lally C, Benson JM, Whitsett C, Hooper WC, Key NS. Hormonal contraception, sickle cell trait, and risk for venous thromboembolism among African American women. Am J Obstet Gynecol. 2009;200(620):e621–3.
50. Thomas RM, Skalicka AE. Successful pregnancy in transfusion-dependent thalassaemia. Arch Dis Child. 1980;55:572–4.

51. Kumar RM, Rizk DE, Khuranna A. ß-thalassemia major and successful pregnancy. J Reprod Med. 1997;42:294–8.
52. Martin K. Successful pregnancy in ß-thalassaemia major. Aust Paediatr J. 1983;19:182–3.
53. Meadows K. A successful pregnancy outcome in transfusion dependent thalassaemia major. Aust N Z J Obstet Gynaecol. 1984;24:43–4.
54. Tampakoudis P, Tsatalas C, Mamopoulos M, Tantanassis T, Christakis JI, Sinakos Z, Mantalenakis S. Transfusion-dependent homozygous ß-thalassaemia major: successful pregnancy in five cases. Eur J Obstet Gynecol Reprod Biol. 1997;74:127–31.
55. Mordel N, Birkenfeld A, Goldfarb AN, Rachmilewitz EA. Successful full-term pregnancy in homozygous ß-thalassemia major: case report and review of the literature. Obstet Gynecol. 1989;73:837–40.
56. Seracchioli R, Porcu E, Colombi C, Ciotti P, Fabbri R, De Sanctis V, Flamigni C. Transfusion-dependent homozygous ß-thalassaemia major: successful twin pregnancy following in-vitro fertilization and tubal embryo transfer. Hum Reprod. 1994;9: 1964–5.
57. Bajoria R, Chatterjee R. Current perspectives of fertility and pregnancy in thalassemia. Hemoglobin. 2009;33 Suppl 1:S131–5.
58. Farmaki K, Gotsis E, Tzoumari I, Berdoukas V. Rapid iron loading in a pregnant woman with transfusion-dependent thalassemia after brief cessation of iron chelation therapy. Eur J Haematol. 2008; 81:157–9.
59. Origa R, Piga A, Quarta G, Forni GL, Longo F, Melpignano A, Galanello R. Pregnancy and ß-thalassemia: an Italian multicenter experience. Haematologica. 2010;95:376–81.
60. Chatterjee R, Katz M, Cox TF, Porter JB. Prospective study of the hypothalamic-pituitary axis in thalassaemic patients who developed secondary amenorrhoea. Clin Endocrinol (Oxf). 1993;39:287–96.
61. Skordis N, Petrikkos L, Toumba M, Hadjigavriel M, Sitarou M, Kolnakou A, Skordos G, Pangalou E, Christou S. Update on fertility in thalassaemia major. Pediatr Endocrinol Rev. 2004;2 Suppl 2:296–302.
62. Jensen CE, Tuck SM, Old J, Morris RW, Yardumian A, De Sanctis V, Hoffbrand AV, Wonke B. Incidence of endocrine complications and clinical disease severity related to genotype analysis and iron overload in patients with ß- thalassaemia. Eur J Haematol. 1997;59:76–81.
63. Borgna-Pignatti C, Rugolotto S, De Stefano P, Piga A, Di Gregorio F, Gamberini MR, Sabato V, Melevendi C, Cappellini MD, Verlato G. Survival and disease complications in thalassemia major. Ann N Y Acad Sci. 1998;850:227–31.
64. Borgna-Pignatti C, Rugolotto S, De Stefano P, Zhao H, Cappellini MD, Del Vecchio GC, Romeo MA, Forni GL, Gamberini MR, Ghilardi R, Piga A, Cnaan A. Survival and complications in patients with thalassemia major treated with transfusion and deferoxamine. Haematologica. 2004;89:1187–93.
65. Chatterjee R, Wonke B, Porter JB, Katz M. Correction of primary and secondary amenorrhoea and induction of ovulation by pulsatile infusion of gonadotrophin releasing hormone (GnRH) in patients with ß thalassaemia major. In: Beuzard Y, Lubin B, Rosa J, editors. Sickle cell disease and thalassaemia: new trends in therapy, Colloquium Inserm, vol. 234. 1995. p. 451–5.
66. El-Toukhy T, Bickerstaff H, Meller S. Preimplantation genetic diagnosis for haematologic conditions. Curr Opin Pediatr. 2010;22:28–34.
67. De Sanctis V, Vullo C, Katz M, Wonke B, Hoffbrand VA, Di Palma A, Bagni B. Endocrine complications in thalassaemia major. Prog Clin Biol Res. 1989;309:77–83.
68. Singh N, Deka D, Dadhwal V, Gupta N, Mittal S. Optimizing antenatal care and delivery in thalassemic mothers: single center experience. Arch Gynecol Obstet. 2008;278:101–2.
69. Tsironi M, Karagiorga M, Aessopos A. Iron overload, cardiac and other factors affecting pregnancy in thalassemia major. Hemoglobin. 2010;34:240–50.
70. Tsironi M, Ladis V, Margellis Z, Deftereos S, Kattamis C, Aessopos A. Impairment of cardiac function in a successful full-term pregnancy in a homozygous ß-thalassemia major: does chelation have a positive role? Eur J Obstet Gynecol Reprod Biol. 2005;120:117–8.
71. Casanueva E, Jimenez J, Meza-Camacho C, Mares M, Simon L. Prevalence of nutritional deficiencies in Mexican adolescent women with early and late prenatal care. Arch Latinoam Nutr. 2003;53:35–8.
72. Daskalakis GJ, Papageorgiou IS, Antsaklis AJ, Michalas SK. Pregnancy and homozygous ß thalassaemia major. Br J Obstet Gynaecol. 1998;105: 1028–32.
73. Karagiorga-Lagana M. Fertility in thalassemia: the Greek experience. J Pediatr Endocrinol Metab. 1998;11 Suppl 3:945–51.
74. Perniola R, Magliari F, Rosatelli MC, De Marzi CA. High-risk pregnancy in ß-thalassemia major women. Report of three cases. Gynecol Obstet Invest. 2000;49:137–9.
75. Berdoukas V, Bentley P, Frost H, SchnEßli HP. Toxicity of oral iron chelator L1. Lancet. 1993;341:1088.
76. Porter JB, Rafique R, Srichairatanakool S, Davis BA, Shah FT, Hair T, Evans P. Recent insights into interactions of deferoxamine with cellular and plasma iron pools: implications for clinical use. Ann N Y Acad Sci. 2005;1054:155–68.
77. Blanc P, Hryhorczuk D, Danel I. Deferoxamine treatment of acute iron intoxication in pregnancy. Obstet Gynecol. 1984;64:12S–4.
78. Bosque MA, Domingo JL, Corbella J. Assessment of the developmental toxicity of deferoxamine in mice. Arch Toxicol. 1995;69:467–71.
79. Khoury S, Odeh M, Oettinger M. Deferoxamine treatment for acute iron intoxication in pregnancy. Acta Obstet Gynecol Scand. 1995;74:756–7.

80. McElhatton PR, Roberts JC, Sullivan FM. The consequences of iron overdose and its treatment with desferrioxamine in pregnancy. Hum Exp Toxicol. 1991;10:251–9.
81. Rayburn WF, Donn SM, Wulf ME. Iron overdose during pregnancy: successful therapy with deferoxamine. Am J Obstet Gynecol. 1983;147:717–8.
82. Singer ST, Vichinsky EP. Deferoxamine treatment during pregnancy: is it harmful? Am J Hematol. 1999;60:24–6.
83. Turk J, Aks S, Ampuero F, Hryhorczuk DO. Successful therapy of iron intoxication in pregnancy with intravenous deferoxamine and whole bowel irrigation. Vet Hum Toxicol. 1993;35:441–4.
84. Vaskaridou E, Konstantopoulos K, Kyriakou D, Loukopoulos D. Deferoxamine treatment during early pregnancy: absence of teratogenicity in two cases. Haematologica. 1993;78:183–4.
85. Borgna-Pignatti C, Carnelli V, Caruso V, Dore F, De Mattia D, Di Palma A, Di Gregorio F, Romeo MA, Longhi R, Mangiagli A, Melevendi C, Pizzarelli G, Musumeci S. Thromboembolic events in ß thalassemia major: an Italian multicenter study. Acta Haematol. 1998;99:76–9.
86. Moratelli S, De Sanctis V, Gemmati D, Serino ML, Mari R, Gamberini MR, Scapoli GL. Thrombotic risk in thalassemic patients. J Pediatr Endocrinol Metab. 1998;11:915–21.
87. Taher A, Isma'eel H, Mehio G, Bignamini D, Kattamis A, Rachmilewitz EA, Cappellini MD. Prevalence of thromboembolic events among 8,860 patients with thalassaemia major and intermedia in the Mediterranean area and Iran. Thromb Haemost. 2006;96:488–91.
88. O'Driscoll A, Mackie IJ, Porter JB, Machin SJ. Low plasma heparin cofactor II levels in thalassaemia syndromes are corrected by chronic blood transfusion. Br J Haematol. 1995;90:65–70.
89. Porter JB, Young L, Mackie IJ, Marshall L, Machin SJ. Sickle cell disorders and chronic intravascular haemolysis are associated with low plasma heparin cofactor II. Br J Haematol. 1993;83:459–65.
90. Veille JC, Hanson R, Sivakoff M, Swain M, Henderson L. Effects of maternal ingestion of low-dose aspirin on the fetal cardiovascular system. Am J Obstet Gynecol. 1993;168:1430–7.
91. Aessopos A, Karabatsos F, Farmakis D, Katsantoni A, Hatziliami A, Youssef J, Karagiorga M. Pregnancy in patients with well-treated ß-thalassemia: outcome for mothers and newborn infants. Am J Obstet Gynecol. 1999;180:360–5.
92. Surbek DV, Glanzmann R, Holzgreve W. Pregnancy and homozygous ß thalassemia major. Br J Obstet Gynaecol. 1999;106:87.
93. Konstantopoulos K, Plataniotis G, Maris T, Voskaridou E, Rekoumi L, Stratigaki M, Loukopoulos D. Extramedullary haemopoiesis in thalassaemia intermedia: an unusual case of relapsing paraparesis in pregnancy. Haematologia (Budap). 1995;27:29–32.
94. Esfandbod M, Malekpour M. Thalassemia and spinal cord compression in pregnancy. CMAJ. 2010;182:E798.
95. Nassar AH, Naja M, Cesaretti C, Eprassi B, Cappellini MD, Taher A. Pregnancy outcome in patients with ß-thalassemia intermedia at two tertiary care centers, in Beirut and Milan. Haematologica. 2008;93:1586–7.
96. Traisrisilp K, Luewan S, Tongsong T. Pregnancy outcomes in women complicated by thalassemia syndrome at Maharaj Nakorn Chiang Mai Hospital. Arch Gynecol Obstet. 2009;279:685–9.
97. Luewan S, Srisupundit K, Tongsong T. Outcomes of pregnancies complicated by ß-thalassemia/hemoglobin E disease. Int J Gynaecol Obstet. 2009;104:203–5.
98. Levy A, Fraser D, Katz M, Mazor M, Sheiner E. Maternal anemia during pregnancy is an independent risk factor for low birthweight and preterm delivery. Eur J Obstet Gynecol Reprod Biol. 2005;122:182–6.
99. Taher AT, Otrock ZK, Uthman I, Cappellini MD. Thalassemia and hypercoagulability. Blood Rev. 2008;22:283–92.
100. Nassar AH, Usta IM, Taher AM. ß-thalassemia intermedia and pregnancy: should we anticoagulate? J Thromb Haemost. 2006;4:1413–4.
101. Androutsopoulos G, Karakantza M, Decavalas G. Thalassemia intermedia, inherited thrombophilia, and intrauterine growth restriction. Int J Gynaecol Obstet. 2007;99:146.
102. Borgna-Pignatti C. Modern treatment of thalassaemia intermedia. Br J Haematol. 2007;138:291–304.
103. White JM, Richards R, Byrne M, Buchanan T, White YS, Jelenski G. Thalassaemia trait and pregnancy. J Clin Pathol. 1985;38:810–7.

Peri-delivery Analgesia and Anesthesia in Women with Hemostatic or Thrombotic Disorders

21

A. Lola Emanuel-Kole and Rory Bell

Abstract

It is well recognised that labor is painful. Analgesia is therefore required by the vast majority of parturients during labor and delivery. Central neuraxial blockade is the most effective form of analgesia in labor and also the most desirable type of anesthesia for peripartum operative interventions. Inadequate hemostasis is a contraindication to central neuraxial blockade. This chapter will discuss all forms of analgesia available to the laboring woman with a hemostatic or thrombotic disorder, and the implications of abnormalities of hemostasis, with particular emphasis on central neuraxial blockade.

Keywords

Labor analgesia • Central neuraxial blockade • Spinal hematoma • Anesthesia • Delivery

21.1 Introduction

When compared with other causes of pain using the McGill Pain Questionnaire, the pain of labor scores high and is exceeded only by that of amputation of a digit or causalgia [1]. A survey of over 10,000 parturients by the National Birthday Trust in the United Kingdom (UK) found that 93 % experienced severe or unbearable pain at some point during their labor [2]. Analgesia is therefore required by the vast majority of parturients during labor and delivery, with only 6 % requiring no pain relief in a survey of all units in the UK [3]. Central neuraxial blockade is the most effective form of analgesia in labor and also the most desirable type of anesthesia for peripartum operative interventions.

Central neuraxial blockade in the obstetric population provides several advantages over systemic analgesia or general anesthesia. These benefits include improved pain relief and patient satisfaction [4, 5] as well as significant reductions in maternal morbidity and mortality, and better fetal safety [6–8]. The 2000–2002 Confidential

A.L. Emanuel-Kole, MBBS, FRCA (✉)
Department of Anaesthesia,
The Royal Free Hospital NHS Foundation Trust,
Pond Street, London NW3 2QG, UK
e-mail: l_eman@yahoo.com

R. Bell, MBBS, FRCA
Department of Anaesthesia, University College
London Hospitals NHS Foundation Trust,
235 Euston Road, London NW1 2BU, UK
e-mail: rorybell@aol.com

H. Cohen, P. O'Brien (eds.), *Disorders of Thrombosis and Hemostasis in Pregnancy: A Guide to Management*, DOI 10.1007/978-3-319-15120-5_21, © Springer-Verlag London 2015

Enquiry into Maternal and Child Health in the UK showed that all 6 deaths attributed directly to anesthesia were associated with the use of general anesthesia [9], as were 4 of 7 deaths in the most recent (2006–2008) Confidential Enquiry [10]. The development of a spinal hematoma following neuraxial blockade is a source of major concern to the anesthetist. This serious complication can result in compression of neural tissue requiring urgent surgical decompression and carries a high risk of permanent neurological injury.

The incidence of spinal or epidural hematoma in the general surgical population remains low with rates up to 4.2:100,000 [11–14] and up to 2:100,000 in the general obstetric population [15, 16]. An analysis of the information from the American Society of Anesthesiologists Closed Claims Project [17] demonstrated more claims for neuraxial injuries due to hematoma in the non-obstetric group (non-obstetric, 33 claims; obstetric, 3 claims). The incidence among patients or parturients with bleeding disorders is more difficult to determine due to the lack of and nature of the published literature. Since these patients represent such a small proportion of the general population, many source articles included in review papers are limited to case reports and case series with relatively few patients. Consideration must also be given to the fact that there is publication bias towards reporting favorable outcomes, which may hide the true frequency of bleeding outcomes. In order to determine the true incidence of epidural or spinal hematoma and to support or refute the safety of neuraxial blocks in patients with bleeding disorders, much larger patient numbers are required.

The management of anesthesia and analgesia in parturients with hemostatic and thrombotic disorders is discussed below. More detailed description of the conditions considered can be found in their relevant chapters.

21.2 Labor Analgesia

Several strategies are available to provide analgesia during labor, including both pharmacological and non-pharmacological techniques.

21.2.1 Non-pharmacological Techniques

There is a wide range of comfort measures and relaxation techniques that can be offered to the woman in labor. These include close emotional and physical support by a trained person during labor and delivery, relaxation and breathing techniques, adopting positions of comfort, massage, hydrotherapy and thermal therapy. Complementary therapies such as aromatherapy, homeopathy, acupuncture and hypnosis may also be of benefit.

Transcutaneous Electrical Nerve Stimulation (TENS) is a safe, non-invasive, technique where two pairs of electrodes are placed either side of the spinous processes around the levels of T10/L1 and S2/S4 in the lower back. Electrical impulses are generated by a battery-powered device and transmitted via the electrodes. The physiological mechanisms by which pain is relieved by TENS remain uncertain; however, it is thought that pain transmission to the brain is blocked through stimulation of inhibitory ascending pathways. It may also induce release of endogenous endorphins, although this has been disputed. TENS has minimal side-effects and may be appropriate in women who have contraindications to other modes of analgesia. Hemostatic disorders are not a contraindication to TENS; however, TENS is not recommended in those with a cardiac pacemaker or epilepsy. A systematic review evaluating 19 studies including over 1,600 patients showed limited evidence that TENS reduced pain in labor [18] although the majority of women using TENS indicated their willingness to use TENS again in a future labor.

21.2.2 Pharmacological Techniques: Systemic Analgesia

Systemic analgesia can be administered via oral (PO), inhalational, intramuscular (IM) or intravenous (IV) routes. The only implication of abnormal hemostasis in this category is the necessity to avoid intramuscular injections in parturients with a significant bleeding tendency.

21.2.2.1 Paracetamol

Paracetamol PO may be offered to the woman in the very early stages of labor but does not generally provide effective analgesia for labor pain.

21.2.2.2 Entonox (*50 % Nitrous Oxide, 50 % Oxygen*)

This is the most common method of labor analgesia in the United Kingdom (UK) where it is available in 99 % of consultant units [2]. It is inexpensive, easy to deliver via self-administration by the patient and can be used throughout labor. It provides rapid reliable analgesia for labor and may be superior to intramuscular meperidine [19]. Analgesia is provided within 20–30 s of commencement of inhalation, with maximum therapeutic effect occurring after 45–50 s, and its effects are non-cumulative. Entonox does not appear to have any effect on the fetus. Inhalation is encouraged from the start of a uterine contraction until the end. Disadvantages include incomplete analgesia, nausea, vomiting, dizziness, drowsiness, poor recall of labor and loss of consciousness from prolonged inhalation. Entonox is not widely available in many countries including North America due to concerns about long-term environmental exposure of healthcare workers to nitrous oxide.

21.2.2.3 Halogenated Agents

Several volatile halogenated inhalational agents in low concentrations including enflurane, halothane, isoflurane and most recently sevoflurane have been compared with entonox for analgesia during labor. Studies have reported more favourable outcomes in terms of maternal satisfaction and improved pain relief in the volatile agent groups. Unfortunately, the use of these agents has been limited by incomplete analgesia, sedation and technical difficulties in providing safe administration such as the need for specialised vapourisers, adequate monitoring and scavenging to prevent environmental pollution [20].

21.2.2.4 Opioids

Some of the more commonly used opioids include meperidine (pethidine), morphine, diamorphine, fentanyl and remifentanil. The effect of opioids on labor pain has been described as modest at best; however, the sedative effects may benefit some women. A recent overview of systematic reviews found insufficient evidence of effective labor analgesia with opioids [21].

Maternal side-effects of opioid analgesia include nausea, vomiting, sedation, dysphoria, pruritis, amnesia in high doses and respiratory depression. The administration of parenteral opioids is associated with delayed gastric emptying which may lead to an increased risk of regurgitation and aspiration during general anesthesia. Caution should therefore be exercised when administering systemic opioids to women at high risk of Cesarean delivery. All opioids readily cross the placenta and adverse effects on the neonate include depressed respiratory function and neurobehavioural activity. Close monitoring of the neonate is therefore essential, and ready access to supplementary oxygen and naloxone is mandatory. With the exception of meperidine (see below), there is no clear evidence to support the use of one opioid over another in terms of analgesic and side-effect profile [22].

21.2.2.5 Meperidine (Pethidine)

This drug is a synthetic phenylpiperidine derivative that may be administered IV but is more commonly given IM at a dose of 1 mg/kg. While its duration of effect is 2–3 h, it has a maternal half-life ($t^{1/2}$) of 8 h and a neonatal $t^{1/2}$ of 22 h. When compared to other opioids such as morphine, fentanyl and remifentanil, it is associated with increased maternal nausea and higher pain scores [23–25] in addition to the side-effects mentioned above. Other effects on the neonate include depressed Apgar scores and impaired breastfeeding for up to 5 days postnatally. Normeperidine is the active metabolite and has a maternal $t^{1/2}$ of 22 h and neonatal $t^{1/2}$ of 62 h. It is a neurotoxin with convulsant effects that can be exacerbated by naloxone and it can also lower the seizure threshold in the neonate. Despite these disadvantages, meperidine continues to be offered as an option for analgesia in labor.

21.2.2.6 Morphine

This is a derivative of the opium poppy with a duration of effect of 3–4 h. It has a $t^{1/2}$ of 1 and 6 h in the mother and neonate, respectively. It has fewer maternal and neonatal side-effects when compared to meperidine. However, it is more sedating and has a longer half-life than fentanyl. It can be administered IV or, more commonly, IM at a dose of 10–20 mg.

21.2.2.7 Diamorphine

This is an opium derivative similar to morphine but more potent and with a more rapid onset. It is usually given by IM injection at a dose of 5–7.5 mg but may be administered IV with caution. One study suggested improved analgesia when compared to meperidine although this was underpowered [26]. Diamorphine is used in 34 % of UK units and is now the second most common opioid used for labor analgesia after meperidine [27].

21.2.2.8 Fentanyl

This is a highly potent phenylpiperidine derivative with a rapid onset of action (3–5 min, peak effect 5–20 min), a short duration of action (<1 h) due to its rapid re-distribution and no active metabolites. It produces less sedation, nausea and vomiting than morphine and meperidine. It is administered IV more commonly as patient controlled analgesia (PCA) with a suggested regimen of 20 μg bolus and a 5-min lockout. Repeated drug dosing can, however, result in drug accumulation in the mother due to its long elimination half-life, and ion trapping in the fetus. As with morphine it can depress maternal and neonatal respiration. Studies have shown increased use of naloxone when IV fentanyl has been used [28], with approximately 20 % of neonates requiring the opioid antagonist [29]. For these reasons, fentanyl is not commonly used in labor.

21.2.2.9 Remifentanil

This is an ultra-short acting opioid that is rapidly metabolised by non-specific blood and tissue esterases, and it does not accumulate even after prolonged infusion. It has a rapid onset (peak effect 60–90 s) and a short $t^{1/2}$ (3 min). Because of its pharmacokinetic profile, remifentanil delivered via IV PCA can be seen as an attractive alternative for analgesia during labor, particularly when neuraxial blockade is contraindicated or unavailable. There are, however, several cautionary issues with regard to remifentanil. Studies have shown that it provides better pain relief than meperidine and nitrous oxide but it remains inferior to neuraxial blockade [30]. The ideal dosing regimen remains unclear (0.25–0.5 μg/kg bolus doses has been suggested). Timing the peak effect of the drug to coincide with the peak of painful contractions has proved problematic for some women. Remifentanil can cause rapid maternal respiratory depression with oxygen desaturation and sedation, making continuous oxygen saturation monitoring and one-to-one midwifery care mandatory. This cannot be achieved in most obstetric units. Its potent effects on the fetus include bradycardia and loss of fetal heart rate variability, which have resulted in emergency Cesarean delivery. One unit has reported the successful introduction of a midwife based remifentanil PCA service which has significantly reduced the epidural rate [31]. In summary, remifentanil PCA probably represents the most effective labor analgesia available to those parturients in whom central neuraxial blockade is contraindicated.

21.2.3 Neuraxial Blockade

Neuraxial blockade includes epidural, spinal and combined spinal epidural (CSE) techniques for labor analgesia. It is used by approximately 30 % of parturients in the UK [32], the majority of whom receive epidural analgesia.

Epidural analgesia is considered the gold standard for effective pain relief in labor. Meta-analysis indicated better pain relief in those receiving epidural labour analgesia but an increased risk of hypotension, motor block and urinary catheterisation. Epidural analgesia was also associated with an increase in assisted vaginal birth and an increased duration of the first and second stages of labor by 40–60 and 14–23 min, respectively. There was no significant difference in Cesarean section rate, maternal satisfaction with pain relief, long-term backache or Apgar scores between those who had epidurals compared with those who did not [28, 33].

Indications for this method of pain relief include maternal request, prolonged or difficult labor, pregnancy induced hypertension and a high risk of Cesarean birth (e.g. obesity). Absolute contraindications include patient objection, local sepsis, allergy to the drugs used, lack of trained staff or resuscitation equipment, and of course coagulopathy. Relative contraindications include some forms of anti-coagulant therapy, a history of active neurological disease, spinal deformity, ongoing hemorrhage and systemic sepsis.

Neuraxial blockade for labor analgesia is commonly sited using a lumbar epidural technique, and placed in one of the interspaces between the L1 and L5. Analgesia is achieved using a "low-dose" mixture of local anesthetic, typically bupivacaine 0.0625–1 %, and an opioid, for example fentanyl 2 μg/mL. Low-dose mixtures were designed to provide sensory blockade while maintaining motor function, thus allowing the parturient to be mobile. The CSE technique, similar to lumbar epidural analgesia, may also be used to provide labor analgesia. The difference is that low-dose local anesthetic combined with a short acting lipid-soluble opioid is first injected into the intrathecal space via a spinal needle passed through the epidural needle. This provides a more rapid onset of pain relief, usually in 5–10 min, and analgesia can be extended using the epidural catheter. This method may be used in advanced or difficult labor when there is significant maternal distress such that rapid pain relief is required. Techniques to maintain epidural analgesia include intermittent top-ups, continuous epidural infusion (CEI) and patient-controlled epidural analgesia (PCEA) with or without a background infusion. Each technique has its advantages and disadvantages that are beyond the scope of this chapter.

21.3 Anesthesia for Delivery

Anesthesia may be required for Cesarean section or for other obstetric peri-delivery indications such as the delivery of retained placenta, trial of instrumental delivery or repair of perineal tears. Anesthesia may be provided by neuraxial blockade or general anesthesia. The decision as to which technique to adopt is dependent on maternal factors (medical conditions, obesity, anticipated airway problems, maternal preference), obstetric urgency and the skills of the anesthetist.

21.3.1 Neuraxial Blockade for Anesthesia

The benefits of neuraxial blockade over general anesthesia have made this the preferred technique for the provision of anesthesia for Cesarean section. Advantages in addition to those mentioned in the introduction include:

- The avoidance of the potentially hazardous complications associated with general anesthesia such as the inability to ventilate, intubate and aspiration pneumonitis
- The avoidance of potential awareness during general anesthesia
- Less neonatal exposure to potentially depressant drugs
- The participation of the both the mother and father in the birth
- A reduction in blood loss
- A reduction in venous thromboembolism
- The option of using epidural or spinal opioids for postoperative analgesia.
- The disadvantages include:
- Time to establish the neuraxial block, particularly when the condition of the mother or fetus is critical
- Hypotension due to vasodilation secondary to the sympathetic block, especially in the presence of aortocaval compression
- Nausea and vomiting during surgery as a result of hypotension
- When used for instrumental vaginal delivery, interference with the mother's ability to push effectively
- Pain during surgery due to inadequate or receding block

The options for neuraxial anesthesia are single shot spinal (SSS), combined spinal epidural (CSE), and epidural techniques. Continuous spinal anesthesia provides a further option following unintentional dural puncture during placement of an epidural catheter. Anesthesia is achieved using a combination of local anesthetic and opioid. Local anesthetic agents commonly in use include bupivacaine 0.5 %, levobupivacaine 0.5 %, lignocaine 2 % and ropivacaine 0.5–0.75 %. Opioids commonly used are fentanyl, diamorphine and morphine.

The spinal technique is the easiest to perform, has a more rapid and predictable onset, may produce a more dense block than an epidural and lacks the potential for serious systemic drug toxicity. It can be used to provide anesthesia in both elective and emergency situations. Its disadvantages are hypotension, a high or total spinal block and an inability to prolong anesthesia in the event of intra-operative pain or an extended procedure.

Anesthesia using an epidural technique may be preferred as the catheter facilitates achieving an adequate block, allows for supplementation if required for prolonged surgery and provides a good option for post-operative analgesia. In addition, it allows for a graduated onset of neuraxial block and more gradual decrease in blood pressure compared with the spinal technique. Anesthesia may be achieved with an epidural catheter placed at the time of the procedure or, more commonly, an effective epidural already in use for labor analgesia may be topped-up with stronger doses of local anesthetic. Compared with the spinal technique, larger doses of local anesthetic are required to achieve a block to an adequate sensory level (15–20 ml in the epidural space versus 2–2.5 ml intrathecally). Safe administration of epidural anesthesia with local anesthetic drugs is therefore critical in order to prevent the hazardous and potentially fatal complications of unintended intravascular or intrathecal injection. Combined Spinal Epidural is our preferred technique for elective Cesarean section as it combines the benefit of rapid, reliable intense blockade of spinal anesthesia with the flexibility and advantages of an epidural catheter. This is commonly performed by passing a spinal needle through an epidural needle to pierce the dura prior to inserting the epidural catheter.

21.3.2 General Anesthesia

General anesthesia is usually performed only in the emergency setting or when regional anaesthesia is contraindicated. This is because of the increased morbidity and mortality associated with general anesthesia in the obstetric population. Deaths attributed to general anesthesia are related to airway problems such as failure to intubate and ventilate the patient, and to aspiration pneumonitis. The incidence of failed endotracheal intubation in the obstetric population is approximately 1:300 vs. 1:2,000 in the general population. The incidence of pulmonary aspiration of gastric contents is 1:400–500 in the obstetric population versus 1:2,000 for all patients. Despite these potential hazards, general anesthesia:

- offers very rapid and reliable onset
- allows control over the airway and ventilation
- potentially causes less hypotension than regional anesthesia
- facilitates management in the event of severe hemorrhagic complications.

21.4 Disorders of Haemostasis

21.4.1 Platelet Disorders

21.4.1.1 Gestational Thrombocytopenia

The incidence of gestational thrombocytopenia (GT) is approximately 8 % of all pregnancies [34] and it is essentially a diagnosis of exclusion. The features are a usually mild thrombocytopenia (platelet count >90×10^9/L) occurring in the third trimester in an asymptomatic woman with no history of bleeding or low platelets pre-pregnancy. This condition does not usually present a contraindication to neuraxial blockade. Several studies have highlighted the safety of neuraxial blockade in parturients with platelet counts >70×10^9/L [35–37].

21.4.1.2 Idiopathic/Immune Thrombocytopenic Purpura

In idiopathic thrombocytopenic purpura (ITP), the platelet count may fall as low as 20×10^9/L or less, and whether treatment is administered to the asymptomatic patient varies at different institutions. It is recommended that treatment may be given to improve platelet levels in the symptomatic woman prior to performing invasive techniques or peri-delivery.

Neuraxial techniques can be administered to patients with ITP and several authors have demonstrated its safety in parturients with low platelet counts [36, 38, 39]. Previous guidelines for the minimum platelet count required to allow neuraxial blockade differed between the British and American Societies of Hematology. The British Committee for Standards in Haematology (BCSH) recommended that the platelet count be no lower than 80×10^9/L (40 [now archived]), while the American Society of Hematology (ASH) set the threshold at 50×10^9/L [41]. An epidural catheter has been placed without any complications unknowingly in a parturient with ITP and a platelet count of 26×10^9/L [38]. A suggested platelet count of $>50 \times 10^9$/L has been deemed sufficient to provide neuraxial anesthesia provided laboratory tests of coagulation are normal and there is no history of bleeding or other existing comorbidities [42]. This concurs with the 2010 International consensus report which states that a small consensus of obstetric anaesthetists agree that the minimum required platelet count is 50×10^9/L, in the absence of bruising, bleeding history, and recent anticoagulation. The international normalized ratio (INR) and the activated partial thromboplastin time (APTT) should be within normal values (evidence grade IV) [43].

21.4.1.3 Congenital Platelet Defects

Bernard-Soulier syndrome (BSS), Glanzmann thrombasthenia, Chediak-Higashi syndrome, the platelet storage pool deficiency group of disorders and the MYH9-related group of disorders are rare disorders of platelet function (see Chap. 13). It is important to liaise closely with the hematologists and obstetricians in the anesthetic management of the parturient with these conditions. There are several reports of pregnancy and delivery in these patients, but few reports of neuraxial blockade in the anesthetic management [44, 45]. Spinal anesthesia has been used following platelet transfusion in parturients with May-Hegglin anomaly [46, 47] and unknowingly in a parturient with grey platelet syndrome [48]. In general, neuraxial blockade and other nerve blocks, invasive procedures and IM injections should be avoided in these patients. Intravenous analgesia and entonox can be administered for pain, and general anesthesia for Cesarean section.

21.4.1.4 Pre-eclampsia

Pre-eclampsia is often associated with disorders of hemostasis including thrombocytopenia and rarely coagulopathy. Thrombocytopenia (platelet count $<150 \times 10^9$/L) is a feature of many affected women, with platelet counts of $<100 \times 10^9$/L occurring in up to 50 % of those with severe disease [49]. In addition, there may be associated platelet dysfunction with or without a low platelet count.

In the pre-eclamptic woman with a platelet count $<100 \times 10^9$/L, a coagulation screen (prothrombin time (PT), activated partial thromboplastin time (APTT) and fibrinogen) should be requested, as there is a strong correlation between counts below this level and coagulopathy [50]. Limited data suggest that the risk of platelet dysfunction is also increased [51, 52]. However, a definitive test used to evaluate primary haemostasis prior to regional analgesia has not been agreed. Measurement of the bleeding time has been found to be unreliable and operator dependent [53]. Studies of the use of thromboelastography (TEG) have been promising [54–56].

The multidisciplinary approach to the management of parturients with pre-eclampsia requires participation of the anesthetist, obstetric team and hematologists if there are significant abnormalities of hemostasis. The principles of anesthetic management include a thorough preassessment of the patient's condition with close attention to the airway. Adequate intravenous access should be established; however, fluid restriction is usually required to reduce the risk of pulmonary edema. Invasive arterial BP and central venous pressure monitoring may be required for women with severe disease. Abnormal hemostasis increases the risk of hemorrhagic complications from both procedures.

Neuraxial blockade is not contraindicated in pre-eclampsia unless there is an accompanying coagulopathy and it has been employed safely in pre-eclamptic women with a platelet count $>100 \times 10^9$/L [57]. The lower limit of platelet count at which neuraxial blockade can be performed safely in preeclampsia remains unclear. Although these techniques have been used without neurological sequelae in patients with a platelet count between 70 and 100×10^9/L [36, 37, 58], there is a general reluctance among anesthetists to perform these techniques when the platelet count is below 100×10^9/L [59], and certainly when the count is less than 50×10^9/L. For a platelet count between $50–100 \times 10^9$/L, central neuraxial block may be considered but the risks must be balanced against the other risks of the clinical situation (i.e. general anesthesia, possible platelet dysfunction). An epidural placed when the platelet count is $<100 \times 10^9$/L requires close monitoring for any neurological signs which may indicate the development of a spinal hematoma. The establishment of an epidural for labor analgesia is the technique of choice in preeclampsia, if not contraindicated. Its benefits include superior pain relief, assisting in blood pressure control and increasing the intervillous blood supply in the utero-placental circulation [60–63]. It may subsequently be used to provide anesthesia for Cesarean section, thus avoiding potential complications associated with general anesthesia [64].

General anesthesia in pre-eclampsia can be associated with many hazards. Maternal mortality is 16 times greater than in healthy pregnant women [65]. There is an increased risk of difficult or failed endotracheal intubation. There may also be uncontrolled hypertension during both intubation and extubation, which carries a risk of cerebral hemorrhage. Drug therapy with antihypertensives and/or opiates can be used to obtund this response but may be complicated by hypotension. Laryngeal edema may necessitate a smaller diameter endotracheal tube and precipitate airway obstruction at extubation. There is an increased risk of airway and pulmonary edema due to the preeclamptic process, which may be exacerbated by IV fluid administration. Monitoring of neuromuscular blockade is essential if magnesium has been given.

21.4.2 Congenital Coagulation Factor Defects

In pregnancy, the physiological changes in the coagulation system result in a hypercoagulable state. With some exceptions, most of the coagulation factors increase by term. Importantly, factor IX (FIX) levels remain unchanged and factor XI (FXI) levels may decrease to 62 % of normal at term. For some women with reduced factor levels pre-pregnancy, levels may increase to within normal parameters by term. Further discussion on coagulation factor deficiencies is considered in Chaps. 11 and 12.

Good liaison and multidisciplinary antenatal assessment and planning between the hemophilia unit, obstetricians and anesthetists are essential, and management decisions, particularly a peri-delivery plan, documented. Options for the anesthetic management during labor and delivery of these women is dependent on measured factor levels and normal laboratory monitoring of hemostasis (APTT, PT/PT ratio, fibrinogen), and the clinical situation. Neuraxial blockade may be considered when factor levels have normalised (with either pregnancy or replacement therapy) and laboratory testing reflects normal coagulation. In cases where the bleeding disorder is uncorrected, neuraxial blockade is contraindicated and alternative methods of labor analgesia such as entonox or IV opioids should be employed. Intramuscular injections are contraindicated when there is a bleeding disorder. Similarly, general anesthesia will be required for Cesarean section.

Some authors [66, 67] recommend that, even when factor levels have normalised, neuraxial block should be performed by an experienced anesthetist, and that a midline approach should be employed. Whenever possible, the smallest needle should be used and consideration given to the use of a spinal versus epidural technique for Cesarean section.

A low-dose local anesthetic should be used so as to preserve motor function for labor analgesia. The extent of any motor block should be assessed regularly and should continue until at least 24 h after the anesthetic has worn off and the epidural catheter removed. Epidural or spinal hematoma must be suspected if the motor block is more pronounced or more prolonged than expected, and prompt imaging should be carried out to aid diagnosis. Since catheter removal is as critical as needle puncture in the development of epidural hematoma [68], care should be taken to remove the catheter when hemostasis and coagulation factor levels are normal, particularly as any pregnancy-induced rise in clotting factor levels may rapidly revert to pre-pregnancy levels postpartum.

21.4.2.1 von Willebrand Disease (VWD), Factor XI (FXI) Deficiency and Carriers of Hemophilia A (Factor VIII Deficiency) and Hemophilia B (Factor IX Deficiency)

These bleeding disorders make up approximately 90 % of all inherited bleeding disorders, with vWD being the most common (prevalence of 1 % in the general population). In the past, neuraxial blockade for analgesia or anesthesia was not performed on women with inherited bleeding disorders, and some anesthetists remain reluctant to perform central neuraxial block in these patients. There have since been several reported cases of successful uncomplicated neuraxial blockade as part of the anesthetic management of labor and delivery [67, 69–72].

The commonly accepted criteria for neuraxial block in these patients are a normal coagulation screen and relevant factor level >50 IU/dL prior to needle puncture. When factor levels lie below 50 IU/dl or the bleeding disorder is severe, neuraxial block should not be attempted. This principle applies to women with type 2 and type 3 vWD, severe hemophilia A and B due to lyonisation of the X chromosome, and FXI deficiency homozygotes or compound heterozygotes. It is important to note that there is no consensus on the safe level of FXI necessary for neuraxial anesthesia.

As ever, the risks versus benefits of appropriate replacement therapy must be balanced against the risks versus benefits of the anesthetic technique; the woman should be appropriately counselled and adequate hemostatic cover must be available. These decisions should ideally be made in advance in conjunction with a hematologist and obstetrician experienced in the management of women with these disorders.

Dhar et al. [67] reported a case where neuraxial block for labor analgesia was given without complications to a woman with severe hemophilia A. She had received replacement therapy with recombinant factor VIIIC. Patients with hemophilia B may require FIX replacement to increase levels. A case series [73] reported nine women with FXI deficiency who were safely managed with a range neuraxial techniques (spinal, epidural and CSE) during labor and delivery. Most received factor replacement with FFP. FXI concentrate may also be considered.

21.4.2.2 Other Coagulation Factor Defects

The remaining factor deficiencies are rare and make up only about 10 % of those with inherited bleeding disorders. With the exception of factor XII deficiency, which in its homozygous state is associated with thrombosis, the remaining factor deficiencies are associated with an increased risk of bleeding. Treatment when required is with factor replacement therapy, either with factor concentrate where available or with blood components such as FFP or cryoprecipitate, and should be under expert hematological guidance. As these conditions are so rare and the outcome of pregnancies may be poor, the published literature regarding their anesthetic management is sparse. The anesthetic management should be formulated with a multidisciplinary team. Particular attention should be paid to correcting factor levels in order to achieve normal laboratory analysis of hemostasis, and to preparation for possible hemorrhage around the time of delivery.

Fibrinogen (Factor I) Deficiency

Although fibrinogen deficiency has been regarded as a contraindication to neuraxial blockade, there have been three case reports of their use in labor and delivery in women with afibrinogenemia [74–76]. In the first two cases, the women received replacement therapy to correct fibrinogen levels prior to needle placement. In the case described by Meldrum and colleagues, neuraxial block for elective Cesarean section was performed before the woman's dysfibrinogenemia was recognized. The woman suffered a severe post partum hemorrhage (PPH). This case report also highlighted the importance of documenting and communicating a plan formulated jointly between the obstetricians, anesthetists and hematologists.

Prothrombin (Factor II, FII) Deficiency

The main complication in women with prothrombin deficiency is bleeding, particularly post partum haemorrhage (PPH).

Factor V (FV) Deficiency

Patients with homozygous factor V deficiency may suffer moderate to severe bleeding, with PPH being a significant feature. Case studies of parturients with this disorder have presented information on the anesthetic management. Women who underwent Cesarean section did so under general anesthesia with FFP administered to raise factor levels [77].

Factor VII (FVII) Deficiency

Patients with FVII deficiency are at risk of bleeding; however, clinical history is a better indicator of bleeding risk than factor levels.

21.4.3 Acquired Coagulation Factor Deficiencies

21.4.3.1 Acquired Factor VIII Deficiency (Acquired Haemophilia A)

Acquired Factor VIII (FVIII) deficiency arises from the development of autoantibodies to FVIII. The majority of patients are healthy; however, the condition is associated with autoimmune diseases such as systemic lupus erythematosus (SLE), rheumatoid arthritis and inflammatory bowel disease. Clinical manifestations range from spontaneous bruising to life-threatening hemorrhage. The management of acquired hemophilia A requires close collaboration with the haematologist/hemophilia center. Prompt diagnosis enables early hemostatic treatment and prevention of non-essential invasive procedures. Recombinant activated factor VII (rtVIIa) and activated prothrombin complex concentrate (Factor Eight Inhibitor Bypassing Activity, or FEIBA) are equally effective but both associated with thrombotic events in this setting. Immunosuppression with steroids and cyclophosphamide is probably more effective than steroids alone. Rituximab does not appear to result in better outcomes. Up to 20 % of patients relapse in the first 6 months after immunosuppression is stopped, and so follow up is required [78]. The anesthetic approach to management of parturients with this condition should follow similar management principles recommended for those with congenital factor deficiencies.

21.4.3.2 Disseminated Intravascular Coagulation

Disseminated intravascular coagulopathy (DIC) is characterised by an acquired consumptive coagulopathy, platelet consumption and secondary activation of fibrinolysis, as a result of pathological widespread uncontrolled activation of the haemostatic system. During pregnancy, any one of multiple disease processes may act as a triggering event. These include placental abruption, amniotic fluid embolism (AFE), HELLP syndrome, sepsis, massive hemorrhage and transfusion, acute fatty liver of pregnancy, intrauterine death with retained fetus, and miscarriage.

Diagnosis is by recognition of the pathological precipitant with concomitant hemorrhage and diagnostic laboratory findings (low fibrinogen and prolonged PT and APTT as a result of generalised consumption of coagulation factors; low platelet count ($<100\times10^9$/L); and raised fibrin/

fibrinogen degradation product levels – the usual parameter measured is D-dimer, a marker of breakdown of cross-linked fibrin). The approach to management is to treat the underlying cause, which often includes prompt delivery of the fetus and placenta, and timely replacement of red cells, platelets and coagulation factors with appropriate blood components.

Anesthetic management involves ensuring that the woman has adequate IV access and providing supportive resuscitation with blood components. DIC is an absolute contraindication to neuraxial blockade. Often, DIC occurs after an epidural catheter has already been sited. Authors differ in their opinions as to the correct timing of catheter removal. Some advocate that the catheter may be removed in a patient with DIC provided there is no bleeding around the epidural insertion site [68]. Others recommend that the catheter is removed only after resolution of the coagulopathy [79]. As epidural catheter removal has been demonstrated to be as critical as catheter placement in the development of epidural hematoma in the anticoagulated patient [68, 80], the most cautionary action would be to keep the epidural catheter in situ until the coagulopathy has fully resolved or has been corrected.

21.4.3.3 Acute Fatty Liver of Pregnancy

Acute fatty liver of pregnancy (AFLP) is a condition often of unknown aetiology affecting 1:7,000–1:10,000 pregnancies [81]. It occurs most commonly in primiparous women during the third trimester. The overall clinico-pathological picture is of markedly increased liver enzymes; reduced synthesis of coagulation factors resulting in prolonged APTT and prothrombin times; reduced fibrin and antithrombin levels; and thrombocytopenia, less severe than is observed in HELLP, TTP and HUS syndromes. A profound hypoglycemia helps to distinguish AFLP from HELLP. The clinical picture of AFLP can range from a mild clinico-pathological presentation to fulminant hepatic failure with resulting fetal and maternal death. Management involves the prompt delivery of the fetus with aggressive supportive therapy similar to that of hepatic failure from other causes. Coagulopathy should be reversed with intravenous vitamin K, FFP, cryoprecipitate and platelet transfusion. Careful fluid resuscitation and electrolyte replacement should be administered along with the reversal of any hypoglycemia and management of seizures. Intramuscular injections, NSAIDs and aspirin are contraindicated if there is thrombocytopenia. Anesthetic management includes assisting with supportive care within a multidisciplinary team, and often requires transfer to a critical care setting. Acute coagulopathy contraindicates neuraxial blockade. Neuraxial techniques have been employed to provide anesthesia for Cesarean section where the symptoms were mild or where coagulation was normal or corrected [82, 83].

In AFLP, general anesthesia is often required for Cesarean section. The challenges for the anesthetist include preserving hepatic and renal blood flow and avoiding hepatotoxicity. The altered pharmacokinetic profile of drugs metabolized by the liver must be considered. Induction with propofol may be preferable to thiopentone as it has a normal pharmacokinetic profile in the presence of cirrhosis [84]. Suxamethonium remains the muscle relaxant of choice for rapid sequence induction; however, reduced levels of plasma cholinesterase exacerbated by liver disease may lead to prolonged neuromuscular block. Atracurium or rocuronium are the non-depolarizing neuromuscular blocking agents of choice. Desflurane may be preferred over sevoflurane and isoflurane as it has negligible hepatic metabolism. The choice of opioids should also be considered in view of the potential increased opioid sensitivity and increased risk of encephalopathy. Unlike other opioids, remifentanil elimination is independent of liver function as it is metabolised by non-specific plasma esterases and may be considered both as an induction agent and for IV analgesia. When fentanyl and morphine are used, dosing frequencies may need to be reduced in order to prevent accumulation of the drug.

21.5 Thrombotic Microangiopathy in Pregnancy

21.5.1 Preeclampsia: Hemolysis, Elevated Liver Enzymes, and Low Platelets (HELLP) Syndrome

The syndrome of hemolysis, elevated liver enzymes and low platelets (HELLP) may develop as a variant of pre-eclampsia in 5–10 % of cases [85]. A multidisciplinary approach to management of these women should be adopted, preferably at a tertiary care centre. In general, the anesthetic management of women with HELLP syndrome follows the same principles suggested for the management of those with preeclampsia. The decision to use neuraxial techniques for analgesia or delivery is dependent on the clinical progression of the disease, the fetal condition and the urgency of the situation. Neuraxial blockade is not advised in patients with severe disease or where the platelet count is falling rapidly. These techniques are contraindicated in the presence of disseminated intravascular coagulopathy (DIC) or active bleeding. A retrospective study [86] reported no neurological or hematological problems in the patients who received neuraxial anesthesia. Thrombocytopenia may be severe with the platelet count falling as low as 10×10^9/L. A few studies have demonstrated the use of steroid therapy to improve the platelet count to a sufficient level (>100×10^9/L) so as to permit neuraxial blockade [87, 88].

21.5.2 Thrombotic Thrombocytopenic Purpura; Hemolytic Uremic Syndrome

Thrombotic thrombocytopenic purpura (TTP) and hemolytic uremic syndrome (HUS) are rare but potentially life-threatening disorders that can occur in pregnancy or postpartum. These disorders are characterised by thrombocytopenia and microangiopathic hemolytic anemia with classically multiorgan failure in TTP and mainly renal involvement in HUS (see Chap. 17).

There is little information in the published literature about the anesthetic management of these rare disorders in pregnancy, with the principles guiding management based on a few non-pregnant case reports with literature reviews by the authors [89, 90]. A management plan should be formulated in conjunction with the hematologists and obstetricians. General anaesthetic care should involve establishing wide bore intravenous access, careful management of fluids to maintain adequate urine output and treatment of hemorrhage with replacement of blood components. Patients often present with a platelet count <100×10^9/L, hence neuraxial blockade is contraindicated. Intramuscular injections should also be avoided and other methods of administering analgesia in labor such as IV opiates employed. Sedative drugs should also be avoided due to concerns about neurological dysfunction. During general anesthesia, care should be taken during manipulation of the airway and intubation to avoid bleeding and edema due to airway trauma. Measures should be taken to avoid hypertension and to maintain the mean arterial pressure within normal limits in order to prevent organ hypoperfusion, while reducing the risk of intracranial hemorrhage.

A case report has described the anesthetic management in a series of pregnancies affected by TTP [91]. This woman was delivered by Cesarean section in all of her four pregnancies. The first two were under general anesthesia prior to her diagnosis and the last two under spinal anesthesia after the diagnosis of her condition had come to light. Prior to three of the deliveries, treatment was administered to improve her platelet count. Therapies used included platelet transfusion (it should be noted that guidance from the British Committee for Standards in Haematology state that due to the risk of precipitating further thrombotic events, platelet transfusions are contraindicated in TTP unless there is life-threatening haemorrhage [92]), fresh frozen plasma (FFP), steroids and immunoglobulin. The platelet counts prior to spinal anesthesia were 94×10^9/L and 71×10^9/L, and no complications were reported.

21.6 Anesthetic Management of Parturients with Thrombotic Disorders

21.6.1 Venous Thromboembolism and Thrombophilias

During pregnancy in normal women, the net effect of changes in the coagulation system is to produce a hypercoagulable state, thus increasing the risk of thrombosis. This thrombogenic potential is increased in women with inherited thrombophilias (protein C, S or antithrombin deficiency; factor V Leiden; or the prothrombin gene mutation G2010A) and those with antiphosphlipid antibodies (lupus anticoagulant, anticardiolipin and/or anti-beta 2 glycoprotein 1 antibodies). Women are treated during pregnancy with thromboprophylactic or treatment dose anticoagulation, generally low molecular weight heparin (LMWH), sometimes in combination with low-dose aspirin or low dose aspirin alone. Postpartum, women are recommenced on LMWH, with a switch to warfarin or another vitamin K antagonist (VKA) if appropriate. The regimens used for venous thromboembolism are summarised in Chaps. 4 and 5.

Regional anesthesia remains desirable in this group of women because of the protective effect against VTE combined with a reduction in blood loss [93]. The challenge for the anesthetist is the timing for performing neuraxial techniques with respect to heparin administration, in order to minimise the risk of spinal hematoma. Guidance on timing is discussed in the section on antithrombotic therapy.

21.6.2 Women with Cardiac Disorders

For many years standard anaesthetic management of patients with cardiac disease mandated general anaesthesia over central neuraxial blockade. Vasodilation secondary to sympathetic block was perceived as a contraindication particularly in severe obstructive cardiac disease. More recently, however, obstetric anaesthetists have successfully used incremental central neuraxial blockade (spinal catheter or CSE techniques) in women with advanced cardiac disease requiring anaesthesia for cesarean section. These techniques impart all the advantages of regional anaesthesia which may be of particular benefit to this group of parturients. Similarly epidural labour analgesia may be beneficial for women in labour with cardiac disease by reducing heart rate, preload and afterload.

Many women with cardiac disease require either prophylactic or therapeutic anticoagulation, which may complicate administration of central neuraxial blockade. The benefits of maintaining anticoagulation need to be balanced against those of central neuraxial blockade (see Sect. 21.7) and timing of antithrombotic therapy needs to be managed to facilitate central neuraxial blockade where appropriate [94].

21.7 Antithrombotic Therapy

Several studies support the safe use of central neuraxial blockade for providing anesthesia and analgesia in the anticoagulated patient. Following a period in the 1990s when spinal haematomas leading to serious neurological sequelae were being reported with increased frequency in patients treated concurrently with low molecular weight heparins [95], the German Society for Anaesthesiology and Intensive Care published the first recommendations on neuraxial anesthesia and antithrombotic drugs in 1997 [96]. This was followed by recommendations published by the American Society of Regional Anesthesia (ASRA) consensus group in 1998 [97] with the most recent update published in 2010 [98]. Other guidelines exist in Europe, the most recent of which was published by the European Society of Anaesthesiology (ESA) [99]. Due to the rarity of spinal haematomas, case reports, expert opinion and an understanding of the pharmacokinetic and pharmacodynamic properties of drugs that alter hemostasis, have formed the basis of published guidance for managing neuraxial blockade in the anticoagulated patient [98, 99]. Knowledge of the dosing time intervals has helped to indicate appropriate times for central neuraxial blockade and catheter removal, the aim being for the procedures to coincide with drug trough levels when there is least risk of haemorrhage. It is important to note that catheter removal is equally significant to catheter placement as a risk of developing spinal haematomas [68].

Challenges emerge as newer antithrombotic agents are introduced, with generally limited information on their safety when combined with regional anesthesia. In case reports where central neuraxial blockade has been successfully used in patients treated with newer antithrombotic drugs, similar principles of using knowledge of the drug pharmacology to guide timing of needle placement, along with careful clinical consideration and vigilant follow-up following catheter removal, have been employed.

There are no published cases of spinal haematoma in a parturient receiving antithrombotic prophylaxis or treatment for venous thromboembolism. The incidence of spinal haematoma following obstetric epidural blockade has been widely reported as being lower than in the elderly. For example, Moen et al. [100] showed an incidence of 1:200,000 in the obstetric compared with 1:3,600 in the elderly populations. Due to a lack of data derived from a large series of neuraxial techniques in the obstetric population receiving thromboprophylaxis or treatment of venous thromboembolism, it has been suggested that guidelines (derived mainly from surgical patients) be applied to parturients [98]. Table 21.1 lists the time intervals recommended by both the ESA and ASRA, before and after neuraxial puncture or catheter removal for the administration of a range of antithrombotic drugs. The guidance below summarises key principles in the management of patients on antithrombotic drugs before and after neuraxial puncture or catheter removal, based on recommendations by ESA and ASRA. The reader should refer to Chap. 2 for further details on the antithrombotic agents covered below.

21.7.1 Parenteral Anticoagulants

21.7.1.1 Unfractionated Heparin

Unfractionated Heparin (UFH) has a half-life of 1–2 h when administered intravenously. The anticoagulant effect is monitored using the activated partial thromboplastin time (APTT). Key recommendations for the anesthetic management of patients treated with UFH are as follows:

- ASRA advocates no contraindication to the use of neuraxial techniques for patients on prophylactic subcutaneous UFH (5,000 IU twice a day). However, the ESA recommends a delay of 4–6 h between drug administration and neuraxial puncture or catheter manipulation/withdrawal.
- Patients treated for more than 4 days (according to ASRA) or more than 5 days (according to ESA) should have a platelet count prior to central neuraxial block due to the risk of heparin induced thrombocytopenia (HIT).
- Confirmation that the APTT is within normal range prior to removal of the catheter may be warranted.
- When the patient is treated with IV heparin, neuraxial placement or epidural catheter removal should occur 1 h before any subsequent heparin administration; or 4–6 h (ESA) or 2–4 h (ASRA) after the last heparin dose. The APTT should be checked prior to performing the neuraxial block

21.7.1.2 Low Molecular Weight Heparins

Low Molecular Weight Heparins (LMWHs) differ from UFH in that the molecular chain length is shorter resulting in greater anti-Factor Xa (FXa) activity than anti-thrombin activity. They also have greater bioavailability and a longer half-life. The time to peak anti-coagulant activity for subcutaneous LMWHs is 3–6 h and it is during this period after dosing that neuraxial procedures should be avoided. Activity falls to around 50 % after 10–12 h. Although anti-FXa levels measure its anticoagulant effect, monitoring the level in patients undergoing neuraxial block is

Table 21.1 Recommended time intervals for regional anaesthesia in the patient receiving anti-thrombotic agents from the European Society of Anaesthesiology [99] and The American Society of Regional Anesthesia and Pain Medicine [98]

	Time between drug administration and neuraxial puncture, catheter manipulation or withdrawal		Time between neuraxial puncture, catheter manipulation or withdrawal and drug administration		Laboratory tests
	ESA	ASRA	ESA	ASRA	
Unfractionated heparin (prophylaxis)	4–6 h	No time interval	1 h	1 h	Check platelets if treatment >5 days[a]/>4 days[b]
Unfractionated heparin (treatment)	IV 4–6 h	2–4 h	1 h	1 h	Check APTT, ACT, platelets
	SC 8–12 h	–	1 h	–	
LMWH (prophylaxis)	12 h	10–12 h	4 h	6–8 h (NP)/>2 h (CW)	Check platelets if treatment >5 days[a]
LMWH (treatment)	24 h	24 h	4 h	24 h (NP)/>2 h (CW)	Check platelets if treatment >5 days[a]
Fondaparinux (prophylaxis, 2.5 mg per day)	36–42 h	36 h[c]	6–12 h	12 h[c]	(anti-Xa standardised for specific agent[a])
Rivaroxaban (prophylaxis, 10 mg o.d.)	22–26 h (CW)	–	4–6 h	–	(PT standardised for specific agent)
Aspirin/acetylsalicylic acid	None	None	None	None	
NSAIDs	None	None	None	None	
Clopidogrel	7 days	7 days	After CW	–	
Ticlopidine	10 days	14 days	After CW	–	
Abciximab	48 h (CW)	24–48 h	–	–	Check platelets
Eptifibatide	8–10 h (CW)	4–8 h	–	–	Check platelets
Tirofiban	8–10 h (CW)	4–8 h	–	–	Check platelets
Warfarin/Coumarins	INR ≤1.4	4–5 days + normal INR (NP)/INR <1.5 (CW)	After CW	After CW	INR
Hirudins (desirudin, lepirudin)	8–10 h	C/I	2–4 h	C/I	APTT/ECT[a]
Argatroban[d]	4 h	C/I	2 h	C/I	APTT, /ECT, ACT[a]
Dabigatran (prophylaxis, 75 mg b.d., 110 mg b.d.)	C/I by manufacturer	–	6 h	–	

All time intervals refer to patients with normal renal function

ESA European Society of Anaesthesiology, *ASRA* American Society of Regional Anesthesia, *APTT* activated partial thromboplastin time, *ACT* activated clotting time, *LMWH* low molecular weight heparin, *IV* intravenous, *SC* subcutaneous, *NP* neuraxial puncture, *CW* catheter withdrawal, *PT* prothrombin time, *NSAIDs* non-steroidal anti-inflammatory drugs, *INR* international normalised ratio, *ECT* ecarin clotting time, *C/I* contraindicated

[a]According to ESA guidelines

[b]According to ASRA guidelines

[c]Performance of neuraxial techniques should be under conditions used in clinical trials (single-needle pass, atraumatic needle placement, avoidance of indwelling neuraxial catheters). If this is not feasible, an alternate method of prophylaxis should be considered

[d]Time interval refers to patients with normal hepatic function

not recommended as it does not predict the risk of bleeding [101].

Key recommendations with regard to patients receiving LMWH therapy according to the ESA and ASRA are as follows:

- For patients receiving LMWH thromboprophylaxis (e.g. dalteparin 5,000 IU or enoxaparin 40 mg once a day), neuraxial placement should be delayed for at least 10–12 h after the last LMWH dose.
- For patients receiving higher (treatment) doses of LMWH (i.e. enoxaparin 1 mg/kg every 12 h, enoxaparin 1.5 mg/kg daily, dalteparin 120 IU/kg every 12 h, dalteparin 200 IU/kg daily or tinzaparin 175 IU/kg daily), needle placement should be avoided for at least 24 h after the last dose of LMWH, in order to ensure normal haemostasis at the time of needle insertion.
- For patients on a once a day dosing regimen with an indwelling epidural catheter, the catheter can be removed after a minimum of 10–12 h after the last dose.
- Post-operative LMWH dosing should occur a minimum of 4 h according to the ESA (or a minimum of 24 h according to the ASRA) after epidural catheter insertion or removal

21.7.1.3 Fondaparinux

Fondaparinux produces its antithrombotic effect by inhibition of FXa activity without inhibition of Factor IIa [102, 103]. It has a long half-life (17–21 h) and is renally excreted [102]. There is limited data in pregnancy (see Chap. 2) and the risk of spinal haematoma associated with this drug is unknown. There also appears to be limited data and no consensus as to the ideal time interval between last administration of fondaparinux and neuraxial placement. Due to the lack of clinical experience at the time, the ASRA Consensus advised limiting the performance of central neuraxial block to clinical trial conditions. In Europe, however, the ESA has recommended a time interval of 22–42 h between the last administration of the drug and neuraxial placement. There are case reports of parturients managed successfully using neuraxial techniques [104, 105].

21.7.1.4 Parenteral Direct Thrombin Inhibitors

Thrombin inhibitors inhibit any further growth of a thrombus by inactivating fibrin already bound to thrombin. The thrombin inhibitors available include the recombinant hirudins (desirudin and lepirudin) and argatroban. They are commonly used for prophylaxis against thrombosis (desirudin) and to treat patients with type-II heparin-induced thrombocytopenia (HIT II) (lepirudin, argatroban). Their action on hemostasis can be monitored using the APTT. These drugs are, however, associated with an increased bleeding tendency, particularly at higher doses, and their actions cannot be reversed (dialysis aids elimination). Although recombinant hirudins are not recommended for use in pregnancy due to evidenced transplacental transfer of the drug [106], there have been case reports of its successful use in pregnant women for the management of HIT II and recurrent VTEs [107–109]. None of these cases reported any adverse effects on the neonate, however, its use in pregnancy remains rare.

While the ASRA has stated that the use of direct thrombin inhibitors is a contraindication to neuraxial blockade, the ESA has not and provides some guidance for the use of these drugs. They advise:

Recombinant Hirudins

- A time interval of 8–10 h between administration of the prophylactic dose hirudin and central neuraxial blockade or epidural catheter removal in patients with normal renal function
- Administration of these drugs following neuraxial procedure should be delayed for 2–4 h
- Avoid combining hirudins with other antithrombotic agents

Like most antithrombotic agents, the hirudins are renally excreted, hence they can accumulate in patients with renal impairment, causing prolonged drug activity; in this situation, monitoring of the APTT is advisable.

Argabatroban

Argatroban is administered as an IV infusion and the APTT returns to normal 2–4 h after the infusion is stopped. It is eliminated exclusively through the liver and dose reduction is necessary in the presence of impaired liver function. The guidelines reviewed do not suggest a time interval between cessation of the infusion and performing a neuraxial block. However, in a recent case report, a woman treated with an argatroban infusion was successfully managed with neuraxial analgesia during labor without any complications [105].

However, there is very limited experience of its use in conjunction with central neuraxial blockade. Even though there have been no reports of spinal haematoma to date, both the ESA and ASRA advise extreme caution when using central neuraxial blockade in patients taking this drug. At present, the ASRA does not provide any guidelines for Rivaroxaban; however, the ESA suggests a 22–26 h interval between the last drug dose and epidural catheter withdrawal, and a delay of 4–6 h between catheter withdrawal and the next dose.

21.7.2 Oral Anticoagulants

21.7.2.1 Warfarin and Other Vitamin K Antagonists

Despite the concerns about fetal safety (see Chap. 2), warfarin therapy may be encountered in the parturient, for example with a mechanical heart valve where it may be deemed a more effective treatment than heparin to prevent valve thrombosis and systemic emboli.

The use of warfarin or other oral VKA is an absolute contraindication to central neuraxial blockade. Key principles in the management of patients on these drugs include:

- Cessation of warfarin 4–5 days prior to initiation of neuraxial block if on therapeutic dose (INR (International Normalised Ratio) >1.4 (ASRA), INR >1.5 (ESA)). The INR should also be checked prior to needle placement to ensure that it is within normal reference limits, indicating the return of adequate levels of factor II, VII, IX and X for safe neuraxial blockade.
- When the woman has received an initial dose of warfarin more than 24 h prior to surgery, or if a second dose has been administered (ASRA), the INR should be checked prior to central neuraxial blockade
- The neuraxial catheter should be removed only when the INR is ≤1.4 Neurological testing of motor and sensory function should be continued for 24 h after catheter removal and longer if the INR was >1.4 at the time of catheter removal.

21.7.2.2 New Oral Anticoagulants/Oral Direct Inhibitors of Coagulation

The non-vitamin K antagonist oral anticoagulants (NOAC) include dabigatran, a direct thrombin inhibitor, and rivaroxaban and apixaban (Pradaxa®, Xarelto®, Eliquis®)[110–112], direct factor Xa inhibitors. Dabigatran, rivaroxaban and apixaban are approved by the National Institute for Health and Care Excellence in England (NICE) and the US Food and Drug Administration (FDA) for the prevention of venous thromboembolism (VTE) in patients undergoing hip or knee replacement, and the prevention of stroke or systemic embolization in patients with atrial fibrillation. These agents have also undergone phase III trials for the treatment of acute deep venous thrombosis (DVT) and pulmonary embolism (PE) and secondary prevention of VTE, and have been licensed for these indications. All three agents have been approved for VTE treatment by the FDA and rivaroxaban and dabigatran are approved by NICE, with NICE review of apixaban underway. The manufacturers recommend that all are contraindicated during pregnancy and breastfeeding.

Rivaroxaban

There is very limited experience of rivaroxaban use in conjunction with central neuraxial blockade. Even though there have been no reports of spinal haematoma to date, both the ESA and ASRA advise extreme caution when using central neuraxial blockade in patients taking this drug. At present, the ASRA does not provide any guidelines for Rivaroxaban; however, the ESA suggests a 22–26 h interval between the last drug dose and epidural catheter withdrawal, and a delay of 4–6 h between catheter withdrawal and the next dose. The ESA guidance applies to prophylactic dose rivaroxaban (10 mg daily), where rivaroxaban has been has been shown to provide superior prevention of VTE when compared with enoxaparin (40 mg once daily) in patients undergoing hip or knee replacement [113].

Dabigatran Etexilate

The ESA has suggested a time interval of at least 34 h between the last dose of dabigatran and epidural catheter manipulation or withdrawal. This guidance applies to prophylactic dose dabigatran (75 and 110 mg BD respectively), where dabigatran has been found at a dose of 110 mg BD to be comparable in efficacy to enoxaparin (40 mg once daily) in patients undergoing hip or knee replacement [114]. Although there have been no reported spinal haematomas in the initial studies where thromboprophylaxis with dabigatran was initiated 4–6 h after epidural catheter removal, the manufacturer advises against its use in conjunction with central neuraxial blockade. For this reason, the medicolegal consequences should a spinal haematoma develop, must be considered where central neuraxial blockade is to be employed in a woman taking this drug.

21.7.2.3 Antiplatelet Drugs

Evidence from the Collaborative Low-Dose Aspirin Study in Pregnancy (CLASP) [115] and from studies by Horlocker et al. [116, 117] has concluded that low-dose aspirin and non-steroidal anti-inflammatory drugs (NSAIDs) do not represent a contraindication to central neuraxial blockade, provided they are not combined with other anti-thrombotic agents.

Thienopyridines, which include clopidogrel and ticlopidine, inhibit platelet aggregation. This group of drugs irreversibly inhibit platelet function. Platelet levels are restored 6–14 days after withdrawal of the drug. The guidelines recommend that a minimum interval of 7 days for clopidogrel and 10 (ESA) to 14 (ASRA) days for ticlopidine between the last drug dose and neuraxial puncture.

Glycoprotein IIb/IIIa antagonists reversibly inhibit the binding of Von Willebrand Factor and fibrinogen to receptor sites. Abciximab should be stopped for 48 h while eptifibatide and tirofiban for 8–10 h prior to neuraxial placement according to ESA. The ASRA advocates a similar approach, recommending intervals of 24–48 h for Abciximab and 4–8 h for eptifibatide and tirofiban. Neuraxial block should be avoided until platelet function has recovered, and is contraindicated when glycoprotein IIb/IIIa inhibitors are used in conjunction with other anticoagulants or aspirin.

21.8 Ehlers-Danlos Syndrome and Other Blood Vessel Wall Disorders

21.8.1 Ehlers-Danlos Syndrome

Ehlers-Danlos syndrome (EDS) is a heterogeneous group of inherited connective tissue disorders with differing clinical, biochemical and genetic findings. The prevalence in the population is around 1:5,000 [118, 119]. The mutated genes coding for structural collagens and for enzymes associated with normal collagen synthesis are either deficient or defective, resulting predominantly in weakness in the supporting structure of skin, the musculoskeletal system, vascular wall, and visceral organs. Although 11 different subgroups have been identified, the syndrome has been described within six subtypes [118]. The classical, benign hypermobility, and vascular are the most common subtypes, making up 96 % of the affected population (60, 30 and 6 %, respectively). The other groups include the kyphoscoliosis, arthrochalasia and dermatosparaxia subtypes. All have autosomal dominant inheritance, with the exception of the vascular and dermatosparaxis subtypes, which are autosomal recessive. EDS is associated with an increased risk of miscarriage and antepartum hemorrhage.

21.8.1.1 Clinical Features and Complications in the Puerperium

The main features of EDS are connective tissue fragility, hypermobility and hyperextensibility affecting the skin and musculoskeletal systems. Complications include poor wound healing, scarring, skin friability (skin breakdown, pressure sores), joint hypermobility (subluxation, dislocation, hemarthrosis) and spinal abnormalities (kyphoscoliosis, spondylolisthesis). Pregnant women with the classical and hypermobility subtypes of EDS have an increased risk of separation of the symphysis pubis, fetal malpresentation, intrauterine growth restriction, premature rupture of membranes, preterm birth, and uterine prolapse. Severe, potentially life-threatening hemorrhage due to vessel wall fragility may be encountered and is usually associated with the vascular and hypermobility subtypes. This may present as post-operative hemorrhage, PPH, spontaneous rupture of blood vessels and excessive bleeding from obstetric trauma. Laboratory analysis of hemostasis including clotting screen, platelet count and aggregation are often normal. However, some patients may present with accompanying coagulation factor and platelet disorders [120]. Other serious complications include rupture of viscera such as the uterus or gastrointestinal tract, and spontaneous pneumothorax due to ruptured bullae. For patients with the vascular subtype of EDS, pregnancy can be life-threatening, with a 12 % risk of death from peripartum arterial or uterine rupture [118, 121].

Cardiovascular complications associated particularly with the vascular subtype of EDS include congenital and valvular heart disease (typically mitral valve prolapse and regurgitation), conduction defects, coronary artery disease and aortic dissection or rupture. Dysautonomia is a recognised complication of the hypermobility subtype [122]. If required, a stress echocardiogram or thalium scan may be preferred to cardiac catheterisation because of the risk of possible vessel rupture and hemorrhage with the latter.

21.8.1.2 Anesthetic Management of EDS

Anesthesia during labor and delivery presents unique risks for the woman with EDS. Key points for the anesthetic management of these patients have been highlighted by some authors based on reported cases [123–127]:

- Genetic consultation to assess the type and severity of disease. Knowing this, likely complications can be anticipated and appropriate multidisciplinary antenatal care can be organised. Due to the potentially life-threatening complications in women with the vascular subtype, they should be considered high risk and managed at a tertiary delivery unit
- Careful pre-assessment should include detailed assessment of bleeding history, cardiac function and any spinal abnormalities
- Evaluation of the airway. Patients with the hypermobility subtype may potentially present difficulties with airway management due to an unstable cervical spine and temporomandibular joint dysfunction. The cervical spine and corresponding nerve roots should be thoroughly examined, along with appropriate imaging where necessary
- Specialised tests of hemostasis to exclude a concomitant hemostatic defect
- Ensure adequate cross-matched red cells are available
- Ensure that adequate IV access is carefully established prior to operation. Vascular access may be hindered by scarring and by the inability to feel the needle passing through the vessel wall. Arterial and central venous lines should be avoided unless absolutely essential, in order to avoid the possibility of post-puncture aneurysm and hematoma formation. All cannulation sites should be reviewed regularly for signs of extravasation.
- Careful insertion of neuraxial block where there are no contraindications
- Careful, atraumatic tracheal intubation in the case of general anesthesia
- Maintenance of low airway pressures to reduce the risk of pneumothorax
- Avoid hypertension, particularly during intubation and extubation, in order to prevent exacerbation of blood loss and the rupture of occult aneurysms.

The decision as to whether to perform neuraxial blockade on the parturient with EDS should be made on a case-by-case basis after full evaluation of the potential risks of bleeding and neurological injury. Vascular fragility per se is unlikely to increase the risk of epidural hematoma; however, uncertainty remains regarding the effect of abnormal vascular collagen on primary hemostasis. There are no reports in the literature of spinal hematoma associated with EDS. Different neuraxial techniques have been described in case reports involving the classic, hypermobility and vascular subtypes of EDS [29, 124–126, 128]. Case reports have indicated that patients with hypermobility type EDS may have resistance to local anesthetics [127, 129, 130] although in a series from our unit, central neuraxial blocks worked well, even in those who gave a history of local anesthetic resistance [131].

When deciding on management for Cesarean section, the risks of neuraxial blockade should also be weighed against the risks associated with general anesthesia. During general anesthesia, attention should be paid to careful patient positioning and padding of areas susceptible to the effects of pressure, in order to prevent tissue damage. Sood and colleagues [127] reported a case of difficult intubation during rapid sequence induction in a patient with the hypermobility subtype of EDS. They suggested that when difficult intubation is encountered using this technique, releasing the cricoid pressure may help to alleviate the obstruction that can result from a collapsed trachea. They also suggest minimal cervical spine movement during positioning and intubation and the use of fibreoptic techniques where there is significant cervical spine instability.

21.8.2 Other Blood Vessel Wall Disorders

Blood vessel wall disorders include the rare hereditary conditions hereditary hemorrhagic telangectasia (HHT, also known as Osler-Weber-Rendu syndrome) and pseudoxanthoma elasticum (PXE) and the vasculitis, Henoch-Schönlein purpura (HSP).

Few case reports exist to provide a guide to anesthetic management of parturients with these disorders. Both general anesthesia and neuraxial blockade have been used to provide peri-delivery analgesia and anesthesia for Cesarean section in women with HHT [132, 133]. Similarly, case reports have described the use of peri-delivery neuraxial blockade in women with PXE [134, 135]. Deciding on the appropriate anesthetic care is dependent on careful assessment of the disorder and its anesthetic implications, preferably during the antenatal period. Neuraxial blockade is contraindicated when there is any potential risk of hemorrhage into the vertebral canal due to abnormal arteriovenous malfomations (HHT) or when there is a history of spontaneous bleeding.

For Cesarean section, the risks of neuraxial blockade should be weighed against the risks of general anesthesia. During general anesthesia, care must be taken to prevent hypertension during induction and extubation in order to prevent rupture of, and increased bleeding from, the abnormal vasculature.

21.9 Case Studies

Case Study 1

A 32-year-old low risk nulliparous woman was noted to have a platelet count of 83×10^9/L on routine full blood count at 34 weeks of gestation. As her platelet count at booking had been slightly reduced at 121×10^9/L, a provisional diagnosis of autoimmune thrombocytopenia was considered. She was referred to both the hematology and anesthetic antenatal clinics. A repeat blood count and film the following week confirmed thrombocytopenia with a further downward trend in the platelet count to 78×10^9/L, with the immature platelet fraction (IPF) twice the upper limit of the normal range. The remainder of the blood count was normal, as was a coagulation screen (prothrombin time, activated partial thromboplastin time and fibrinogen). ANA and antiphospholipid antibodies were negative.

The patient was noted to have a potentially difficult airway and was keen to retain the option of regional analgesia for labor. Therefore, although her platelet count was borderline for regional anesthesia, she was commenced on oral Prednisolone 20 mg daily, and had her full blood count checked weekly.

She presented in established labor at 39 weeks +3 days' gestation and a full blood count on admission showed a platelet count of 99×10^9/L. She declined labor epidural analgesia as she was anxious about the possibility of epidural hematoma, despite reassurance that this was extremely unlikely with her current platelet count. She subsequently required a Cesarean delivery for failure to progress and consented to a spinal anesthetic, being aware that any risk of spinal anesthesia was outweighed by those of an emergency general anesthetic.

Case Study 2

A 28 year old woman, G2 P1, with a history of joint hypermobility syndrome (JHS)/Ehlers Danlos Type 3, was referred to the anesthetic antenatal clinic. She gave a history of chronic pain secondary to multiple joint problems, easy bruising and failure of local anesthesia at the dentist. She also reported occasional spontaneous bruising, a previous postpartum hemorrhage requiring blood transfusion, and significant bleeding following a dental extraction as a teenager. Tests of haemostatic function which included the following revealed no abnormality of hemostasis: platelet count and morphology, coagulation screen (prothrombin time, activated partial thromboplastin time and fibrinogen), PFA 100 modified bleeding time, platelet aggregation studies in platelet rich plasma to ADP, collagen, ristocetin, arachidonic acid and epinephrine at various agonist doses, platelet adenine nucleotides, factor VIII/von Willebrand factor activity and antigen, factors IX, XI and XIII.

There is uncertainty regarding the effect of abnormal collagen on primary hemostasis and the significance of vascular fragility as a risk factor for epidural hematoma. In view of this and her significant bleeding history, the patient was counseled that although her laboratory clotting tests were normal, a significant risk of epidural hematoma could not be excluded. It was agreed that she would not have central neuraxial blockade for either labor or Cesarean section. She subsequently had an uncomplicated and rapid labor using entonox analgesia.

Key Learning Points

- Analgesia for women in labour can be provided using non-pharmacological and pharmacological techniques
- Central neuraxial blockade (CNB) is the only technique that provides complete pain relief in labour (where low dose local anaesthetic is often combined with an opioid). In addition, it is the preferred technique for providing anaesthesia for peripartum obstetric procedures due to its significant reductions in maternal morbidity and mortality when compared with general anaesthesia
- The development of a spinal haematoma can present as a serious complication following CNB thus, patient coagulopathy is an absolute contraindication to the procedure
- All pregnant women with underlying bleeding disorders or undergoing anticaogulant therapy should be identified early and managed within a multidisciplinary environment that includes the haematologists, obstetricians and anaesthetist.

References

1. Melzack R. The myth of painless childbirth (the John J. Bonica Lecture). Pain. 1984;19(4):321–37.
2. Chamberlain G, Wraight A, Steer P, editors. Pain and its relief in childbirth: the results of a national survey conducted by the National Birthday Trust. Edinburgh: Churchill Livingstone; 1993.
3. Maternity services survey. 2010. http://www.cqc.org.uk/public/reports-surveys-and-reviews/surveys/maternity-services-survey-2010equalitycommission
4. Sharma SK, SIdawi JE, Ramin SM, Lucas MJ, Leveno KJ, Cunningham FG. Cesarean delivery: a randomised trial of epidural versus patient

controlled-meperidine analgesia during labor. Anesthesiology. 1997;87:487–94.
5. Thorp JA, Hu DH, Albin RM, McNItt J, Meyer BA, Cohen GR, Yeast JD. The effect of intrapartum epidural analgesia on nulliparous labor: a randomized, controlled, perspective trial. Am J Obstet Gynecol. 1993;169:851–8.
6. Barnardo PD, Jenkins JG. Failed tracheal intubation in the obstetrics: a 6-year review in a UK region. Anesthesia. 2000;55:690–4.
7. Hawthorne L, Wilson R, Lyons G, Dresner M. Failed intubation revisited: 17- yr experience in a teaching maternity unit. Br J Anaesth. 1996;76:680–4.
8. Yentis S, Hirsch N, Smith G. Anaesthesia and intensive care. 3rd ed. London: Elsevier Ltd; 2004.
9. Confidential Enquiry into Maternal and Child Health. Why mothers die 2000–2002: the sixth report of the confidential enquiries into maternal death in the United Kingdom. London: RCOG Press; 2004.
10. Centre for Maternal and Child Enquiries. Saving Mothers' Lives: reviewing maternal deaths to make motherhood safer – 2006–2008. The Eighth Report of the Confidential Enquiries into Maternal Death in the United Kingdom. BJOG. 2011;118 Suppl 1:1–203.
11. Wulf H. Epidural anaesthesia and spinal haematoma. Can J Anaesth. 1996;43:1260–71.
12. Auroy Y, Benhamou D, Bargues L, Ecoffey C, Falissard B, Mercier FJ, et al. Major complications of regional anaesthesia in France: The SOS Regional Anesthesia Hotline Service. Anesthesiology. 2002; 97:1274–80.
13. Cameron CM, Scott DA, McDonald WM, Davies MJ. A review of neuraxial epidural morbidity: experience of more than 8,000 cases at a single teaching hospital. Anesthesiology. 2007;106:997–1002.
14. Cook TM, Councell D, Wildsmith JA. Major complications of central neuraxial block: report on the Third National Audit Project of The Royal College of Anaesthetists. Br J Anaesth. 2009;102:179–90.
15. Peach MJ, Godkin R, Webster S. Complications of obstetric epidural analgesia and anesthesia: a prospective analysis of 10,995 cases. Int J Obstet Anesth. 1998;7:5–11.
16. Ruppen W, Derry S, McQuay H, Moore RA. Incidence of epidural haematoma, infection, and neurologic injury in obstetric patients with epidural analgesia/anesthesia. Anesthesiology. 2006;105: 394–9.
17. Lee LA, Posner KL, Domino KB, Caplan RA, Cheney FW. Injuries associated with regional anesthesia in the 1980s and 1990s: a closed claims analysis. Anesthesiology. 2004;101(1):143–52.
18. Dowswell T, Bedwell C, Lavender T, Neilson JP. Transcutaneous electrical nerve stimulation (TENS) for pain relief in labour. Cochrane Database Syst Rev. 2009;(2):CD007214. doi: 10.1002/14651858. CD007214.pub2.
19. Holdcroft A, Morgan M. An assessment of the analgesic effect in labour of pethidine and 50 per cent nitrous oxide in oxygen (ENTONOX). Br J Obstet Gynaecol. 1974;81:603–7.
20. Yeo ST, Holdcroft A, Yentis SM, Stewart A, Bassett P. Analgesia with Sevoflurane during labour II: Sevoflurane compared with Entonox for labour analgesia. Br J Anaesth. 2007;98(1):110–5.
21. Jones L, Othman M, Dowswell T, Alfirevic Z, Gates S, Newburn M, Jordan S, Lavender T, Neilson JP. Pain management for women in labor: an overview of systematic reviews. Cochrane Database Syst Rev. 2012;(3):CD009234. doi:10.1002/14651858. CD009234.pub2.
22. Bricker L, Lavender T. Parenteral opioids for labor pain relief: a systematic review. Am J Obstet Gynecol. 2002;186(5):94–109.
23. Latta K, Ginsberg B, Barkin R. Meperidine: a critical review. Am J Ther. 2002;9:53–68.
24. Elbourne E, Wiseman RA. Types of intramuscular opioids for maternal pain relief in labour. Cochrane Database Syst Rev. 2006;(4):CD001237.
25. Van de Velde M. Remifentanil patient-controlled analgesia should be routinely available for use in labour. Int J Obstet Anesth. 2008;17(4):339–42.
26. Fairlie FM, Marshall L, Walker JJ, Elbourne D. Intramuscular opioids for maternal pain relief in labor: a randomised controlled trial comparing pethidine with diamorphine. Br J Obstet Gynaecol. 1999;106(11):1181–7.
27. Tuckey JP, Prout RE, Wee WY. Prescribing intramuscular opioids for labour analgesia in consultant-led maternity units: a survey of UK practice. Int J Obstet Anesth. 2008;17(1):3–8.
28. Halpern SH, Muir H, Breen TW, Campbell DC, Barrett J, Liston R, et al. A multicentre randomized controlled trial comparing patient-controlled epidural with intravenous analgesia for pain relief in labour. Anesth Analg. 2004;99:1532–8.
29. Campbell N, Rosaeg OP. Anaesthetic management of a patient with Ehlers-Danlos syndrome type IV. Can J Anaesth. 2002;49:493–6.
30. Van de Velde M, Schepers R, Berends N, Vandermeersch E, De Buck F. Ten years of experience with accidental dural puncture and post-dural puncture headache in a tertiary obstetric anaesthesia department. Int J Obstet Anesth. 2008;17(4): 329–35.
31. Gupta N, Hill D, Hughes D, Wallace N. Impact of introduction of remifentanil PCA for labor analgesia on epidural rate and obstetric outcome over a two-year period. Int J Obstet Anesth. 2008;17:s51.
32. Towards better births: a review of maternity services in England. Service Commission for Healthcare Audit and Inspection; 2008.
33. Anim-Somuah M, Smyth RM, Jones L. Epidural versus non-epidural or no analgesia in labour. Cochrane Database Syst Rev. 2011. doi:10.1002/14651858. CD000331.pub3.

34. Burrows RF, Kelton JG. Thrombocytopenia at delivery: a prospective survey of 6715 deliveries. Am J Obstet Gynecol. 1990;162(3):731–4.
35. Rolbin SH, Abbott D, Musclow E, Papsin F, Lie LM, Freedman J. Epidural anesthesia in pregnant patients with low platelet counts. Obstet Gynecol. 1988;71(6 Pt 1):918–20.
36. Rasmus KT, Rottman RL, Kotelko DM, Wright WC, Stone JJ, Rosenblatt RM. Unrecognised thrombocytopenia and regional anesthesia in parturients: a retrospective review. Obstet Gynecol. 1989;73(6):943–6.
37. Beilin Y, Zahn J, Comerford M. Safe epidural analgesia in thirty parturients with platelet counts between 69,000 and 98,000 mm(−3). Anesth Analg. 1997;85(2):385–8.
38. Moeller-Bertram T, Kuczkowski KM, Benumof JL. Uneventful epidural labor analgesia in a parturient with immune thrombocytopenic purpura and a platelet count of 26,000/mm3 which was unknown preoperatively. J Clin Anesth. 2004;16:51–3.
39. Ramos I, Pacreu S, Fernandez C, Gomer C. Obstetric analgesia in 28 women with idiopathic thrombocytopenic purpura. Rev Esp Anestesiol Reanim. 2004;51:378–84.
40. British Committee for Standards in Haematology General Haematology Task Force. Guidelines for the investigation and management of idiopathic thrombocytopenic purpura in adults, children and in pregnancy. Br J Haematol. 2003;120(4):574–96.
41. Diagnosis and treatment of immune thrombocytopenic purpura: recommendations of the American Society of Hematology. Ann Intern Med. 1997; 126(4):319–26.
42. Douglas MJ. Platelets, the parturient and regional anaesthesia. Int J Obstet Anesth. 2001;10:113–20.
43. Provan D, Stasi R, Newland AC, Blanchette VS, Bolton-Maggs P, Bussel JB, et al. International consensus report on the investigation and management of primary thrombocytopenia. Blood. 2010;115:168–86.
44. Saade G, Homsi R, Seoud M. Bernard-Soulier syndrome in pregnancy: a report of four pregnancies in one patient, and review of the literature. Eur J Obstet Gynecol Reprod Biol. 1991;40:149–52.
45. Rahimi G, Relleke S, Mallmann P, Nawroth F. Course of pregnancy and birth in a patient with Bernard-Soulier syndrome: a case report. J Perinat Med. 2005;33(3):264–6.
46. Kotelko DM. Anaesthesia for caesarean delivery in a patient with May-Hegglin anomaly. Can J Anaesth. 1989;36:328–30.
47. Fishman EB, Connors JM, Camann WR. Anesthetic management of seven deliveries in three sisters with the May-Hegglin anomaly. Anesth Analg. 2009;108:1603–5.
48. Laskey AL, Tobias JD. Anesthetic implications of the grey platelet syndrome. Can J Anaesth. 2000;47:1224–9.
49. Burrows RF, Hunter DJF, Andrew M, Kelton JG. A prospective study investigating the mechanisms of thrombocytopenia in preeclampsia. Obstet Gynecol. 1987;70:334–8.
50. Barker P, Callander CC. Coagulation screening before epidural analgesia in preeclampsia. Anaesthesia. 1991;46:64–7.
51. Kelton JG, Hunter DJ, Neame PB. A platelet function defect in preeclampsia. Obstet Gynecol. 1985;65:107–9.
52. Schindler M, Gatt S, Isert P, Morgans D, Cheung A. Thrombocytopenia and platelet functional defects in pre-eclampsia: implications for regional anaesthesia. Anaesth Intensive Care. 1990;18:169–74.
53. Channing Rodgers RP, Levin J. A critical reappraisal of bleeding time. Semin Thromb Hemost. 1990;16:1–20.
54. Wong C, Liu S, Glassenberg R. Comparison of thromboelastography with common coagulation tests in preeclamptic and healthy parturients. Reg Anesth Pain Med. 1995;20:521–7.
55. Orlikowski CEP, Roake DA, Murray WB, Gouws E, Moodley J, Kenoyer DG, Byrne S. Thromboelastography changes in pre-eclampsia and eclampsia. Br J Anaesth. 1996;77:157–61.
56. Beilin Y, Arnold I, Hossain S. Evaluation of the platelet function analyzer (PFA-100) vs. the thromboelastogram (TEG) in the parturient. Int J Obstet Anesth. 2006;15:7–12.
57. Wallace DH, Leveno KJ, Cunningham FG, Giesecke AH, Shearer VE, Sidawi JE. Randomized comparison of general and regional anesthesia for caesarean delivery in pregnancies complicated by severe pre-eclampsia. Obstet Gynecol. 1995;86(2):193–9.
58. Norris LA, Gleeson N, Sheppard BL, Bonnar J. Whole blood platelet aggregation in moderate and severe pre-eclampsia. Br J Obstet Gynaecol. 1993;100:684–8.
59. Woo L, Sinah P, Lewis M. Central nerve block and coagulation: a survey of obstetric anaesthetists. Int J Obstet Anesth. 2002;11:170–5.
60. Lucas MJ, Sharma BK, McIntire DD, Wiley J, Sidawi JE, Ramin SM, Leveno KJ, Cunningham FG. A randomized trail of labor analgesia in women with pregnancy-induced hypertension. Am J Obstet Gynecol. 2001;185:970–5.
61. Jouppila P, Jouppila R, Hollmen A, Koivula A. Lumbar epidural analgesia to improve intervillous blood flow during labor in severe preeclampsia. Obstet Gynecol. 1982;59(2):158–61.
62. Newsome LR, Bramwell RS, Curling PE. Severe preeclampsia: hemodynamic effects of lumbar epidural anesthesia. Anesth Analg. 1986;65:31–6.
63. Ramos-Santos E, Devoe LD, Lawrence D, Wakefield ML, Sherline DM, Metheny WP. The effects of epidural anesthesia on the Doppler velocimetry of umbilical and uterine arteries in normal and hypertensive patients during active term labor. Obstet Gynecol. 1991;77(1):20–6.

64. Hodgkinson R, Farkhana JH, Hayashi R. Systemic and pulmonary blood pressure during caesarean section in parturients with gestational hypertension. Can J Anaesth. 1980;27(4):389–94.
65. Hawkins JL, Koonin LM, Palmer SK, Gibbs CP. Anaesthesia related deaths during obstetric delivery in the United States: 1979–1990. Anesthesiology. 1997;86(2):277–84.
66. Chi C, Kadir RA. Management of women with inherited bleeding disorders in pregnancy. Obstetrician Gynaecologist. 2007;9(1):27–33.
67. Dhar P, Abramovitz S, DiMichele D, Gibb CB, Gadalla F. Management of pregnancy in a patient with severe haemophilia A. Br J Anaesth. 2003;91(3):432–5.
68. Vandermeulen EP, Van Aken H, Vermylen J. Anticoagulants and spinal-epidural anesthesia. Anesth Analg. 1994;79:1165–77.
69. Milaskiewicz RM, Holdcroft A, Letsky E. Epidural anaesthesia and von Willebrand's disease. Anaesthesia. 1990;45(6):462–4.
70. Kadir RA, Economides DL, Braithwaite J, Goldman E, Lee CA. The obstetric experience of carriers of haemophilia. Br J Obstet Gynaecol. 1997;104:803–10.
71. Cohen S, Zada Y. Neuraxial block for von Willebrand's disease (Letter). Anaesthesia. 2001;56:397.
72. Chi C, Lee CA, England D, Hingorani J, Paintsil J, Kadir RA. Obstetric analgesia and anaesthesia in women with inherited bleeding disorders. Thromb Haemost. 2009;101(6):1104–11.
73. Singh A, Harnett MJ, Connors JM, Camann WR. Factor XI deficiency and obstetrical anesthesia. Anesth Analg. 2009;108(6):1882–5.
74. Inamoto Y, Terao T. First report of case of congenital afibrinogenemia with successful delivery. Am J Obstet Gynecol. 1985;153:803–4.
75. Trehan AK, Fergusson IL. Congenital afibrinogenemia and successful pregnancy outcome. Case report. Br J Obstet Gynaecol. 1991;98:722–4.
76. Meldrum DJ, Evans G, Popham P. Spinal anaesthesia and dysfibrinogenemia. Int J Obstet Anesth. 2001;10:64–7.
77. Girolami A, Scandellari R, Lombardi AM. Pregnancy and oral contraceptives in factor V deficiency: a study of 22 patients (5 homozygotes and 17 heterozygotes) and review of the literature. Haemophilia. 2005;11:26–30.
78. Collins PW. Therapeutic challenges in acquired factor VIII deficiency. Hematology Am Soc Hematol Educ Program. 2012;2012:369–74.
79. Sprung J, Cheng EY, Patel S. When to remove an epidural catheter in a parturient with disseminated intravascular coagulation. Reg Anesth. 1992;17:351.
80. Okuda Y, Kitajima T. Epidural haematoma in a parturient who developed disseminated intravascular coagulation after spinal anesthesia. Reg Anesth Pain Med. 2001;26:383.
81. Castro MA, Fassett MJ, Reynolds TB, Shaw KJ, Goodwin TM. Reversible peripartum liver failure: a new perspective on the diagnosis, treatment and cause of acute fatty liver of pregnancy based on 28 consecutive cases. Am J Obstet Gynecol. 1999;181:389–95.
82. Gregory TL, Hughes S, Coleman MA, De Silva A. Acute fatty liver of pregnancy; three cases and discussion of analgesia and anaesthesia. Int J Obstet Anesth. 2007;16:175–9.
83. Antognini JF, Andrews S. Anaesthesia for caesarean section in a patient with acute fatty liver of pregnancy. Can J Anaesth. 1991;38:904–7.
84. Servin F, Cockshott ID, Farinotti R, Haberer JP, Winckler C, Desmonts JM. Pharmacokinetics of propofol infusions in patients with cirrhosis. Br J Anaesth. 1990;65:177–83.
85. Barton JR, Sibai BM. Diagnosis and management of hemolysis, elevated liver enzymes, and low platelets syndrome. Clin Perinatol. 2004;31(4):807–33, vii. Review.
86. Vigil-De Garcia P, Silva S, Montufar C, Carrol I, De Los Rios S. Anesthesia in pregnant women with HELLP syndrome. Int J Obstet Anesth. 2001;74:23–7.
87. O'Brien JM, Shumate SA, Satchwell SL, Milligan DA, Barton JR. Maternal benefit of corticosteroid therapy in patients with HELLP (hemolysis, elevated liver enzymes, and low platelet count) syndrome: impact on the rate of anesthesia. Am J Obstet Gynecol. 2002;186:475–9.
88. Rose CH, Thigpen BD, Bofill JA, Cushman J, May WL, Martin JN. Obstetric implications of the antepartum corticosteroid therapy for HELLP syndrome. Obstet Gynecol. 2004;104:1011–4.
89. Johnson GD, Rosale JK. The haemolytic uraemic syndrome and anesthesia. Can J Anaesth. 1987;34:196–9.
90. Pivalizza EG. Anesthetic management of a patient with thrombotic thrombocytopenic purpura. Anesth Analg. 1994;79:1203–5.
91. Kato R, Shinohara A, Sato J. ADAMTS13 deficiency, an important cause of thrombocytopenia during pregnancy. Int J Obstet Anesth. 2009;18:73–7.
92. Scully M, Hunt BJ, Benjamin S, Liesner R, Rose P, Peyvandi F, et al. British Committee for Standards in Haematology: Guidelines on the diagnosis and management of thrombotic thrombocytopenic purpura and other thrombotic microangiopathies. Br J Haematol. 2012;158:323–35.
93. Roderick P, Ferris G, Wilson K, Halls H, Jackson D, Collins R, Baigent C. Towards evidence-based guidelines for the prevention of venous thromboembolism: systematic reviews of mechanical methods, oral anticoagulation, dextran and regional anaesthesia as thromboprophylaxis. Health Technol Assess. 2005;9:1–78.
94. Langesaeter E, Dragsund M, Rosseland LA. Regional anaesthesia for a Caesarean section in women with cardiac disease. A prospective study. Acta Anaesthesiol Scand. 2010;54(1):46–54.
95. Schroeder DR. Statistics: detecting a rare adverse drug reaction using spontaneous reports. Reg Anesth Pain Med. 1998;23:183–9.

96. Gogarten W, Van Aken H, Wulf H, Klose R, Vandermeulen E, Harenberg J. Regional anesthesia and thromboembolism prophylaxis/anticoagulation. Guidelines of the German Society of Anesthesiology and Intensive Care Medicine (DGAI). Anasthesiol Intensivmed. 1997;12:623–8 [Article in German].
97. Horlocker TT, Wedel DJ. Anticoagulation and neuraxial block: historical perspective, anesthetic implications, and risk management. Reg Anesth Pain Med. 1998;23:129–34.
98. Horlocker TT, Wedel DJ, Rowlingson JC, Enneking FK, Kopp SL, Benzon HT, et al. Regional anesthesia in the patient receiving antithrombotic or thrombolytic therapy: American Society of regional Anesthesia and Pain Medicine Evidence-Based Guidelines (Third Edition). Reg Anesth Pain Med. 2010;35(1):54–101.
99. Gogarten W, Vandermeulen E, Van Aken H, Kozek S, et al. Regional anaesthesia and antithrombotic agents: recommendations of the European Society of Anaesthesiology. Eur J Anaesthesiol. 2010;27:999–1015.
100. Moen V, Dahlgren N, Irestedt L. Severe neurological complications after central neuraxial blockades in Sweden 1990–1999. Anesthesiology. 2004;101:950–9.
101. Paige JT, Gouda BP, Gaitor-Stampley V, Scalla PG, Klainer TE, et al. No correlation between anti-factor Xa levels, low-molecular-weight heparin, and bleeding after gastric bypass. Surg Obes Relat Dis. 2007;3(4):469–75.
102. Keam SJ, Goa KL. Fondaparinux sodium. Drugs. 2002;62(11):1673–85; discussion 1686–7.
103. Samama MM, Gerotziafas GT. Evaluation of the pharmacological properties and clinical results of the synthetic pentasaccharide (fondaparinux). Thromb Res. 2003;109(1):1–11.
104. Tagaloa LA, Carvalho B. Epidural labour analgesia n a patient receiving fondaparinux. Int J Obstet Anesth. 2009;18(1):94–5.
105. Ekbatani A, Asaro LR, Malinow AM. Anticoagulation with argatroban in a patient with heparin-induced thrombocytopenia. Int J Obstet Anesth. 2010;19(1):82–7.
106. Markwardt F, Fink G, Kaiser B, Klöcking HP, Nowak G, Richter M, Stürzebecher J. Pharmacological survey of recombinant hirudin. Pharmazie. 1988;43:202–7.
107. Huhle G, Geberth M, Hoffmann U, Heene DL, Harenberg J. Management of heparin-associated thrombocytopenis in pregnancy with subcutaneous r-hirudin. Gynecol Obstet Invest. 2000;49:67–9.
108. Aijaz A, Nelson J, Naseer N. Management of heparin allergy in pregnancy. Am J Hematol. 2001;67:268–9.
109. Chapman ML, Martinez-Borges AR, Mertz HL. Lepirudin for treatment of acute thrombosis during pregnancy. Obstet Gynecol. 2008;112:432–3.
110. Pradaxa® 75 mg, 110 mg and 150 mg hard capsules. Boehringer-Ingelheim. Summary of Product Characteristics (SPC). The electronic medicines compendium. 2013. Available from: https://www.medicines.org.uk
111. Xarelto® 10 mg, 15 and 20 mg film coated tablets. Bayer HealthCare AG. Summary of Product Characteristics (SPC). The electronic medicines compendium. 2013. Available from: https://www.medicines.org.uk
112. Eliquis® 5 mg film-coated tablets. Bristol-Myers Squibb-Pfizer. Summary of Product Characteristics (SPC). The electronic medicines compendium. 2013. Available from: https://www.medicines.org.uk
113. Eriksson BI, Borris LC, Friedman RJ, Haas S, Huisman MV, Kakkar AK, et al. RECORD1 Study Group. Rivaroxaban versus enoxaparin for thromboprophylaxis after hip arthroplasty. N Eng J Med. 2008;358(26):2765–75.
114. Eriksson BI, Dahl OE, Rosencher N, Kurth AA, van Dijk CN, Frostick SP, et al. RE-MODEL Study Group. Oral dabigatran etexilate vs. subcutaneous enoxaparin for the prevention of venous thromboembolism after knee replacement: the RE-MODEL randomized trial. J Thromb Haemost. 2007;5(11):2178–85.
115. CLASP: a randomised trial of low-dose aspirin for the prevention and treatment of pre-eclampsia among 9364 pregnant women. CLASP (Collaborative Low-dose Aspirin Study in Pregnancy) Collaborative Group. Lancet. 1994;343(8898):619–29.
116. Horlocker TT, Wedel DJ, Schroeder DR, Rose SH, Elliott BA, McGregor DG, Wong GY. Preoperative antiplatelet therapy does not increase the risk of spinal hematoma associated with regional anesthesia. Anesth Analg. 1995;80(2):303–9.
117. Horlocker TT, Bajwa ZH, Ashraf Z, Khan S, Wilson JL, Sami N, et al. Risk assessment of hemorrhagic complications associated with nonsteroidal antiinflammatory medications in ambulatory pain clinic patients undergoing epidural steroid injection. Anesth Analg. 2002;95(6):1691–7.
118. Beighton P, De Paepe A, Steinmann B, Tsipouras P, Wenstrup RJ. Ehlers-Danlos syndromes: revised nosology, Villefranche, 1997. Ehlers-Danlos National Foundation (USA) and Ehlers-Danlos Support Group (UK). Am J Med Genet. 1998;77(1):31–7.
119. Pyeritz RE. Ehlers Danlos syndrome. N Engl J Med. 2000;342(10):730–2.
120. Anstey A, Mayne K, Winter M, Van De Pette J, Pope FM. Platelet and coagulation studies in Ehlers-Danlos syndrome. Br J Dermatol. 1991;125(2):155–63.
121. Pepin M, Schwarze U, Superti-Furga A, Byers P. Clinical and genetic features of Ehlers-Danlos Syndrome type IV, the vascular type. N Engl J Med. 2000;342(10):673–80.
122. Jones TL, Ng C. Anaesthesia for caesarean section in a patient with Ehlers-Danlos syndrome associated with postural orthostatic tachycardia syndrome. Int J Obstet Anesth. 2009;17(4):365–9.

123. Dolan P, Sisko F, Riley E. Anesthetic considerations for Ehlers-Danlos syndrome. Anesthesiology. 1980;52(3):266–9.
124. Brighouse D, Guard B. Anaesthesia for caesarean section in a patient with Ehlers-Danlos syndrome type IV. Br J Anaesth. 1992;69(5): 517–9.
125. Dill-Russell P, Jones LS. Anaesthetic for caesarean section in a patient with Ehlers-Danlos syndrome and mitral valve prolapse. Int J Obstet Anesth. 2001;10(3):192–7.
126. Kuczkowski KM, Benumof JL. Cesarean section and Ehlers-Danlos syndrome: choice of anesthesia. Int J Obstet Anesth. 2002;11(3):222–4.
127. Sood V, Robinson DA, Suri I. Difficult intubation during rapid sequence induction in a parturient with Ehlers-Danlos syndrome, hypermobility type. Int J Obstet Anesth. 2009;18(4):408–12.
128. Abouleish E. Obstetric anaesthesia and Ehlers-Danlos syndrome. Br J Anaesth. 1980;52(12):1283–6.
129. Arendt-Nielsen L, Kaalund S, Bjerring P, Hogsaa B. Insufficient effect of local analgesics in Ehlers-Danlos type III patients (connective tissue disorder). Acta Anaesthesiol Scand. 1990;34(5): 358–61.
130. Glynn JC, Yentis SM. Epidural analgesia in a parturient with classic type Ehlers-Danlos syndrome. Int J Obstet Anesth. 2005;14(1):78–9.
131. Kaskos H, Patel N, Bell R. Anaesthetic management and outcome of parturients with hypermobility type Ehlers-Danlos syndrome: a case series (abstract). Int J Obstet Anesth. 2012;21:26.
132. Wroth RP, Alderson JD. The anaesthetic management of a labouring woman with pulmonary arterio-venous malformations. Int J Obstet Anesth. 1996;5(4):278–82.
133. El Shobary H, Schricker T, Kaufman I. Anaesthetic management of parturients with hereditary haemorrhagic telangiectasia for caesarean section. Int J Obstet Anesth. 2009;18(2):176–81.
134. Douglas MJ, Gunka VB, von Dadelszen P. Anesthesia for the parturient with pseudoxanthoma elasticum. Int J Obstet Anesth. 2003;12(1):45–7.
135. Youngs PJ, Sice P, Harvey P. Labour analgesia and pseudoxanthoma elasticum (PXE). Int J Obstet Anesth. 2003;12(1):48–50.

The Neonate

22

Vidheya Venkatesh, Anna E. Curley,
and Simon Stanworth

Abstract

The development of the hematological system in the neonate is a complex interplay of genetic, prenatal, intrapartum, gestational age-related, and postnatally acquired factors. Increased survival of neonates at lower limits of gestational age coupled with the dynamic changes in neonatal hematological physiology during the transition from fetus to neonate makes diagnosis and management of disorders of neonatal hemostasis and thrombosis challenging. Thrombocytopenia is one of the commonest neonatal hematological problems encountered, but thromboembolism and coagulation defects also contribute to neonatal morbidity and mortality. This chapter will discuss the principal thrombocytopenic, thrombotic, and hemostatic disorders presenting in a neonatal population.

Keywords

Neonatal • Thrombocytopenia • Thromboembolism • Inherited and acquired coagulation disorders

22.1 Thrombocytopenia

The mean fetal platelet count at the end of the first trimester is 150×10^9/L achieving a high of 175×10^9/L at the end of the second trimester [1–3]. Overall, the prevalence of neonatal thrombocytopenia varies between 1 and 5 % of all infants, and more than 98 % of all term babies have a platelet count of 150×10^9/L or more [4–7]. Thrombocytopenia (platelet count $<150 \times 10^9$/L) affects at least a quarter of all babies admitted to the neonatal unit [8], and 5–10 % of admitted neonates will have severe thrombocytopenia ($<50 \times 10^9$/L) [9]. In a cross-

V. Venkatesh, MB ChB, MRCP, MPhil (✉)
A.E. Curley, MB ChB, MRCP, MD, LLB
Neonatal Intensive Care Unit,
Cambridge University Hospitals NHS Trust,
Hills Road 226, Cambridge CB02QQ, UK
e-mail: vidheya.venkatesh@addenbrookes.nhs.uk;
annacurley@gmail.com

S. Stanworth, BM BCh, BA, DPhil, MRCP
NHS Blood and Transplant, John Radcliffe Hospital,
Oxford University Hospitals NHS Foundation Trust,
Headington Road, Oxford OX3 9BQ, UK
e-mail: simon.stanworth@nhsbt.nhs.uk

H. Cohen, P. O'Brien (eds.), *Disorders of Thrombosis and Hemostasis in Pregnancy: A Guide to Management*, DOI 10.1007/978-3-319-15120-5_22,

Table 22.1 Classification of fetal and neonatal thrombocytopenia

	Condition
Fetal	Alloimmune
	Congenital infection (e.g. CMV, toxoplasma, rubella, HIV) Aneuploidy (e.g. trisomies 13, 18, 21) Autoimmune (e.g. ITP, SLE) Severe rhesus hemolytic disease Inherited (e.g. Wiskott-Aldrich syndrome)
Early-onset neonatal (<72 h)	Chronic fetal hypoxia (e.g. pre-eclampsia, IUGR, diabetes)
	Perinatal asphyxia Perinatal infection (e.g. E. Coli, GBS, Hemophilus influenzae) DIC Alloimmune Autoimmune (e.g. ITP, SLE) Congenital infection (e.g. CMV, toxoplasma, rubella, HIV) Thrombosis (e.g. aortic, renal vein) Bone marrow replacement (e.g. congenital leukemia) Kasabach-Merritt syndrome Metabolic disease (e.g. propionic and methylmalonic acidemia) Inherited (e.g. TAR, CAMT)
Late-onset neonatal (>72 h)	Late-onset sepsis NEC
	Congenital infection (e.g. CMV, toxoplasma, rubella, HIV) Autoimmune Kasabach-Merritt syndrome Metabolic disease (e.g. propionic and methylmalonic acidemia) Inherited (e.g. TAR, CAMT)

Table from Roberts et al. [9]
CMV cytomegalovirus, *HIV* human immunodeficiency virus, *ITP* idiopathic thrombocytopenic purpura, *SLE* systemic lupus erythematosus, *IUGR* intrauterine growth restriction, *E. coli* Escherichia coli, *GBS* group B Streptococcus, *TAR* thrombocytopenia with absent radius syndrome, *CAMT* congenital amegakaryocytic thrombocytopenia, *NEC* necrotizing enterocolitis

sectional observational prospective study, 20 % of babies admitted to the neonatal unit at less than 28 weeks' gestation had a platelet count $<60 \times 10^9$/L [10].

22.1.1 Causes of Thrombocytopenia

Thrombocytopenia can occur during the fetal or early or late postnatal period. Fetal thrombocytopenia can occur as a result of neonatal autoimmune and alloimmune conditions, and is dealt with in Chaps. 11 and 12 respectively. Early-onset thrombocytopenia is most frequently associated with chronic fetal hypoxia secondary to intrauterine growth restriction (IUGR) due to placental insufficiency, pre-eclampsia or maternal diabetes [11, 12]. Typically, such thrombocytopenia is benign and resolves spontaneously within the first 10 days of life [10]. Other causes of fetal-onset/early thrombocytopenia include congenital infections, perinatal bacterial infections, aneuploidies, and perinatal asphyxia (Table 22.1). Inherited thrombocytopenia is rare. The most common causes of late-onset thrombocytopenia are sepsis and necrotizing enterocolitis (NEC), which account for over 80 % of cases [8, 13].

22.1.2 Clinical and Laboratory Features of Thrombocytopenia

22.1.2.1 Alloimmune

Neonatal alloimmune thrombocytopenia (NAIT) constitutes less than 5 % of cases of neonatal thrombocytopenia but is important to exclude due to its associated morbidity and mortality [13], and the requirement for specific platelet transfusion components matched for the alloantibodies. The diagnosis and management of this condition is dealt with in Chap. 16.

22.1.2.2 Congenital Infection

The toxoplasma, rubella, cytomegalovirus, herpes (TORCH) viral infections can cause thrombocytopenia although the exact mechanism is unclear. Parvovirus can also cause thrombocytopenia through suppression of bone marrow and megakaryocyte colony formation [14]. Other viruses known to cause thrombocytopenia include enterovirus, Coxsackie virus, adenovirus, Epstein-Barr virus, and dengue virus. HIV is known to infect megakaryocytes and suppress colony growth [15] and is so frequently associated with neonatal thrombocytopenia that it has been suggested as a screening tool [16].

22.1.2.3 Aneuploidies

Thrombocytopenia is common although rarely severe in the trisomies 18 (86 %), 13 (31 %), and 21 (6 %), as well as in Turner syndrome (31 %) [17]. The mechanism of thrombocytopenia in trisomies 13 and 18 is unknown although it may have its etiology in chronic fetal hypoxia. Thrombocytopenia in trisomy 21 is similar to that seen in growth-restricted infants: neutropenia, polycythemia and increased circulating normoblasts. Ten percent of infants with Down syndrome, however, develop a clonal preleukemic disorder showing increased myeloblasts and variable levels of thrombocytopenia, and 20–30 % of these babies will develop acute megakaryoblastic leukemia within the first 5 years of life [18]. It is thought that trisomy of chromosome 21 disturbs fetal hemopoiesis and predisposes to mutations in the GATA1 gene, a key megakaryocyte/erythroid transcription factor [19].

22.1.2.4 Autoimmune

Autoimmune conditions such as maternal idiopathic thrombocytopenic purpura, which may occur in association with systemic lupus erythematosus, can also cause thrombocytopenia in the fetus and neonate. This is dealt with in Chap. 15.

In addition to anemia, neutropenia and reticulocytosis, thrombocytopenia is common in severe rhesus hemolytic disease, especially after intrauterine or exchange transfusions; this is due to platelet-poor blood product and suppression of platelet production in favor of erythropoiesis.

22.1.2.5 Inherited Thrombocytopenias

These are caused by reduced platelet production due to abnormal hemopoietic stem or progenitor cell development. They may be associated with defective platelet function. Many of these disorders will be diagnosed by their associated congenital anomalies.

Bernard-Soulier Syndrome

This syndrome can lead to fetal or early neonatal thrombocytopenia although severe bleeding is not often seen in neonates. It is characterized by mild thrombocytopenia with giant megakaryocytes. It has an autosomal recessive pattern of inheritance and leads to defects in the glycoprotein 1b-IX-V complex [20, 21], which results in defective platelet adhesion (see Chap. 13). Neonates can develop alloantibodies following platelet transfusions, so transfusions should be restricted to cases of severe hemorrhage.

Wiskott-Aldrich Syndrome and X-Linked Thrombocytopenia

These syndromes form part of a spectrum of disorders caused by a mutation in the WAS protein of the X chromosome [22] which leads to disorders of platelet function and survival. X-linked thrombocytopenia can present in the neonatal period with a mild thrombocytopenia. These conditions are characterized by microthrombocytopenia, eczema, immunodeficiency, and recurrent bacterial and viral infections [23].

22.1.3 Timing of Onset of Thrombocytopenia

22.1.3.1 Early-Onset Thrombocytopenia

Chronic Fetal Hypoxia

Placental insufficiency is associated with early-onset thrombocytopenia in preterm neonates. Impaired delivery of oxygen and essential nutrients is implicated in its development. Platelets are initially produced in the fetal liver, with production transferred to the bone marrow in the third trimester [11]. In hypoxia, blood flow to the liver falls. Previous studies have also demonstrated a reduction in circulating megakaryocyte progenitors, suggesting decreased platelet production as a cause [11, 12, 14]. Typically, thrombocytopenia is mild to moderate and self-limiting, resolving in the majority of cases before 10 days of age [12]. Additional hematological abnormalities which can help to confirm growth restriction and hypoxia as causative factors include transient neutropenia, increased circulating nucleated red cells, and evidence of hyposplenism (spherocytes, target cells, and Howell-Jolly bodies) [12, 24].

Perinatal Asphyxia

Thrombocytopenia can occur after perinatal asphyxia as a result of bone marrow suppression and reduced platelet production. Asphyxia-related liver dysfunction also causes decreased production of coagulation factors. Increased consumption of platelets often follows severe acidosis, hypoxia, and endothelial damage and disseminated intravascular coagulation (DIC).

Perinatal Infection

Group B streptococcus (GBS) and gram-negative enteric organisms (predominantly *Escherichia coli*) account for 70 % of early-onset sepsis. Non-typeable Haemophilus influenzae sepsis has been increasingly identified in neonates, particularly those that are premature. Other gram-negative enteric bacilli such as *Klebsiella* sp. and gram-positive organisms such as Listeria monocytogenes, enterococci, group D streptococci, α-hemolytic streptococci, and staphylococci have also been implicated. The thrombocytopenia in sepsis is most likely due to increased platelet destruction; platelet levels drop quickly after onset of symptoms of infection [25, 26]. The mean duration of thrombocytopenia is 5–6 days [25, 26]. Platelet transfusions given to septic infants have a shortened life span [26].

Thrombotic Disorders

Thrombotic thrombocytopenic purpura (TTP), hemolytic-uremic syndrome (HUS), and heparin-induced thrombocytopenia (HIT) have all been reported in neonates [27–29]. Thrombocytopenia may also occur secondary to thrombosis of a major vessel.

Bone Marrow Infiltration

Congenital leukemia, osteopetrosis, and histiocytoses can also cause thrombocytopenia secondary to bone marrow infiltration.

Kasabach-Merritt Syndrome

Thrombocytopenia in this condition is associated with sequestration of platelets on the endothelium of hemangiomas, either cutaneous (80 %) or visceral [30]. Thrombocytopenia may be associated with DIC and microangiopathic anemia. Treatment options include corticosteroids, antifibrinolytic agents (e-aminocaproic acid and tranexamic acid), interferon alpha-2a, cytotoxic chemotherapy, intralesional steroids, embolization, and laser therapy.

Metabolic Disease

The organic acidemias, propionic, methylmalonic, and isovaleryl academia, can also present with neonatal thrombocytopenia and neutropenia, mimicking neonatal sepsis [31]. The clinical finding is of a healthy newborn at birth that rapidly becomes ill after the first day of life. Urine organic acid analysis is diagnostic.

Lysosomal storage diseases such as Gaucher's disease can also present with thrombocytopenia [32]. These disorders are characterized by mutations in one of a series of enzymes involved in the degradation of glycosphingolipids. Patients can present with hepatosplenomegaly, cardiomyopathy, renal dysfunction, anemia, thrombocytopenia, and neurological degeneration. Thrombocytopenia associated with splenomegaly may also be secondary to infiltrative metabolic disorders such as the mucolipidoses and mucopolysaccharidoses.

Inherited Disorders

Inherited disorders typically presenting in the early to late neonatal period with variable severity of onset include Bernard-Soulier syndrome, X-linked thrombocytopenia, thrombocytopenia-absent radius syndrome, amegakaryocytic thrombocytopenia with radioulnar synostosis, and congenital amegakaryocytic thrombocytopenia.

Fanconi anemia is characterized by short stature, skeletal anomalies, increased incidence of solid tumors and leukemias, and aplastic anemia. It is rare to present with thrombocytopenia in the neonatal period although it should be considered in the presence of dysmorphic features and unexplained thrombocytopenia. The diepoxybutane test is almost always diagnostic of this disorder [33].

Thrombocytopenia-Absent Radius (TAR) Syndrome

Thrombocytopenia-absent radius (TAR) syndrome is a rare autosomal recessive condition in which thrombocytopenia is associated with bilateral radial aplasia, although thumbs may be present and normal. It can also be associated with lower limb abnormalities (47 %), renal anomalies (27 %) and cardiac defects (15 %) [34]. Episodes of thrombocytopenia begin in the neonatal period, and around 50 % of affected infants are symptomatic (showing evidence of bleeding) in the first week of life, with a further 40 % becoming symptomatic by the age of 4 months [35]. The platelet count improves spontaneously after the first year of life. The therapy of TAR syndrome is supportive with platelet transfusions for hemorrhage, red cell transfusions for anemia, and avoidance of stressors, such as cow's milk, which may induce thrombocytopenia.

Amegakaryocytic thrombocytopenia with radioulnar synostosis (ATRUS) is caused by mutations in the HOXA11 gene and is characterized by severe thrombocytopenia from birth, radioulnar synostosis, clinodactyly, and shallow acetabula [36].

Congenital amegakaryocytic thrombocytopenia (CAMT) is an autosomal recessive condition that almost always presents early in the neonatal period with severe thrombocytopenia; 50 % of affected infants will have evidence of bleeding [37]. Although there is isolated thrombocytopenia in the newborn period, 50 % will go on to develop aplastic anemia in childhood. Stem cell transplantation is curative in cases of severe disease [38].

22.1.3.2 Late-Onset Thrombocytopenia

Thrombocytopenia occurring after 72 h of age is due to sepsis or NEC in more than 80 % of cases [14].

Late-Onset Sepsis

The vast majority of late-onset infections are caused by gram-positive organisms, with coagulase-negative staphylococci accounting for almost half of infections [39]. The rate of infection is inversely related to birthweight and gestational age. Candida species are increasingly important causes of late-onset sepsis, occurring in 12 % of very low birthweight infants [40]. Thrombocytopenia occurs in 79–100 % of these infants [41, 42]. In late-onset sepsis, thrombocytopenia is often more severe ($<30\times10^9$/L) and of rapid onset, and can take several weeks to resolve [8].

Necrotizing Enterocolitis

This is the most common neonatal gastrointestinal illness, affecting predominantly preterm infants (90 % of cases occur in premature infants). Surgery is required in 20–60 %, and there is a mortality rate of 20–28 % [42]. In one study, 90 % of infants with NEC had thrombocytopenia ($<150\times10^9$/L), with 55 % of these infants having platelet counts below 50×10^9/L [43]. Within the group with severe thrombocytopenia, 55 % had severe bleeding complications. Severe thrombocytopenia had an 89 % positive predictive value for intestinal gangrene in one study [44]. The most likely reason for low platelets is increased platelet destruction although there may be suppression of platelet production by pro-inflammatory cytokines.

22.1.4 Treatment of Neonatal Thrombocytopenia

Neonatal thrombocytopenia and bleeding are common and important clinical problems for preterm neonates. The main specific treatment for thrombocytopenia in the neonate is platelet transfusion, but intravenous immunoglobulin (IVIg) may be used for maternal ITP-associated thrombocytopenia. Current national guidance recommends platelet transfusion thresholds of $20–30 \times 10^9/L$ and $50 \times 10^9/L$ for neonates depending on the clinical situation [45], but policies and protocols for neonatal platelet transfusion therapy vary widely among clinicians and institutions [46, 47]. This variation reflects the generally broad nature of recommendations in national guidelines, which themselves are based largely on consensus rather than evidence, and often extrapolated from data on adults [48, 49].

Platelet transfusions are frequently used in modern neonatal clinical practice as prophylaxis in thrombocytopenic neonates [49]. Previous studies estimate that 25 % of neonates and 50 % of extremely low birthweight neonates whose platelet counts fall below $150 \times 10^9/L$ receive one or more transfusions [50, 51]. In the only randomized controlled trial to assess a threshold level for the effectiveness of neonatal prophylactic platelet transfusions, moderate thrombocytopenia ($50–150 \times 10^9/L$) was not detrimental to short-term neonatal outcome. However, neonates with severe thrombocytopenia (platelet count less than $50 \times 10^9/L$) were excluded from the study because of their perceived high risk of hemorrhage [52]. Benefits of transfusion need to be weighed against possible risks.

22.1.5 Conclusions

The most common cause of early thrombocytopenia in neonates is chronic hypoxia. NAIT accounts for less than 5 % of all cases of neonatal thrombocytopenia. Sepsis and NEC account for more than 80 % of the late-onset thrombocytopenia. Inherited causes of thrombocytopenia are rare. Infants with severe thrombocytopenia and evidence of bleeding should receive platelets, but the role of prophylactic platelets in the neonate with asymptomatic thrombocytopenia is unclear.

Key Learning Points

- The underlying cause of thrombocytopenia is predicted by the timing of onset.
- Chronic fetal hypoxia is the most common cause of early-onset thrombocytopenia and is mild and self-limiting.
- Sepsis and/or NEC is the most common cause of late-onset thrombocytopenia.
- Bleeding risk is greater in NAIT than in sepsis/NEC and greater in sepsis/NEC than in chronic fetal hypoxia.
- The role of prophylactic platelet transfusions and the optimal platelet count thresholds are not known.

22.2 Neonatal Thromboembolism

22.2.1 Introduction

Neonatal thromboembolism is a rare but increasingly reported condition in the neonatal unit that can cause significant neonatal mortality and morbidity. Ninety percent of thromboembolism is associated with thrombosis of arterial or venous catheters and central venous lines, but stroke is also prevalent, and the incidence of perinatal stroke ranks second only to the strokes of the elderly population (1 in 2,300 to 1 in 5,000 births) [53].

22.2.2 Etiology of Neonatal Thromboembolism

Idiopathic thromboembolism accounts for less than 1 % of cases of newborn thromboembolism as compared to 40 % in the adult population [54]. Usually at least one risk factor can be identified, either maternal or fetal, including maternal diabetes or SLE with antiphospholipid syndrome, pre-eclampsia, IUGR, maternal autoimmune conditions, maternal thrombophilia, placental vasculopathy, infection, hypovolemia, dehydration, hypoxia, acidosis, and neonatal prothrombotic disorders [55–62].

The prothrombotic disorders that have been linked with neonatal thromboembolism include deficiencies in protein C, protein S, antithrombin, and plasminogen [63–66]. Homozygous deficiencies of these factors usually present with severe clinical symptoms and require urgent management. However, diagnosing heterozygous states can be difficult in the neonate because physiological values are lower than in older children and adults [67]. Diagnosis can also be complicated by the coexistence of acquired disorders – present in over 80 % of newborns with systemic thromboembolism [68]. Of note, homozygous plasminogen deficiency is associated with ligneous conjunctivitis, and in some cases with occlusive hydrocephalus [66], the pathogenesis of which is unclear. Both homozygous and heterozygous plasminogen deficiency do not appear to be associated with spontaneous thrombotic events, although repeated thrombotic occlusion of implanted catheters has been described [66, 69, 70]. It has been suggested that patients with heterozygous type I plasminogen deficiency who develop thrombosis may have additional risk factors such as deficiency or protein C or S or antithrombin deficiencies [70].

The clinical presentation of homozygous protein C deficiency in the neonatal period is purpura fulminans, cerebral stroke, and/or large-vessel thrombosis. The diagnosis is confirmed in the presence of these clinical features with an undetectable protein C level and both parents testing as heterozygotes for protein C deficiency. Heterozygous protein C deficiency does not normally present with thrombosis in early infancy [71], but cohort studies have indicated an increased prevalence of protein C heterozygosity in neonates with thromboembolism and additional risk factors [72]. Babies with homozygous protein S deficiency also present with purpura fulminans, but like protein C deficiency, the heterozygous state is only uncommonly associated with thromboembolic phenomena in infancy or childhood [73]. Homozygous antithrombin (AT) deficiency, where levels are less than 10 % of normal, is rare but can be associated with severe thromboembolic events, venous or arterial [74]. Heterozygous AT deficiency is associated with diverse but less severe thrombotic events.

The presence of Factor V Leiden or the prothrombin G20210A mutation have also been linked to neonatal thromboembolism [61, 62, 75, 76]. Approximately 5 % of Caucasians are heterozygous for the factor V Leiden mutation (R506Q) at the cleavage site for activated protein C (APC), which decreases the rate of inactivation of factor V, leading to a reduced anticoagulant effect of APC (APC resistance [77]); and 2 % for the prothrombin G20210A mutation, that is associated with increased prothrombin levels possibly due to increased mRNA stability [78]. A homozygous polymorphism in the C677T methylene tetrahydrofolate reductase (MTHFR) gene has been linked to an increased thrombotic risk in infants with perinatal arterial stroke [79]. Homozygosity for this polymorphism, in the presence of folate deficiency, may predispose to hyperhomocystinaemia, with the phenotypic expression silenced by folic acid supplementation. An elevated homocysteine level has also been associated with an increased thrombotic risk [80], but the contribution of these risk factors to neonatal thrombosis is unclear.

22.2.3 Clinical Presentation

22.2.3.1 Thrombosis Following Umbilical Catheterization

Studies have identified central venous lines as an important risk factor for neonatal thrombosis [81]. Clinical studies have shown an incidence of 13 % [82] and autopsy studies a 20–65 % incidence of venous thromboembolism in infants with an umbilical venous catheter (UVC) in situ [83, 84]. UVCs have been associated particularly with portal venous thrombosis. Major venous thrombosis due to umbilical artery catheters (UAC) occurs in 1–3 % of all infants [85]. High position of the UAC (UAC tip between T6–T10) may be associated with fewer complications compared to low position (UAC tip L3–L5) [86].

Many factors contribute to catheter-related thrombosis, including vessel caliber, blood flow, and catheter type. Use of a heparin infusion [87] or heparin-bonded lines [88] prolongs the duration of catheter patency but has not been shown to alter the rate of catheter-related thrombus. In order to reduce the incidence of catheter-related thrombosis, catheter use should be restricted to those situations in which it is truly necessary.

The majority of babies with UAC-related thrombosis remain asymptomatic, but some babies can show evidence of loss of patency of the catheter, limb ischemia, and NEC secondary to mesenteric artery occlusion, or hypertension secondary to renal artery occlusion. Contrast angiography is the gold standard diagnostic method but rarely available in neonates. Ultrasound may not pick up all cases of arterial obstruction [89]. Long-term morbidity can include hypertension, impaired renal function and paraplegia.

Clinical features of venous catheter-related thromboembolism include loss of central venous line patency, venous congestion, and/or discoloration of the limbs. Superior vena caval obstruction leads to facial and venous congestion of the upper chest. Pulmonary thromboembolism presents with respiratory compromise. Long-term complications of thromboembolism include prominent collateral circulation, catheter-related sepsis, chylothorax, portal hypertension, and post-thrombotic syndrome.

22.2.3.2 Renal Vein Thrombosis

Renal vein thrombosis is the most common non-catheter-related thromboembolism in neonates and is responsible for around 10 % of all thromboembolism. It is commonest in the first week of life, and almost 80 % of all renal vein thromboses occur in the first month of life [90, 91]. Reduced renal blood flow, increased blood viscosity, hyperosmolarity, hypercoagulability due to perinatal asphyxia, polycythemia, dehydration, septicemia, and maternal diabetes have been suggested as possible pathophysiological mechanisms. Newborns usually present with hematuria, proteinuria and a flank mass. Bilateral renal vein thrombosis is present in 24 % of newborns [92]. Ultrasound is the diagnostic method of choice. There are no recent studies on long-term morbidity of this condition.

22.2.3.3 Perinatal Stroke

Perinatal ischemic stroke is defined as "a group of heterogeneous conditions in which there is a focal disruption of cerebral blood flow secondary to arterial or venous embolization between 20 weeks of fetal life and the 28th day of postnatal life, confirmed by neuroimaging or neuropathologic studies" [93]. The incidence of ischemic perinatal stroke is 0.25–1 infants per 1,000 live births and accounts for 30 % of all children with hemiplegic cerebral palsy born at term or late preterm [53, 55, 94].

Early neonatal stroke typically presents in the first 3 days and can occur as a result of placental embolism, infection, birth trauma, or hypoxic ischemic encephalopathy (HIE). Late neonatal stroke occurs between 4 and 28 days of age and can be secondary to infection, cardiac disease, or venous thrombosis with paradoxical embolism. Neonates with stroke may present with focal or generalized neonatal seizures, or with non-specific features such as apnea, poor feeding, irritability, abnormalities in tone, or cyanosis. The differential diagnosis includes kernicterus, bacterial and viral encephalitis, mitochondrial disorders, tumors, or hypoglycemia.

Several classifications of neonatal stroke have been suggested, based either on distribution of these events [95] or on the proposed underlying etiological mechanism [96]. In the neonatal period, two common subtypes of stroke are arterial ischemic stroke (AIS) and cerebral sinovenous thrombosis. In AIS it is thought that emboli originating in the placenta pass through the foramen ovale and occlude the intracerebral vessel. Neonatal AIS is characterized by documented complete or incomplete occlusion of an intracerebral vessel causing a focal lesion in the brain, or a documented lesion that can be explained only by occlusion of a particular vessel [97]. Studies have shown that middle cerebral artery infarction accounted for between 50 and 83 % of focal events [95].

Sinovenous thrombosis accounted for 45 % of all neonatal stroke cases registered in the Canadian registry, with an incidence of 41 per 100,000 births [53]. Risk factors such as maternal diabetes, hypertension, infection, asphyxia, complicated delivery, and congenital cardiac disorders have been commonly identified [98].

Additional forms of vaso-occlusive ischemic events unique to the perinatal period are periventricular venous infarction and presumed fetal stroke detected in later infancy. Less common types of neonatal stroke are multifocal infarctions, subcortical infarctions, and infarctions caused by meningitis, thrombophilia, and arteriopathy. Maternal cocaine abuse has also been associated with cortical infarction in up to 17 % of exposed infants [99].

Neuroimaging remains the mainstay in the diagnosis of stroke. Cranial ultrasound may miss the cerebral ischemic lesions, in particular more anterior or posterior lesions [100, 101]. Appropriately timed conventional T2-weighted magnetic resonance imaging (MRI), diffusion-weighted imaging, and magnetic resonance angiography remain the principal methods of diagnosing neonatal stroke [102, 103]. Infants diagnosed with stroke should be investigated for thrombophilia.

Outcome data vary but, overall, neurological deficits or epilepsy occur in two thirds of survivors of acute ischemic stroke, with sensori-motor deficit being the most common. Lesions involving the motor cortex, basal ganglia, and internal capsule together are more likely to be associated with motor disability than lesions limited to the cortex or basal ganglia alone [104]. Seizure disorders have been shown to occur in 15 % of long-term survivors of AIS [82]. However, fewer than 5 % of neonates with AIS have recurrent systemic or cerebral thrombosis [53]. A follow-up study of survivors of cerebral sino-venous thrombosis showed that, in contrast to AIS, 77 % of survivors had no neurological sequelae [105].

22.2.4 Treatment of Neonatal Thrombosis

Treatment options for neonatal thrombosis include supportive care, anticoagulation and thrombolysis. In the past, clinicians have been reluctant to use anticoagulant therapy in neonates due to the possible risks of bleeding. The German registry of neonatal thrombosis reported rates of major hemorrhage of 2 % for heparin anticoagulation and 15 % for thrombolysis [90]. The American College of Chest Physicians (ACCP) guidelines suggest that where possible, pediatric hematologists with experience in thromboembolism manage pediatric patients with thromboembolism; and when this is not possible, a combination of a neonatologist/pediatrician and adult hematologist supported by consultation with an experienced pediatric haematologist [106].

Possible anticoagulants for use in neonates include unfractionated heparin (UFH), low molecular weight heparin (LMWH). However, target therapeutic ranges are based on adult rather than neonatal ranges. Neonates often require high doses of UFH to maintain the target therapeutic range; this is because of physiologically decreased levels of antithrombin, increased volume of distribution, rapid heparin clearance, and non-specific protein binding in plasma [107, 108]. Advantages of LMWH in this population relates mostly to its subcutaneous administration and reduced requirement for monitoring compared with UFH, particularly given that venous access is often limited in infants. There is limited dosing data regarding LMWH use in neonates. Small pharmacokinetic studies of enoxaparin and dalteparin in pediatric patients demonstrate wide ranges of dose requirements, with neonates requiring the highest doses [109–111]. The majority of neonates reach a therapeutic anti-Xa activity level using 1.625 mg/kg/dose. Anti-Xa activity levels effectively monitor LMWH therapy in neonates [112].

Thrombolytic therapy should be considered for neonates with acute thrombosis, such as aortic, atrial or peripheral arterial thrombosis, that is life-threatening or that could potentially lead to loss of a limb, that presents within 2 weeks of symptomatic onset. Thrombolytic agents can be administered systemically or locally. Systemic thrombolysis avoids the requirement for interventional radiologic procedures (often challenging in small children), a requirement for anesthesia, and the delay to therapy potentially encumbered during the organization of local invasive thrombolysis. Higher-dose recombinant tissue plasminogen activator (rt-PA, alteplase) (0.1–0.5 mg/kg/h) in short courses of 6–48 h are generally chosen for arterial clots and can also be used for venous thrombi. Low-dose (0.03–0.06 mg/kg/h) longer duration systemic infusions of t-PA for 12–96 h have been shown to be effective for lysis of venous thrombi [112–114]. Coagulation screening tests including PT, APTT, fibrinogen, plasminogen and D-dimer or FDP levels, should be monitored during therapy to ensure hemostatic levels of platelets and fibrinogen and to determine baseline fibrinolytic potential (plasminogen concentration) and activation (D-dimer levels). The therapeutic action of t-PA requires plasminogen and therefore its effect may be improved by the administration of fresh frozen plasma (FFP) 10 mL/kg daily for plasminogen concentrations less than 50 %. Infusions of thrombolytic agents should be discontinued as soon as clot lysis has been achieved, as there is no potential for further improvement and bleeding complications increase with increasing dose and duration of thrombolytic therapy. Therefore repeated imaging should be undertaken. In addition, cranial ultrasound imaging is recommended prior to initiation of therapy and daily thereafter [114].

Supportive care is usually provided to infants with renal vein thrombosis, and anticoagulant and thrombolytic therapy are controversial in the treatment of this condition. Unilateral renal vein thrombosis with thrombus extending into the inferior vena cava may warrant treatment with LMWH. In bilateral renal vein thrombosis, thrombolysis should be considered [115].

In neonates with clinical presentations of homozygous protein C deficiency, the ACCP recommends administration of either 10–20 mL/kg of FFP every 12 h or protein C concentrate, when available, at 20–60 units/kg until the clinical lesions resolve. For neonates with homozygous protein C deficiency, after initial stabilization, the ACCP recommends long-term treatment with a vitamin K antagonist (VKA) such as warfarin, LMWH, protein C replacement, or liver transplantation [106].

There are no trials supporting the efficacy or safety of anticoagulant therapy for treatment of stroke in the neonate, and currently there are no recommendations for anticoagulation or aspirin for this condition. For neonates with a first arterial ischemic stroke (AIS), in the absence of a documented, ongoing cardioembolic source, the ACCP suggests supportive care over anticoagulation or aspirin therapy. For AIS secondary to cardioembolic causes, the ACCP suggests anticoagulant therapy with LMWH or VKA for at least 3 months. For AIS secondary to cardioembolic causes in children with demonstrated right-to-left shunts (e.g. patent foramen ovale, PFO), the ACCP suggests surgical closure of the shunt [106].

Further studies are required to define optimal antithrombotic therapy, neonatal therapeutic ranges for antithrombotic therapy, and long-term clinical outcome in neonates with evidence of thrombosis.

Key Learning Points

- Thromboembolic events are relatively common in the perinatal period compared to later childhood.
- There is little information on the most appropriate diagnostic methods, treatment, and outcome in this age group.
- Anticoagulation should be considered in bilateral renal vein thrombosis, cardioembolic stroke, and arterial occlusive events threatening life or limb.
- Thrombolytic therapy should be considered for neonates with acute thrombosis, such as aortic, atrial or peripheral arterial thrombosis, that is life-threatening or that could potentially lead to loss of a limb, that presents within 2 weeks of symptomatic onset.

22.3 Disorders of Hemostasis

This section deals with the etiology, clinical presentation, diagnosis, management, and prognosis of these disorders. The majority are secondary to acquired conditions, but inherited coagulation disorders can also present in the perinatal period.

22.3.1 Introduction

Hemostasis describes the process by which coagulation factors, platelets, naturally occurring anticoagulants, and the fibrinolytic system combine to prevent excessive bleeding or thrombosis. Coagulation factors in the fetus begin to appear at 10 weeks' gestational age. At birth, concentrations of the vitamin K-dependent factors (FII, FVII, FIX, FX) and contact factors (FXI, FXII), naturally occurring anticoagulants (antithrombin, protein C, protein S), and plasminogen, are reduced and further reduced in preterm infants [116–118]. At birth, concentrations of FV and FXIII are similar to those in adults; in contrast, levels of FVIII and von Willebrand factor (VWF) are increased at birth [114–116]. Reference ranges for a coagulation profile must therefore take into account both gestational age and postnatal age. The most frequently quoted reference range data are based on work by Maureen Andrews and colleagues who used a standardized protocol, taking venous blood samples from healthy term and preterm neonates above 30 weeks' gestational age who had received vitamin K [117, 118].

Commonly used tests of coagulation status, the prothrombin time (PT) and activated partial thromboplastin time (APTT) can be prolonged in the newborn compared to the adult, as they depend on the amount of coagulation factor present. As these are less than 50 % of the adult mean and have a wide range, a longer PT and APTT are normal findings in the term, and particularly the preterm, neonate [119]. Although absolute values of fibrinogen in the neonate are similar to those in the adult, the fibrinogen is present in a fetal form that differs from adult fibrinogen, so the thrombin clotting time can again be prolonged in neonates, although the exact physiological significance of the fetal type of fibrinogen is not known. Levels of antithrombin, protein C, protein S, and plasminogen are also reduced in the neonate [119].

22.3.2 Inherited Coagulation Disorders

The reader should also refer to Chaps. 11 and 12.

22.3.2.1 Hemophilia

The most common inherited coagulation disorders in the neonatal period are hemophilia A and B resulting from deficiencies of FVIII and FIX, respectively. Hemophilia occurs in 1 in 5,000 male births, and the clinical presentation and severity of bleeding are variable. Eighty to eighty-five percent of cases are hemophilia A and 15–20 % hemophilia B [119]. Two thirds of cases have a positive family history. Forty to sixty percent of infants with severe hemophilia A (FVIII levels <1 %) will be clinically symptomatic as newborns; a further 40 % present by 1 year of age; and 50 % have had a major bleed by 18 months of age [119–121]. Common clinical presentations of FVIII deficiency include hematoma formation following venepuncture, intracranial hemorrhage (41 % of cases reported in the first month of life), cephalhematoma, and bleeding from the umbilicus or post-circumcision [122–124]. Intracranial hemorrhage is usually related to trauma at delivery and is associated with a poor outcome [122]. Although rare, severe hemophilia A may occur in females and present at birth [119]. Bleeding due to severe FIX deficiency (<1 % FIX levels) presents in a similar way to FVIII deficiency in the newborn.

Isolated prolongation of the APTT in an otherwise healthy neonate is highly suggestive of hemophilia A or B. The diagnosis is confirmed by measuring levels of FVIII and FIX, respectively. The diagnosis of mild hemophilia B may be difficult due to physiologically low levels of FIX in the newborn, and there can be a delay of 3–6 months after birth before the diagnosis can be confirmed.

If available, recombinant factor VIII or FIX concentrate is the treatment of choice for hemophilia A and B, respectively. Highly purified derived factor concentrates are the next best alternative. DiMichele et al. have provided guidelines for FVIII and FIX replacement for specific acute hemorrhages [125]. There are no data to support the use of prophylactic doses of FVIII, either intrauterine or immediately after birth, to reduce bleeding complications.

22.3.2.2 von Willebrand Disease

von Willebrand disease (VWD) is a relatively common inherited bleeding disorder which results from either quantitative or qualitative abnormalities in the VWF protein. The VWF glycoprotein mediates the adhesion of platelets to the injured vascular wall and also acts as a plasma carrier and stabilizing protein for FVIII. Bleeding due to VWF deficiency is rare in the newborn period as plasma concentrations of VWF are increased at birth with an increased proportion of high molecular weight multimers.

VWF deficiency is divided into three broad subtypes: partial or complete deficiency of VWF (types I and III) and qualitative defects in VWF (type II). Type 1 VWD is the commonest and occurs as a mild clinical phenotype. Type II VWD can be associated with neonatal thrombocytopenia and may present with bleeding. Type III VWD is a rare autosomal recessive condition characterized by markedly reduced or absent VWF levels, resulting in a severe bleeding tendency, especially from the mucous membranes.

Diagnosis

Type I VWF deficiency is not usually diagnosed in the neonatal period due to the higher levels of VWF normally present at birth. Subtypes of type II may present in association with thrombocytopenia which is apparent in the neonatal period. Type III VWD usually results in an isolated prolongation of the APTT, and the diagnosis is confirmed by measuring FVIII and VWF antigen and activity levels, and VWF multimer analysis.

Treatment

Management of bleeding in type III VWD is usually with factor replacement using an intermediate purity FVIII concentrate containing the high molecular weight VWF multimers.

22.3.3 Rare Coagulation Disorders

This group of autosomal recessive deficiencies in the homozygous or compound heterozygous state can give rise to major clinical bleeding which may manifest in the first few days of life. Severe deficiencies of fibrinogen, FVII, FX, and FXIII are the conditions most likely to present neonatally.

Afibrinogenemia/Hypofibrinogenemia

Fibrinogen deficiency is rare but may present with bleeding in the newborn period, usually in the form of bleeding from the umbilicus or soft tissue hemorrhage. Fresh frozen plasma can be used as initial treatment, but cryoprecipitate (both methylene blue-treated in the UK) or fibrinogen concentrates are preferable.

Factor VII Deficiency

This coagulation factor is a component of the extrinsic pathway of blood coagulation. Activated factor VII activates further FVIII, FIX and FX. Severe deficiency presents similarly to severe hemophilia. The most common presentation of FVII deficiency is intracranial hemorrhage [126]. Deficiencies in factor VII result in an abnormal baseline coagulation screen. Specific factor assays are then required to confirm the diagnosis.

Factor X Deficiency

Activated factor X converts prothrombin to thrombin in the presence of activated factor V, phospholipids and calcium. The most common clinical presentation of FX deficiency in the neonate is intracranial hemorrhage, but bleeding from the umbilicus, heel-prick sites, and the gastrointestinal tract, and spontaneous bruising have been reported [127]. Deficiencies in factor X result in an abnormal coagulation screen; specific factor assays are then required to confirm the diagnosis.

Management of bleeding episodes in FVII and FX deficiency should be with a specific factor concentrate where this is available. Because of the high risk of intracranial hemorrhage, regular prophylaxis should be considered for both severe FVII and FX deficiency.

Factor XIII Deficiency

Factor XIII deficiency leads to reduced cross-linking of clot fibrin polymer and weak clot formation. FXIII deficiency is extremely rare (<1 in one million) and in 80 % of homozygous cases is associated with umbilical bleeding after the umbilical cord separates [128]. It may also be associated with intracranial hemorrhage or bleeding post-circumcision. Heterozygous neonates are not clinically affected. The time taken to clot is normal, so PT and APTT will be normal in this condition. It can be diagnosed using the clot solubility test. The FXIII screening test is sensitive to only the most severe forms of the deficiency, however, and there is currently debate about optimal testing strategies (see Chap. 9). Treatment of FXIII deficiency is with plasma-derived FXIII concentrate (where available), cryoprecipitate, or FFP.

22.3.4 Acquired Coagulation Disorders

22.3.4.1 Vitamin K-Deficiency Bleeding

Vitamin K deficiency bleeding (VKDB), previously known as hemorrhagic disease of the newborn, is now rare due to routine administration of prophylactic vitamin K to neonates. Vitamin K-dependent factors (FII, FVII, FIX and FX) are functionally inactive and reduced in the newborn period in VKDB. The classification of VKDB as early, classical and late, depending on the timing of the presentation, reflects the differing risk factors associated with this condition. Early VKDB (<24 h) is rare and typically associated with antenatal ingestion of drugs that cross the placenta and interfere with vitamin K metabolism (carbamazepine, phenytoin, barbiturates, cephalosporins, rifampicin, isoniazid) and vitamin K antagonists (warfarin). Classical (2–7 days) and late (week 1–week 12) forms are associated with breast-feeding and malabsorption. Presentation is often with melaena, but neonates can also present with intracranial hemorrhage or internal hemorrhage.

Diagnosis

Isolated prolongation of the PT, followed by prolongation of the APTT, in association with a normal fibrinogen concentration and a normal platelet count, suggest the diagnosis of VKDB. This is confirmed by the measurement of the specific vitamin K-dependent factors (II, VII, IX, X), deficiency of which is corrected by the administration of vitamin K.

Prophylaxis and Treatment

Intramuscular (IM) administration of 1 mg of vitamin K at birth provides complete protection against VKDB. The only infants not fully protected in this way are those with yet unrecognised liver disease [129]. Oral administration of a single dose of 1 mg of vitamin K at birth protects against early and classical VKDB but may not be effective against late-onset bleeding [130, 131]. Repeated doses of oral vitamin K have been shown to be as effective as IM vitamin K but may not protect infants with cholestatic disease against late-onset VKDB [130, 132, 133]. For treatment of established or suspected VKDB, vitamin K (1 mg IM) should be administered to correct the existing deficiency. In the presence of major bleeding, factor replacement therapy may also be required with FFP, prothrombin complex concentrate (PCC; FII, FIX, and FX±FVII), preferably a four-factor PCC containing all the vitamin K-dependent coagulation factors.

22.3.4.2 Disseminated Intravascular Coagulation

In the sick neonate, DIC is a relatively common problem. It can occur secondary to birth asphyxia, acidosis, meconium aspiration, amniotic fluid aspiration syndromes, hypothermia, respiratory distress syndrome, viral or bacterial sepsis, and necrotizing enterocolitis [134]. Once established, DIC is often associated with increased mortality.

Clinical Presentation

Clinically, both bleeding and thrombotic problems may occur, and microvascular thrombosis in particular contributes to multi-organ damage. Failure to regulate the coagulation process results in massive uncontrolled thrombin generation, with widespread fibrin deposition and consumption of coagulation proteins and platelets.

Diagnosis

Early DIC can be difficult to diagnose. The laboratory diagnosis of DIC in the neonate is often but not invariably characterized by a prolonged PT and APTT, low fibrinogen, low platelet count, and increased D-dimers (or other markers of fibrin or fibrinogen degradation) [135]. There may be difficulty distinguishing what represents an abnormal result, particularly in preterm infants due to, for example, the frequent presence of thrombocytopenia in infants without DIC, the lack of reliable normal ranges for D-dimers, and increased baseline D-dimer concentrations in the neonatal period [136]. Fibrinogen concentrations are also increased in the first few days of life and may initially be preserved.

Treatment

The management of DIC is prompt and effective treatment of sepsis, hypoxia, and acidosis, and support of oxygenation and perfusion. Treatment continues to center around the use of supportive treatment with fresh frozen plasma, cryoprecipitate and platelets to try to maintain adequate hemostasis. British Committee for Standards in Haematology (BCSH) transfusion guidelines for neonates and older children suggest that the platelet count in a bleeding preterm or term neonate should be maintained above 50×10^9/L by the transfusion of platelet concentrates (10–20 mL/kg) [45]. Fresh frozen plasma (10–20 mL/kg) can be used to replace coagulation factors, although cryoprecipitate (5–10 mL/kg) or fibrinogen concentrates are better sources of fibrinogen, which should be kept above 1 g/L [133].

22.4 Case Study

A 570-g infant was born at 26 weeks' gestation by Cesarean section. Growth restriction was noted antenatally from his 20-week ultrasound scan. By 26 weeks' gestation, fetal growth was below the fifth centile, and Doppler studies showed reversed end-diastolic flow in the umbilical artery, with maximal cerebral redistribution, prompting delivery due to the risk of intrauterine demise.

The infant developed respiratory distress syndrome and was ventilated for 5 days. He had polycythemia on full blood count, normal white cell count and platelets of 90×10^9/L. C-reactive protein was normal, and initial blood and cerebrospinal fluid cultures were negative for infection. He had no evidence of hemorrhage.

The infant was extubated on day 6 and remained stable until day 19. Feeding was commenced slowly on day 2, and he reached full feeds by day 14. On day 19, he had apneic episodes requiring re-ventilation. Associated signs were abdominal distension, bilious aspirates, and hypotension requiring dopamine. Abdominal X-ray showed dilated bowel loops but no pneumatosis intestinalis or evidence of bowel perforation. A blood profile showed a low white cell count, thrombocytopenia (platelet count 40×10^9/L), and a C-reactive protein of 70.

What is the most likely cause and duration of this infant's first and second episodes of thrombocytopenia? The most likely cause of the first episode of thrombocytopenia is chronic hypoxia as a result of placental insufficiency leading to intrauterine growth restriction. The most likely cause of the second episode of thrombocytopenia is necrotizing enterocolitis (NEC).

Would you perform any additional investigations? A coagulation screen should be performed to look for evidence of disseminated intravascular coagulation (DIC), which may require supportive treatment with transfusion of fresh frozen plasma and cryoprecipitate/fibrinogen concentrate. A sepsis screen should also be performed as sepsis together with NEC account for more than 80 % of late onset neonatal thrombocytopenia. An urgent pediatric surgical opinion should be sought.

Would you transfuse this infant? Current guidance in this situation is based on consensus rather than evidence. Platelet transfusion would be appropriate in this situation, in view of the high risk of bleeding in thrombocytopenic infants with NEC, and the potential for DIC, as DIC would exacerbate the thrombocytopenia and DIC-related coagulopathy would further increase the risk of bleeding.

Key Learning Points

- Coagulation reference ranges vary according to gestational age and postnatal age. The PT and APTT can be markedly prolonged in premature neonates.
- Hemophilia A and B are the most common inherited coagulation disorders in the neonatal period: an isolated prolongation of APTT is highly suggestive of hemophilia.
- Isolated prolongation of the PT, followed by prolongation of the APTT, with a normal fibrinogen concentration and platelet count, suggests VKDB. Neonates should be given intramuscular (IM) administration of 1 mg of vitamin K at birth to provide protection against VKDB. Repeated doses of oral vitamin K have been shown to be as effective as IM vitamin K but may not protect infants with cholestatic disease against late-onset VKDB.
- The management of DIC is prompt and effective treatment of the underlying condition, and supportive treatment with blood components/products to maintain adequate hemostasis.

References

1. Holmberg L, Gustavii B, Jonsson A. A prenatal study of fetal platelet count and size with application to the fetus at risk of Wiskott Aldrich syndrome. J Pediatr. 1983;102:773–81.
2. Forestier F, Daffos F, Galacteros F. Haematological values of 163 normal fetuses between 18 and 30 weeks of gestation. Pediatr Res. 1986;20:342–6.
3. Forestier F, Daffos F, Catherine N, Renard M, Andreux JP. Developmental hematopoiesis in normal human fetal blood. Blood. 1991;77:2360–3.
4. Burrows RF, Kelton JG. Incidentally detected thrombocytopenia in healthy mothers and their infants. N Engl J Med. 1988;319:142–5.
5. Burrows RF, Kelton JG. Thrombocytopenia at delivery: a prospective survey of 6715 deliveries. Am J Obstet Gynecol. 1990;162:731–4.
6. Burrows RF, Kelton JG. Fetal thrombocytopenia and its relation to maternal thrombocytopenia. N Engl J Med. 1993;329:1463–6.
7. Sainio S, Järvenpää AL, Renlund M, Riikonen S, Teramo K, Kekomäki R. Thrombocytopenia in term infants: a population-based study. Obstet Gynecol. 2000;95(3):441–6.
8. Murray NA, Howarth LJ, McCloy MP, Letsky EA, Roberts IA. Platelet transfusion in the management of severe thrombocytopenia in neonatal intensive care unit patients. Transfus Med. 2002;12(1):35–41.
9. Roberts I, Stanworth S, Murray N. Thrombocytopenia in the neonate. Blood Rev. 2008;22(4):173–86.
10. Stanworth SJ, Clarke P, Watts T, Ballard S, Choo L, Morris T, Murphy MF, Roberts I, Platelets and Neonatal Transfusion Study Group. Prospective, observational study of outcomes in neonates with severe thrombocytopenia. Pediatrics. 2009;124(5):e826–34.
11. Murray NA, Roberts IAG. Circulating megakaryocytes and their progenitors in early thrombocytopenia in preterm neonates. Pediatr Res. 1996;40:112–9.
12. Watts TL, Roberts IAG. Haematological abnormalities in the growth-restricted infant. Semin Neonatol. 1999;4:41–54.
13. Ghevaert C, Campbell K, Walton J, Smith GA, Allen D, Williamson LM, et al. Management and outcome of 200 cases of fetomaternal alloimmune thrombocytopenia. Transfusion. 2007;47(5):901–10.
14. Srivastava A, Bruno E, Briddell R, Cooper R, Srivastava C, van Besien K, Hoffman R. Parvovirus B19 induced perturbation of human megakaryocytopoiesis in vitro. Blood. 1990;76(10):1997–2004.
15. Cole JL, Marzec UM, Gunthel CJ, Karpatkin S, Worford L, Sundell IB, et al. Ineffective platelet production in thrombocytopenic human immunodeficiency virus infected patients. Blood. 1998;91:3239–46.
16. Roux W, Pieper C, Cotton M. Thrombocytopenia as marker for HIV exposure in the neonate. J Trop Pediatr. 2001;47:208–10.
17. Hohlfeld P, Forestier F, Kaplan C, Tissot JD, Daffos F. Fetal thrombocytopenia: a retrospective survey of 5,194 fetal blood samplings. Blood. 1994;84:1851–6.
18. Webb D, Roberts I, Vyas P. The haematology of Down syndrome. Arch Dis Child. 2007;92:F503–7.
19. Wechsler J, Greene M, McDevitt MA, Anastasi J, Karp JE, LeBeau MM, et al. Acquired mutations in GATA1 in the megakaryoblastic leukemia of Down syndrome. Nat Genet. 2002;32:148–52, 1013.
20. Lopez JA, Andrews RK, Afshar-Kharghan V, Berndt MC. Bernard-Soulier syndrome. Blood. 1998;91:4397–418.
21. Kunishima S, Kamiya T, Saito H. Genetic abnormalities of Bernard-Soulier syndrome. Int J Hematol. 2002;76:319–27.

22. Villa A, Notarangelo L, Macchi P, Mantuano E, Cavagni G, Brugnoni D, et al. X-linked thrombocytopenia and Wiskott-Aldrich syndrome are allelic diseases with mutations in the WASP gene. Nat Genet. 1995;9:414–7.
23. Dupuis-Girod S, Medioni J, Haddad E, Quartier P, Cavazzana-Calvo M, Le Deist F, et al. Autoimmunity in Wiskott-Aldrich syndrome: risk factors, clinical features, and outcome in a single center cohort of 55 patients. Pediatrics. 2003;111(5):e622–7.
24. Salvesen DR, Brudenell JM, Snijders RJ, Ireland RM, Nicolaides KH. Fetal plasma erythropoietin in pregnancies complicated by maternal diabetes mellitus. Am J Obstet Gynecol. 1993;168:88–94.
25. Mondanlou HD, Ortiz OB. Thrombocytopenia in neonatal infection. Clin Pediatr. 1981;20:402–7.
26. Zipursky A, Jaber HM. The haematology of bacterial infection in newborn infants. Clin Haematol. 1978;7:175–93.
27. Jubinsky PT, Moraille R, Tsai HM. Thrombotic thrombocytopenic purpura in a newborn. J Perinatol. 2003;23:85–7.
28. Berner R, Krause MF, Gordjani N, Zipfel PF, Boehm N, Krueger M, et al. Hemolytic uremic syndrome due to an altered factor H triggered by neonatal pertussis. Pediatr Nephrol. 2002;17(3):190–2.
29. Spadone D, Clark F, James E, Laster J, Hoch J, Silver D. Heparin induced thrombocytopenia in the newborn. J Vasc Surg. 1992;15:306–11.
30. Hall GW. Kasabach Merritt syndrome: pathogenesis and management. Br J Haematol. 2001;112:851–62.
31. Burtina AB, Bonafe L, Zacchello F. Clinical and biochemical approach to the neonate with a suspected inborn error of amino acid and organic acid metabolism. Semin Perinatol. 1999;23:162–73.
32. Roth P, Sklower Brooks S, Potaznik D, Cooma R, Sahdev S. Neonatal Gaucher disease presenting as persistent thrombocytopenia. J Perinatol. 2005;25(5):356–8.
33. Faivre L, Guardiola P, Lewis C, Dokal I, Ebell W, Zatterale A, Altay C, et al. Association of complementation group and mutation type with clinical outcome in Fanconi anaemia. Blood. 2000;96(13):4064–70.
34. Greenhalgh KL, Howell RT, Bottani A, Anclif PJ, Brunner HG, Verschuuren-Bemelmans CC, et al. Thrombocytopenia-absent radius syndrome: a clinical genetic study. J Med Genet. 2002;39(12):876–81.
35. Hall JG, Levin J, Kuhn JP, Ottenheimer EJ, van Berkum KA, McKusick VA. Thrombocytopenia with absent radius (TAR). Medicine (Baltimore). 1969;48(6):411–39.
36. Thompson AA, Nguyen LT. Amegakaryocytic thrombocytopenia and radio-ulnar synostosis are associated with HOXA11 mutation. Nat Genet. 2000;26:397–8.
37. Freedman MH, Doyle JJ. Inherited bone marrow failure syndromes. In: Lilleyman JS, Hann IM, Blanchette VS, editors. Pediatric hematology. London: Churchill Livingstone; 1999. p. 23–49.
38. Lackner A, Basu O, Bierings M, Lassay L, Schaefer UW, Révész T, et al. Haematopoietic stem cell transplantation for amegakaryocytic thrombocytopenia. Br J Haematol. 2000;109(4):773–5.
39. Stoll BJ, Hansen N, Fanaroff A, Wright LL, Carlow WA, Ehrnekranz RA, et al. Late onset sepsis in very low birth weight neonates: the experience of the NICHD neonatal research network. Pediatrics. 2002;110(2):285–91.
40. Warris A, Semmekrot BA, Voss A. Candidal and bacterial bloodstream infections in premature neonates: a case control study. Med Mycol. 2001;39:75–9.
41. Dyke MP, Ott K. Severe thrombocytopenia in extremely low birth weight infants with systemic candidiasis. J Paediatr Child Health. 1993;29:298–301.
42. Hsueh W, Caplan MS, Qu XW, Tan XD, De Plaen IG, Gonzalez-Crussi F. Neonatal necrotising enterocolitis: clinical considerations and pathogenetic concepts. Pediatr Dev Pathol. 2003;6(1):6–23.
43. Hutter JJ, Hathaway WE, Wayne ER. Hematologic abnormalities in severe neonatal necrotising enterocolitis. J Pediatr. 1976;88:1026–31.
44. Ververidis M, Kiely EM, Spitz L, Drakek DP, Eaton S, Pierro A. The clinical significance of thrombocytopenia in neonates with necrotising enterocolitis. J Pediatr Surg. 2001;36(5):799–803.
45. Gibson BE, Todd A, Roberts I, Pamphilon D, Rodeck C, Bolton-Maggs P, et al. British Committee for Standards in Haematology Transfusion Task Force: Writing group. Transfusion guidelines for neonates and older children. Br J Haematol. 2004;124(4):433–53.
46. Chaudhary R, Clarke P. Current transfusion practices for platelets and fresh, frozen plasma in UK tertiary level neonatal units. Acta Paediatr. 2008;97(1):135.
47. Strauss R. How do I transfuse red blood cells and platelets to infants with the anaemia and thrombocytopenia of prematurity. Transfusion. 2008;48:209–17.
48. Saxonhouse M, Slayton W, Sola MC. Platelet transfusions in the infant and child. In: Hillyer CD, Luban NLC, Strauss RG, editors. Pediatric handbook of transfusion medicine. San Diego: Elsevier; 2004. p. 253.
49. Josephson CD, Su LL, Christensen RD, Hillyer CD, Castillejo MI, Emory MR, et al. Platelet transfusion practices among neonatologists in the United States and Canada: results of a survey. Pediatrics. 2009;123(1):278–85.
50. Roberts IAG, Murray NA. Thrombocytopenia in the newborn. Curr Opin Pediatr. 2003;15:17–23.
51. Baer VL, Lambert DK, Henry E, Snow GL, Sola-Visner MC, Christensen RD. Do platelet transfusions in the NICU adversely affect survival? Analysis of 1600 thrombocytopenic neonates in a multihospital healthcare system. J Perinatol. 2007;27(12):790–6.
52. Kenton AB, Hegemier S, Smith EO, O'Donovan DJ, Brandt ML, Cass DL, et al. Platelet transfusions in infants with necrotizing enterocolitis do not lower

mortality but may increase morbidity. J Perinatol. 2005;25(3):173–7.
53. De Veber G, Canadian Pediatric Ischaemic Stroke Study Group. Canadian Pediatric Ischaemic Stroke Registry: analysis of children with ischemic arterial stroke (Abstract). Ann Neurol. 2000;48:526.
54. Albisetti M, Andrew M, Monagle P. Hemostaric abnormalities. In: De Alarcon PA, Werner EJ, editors. Neonatal hematology. New York: Cambridge University Press; 2005. p. 310–48.
55. Chalmers EA. Perinatal stroke: risk factors and management. Br J Haematol. 2005;130:333–43.
56. Benders MJ, Groenendaal F, Uiterwaal CS, Nikkels PG, Bruinse HW, Nievelstein RA, et al. Maternal and infant characteristics associated with perinatal arterial stroke in the preterm infant. Stroke. 2007;38:1759–65.
57. Günther G, Junker R, Sträter R, et al. Symptomatic ischemic stroke in full-term neonates: role of acquired and genetic prothrombotic risk factors. Stroke. 2000;31(10):2437–41. *Erratum*: Stroke. 2001;32(1):279.
58. Heller C, Becker S, Scharrer I, Kreuz W. Prothrombotic risk factors in childhood stroke and venous thrombosis. Eur J Pediatr. 1999;158 Suppl 3:S117–21.
59. Kenet G, Sadetzki S, Murad H, Martinowitz U, Rosenberg N, Gitel S, Inbal A. Factor V Leiden and antiphospholipid antibodies are significant risk factors for ischemic stroke in children. Stroke. 2000;31(6):1283–8.
60. Manco-Johnson MJ, Nuss R, Key N, Moertel C, Jacobson L, Meech S, et al. Lupus anti-coagulant and protein S deficiency in children with postvaricella purpura fulminans or thrombosis. J Pediatr. 1996;128:319–23.
61. McColl MD, Chalmers EA, Thomas A, Sproul L, Healey C, Rafferty I, et al. Factor V Leiden prothrombin 20210G→A and the MTHFR C677T mutations in childhood stroke. Thromb Haemost. 1999;81(5):690–4.
62. Zenz W, Bodo Z, Plotho J, Streif W, Male C, Bernert G, et al. Factor V Leiden and prothrombin gene G20210A variant in children with stroke. Thromb Haemost. 1998;80(5):763–6.
63. Bauer K. Rare hereditary coagulation factor abnormalities. In: Nathan DG, Oski FA, editors. Hematology of infancy and childhood. Philadelphia: WB Saunders; 1998. p. 1660–5.
64. Pegelow CH, Ledford M. Severe protein S deficiency in a newborn. Pediatrics. 1992;89:674–5.
65. Brenner B, Fishman A, Goldsher D, Schreibman D, Tavory S. Cerebral thrombosis in a newborn with congenital deficiency of antithrombin III. Am J Hematol. 1988;27:209–11.
66. Schuster V, Mingers AM, Seidenspinner S, Nussgens Z, Pukrop T, Kreth HW. Homozygous mutations in the plasminogen gene of two unrelated girls with ligneous conjunctivitis. Blood. 1997;90:958–66.
67. Andrew M, Vegh P, Johnston M, Bowker J, Ofosu F, Mitchell L. Maturation of the hemostatic system during childhood. Blood. 1992;80:1998–2005.
68. Andrew MA, Monagle P, de Veber G, Chan AKC. Thromboembolic disease and antithrombotic therapy in newborns. Hematology Am Soc Hematol Educ Program. 2001:358–74.
69. Shigekiyo T, Uno Y, Tomanari A, Satoh K, Hondo H, Ueda S, Saito S. Type I congenital plasminogen deficiency is not a risk factor for thrombosis. Thromb Haemost. 1992;67(2):189–92.
70. Tait RC, Walker ID, Conkie JA, Islam SI, McCall F. Isolated familial plasminogen deficiency may not be a risk factor for thrombosis. Thromb Haemost. 1996;76(6):1004–8.
71. De Stefano V, Finazzi G, Mannucci PM. Inherited thrombophilia: pathogenesis, clinical syndromes and management. Blood. 1996;87:3531–44.
72. Toumi NH, Khaldi F, Ben Becheur S, Hammou A, Bouttière B, Sampol J, Boukef K. Thrombosis in congenital deficiencies of AT III, protein C or protein S: a study of 44 children. Hematol Cell Ther. 1997; 39(6):295–9.
73. Blanco A, Bonduel M, Penalva L, Hepner M, Lazzari M. Deep vein thrombosis in a 13 year old boy with hereditary protein S deficiency and a review of the pediatric literature. Am J Hematol. 1994;45:330–4.
74. Olds RJ, Lane DA, Ireland H, Ireland H, Leone G, De Stefano V, et al. Novel point mutations leading to type 1 antithrombin deficiency and thrombosis. Br J Haematol. 1991;78(3):408–13.
75. Dilley A, Austin H, Hooper WC, El-Jamil M, Whitsett C, Wenger NK, et al. Prevalence of the prothrombin 20210G to A variant in blacks: infants, patients with venous thrombosis, patients with suspected myocardial infarction, and control subjects. J Lab Clin Med. 1998;132(6):452–5.
76. Pipe SW, Schmaier AH, Nichols WC, Ginsburg D, Bozynski ME, Castle VP. Neonatal purpura fulminans in association with factor V R506Q mutation. J Pediatr. 1996;128(5 Pt 1):707–9.
77. Bertina RM, Koeleman RPC, Koster T, Rosendaal FR, Dirven RJ, de Ronde H, et al. Mutation in blood coagulation factor V associated with resistance to activated protein C. Nature. 1994;369(6475):64–7.
78. Poort SR, Rosendaal FR, Reitsma PH, Bertina RM. A common genetic variation in the 3′-untranslated region of the prothrombin gene is associated with elevated plasma prothrombin levels and an increase in venous thrombosis. Blood. 1996;88(10): 3698–703.
79. Curry CJ, Bhullar S, Holmes J, Delozier CD, Roeder ER, Hutchinson HT. Risk factors for perinatal arterial stroke: a study of 60 mother-child pairs. Pediatr Neurol. 2007;37:99–107.
80. Ehrenforth S, Junker R, Koch HG, Kreuz W, Münchow N, Scharrer I, Nowak-Göttl U. Multicentre evaluation of combined prothrombotic defects associated with thrombophilia in childhood. Childhood Thrombophilia Study Group. Eur J Pediatr. 1999;158 Suppl 3:S97–104.

81. Hermansen MC, Hermansen MG. Intravascular catheter complications in the neonatal intensive care unit. Clin Perinatol. 2005;32:141–56.
82. Tanke RB, van Megen R, Daniels O. Thrombus detection on central venous catheters in the neonatal intensive care unit. Angiology. 1994;45:477–80.
83. Khilnani P, Goldstein B, Todres ID. Double lumen umbilical venous catheters in critically ill neonates: a randomised prospective study. Crit Care Med. 1991;19:1348–51.
84. Roy M, Turner Gomes S, Gill G. Incidence and diagnosis of neonatal thrombosis associated with umbilical venous catheters (abstract). Thromb Haemost. 1997;78:724.
85. Cohen RS, Ramachandran P, Kim EH, Glasscock GF. Retrospective analysis of risks associated with an umbilical artery catheter system for continuous monitoring of arterial oxygen tension. J Perinatol. 1995;15:195–8.
86. Barrington KJ. Umbilical arterial catheters in the newborn: effect of position of the catheter tip. Cochrane Database Syst Rev. 2000;(2):CD000505.
87. Barrington KJ. Umbilical artery catheters in the newborn: effects of heparin. Cochrane Database Syst Rev. 2000;(2):CD000507.
88. Barrington KJ. Umbilical artery catheters in the newborn: effects of catheter materials. Cochrane Database Syst Rev. 2000;(2):CD000949.
89. Vailas GN, Brouillette RT, Scott JP, Shkolnik A, Conway J, Wiringa K. Neonatal aortic thrombosis: recent experience. J Pediatr. 1986;109:101–8.
90. Nowak-Gottl U, Von Kries R, Gobel U. Neonatal symptomatic thromboembolism in Germany: two year survey. Arch Dis Child Fetal Neonatal Ed. 1997;76:F163–7.
91. Mocan H, Beattie TJ, Murphy AV. Renal venous thrombosis in infancy: long term follow up. Pediatr Nephrol. 1991;5:45–9.
92. Andrew M, Monagle P, Brooker L. Thromboembolic complications in specific organ sites and pediatric diseases. In: Thromboembolic complications during infancy and childhood. Hamilton: Decker Inc; 2000. p. 231–76.
93. Raju TNK, Nelson KB, Ferriero D, Lynch JK, NICHD-NINDS Perinatal Stroke Workshop Participants. Ischaemic perinatal stroke: a summary of a workshop sponsored by the National Institute of Child Health and Development and the National Institute of Child Health and Human Development and the National Institute of Neurological Disorders and Stroke. Pediatrics. 2007;120:609–16.
94. Lee J, Croen LA, Backstrand KH, Yoshida CK, Henning LH, Lindan C, et al. Maternal and infant characteristics associated with perinatal arterial stroke in the infant. JAMA. 2005;293(6):723–9.
95. Govaert P, Dudink J, Visser G, Breukhoven P, Vanhatalo S, Lequin M. Top of the basilar artery embolic stroke and neonatal myoclonus. Dev Med Child Neurol. 2009;51:324–7.
96. Mercuri E, Cowan F. Cerebral infarction in the newborn infant: review of the literature and personal experience. Eur J Paediatr Neurol. 1999;3(6):255–63.
97. Govaert P, Ramenghi L, Taal L, de Vries L, de Veber G. Diagnosis of perinatal stroke I: definitions, differential diagnosis and registration. Acta Paediatr. 2009;98:1556–67.
98. Wu YW, Lynch JK, Nelson KB. Perinatal arterial stroke: understanding mechanisms and outcomes. Semin Neurol. 2005;25:424–34.
99. Dominguez R, Aguirre Vila-Coro A, Slopis JM, Bohan TP. Brain and ocular abnormalities in infants with in utero exposure to cocaine and other street drugs. Am J Dis Child. 1991;145:688–95.
100. Golomb MR, Dick PT, MacGregor DL, Armstrong DC, de Veber GA. Cranial ultrasonography has a low sensitivity for detecting arterial ischemic stroke in term neonates. J Child Neurol. 2003;18:98–103.
101. Cowan F, Mercuri E, Groenendaal F, Bassi L, Ricci D, Rutherford M, de Vries L. Does cranial ultrasound imaging identify arterial cerebral infarction in term neonates? Arch Dis Child Fetal Neonatal Ed. 2005;90(3):F252–6.
102. Roelants-van Rijn AM, Nikkels PG, Groenendaal F, van Der Grond J, Barth PG, Snoeck I, et al. Neonatal diffusion weighted MR imaging: relation with histopathology or follow up MR examination. Neuropediatrics. 2001;32(6):286–94.
103. Bydder GM, Rutherford MA, Cowan FM. Diffusion weighted imaging in neonates. Childs Nerv Syst. 2001;17:190–4.
104. Mercuri E, Rutherford M, Cowan F, Pennock J, Counsell S, Papadimitriou M, et al. Early prognostic indicators of outcome in infants with neonatal cerebral infarction: a clinical electroencephalogram and magnetic resonance imaging study. Pediatrics. 1999;103(1):39–46.
105. de Veber GA, MacGregor D, Curtis R, Mayank S. Neurologic outcome in survivors of childhood arterial ischemic stroke and sinovenous thrombosis. J Child Neurol. 2000;15:316–24.
106. Monagle P, Chan AK, Goldenberg NA, Ichord RN, Journeycake JM, Nowak-Göttl U, Vesely SK, American College of Chest Physicians. Antithrombotic therapy in neonates and children: Antithrombotic Therapy and Prevention of Thrombosis, 9th ed: American College of Chest Physicians Evidence-Based Clinical Practice Guidelines. Chest. 2012;141(2 Suppl):e737S–801.
107. McDonald MM, Jacobson LJ, Hay Jr WW, Hathaway WE. Heparin clearance in the newborn. Pediatr Res. 1981;15(7):1015–8.
108. McDonald MM, Hathaway WE. Anticoagulant therapy by continuous heparinisation in newborn and older infants. J Pediatr. 1982;101:451–7.

109. Punzalan RC, Hillery CA, Montgomery RR, Scott CA, Gill JC. Low-molecular weight heparin in thrombotic disease in children and adolescents. J Pediatr Hematol Oncol. 2000;22(2):137–42.
110. Massicotte P, Adams M, Marzinotto V, Brooker L, Andrew M. Low molecular weight heparin in pediatric patients with thrombotic disease: a dose finding study. J Pediatr. 1996;138(3):313–8.
111. Nohe N, Flemmer A, Rümler R, Praun M, Auberger K. The low molecular weight heparin dalteparin for prophylaxis and therapy of thrombosis in childhood: a report on 48 cases. Eur J Pediatr. 1999;158 Suppl 3:S134–9.
112. Manco-Johnson MJ. How I, treat venous thrombosis in children. Blood. 2006;107:21–9.
113. Wang M, Hays T, Balasa V, Bagatell R, Grupp RO, Grabowski EF, et al. Low dose tissue plasminogen activator thrombolysis in children. J Pediatr Hematol Oncol. 2003;25(5):379–86.
114. Saxonhouse MA, Manco-Johnson MJ. The evaluation and management of neonatal coagulation disorders. Semin Perinatol. 2009;33:52–65.
115. Vogelzang RL, Moel DI, Cohn RA, Donaldson JS, Langman CB, Nemcek Jr AA. Acute renal vein thrombosis: successful treatment with intraarterial urokinase. Radiology. 1988;169(3):681–2.
116. Andrew M, Paes B, Milner R, Johnston M, Mitchell L, Tollefsen DM, Powers P. Development of the coagulation system in the full-term infant. Blood. 1987;70(1):165–72.
117. Andrew M, Paes B, Milner R, Johnston M, Mitchell L, Tollefsen DM, et al. Development of the human coagulation system in the healthy premature infant. Blood. 1988;72(5):1651–7.
118. Andrew M, Paes B, Johnston M. Development of the haemostatic system in the neonate and young infant. Am J Pediatr Hematol Oncol. 1990;12:95–104.
119. Moskowitz NP, Karpatkin M. Coagulation problems in the newborn. Curr Paediatr. 2005;15:50–6.
120. Pollman H, Richter H, Ringkamp H, Jurgens H. When are children diagnosed as having severe haemophilia and when do they start to bleed? A 10 year single centre PUP study. Eur J Pediatr. 1999;158:S166–70.
121. Kulkarni R, Lusher J. Perinatal management of neonates with haemophilia. Br J Haematol. 2001; 112:264–74.
122. Yoffe G, Buchanan GR. Intracranial hemorrhage in newborn and young infants with hemophilia. J Pediatr. 1988;113:333–6.
123. Myles LM, Massicotte P, Drake J. Intracranial hemorrhage in neonates with unrecognised hemophilia A: a persisting problem. Pediatr Neurosurg. 2001; 34:94–7.
124. United Kingdom Haemophelia Centre Doctors' Organisation. Guideline for the selection and use of therapeutic products to treat haemophilia and other hereditary bleeding disorders. Haemophilia. 2003;9(1):1–23.
125. DiMichele D, Neufeld EJ. Hemophilia: a new approach to an old disease. Hematol Oncol Clin North Am. 1998;12:1315–44.
126. Matthay K, Koerper M, Ablin AR. Intracranial hemorrhage in congenital factor VII deficiency. J Pediatr. 1979;94:413–5.
127. Machin S, Winter M, Davies S, Mackie I. Factor X deficiency in the neonatal period. Arch Dis Child. 1980;55:406–8.
128. Anwar R, Minford A, Gallivan L, Trinh CH, Markham AF. Delayed umbilical bleeding-a presenting feature for Factor XIII deficiency: clinical features, genetics and management. Pediatrics. 2002;109(3):E32.
129. Van Winckel M, De Bruyne R, Van De Velde S, Van Biervliet S. Vitamin K, an update for the paediatrician. Eur J Pediatr. 2009;168(2):127–34.
130. Von Kries R, Gobel U. Vitamin K prophylaxis and vitamin K deficiency bleeding (VKDB) in early infancy. Acta Paediatr. 1992;81:655–7.
131. Tonz O, Schubiger G. Neonatal vitamin K prophylaxis and vitamin K deficiency haemorrhages in Switzerland 1986–1988. Schweiz Med Wochenschr. 1988;118:1747–52.
132. Suzuki S, Iwata G, Sutor A. Vitamin K deficiency bleeding during the perinatal and infantile period. Semin Thromb Hemost. 2001;27:93–8.
133. Cornelissen EAM, Kollee AA, van Lith TGPJ, Motohar K, Monnens LAH. Evaluation of a daily dose of 25 micrograms vitamin K to prevent vitamin K deficiency bleeding in breastfed infant. J Pediatr Gastroenterol Nutr. 1993;16:301–5.
134. Cornelissen M, von Kries R, Loughnan P, Schubiger G. Prevention of vitamin K deficiency bleeding: efficacy of different multiple oral dose schedules of vitamin K. Eur J Pediatr. 1997;156:126–30.
135. Williams MD, Chalmers EA, Gibson BE, Haemostasis and Thrombosis Task Force, British Committee for Standards in Haematology. The investigation and management of neonatal haemostasis and thrombosis. Br J Haematol. 2002;119(2):295–309.
136. Hudson IRB, Gibson BE, Brownlie J, Holland BM, Turner TL, Webber RG. Increased concentrations of D-dimers in newborn infants. Arch Dis Child. 1990;65(4 Spec No):383–4.

Thrombotic and Hemostatic Aspects of Assisted Conception

23

Irfana Koita-Kazi, Maria Efthymiou, Hannah Cohen, and Paul Serhal

Abstract

Assisted conception is a women's health issue of growing importance, with the number of women undergoing *in vitro* fertilization (IVF) increasing worldwide. IVF treatment involves ovarian stimulation that can result in a hyperestrogenic state, and in turn can lead to ovarian hyperstimulation syndrome (OHSS), which is associated with both venous and arterial thromboembolism. This chapter addresses clinically relevant thrombotic and hemostatic aspects of assisted conception, including the diagnosis, treatment and prevention of OHSS-related thromboembolism.

Keywords

Assisted conception • *In vitro* fertilization • Ovarian hyperstimulation syndrome • Thrombosis • Prothrombotic changes • Thrombophilia

I. Koita-Kazi, MB ChB, MRCOG (✉)
P. Serhal, MB ChB, MRCOG
The Centre for Reproductive and Genetic Health, Eastman Dental Hospital, 256 Grays Inn Road, London WC1x 8LD, UK
e-mail: irfana.koita-kazi@crgh.co.uk; paul.serhal@crgh.co.uk

M. Efthymiou, BSc, MSc, PhD
Haemostasis Research Unit, Department of Haematology, University College London Hospitals NHS Foundation Trust, 1st Floor, 51 Chenies Mews, London WC1E 6HX, UK
e-mail: m.efthymiou@ucl.ac.uk

H. Cohen, MB ChB, MD, FCRP, FRCPath
Department of Haematology, University College London Hospitals NHS Foundation Trust, 250 Euston Road, London NW1 2PG, UK
e-mail: hannah.cohen@uclh.nhs.uk

23.1 Introduction

In the UK, one in six couples have difficulty in conceiving. The use of assisted conception is on the rise worldwide, and over 50,000 procedures are performed annually in the UK alone. It is estimated that 4.2 % of babies in Europe are born as a consequence of these techniques [1].

In vitro fertilization (IVF) treatment involves ovarian stimulation with exogenous hormones. This can result in a hyperestrogenic state, which can cause ovarian hyperstimulation syndrome (OHSS). OHSS is a systemic disease resulting from the release of vasoactive products from overstimulated ovaries. The syndrome has a broad spectrum of presentation, ranging from mild illness needing only careful observation to

H. Cohen, P. O'Brien (eds.), *Disorders of Thrombosis and Hemostasis in Pregnancy: A Guide to Management*, DOI 10.1007/978-3-319-15120-5_23, © Springer-Verlag London 2015

severe disease requiring hospitalization and intensive care. OHSS is associated with both venous and arterial thromboembolism [2–6]. The hyperestrogenic state may induce prothrombotic changes, which in turn may be potentially contributory to thromboembolism. Limited evidence suggests that prothrombotic mechanisms may also play a role in implantation failure.

This chapter addresses clinically relevant thrombotic and hemostatic aspects of assisted conception, including the diagnosis, treatment and prevention of OHSS-related thrombosis.

23.2 Hemostatic Changes Associated with Assisted Conception

Ovarian stimulation during IVF treatment results in a dramatic increase in endogenous estradiol levels of as much as 20–50 times baseline estradiol levels [6]. This supra-physiological increase in estradiol may lead to prothrombotic changes in hemostatic parameters.

The supra-physiological increases in baseline estradiol levels observed in these situations have been reported to be associated with increased levels of the procoagulant factors VIII, fibrinogen, and factor V, and von Willebrand factor (vWF). These prothrombotic changes are not balanced by corresponding increases in the naturally occurring anticoagulants antithrombin, protein C and S, which are reported to decrease following ovarian stimulation, with the net result a potentially prothrombotic state [5, 7–11]. Increasing resistance to activated protein C (APCr) appears to correlate with increasing estradiol levels, providing further support for development of a procoagulant phenotype in association with ovarian stimulation. The increased APCr does not appear to be explained by corresponding changes in the protein C/S system, suggesting another mechanism involved during IVF processes that induces acquired APC resistance during hyperstimulation [7, 11].

Fibrinolysis leads to dissolution of fibrin thrombus and enables vessel repair, and defects may predispose to venous and arterial thrombosis [12, 13]. Down-regulation of the fibrinolytic system has been observed as estradiol levels increase following ovarian stimulation. Levels of tissue plasminogen activator (t-PA), the main physiological activator of fibrinolysis, decreased with increasing estradiol levels, however, the major plasminogen activator inhibitor – 1 (PAI-1), the main physiological inhibitor of t-PA also decreased, with levels of both within normal ranges, so that the net clinical effect in terms of increased potential for thrombosis would be minimal. Rice et al. also showed down-regulation of fibrinolysis as estradiol levels increased, and also reported that thrombin-antithrombin complexes, a marker of coagulation activation leading to increased thrombin formation, remained unchanged. These observations suggest that elevated circulating estradiol does not predispose to thromboembolism as a result of hypofibrinolysis [14, 15]. Platelet function appears to remain unchanged [16].

Identification of specific thrombophilic defects does not necessarily aid in establishing overall potential thrombogenecity, and does not appear to have predictive value for recurrent thromboembolism [17–20]. More recently, attention has focused on markers of coagulation activation and global tests of haemostasis. Ovarian stimulation has been linked to increased levels of markers of *in vivo* coagulation activation: prothrombin fragment F1.2, which comes from *in vivo* cleavage of prothrombin by factor Xa, thrombin-antithrombin complexes, and D-dimer, a marker of breakdown of cross-linked fibrin/fibrinogen which rises following secondary activation of fibrinolysis after coagulation activation and fibrin formation.

In contrast to conventional tests of hemostasis which measure specific factor levels, assessment of *ex vivo* thrombin generation test using a calibrated automated thrombogram (CAT) system, can capture the end result of the interaction between proteases and their inhibitors and it is therefore potentially more useful and sensitive as a reflection of a haemorrhagic (low thrombin generation) or thrombotic (high thrombin generation) phenotype [21, 22]. Thrombin generation provides a global measure of thrombotic potential [23]. The thrombin generation test (TGT) provides information about the dynamics of *ex vivo* thrombin generation, with the thrombin generation curve described in terms of: the lag-time; the time to peak; peak thrombin concentration; and thrombin generation, with the area under the thrombin generation curve known as the endogenous thrombin potential (ETP). The ETP, a key parameter of the TGT, has been shown to have predictive value for the development of recurrent venous thromboembolism [18–20]. The ETP has been reported to be increased in women undergoing IVF [24]. This provides some support for a thrombotic phenotype associated with ovarian stimulation. Analysis of whole blood using thromboelastography has suggested changes towards hypercoagulability in women undergoing IVF treatment, although parameters remained within normal limits [25].

Despite the considerable changes in baseline concentrations of estradiol and progesterone, the clinical impact of the induced changes in haemostatic parameters during IVF treatment overall appears to be potentially limited as there is a generally a modest effect on the majority of the parameters detailed above [7, 11, 14, 26]. However, prothrombotic changes induced by a hyperestrogenic state may be potentially contributory to thromboembolism, particularly in the presence of a pre-existing prothrombotic state, and implantation failure. In women with OHSS, prothrombotic changes may be more pronounced. Excessive coagulation activation reflected by raised D-dimer levels and TAT thrombin-antithrombin complexes, or raised tissue factor and low tissue factor pathway inhibitor levels, seen in women with OHSS who do not fall pregnant even with higher oocyte yield suggests that prothrombotic mechanisms play a role in implantation failure [8, 27, 28].

23.3 Ovarian Hyperstimulation Syndrome (OHSS)

OHSS is a recognized complication of assisted conception. Mild forms of OHSS are common, affecting up to 33 % of in IVF cycles and 3–8 % of IVF cycles are complicated by moderate or severe OHSS [29]. It usually develops after the administration of hCG and oocyte retrieval, and lasts for 10–14 days.

Women at high risk of developing OHSS include:

- Those with polycystic ovaries
- Those under 30 years of age
- Those with low body weight
- Use of high doses of gonadotrophins for stimulation
- Use of gonadotrophin releasing hormone (GnRH) agonists, luteinizing hormone (LH), or human chorionic gonadotrophin (hCG)
- Development of multiple follicles during treatment
- High absolute or rapidly rising serum estradiol levels
- Increased number of eggs retrieved
- Previous history of OHSS

Women are classified as having mild, moderate, severe or critical OHSS based on the clinical severity at presentation. Those who develop thromboembolism lie in the critical category.

The drugs used for hormonal manipulation include follicle-stimulating hormone (FSH), human menopausal gonadotrophin (hMG), GnRH, GnRH agonist, clomiphene citrate, and hCG. Clomiphene citrate and GnRH are only rarely associated with OHSS [30].

23.4 Thrombosis Associated with Assisted Conception

The possibility that elevated estradiol levels may be linked to venous and arterial thrombosis stems from a number of studies on oral contraceptive pill use [31] and hormone replacement therapy [32].

23.4.1 Incidence

The incidence of antepartum thromboembolism associated with assisted conception has been estimated to be 0.08–0.11 % [2], an incidence similar to that of pregnancy-associated VTE. The incidence of arterial thromboembolism reported to be several times lower [3], with the ratio of venous to arterial thrombosis estimated to be 3:1 [33]. A Danish study of 30,884 women which compared the incidence rates of venous and arterial thrombosis with previously published estimates of the risk of thrombosis among young Danish women found no evidence that assisted reproduction increased the risk of thrombosis [34]. It can be concluded that although assisted conception appears to be a risk factor for antepartum thromboembolism, the absolute incidence of venous thromboembolism (VTE) associated with this treatment appears to be low.

OHSS is the main predisposing factor for both arterial and venous thrombotic events, with the reported incidence of thrombosis with OHSS ranging between 0.7 and 10 % [2–6, 35], however, the development of thrombosis associated with IVF is not always preceded by OHSS [36].

23.5 OHSS-Related Thrombosis

23.5.1 Pathophysiology of OHSS-Related Thrombosis

Mechanisms contributing to thrombosis in women with OHSS include hemoconcentration, prothrombotic blood changes and reduced venous return secondary to enlarged ovaries, ascites and immobility [4, 28].

The pathophysiology of OHSS is characterized by the release of vasoactive substances, which result in increased capillary permeability, leading to leakage of fluid from the vascular compartment. This causes third-space fluid accumulation and intravascular dehydration.

Factors that have been suggested in the process leading to OHSS include:

- Increased exudation of protein-rich fluid from the ovaries or peritoneal surfaces [37–40]
- Increased levels of prorenin and renin in follicular fluid [41, 42]
- Angiotensin-mediated changes in capillary permeability [42, 43]
- Vascular endothelial growth factor (VEGF)/Vascular permeability factor (VPF): expression and production within the ovary appear critical for normal reproductive function [44]

Arterial thrombosis is most likely due to thromboembolic events. Autopsy findings in a patient who died from stroke revealed small brain thrombi with otherwise normal vessels [45]. Similarly, angiography and MRI studies in several reported cases suggest isolated thrombi within affected vessels [46–49].

Women who have an underlying thrombophilia and who fall pregnant as a result of the assisted conception are more likely to develop venous thrombosis. The supraphysiological estrogenic state secondary to ovarian stimulation may add to the pre-existing hypercoagulability in these patients and result in venous thrombosis. The pathogenesis of the specific, yet unusual, localisation of DVT in OHSS remains elusive. Bauersachs et al. [50] hypothesized that ascitic fluid high in estrogen, particularly in women with OHSS, drained into the thoracic duct. This lymphatic fluid then drains into the left subclavian vein resulting in a local area of high estrogen level leading to thrombosis in these neck veins. Salomon et al. [51] hypothesized that the rudimentary brachial cysts in the neck fill with fluid due to OHSS causing mechanical obstruction at the base of the jugular and subclavian veins leading to upper extremity thrombosis.

Apart from OHSS, other risk factors for VTE include a previous personal or family history of venous thromboembolism, concurrent medical conditions such as chronic infective or inflammatory disorders, and obesity.

23.5.2 Diagnosis of OHSS-Related Thrombosis

The commonest reported site for both arterial and venous thrombotic events is the head and neck region although an underreporting of lower extremity venous thrombosis cannot be excluded. The predominant sites of involvement of venous thromboembolism are the veins in the neck and upper extremities in 80 % of cases [3]. Arterial events most commonly (two-thirds) present as cerebrovascular accidents or stroke; the remaining third present in extremities or with myocardial infarction. This is in stark contrast to the classical left iliofemoral deep vein thrombosis seen in pregnancy. The sites for OHSS-related thrombosis reported in the literature include the superior sagittal sinus, internal jugular vein, superior vena cava, thromboembolism extending from the right ovarian vein to the inferior vena cava, basilar artery, subclavian vein, central retinal vein, and the internal carotid vein.

Arterial thrombotic events invariably present early, that is within 2 weeks after embryo transfer, and occur along with the development of OHSS. Venous thromboembolic events, however, may present at any time from within a week after embryo transfer to approximately 12 weeks of gestation, well beyond the resolution of clinical OHSS.

Almost all cases of OHSS-associated VTE occur in women who are pregnant; in contrast, only half of those who develop arterial thrombosis are pregnant.

The causes of death reported in the literature include acute respiratory distress syndrome, cerebral infarction, and hepatorenal failure (reported in a woman with preexisting hepatitis C) [52].

Symptoms and signs suggestive of thromboembolism demand prompt additional diagnostic measures. These include arterial blood gas measurement and appropriate imaging tailored to the individual situation and may include Doppler/Duplex ultrasound of the vasculature of the site involved, CT pulmonary angiography (CTPA), and brain imaging: CT/CT venography and/or MRI.

Thromboembolic events can occur in the absence of other clinical features of OHSS, particularly in patients with severe prothrombotic abnormalities, for example combined heritable thrombophilias or antiphospholipid syndrome. Neck pain and swelling in a pregnant woman, especially one that has undergone IVF, should be taken seriously and investigated with Duplex scanning and/or MR angiography. Unusual neurological symptomatology following ovarian stimulation should raise the possibility of a thrombotic episode in an uncommon location, prompting referral for expert opinion [52] and appropriate investigation.

23.5.3 Management of OHSS-Related Thrombosis

Women who develop thrombosis secondary to assisted conception treatment should be promptly admitted to hospital and managed by a multidisciplinary team. If there is also severe OHSS, pulmonary embolus or head/neck thrombosis, intensive care admission may be advisable until the woman's condition is controlled.

The treatment of VTE involves the use of therapeutic doses of low molecular weight heparin (LMWH) and thrombolysis if indicated [53]. Anticoagulation should be under the supervision of a hematologist, and continued for an appropriate period depending on the site of thrombosis and presence of pregnancy. The management of arterial thrombosis should be tailored to the clinical presentation of the condition, with input by appropriate specialists, particularly neurologists. The reader should refer to Chaps. 5 and 6 for additional information on diagnosis and management.

It is concerning that some studies have demonstrated thrombosis in association with OHSS despite prophylactic [54, 55] and even therapeutic anticoagulation [56]. It has been suggested that this may be due to localized increase in activation of coagulation and raised concentrations of estradiol resulting in impairment of the endothelium's antithrombotic properties [50].

23.5.4 Prevention of OHSS

Measures that can prevent OHSS include:

(a) Controlled ovarian stimulation using the lowest effective dose, especially in those women with risk factors for OHSS
(b) Coasting, that is, cessation of ovarian stimulation
(c) Delaying administration of hCG until estradiol levels have fallen significantly or plateau
(d) Cycle cancellation prior to hCG administration
(e) A lower dose of hCG, that is 5,000 IU instead of 10,000 IU, or a single bolus of GnRH agonist to trigger ovulation in a GnRH antagonist-based protocol

(f) Use of progesterone instead of hCG for luteal support
(g) Cryopreservation of all embryos

Thromboprophylaxis should be initiated in all women admitted to hospital with OHSS, but is particularly important in those with a personal or family history of thromboembolic events, thrombophilia, or vascular anomalies. Anti-embolism stockings and prophylactic dose LMWH should be used. This should be continued at least until discharge from hospital or resolution of symptoms. The risk of thrombosis appears to persist into the first trimester of pregnancy, so LMWH prophylaxis should be continued until the end of the first trimester and possibly longer, depending on other risk factors and the course of the OHSS [57]. The use of intermittent pneumatic compression devices is useful in patients who are confined to bed.

Routine screening for thrombophilia in all women undergoing assisted conception is not warranted, although testing may be helpful for those with a personal or family history of thrombosis [52]. The British Committee for Standards in Haematology (BCSH) Haemostasis and Thrombosis Task Force states that, as the incidence of severe OHSS is so low, the predictive value of thrombophilia testing would be very low and testing should not be used to influence antithrombotic strategies in women commencing ovarian stimulation [58]. There are limited data on dosage and duration of thromboprophylaxis after assisted reproductive therapy. The American College of Chest Physicians (ACCP) guidelines states the following: if LMWH is used in women who develop ovarian OHSS, extension of prophylaxis for 4–8 weeks post-resolution of hyperstimulation [5] or throughout any resultant pregnancy and into the postpartum period [59] has been suggested, given that most reported thrombotic events have developed days to weeks (range, 2 days–11 weeks) after resolution of ovarian hyperstimulation [59]. However, given the lack of a clear association between assisted reproductive technology and postpartum events [60, 61], continuing anticoagulant prophylaxis after delivery is less likely to be of benefit [62].

In the absence of well-designed trials, a pragmatic approach to the prevention of thromboembolism is needed. Hence, all women undergoing ovarian stimulation should undergo risk assessment for thrombosis. Women with a previous history or additional current risk factors for VTE and with known thrombophilia should be closely monitored. LMWH thromboprophylaxis (e.g. enoxaparin 40 mg or dalteparin 5,000 units daily or 12 hourly) along with anti-embolism stockings should be initiated depending on the clinical situation. Thromboprophylactic measures will generally need to be continued throughout pregnancy and for 6 weeks postpartum in high-risk women. Those on long-term oral anticoagulation should be switched to therapeutic dose LMWH, with hematological follow up during pregnancy.

23.5.5 Reporting of Adverse Incidents

The Human Fertilisation and Embryology Authority (HFEA) is a licensing body that regulates all the fertility units in the UK. All adverse incidents occurring at the treatment center must be reported to the HFEA by telephone within 12 working hours of the identification of the incident and submission of an incident report form is required within 24 working hours.

23.6 Heritable and Acquired Thrombophilia in Assisted Conception

Adverse pregnancy outcome in women with thrombophilia has led to speculation that these conditions may also play a role in subfertility, especially recurrent implantation failure. Proposed mechanisms include local microthrombosis at the site of implantation which impairs invasion of maternal vessels by syncytiotrophoblast and leads to implantation failure [63]. However, due to the low and varying prevalence of inherited thrombophilia, the small studies that have been conducted so far have been unable to confirm whether thrombophilia is contributory to subfertility [1].

An increased incidence of heterozygosity for the Factor V Leiden and G20210 prothrombin gene mutations was reported in women failing to conceive after three or more IVF–embryo transfer cycles [64]. In a larger study, 90 women who failed to fall pregnant after three embryo transfers were compared with two separate control groups containing women who conceived after their first attempt (n = 90) and another group containing women who conceived spontaneously (n = 100). The study group was found to have an increased incidence of homozygosity for the C677TT methylene tetrahydrofolate (MTHFR) polymorphism (and combined thrombophilias but not isolated Factor V Leiden) [65]. The C677T MTHFR polymorphism is a normal variant present in approximately 10 % of the normal population. It may, in the presence of folate deficiency, lead to hyperhomocysteinemia, which in turn may lead to thrombosis, although there is no direct association between this polymorphism and thrombosis. The phenotypic expression is silenced by oral folic acid administration. Folic acid 5 mg daily is usually advised throughout pregnancy and a dose of 400 μg considered long-term. Other studies have replicated the findings of an increased prevalence of heritable thrombophilia in women with recurrent implantation failure [66, 67] compared with those who conceived spontaneously or after their first cycle of IVF treatment. Proteins involved in fibrinolysis are necessary for trophoblast invasion into the endometrium. The precise clinical associations of polymorphisms of the gene for PAI-1, a major physiological inhibitor of fibrinolysis, with VTE and recurrent pregnancy loss remain unclear. The 4G allele is associated with higher levels of PAI-1, and might increase the risk for intravascular thrombosis. However, the contribution of this genetic variant to the risk for thrombosis, both arterial and venous, has not been established [67]. Limited data suggest that the 4G/5G polymorphism may be linked to a higher risk of implantation failure [68]. Heritable hypofibrinolysis, mediated by 4G/4G homozygosity for the PAI-1 gene, may be associated with late placenta-mediated pregnancy complications, postulated to be through thrombotic induction of placental insufficiency [69]. A meta-analysis of the PAI-1 4G/5G polymorphism showed no associations with two or three pregnancy losses [70].

The role of acquired thrombophilia, primarily antiphospholipid syndrome, in subfertility is also debatable. As with heritable thrombophilias, large multicenter trials are needed in order to reach a consensus on which antibodies should be tested for and what level corresponds to a clinically significant result. Women who do not conceive after three embryo transfers may exhibit an increased prevalence of antiphospholipid antibodies (aPL) [65, 71, 72]. In women with thrombotic or obstetric APS [73], therapeutic or prophylactic dose LMWH respectively plus low dose aspirin should be started at the time of ovarian stimulation and anticoagulation continued throughout pregnancy and anticoagulation continued for at least 6 weeks postpartum. Infertile women, and those with recurrent IVF implantation failure, have an increased incidence of aPL (22 and 30 %, respectively) compared with a healthy, fertile population (1–3 %). Despite this increased incidence, aPL are not predictive of an adverse outcome following IVF [74], and treatment of these women with antithrombotic therapy remains empirical.

A systematic review and meta-analysis of studies reporting on thrombophilia in women undergoing assisted reproductive techniques (ART) up to April 2011 yielded 33 studies (23 evaluating anti-PL, 5 inherited thrombophilia, and 5 both) involving 6,092 patients. Overall, methodologic quality of the studies was poor. Combined results from case–control studies showed that factor V Leiden was significantly more prevalent among women with ART failure compared with fertile parous women or those achieving pregnancy after ART (odds ratio = 3.08; 95 % confidence interval, 1.77–5.36). The G20210A prothrombin gene mutation, C677T MTHFR, deficiency of protein S, protein C, or antithrombin were all not associated with ART failure. Women with ART failure tested more frequently positive for aPL (odds ratio = 3.33; 95 % confidence interval, 1.77–6.26) with evidence of a high degree of between-study heterogeneity. Prospective cohort studies did not show significant associations between thrombophilia and ART outcomes. The authors concluded that although case–control studies suggest that women experiencing ART failures are more frequently positive for factor V Leiden and aPL, the evidence is inconclusive and not supported by cohort studies [75].

There is a paucity of substantive data as regards the impact of other potentially prothrombotic states, such as myeloproliferative disorders, haemoglobinopathies, paroxysmal nocturnal haemoglobinuria or a history of thrombotic microangiopathies, such as thrombotic thrombocytopenic purpura or atypical haemolytic uremic syndrome, on implantation.

23.7 The Role of Heparin in Assisted Conception

Heparin can alter the hemostatic response to controlled ovarian stimulation and modify the risk of thrombosis associated with exogenous gonadotrophin use. Vascular endothelial growth factor (VEGF), a proangiogenic factor, plays a major role in the pathogenesis of OHSS, and heparin may have a direct role in OHSS due to its reported action on VEGF [76, 77]. There is increasing evidence that heparin can influence many of the basic physiological processes that are required for blastocyst apposition, adherence and implantation. In addition, heparin seems to have a role in trophoblast differentiation and invasion [78–80]. This is likely to have the potential to improve pregnancy rates, perinatal outcome and live birthrates. However, Nelson and Greer concluded in 2008 that there is little substantive evidence to support its use in assisted conception [1]. More recently, a Cochrane review included three RCTs (386 women) in which LMWH given at embryo transfer (one randomized controlled trial (RCT)) or egg collection (two RCTs) was compared with placebo or no treatment [81–83]. The review reported that participant characteristics varied across studies. One study included women having their first IVF cycle, with no blood clotting disorder; one included women with at least one blood clotting disorder; and the third included women who had undergone at least two previous unsuccessful ART cycles. The conclusions were as follows: it is unclear whether peri-implantation heparin improves livebirth and pregnancy rates in subfertile women undergoing ART, as the evidence is seriously limited by inconsistency and imprecision. No benefit is apparent when a random effects model is used. Adverse events were inadequately reported, and no firm conclusions could be drawn regarding the safety of heparin. The findings do not justify the use of heparin in this context except in well-conducted research trials, and further such studies are recommended. Further investigations could also focus on the effects of local (uterine) heparin during ART [84].

23.8 Conclusions

The increasing use of assisted conception worldwide is testament to its overall success, and has also highlighted challenges particularly as regards an evidence based approach to the optimal management of implantation failure, OHSS and the low but potentially avoidable risk of thrombosis. Improved understanding of the pathophysiological mechanisms involved in these situations, including the role of heritable thrombophilia, antiphospholipid antibodies and other potentially prothrombotic states, would provide further insight into their genesis and guide the development of evidence-based therapeutic approaches. Adequately powered and appropriately designed studies are required to define optimal therapeutic strategies, including the role of LMWH, in women undergoing assisted conception.

23.9 Case Studies

Case Study 1

This is a case of forearm amputation after ovarian stimulation for IVF–ET (embryo transfer) [56].

A 41-year-old woman affected by primary subfertility had ovarian stimulation for IVF treatment in a university hospital. The patient underwent many cycles of IVF–ET with administration of purified FSH (75 IU 10 times per day, for 12 days). Nine oocytes were obtained and seven oocytes were inseminated *in vitro*.

A few days later, the patient exhibited absolute arterial insufficiency and an ischemic hand. She had developed ovarian hyperstimulation syndrome. Angiography confirmed thrombi in the subclavian artery. She was treated with thrombolysis and underwent thromboendarterectomy. The subclavian artery thrombosis recurred twice after thromboendarterectomy and resulted in amputation of her forearm.

Case Study 2

This is a case of lower limb DVT followed by internal jugular vein thrombosis as a complication of IVF in a woman heterozygous for the G20210A prothrombin gene and factor V Leiden mutations [85].

A 30-year-old woman heterozygous for both the G20210A prothrombin gene and factor V Leiden mutations underwent IVF treatment. Two embryos were transferred following ovarian stimulation. She presented with lower limb swelling due to proximal deep vein thrombosis that was diagnosed on Doppler ultrasound. Transvaginal ultrasound at 5 weeks' gestation revealed twin gestational sacs, hyperstimulated ovaries, and free fluid in both adnexa. She was started on therapeutic anticoagulant therapy with subcutaneous LMWH (enoxaparin 0.75 mg/kg b.d.). Despite this, she subsequently developed pain and restricted movements, particularly involving the right side of the neck, due to an internal jugular vein thrombosis extending into the subclavian, axillary and cephalic veins on that side. In view of this patient's history of two DVTs in pregnancy, together with her underlying combined thrombophilia, she remained on therapeutic anticoagulation throughout her pregnancy. She delivered healthy twins by Cesarean section at 38 weeks gestation and had no further thrombotic problems postnatally.

Key Learning Points

- The absolute incidence of venous thromboembolism (VTE) associated with assisted conception appears to be low.
- All women undergoing ovarian stimulation should undergo risk assessment for thromboembolism so that appropriate and timely thromboprophylactic measures can be instituted.
- Ovarian hyperstimulation syndrome (OHSS) is the main predisposing factor in both venous and arterial thrombotic events associated with assisted conception. Thromboprophylaxis should be initiated in all women admitted to hospital with OHSS, but is particularly important in those with a personal or family history of thromboembolic events, thrombophilia, or vascular anomalies. Anti-embolism stockings and prophylactic dose low molecular weight heparin (LMWH) should be used.
- The predominant sites of involvement of OHSS-related venous thromboembolism (VTE) are the veins in the neck and upper extremities in 80 % of cases. Arterial events most commonly (two-thirds) present as cerebrovascular accidents or stroke; the remaining third present in extremities or as myocardial infarction.
- Arterial thrombotic events invariably present early, that is within 2 weeks after embryo transfer, and occur along with the development of OHSS. VTE events, however, may present at any time from within a week after embryo transfer to approximately 12 weeks of gestation, well beyond the resolution of clinical OHSS.
- Women who develop thrombosis secondary to assisted conception treatment should be promptly admitted to hospital

and managed by a multidisciplinary team. If there is also severe OHSS, pulmonary embolus or head/neck thrombosis, intensive care admission may be advisable until the woman's condition is controlled.

- The treatment of VTE involves the use of therapeutic doses of LMWH and thrombolysis if indicated. Anticoagulation should be under the supervision of a hematologist, and continued for an appropriate period depending on the site of thrombosis and presence of pregnancy. The management of arterial thrombosis should be tailored to the clinical presentation of the condition, with input by appropriate specialists, particularly neurologists.
- Limited evidence suggests that prothrombotic mechanisms play a role in implantation failure, and that LMWH thromboprophylaxis may be beneficial. However, definition of the role of LMWH requires further studies.

References

1. Nelson SM, Greer IA. The potential role of heparin in assisted conception. Hum Reprod Update. 2008;14(6): 623–45.
2. Mára M, Koryntová D, Rezábek K, Kaprál A, Drbohlav P, Jirsová S, Zivný J. Thromboembolic complications in patients undergoing in vitro fertilization: retrospective clinical study. Ceska Gynekol. 2004;69(4):312–6. [Article in Czech].
3. Chan WS. The 'ART' of thrombosis: a review of arterial and venous thrombosis in assisted reproductive technology. Curr Opin Obstet Gynecol. 2009;21(3): 207–18.
4. Stewart JA, Hamilton PJ, Murdoch AP. Thromboembolic disease associated with ovarian stimulation and assisted conception techniques. Hum Reprod. 1997;12(10):2167–73.
5. Chan WS, Dixon ME. The "ART" of thromboembolism: a review of assisted reproductive technology and thromboembolic complications. Thromb Res. 2008; 121(6):713–26.
6. Whelan JG, Vlahos NF. The ovarian hyperstimulation syndrome. Fertil Steril. 2000;73(5):883–96.
7. Biron C, Galtier-Dereure F, Rabesandratana H, et al. Hemostasis parameters during ovarian stimulation for in vitro fertilization: results of a prospective study. Fertil Steril. 1997;67(1):104–9.
8. Phillips LL, Gladstone W, Vande Wiele R, et al. Studies of the coagulation and fibrinolytic systems in hyperstimulation syndrome after administration of human gonadotropins. J Reprod Med. 1975;14(4): 138–43.
9. Aune B, Hoie KE, Oian P, et al. Does ovarian stimulation for in-vitro fertilization induce a hypercoagulable state? Hum Reprod. 1991;6(7):925–7.
10. Michelon J, Petracco A, Bruxel DM, Moretto M, Badalotti M. Analysis of coagulation parameters in patients undergoing controlled ovarian hyperstimulation for in vitro fertilization. Rev Assoc Med Bras. 2002;48(4):345–7. [Article in Portuguese].
11. Curvers J, Nap AW, Thomassen MC, Nienhuis SJ, Hamulyak K, Evers JL, Tans G, Rosing J. Effect of in vitro fertilization treatment and subsequent pregnancy on the protein C pathway. Br J Haematol. 2001;115(2):400–7.
12. Lisman T, de Groot PG, Meijers JC, Rosendaal FR. Reduced plasma fibrinolytic potential is a risk factor for venous thrombosis. Blood. 2005;105(3): 1102–5.
13. Guimarães AH, de Bruijne EL, Lisman T, Dippel DW, Deckers JW, Poldermans D, Rijken DC, Leebeek FW. Hypofibrinolysis is a risk factor for arterial thrombosis at young age. Br J Haematol. 2009;145(1): 115–20.
14. Lox C, Canez M, Prien S. The influence of hyperestrogenism during in vitro fertilization on the fibrinolytic mechanism. Int J Fertil Womens Med. 1998;43(1):34–9.
15. Rice VC, Richard-Davis G, Saleh AA, et al. Fibrinolytic parameters in women undergoing ovulation induction. Am J Obstet Gynecol. 1993;169(6): 1549–53.
16. Richard-Davis G, Montgomery-Rice V, Mammen EF, et al. In vitro platelet function in controlled ovarian hyperstimulation cycles. Fertil Steril. 1997;67(5): 923–7.
17. Baglin T, Luddington R, Brown K, Baglin C. Incidence of recurrent venous thromboembolism in relation to clinical and thrombophilic risk factors: prospective cohort study. Lancet. 2003;362(9383): 523–6.
18. Brummel-Ziedins KE, Vossen CY, Butenas S, Mann KG, Rosendaal FR. Thrombin generation profiles in deep venous thrombosis. J Thromb Haemost. 2005;3(11):2497–505.
19. Hron G, Kollars M, Binder BR, Eichinger S, Kyrle PA. Identification of patients at low risk for recurrent venous thromboembolism by measuring thrombin generation. JAMA. 2006;296(4):397–402.
20. Besser M, Baglin C, Luddington R, van Hylckama VA, Baglin T. High rate of unprovoked recurrent venous thrombosis is associated with high

thrombin-generating potential in a prospective cohort study. Thromb Haemost. 2008;6(10):1720–5.
21. Hemker HC, Giesen P, Al Dieri R, Regnault V, de Smedt E, Wagenvoord R, Lecompte T, Béguin S. Calibrated automated thrombin generation measurement in clotting plasma. Pathophysiol Haemost Thromb. 2003;33(1):4–15.
22. Hemker HC, Giesen P, AlDieri R, Regnault V, de Smed E, Wagenvoord R, Lecompte T, Béguin S. The calibrated automated thrombogram (CAT): a universal routine test for hyper- and hypocoagulability. Pathophysiol Haemost Thromb. 2002;32(5–6):249–53.
23. Hemker HC, Al Dieri R, De Smedt E, Béguin S. Thrombin generation, a function test of the haemostatic-thrombotic system. Thromb Haemost. 2006;96(5):553–61.
24. Westerlund E, Henriksson P, Wallén H, Hovatta O, Wallberg KR, Antovic A. Detection of a procoagulable state during controlled ovarian hyperstimulation for in vitro fertilization with global assays of haemostasis. Thromb Res. 2012;130(4):649–53.
25. Harnett MJ, Bhavani-Shankar K, Datta S, Tsen LC. In vitro fertilization-induced alterations in coagulation and fibrinolysis as measured by thromboelastography. Anesth Analg. 2002;95(4):1063–6.
26. Bremme K, Wramsby H, Andersson O, Wallin M, Blombäck M. Do lowered factor VII levels at extremely high endogenous oestradiol levels protect against thrombin formation? Blood Coagul Fibrinolysis. 1994;5:205–10.
27. Kodama H, Fukuda J, Karube H, et al. Status of the coagulation and fibrinolytic systems in ovarian hyperstimulation syndrome. Fertil Steril. 1996;66(4):417–24.
28. Rogolino A, Coccia ME, Fedi S, et al. Hypercoagulability, high tissue factor and low tissue factor pathway inhibitor levels in severe ovarian hyperstimulation syndrome: possible association with clinical outcome. Blood Coagul Fibrinolysis. 2002;14(3): 27–282.
29. Delvigne A, Rozenberg S. Epidemiology and prevention of ovarian hyperstimulation syndrome (OHSS): a review. Hum Reprod Update. 2002;8(6):559–77.
30. Practice Committee of the American Society for Reproductive Medicine. Ovarian hyperstimulation syndrome. Fertil Steril. 2008;90(5 Suppl): S188–93.
31. Douketis JD, Ginsberg JS, Holbrook A, Crowther M, Duku EK, Burrows RF. A reevaluation of the risk for venous thromboembolism with the use of oral contraceptives and hormone replacement therapy. Arch Intern Med. 1997;157(14):1522–30.
32. Rossouw JE, Anderson GL, Prentice RL, Writing Group for the Women's Health Initiative Investigators, et al. Risks and benefits of estrogen plus progestin in healthy postmenopausal women: principal results from the Women's Health Initiative Randomized Controlled Trial. JAMA. 2002;288(3):321–33.
33. Aboulghar MA, Mansour RT, Serour GI, Amin YM. Moderate ovarian hyperstimulation syndrome complicated by deep cerebrovascular thrombosis. Hum Reprod. 1998;13(8):2088–91.
34. Hansen AT, Kesmodel US, Juul S, Hyas AM. No evidence that assisted reproduction increases the risk of thrombosis: a Danish National cohort study. Hum Reprod. 2012;27:1499–503.
35. Delvigne A, Rozenberg S. Review of clinical course and treatment of ovarian hyperstimulation syndrome (OHSS). Hum Reprod Update. 2003;9(1):77–96.
36. Chan WS, Ginsberg JS. A review of upper extremity deep vein thrombosis in pregnancy: unmasking the 'ART' behind the clot. J Thromb Haemost. 2006;4(8): 1673–7.
37. Bergh PA, Navot D. Ovarian hyperstimulation syndrome: a review of pathophysiology. J Assist Reprod Genet. 1992;9(5):429–38.
38. Koninckx PR, Heyns W, Verhoeven G, Van Baelen H, Lissens WD, et al. Biochemical characterization of peritoneal fluid in women during the menstrual cycle. J Clin Endocrinol Metab. 1980;51(6):1239–44.
39. Koninckx PR, Renaer M, Brosens IA. Origin of peritoneal fluid in women: an ovarian exudation product. Br J Obstet Gynaecol. 1980;87(3):177–83.
40. Donnez J, Langerock S, Thomas K. Peritoneal fluid volume and 17 beta-estradiol and progesterone concentrations in ovulatory, anovulatory and postmenopausal women. Obstet Gynecol. 1982;59(6):687–92.
41. Sealey JE, Atlas SA, Glorioso N, Manapat H, Laragh JH. Cyclical secretion of prorenin during the menstrual cycle: synchronization with luteinizing hormone and progesterone. Proc Natl Acad Sci U S A. 1985;82(24):8705–9.
42. Derkx FH, Alberda AT, Zeilmaker GH, Schalekamp MA. High concentrations of immunoreactive renin, prorenin and enzymatically-active renin in human ovarian follicular fluid. Br J Obstet Gynaecol. 1987;94(1):4–9.
43. Lightman A, Tarlatzis BC, Rzasa PJ, Culler MD, Caride VJ, NegroVilar AF, et al. The ovarian reninangiotensin system: renin-like activity and angiotensin II/III immunoreactivity in gonadotropin-stimulated and unstimulated human follicular fluid. Am J Obstet Gynecol. 1987;156(4):808–16.
44. Geva E, Jaffe RB. Role of vascular endothelial growth factor in ovarian physiology and pathology. Fertil Steril. 2000;74(3):429–38.
45. Cluroe AD, Synek BJ. A fatal case of ovarian hyperstimulation syndrome with cerebral infarction. Pathology. 1995;27(4):344–6.
46. Togay-Isikay C, Celik T, Ustuner I, Yigit A. Ischaemic stroke associated with ovarian hyperstimulation syndrome and factor V Leiden mutation. Aust N Z J Obstet Gynaecol. 2004;44(3):264–6.
47. Demirol A, Guven S, Gurgan T. Aphasia: an early uncommon complication of ovarian stimulation without ovarian hyperstimulation syndrome. Reprod Biomed Online. 2007;14(1):29–31.

48. Song TJ, Lee SY, Oh SH, Lee KY. Multiple cerebral infarctions associated with polycystic ovaries and ovarian hyperstimulation syndrome [letter]. Eur Neurol. 2008;59(1–2):76–8.
49. Bartkova A, Sanak D, Dostal J, et al. Acute ischaemic stroke in pregnancy: a severe complication of ovarian hyperstimulation syndrome. Neurol Sci. 2008;29(6): 463–6.
50. Bauersachs RM, Manolopoulos K, Hoppe I, et al. More on: the 'ART' behind the clot – solving the mystery. J Thromb Haemost. 2007;5(2):438–9.
51. Salomon O, Schiby G, Heiman Z, et al. Combined jugular and subclavian vein thrombosis following assisted reproductive technology: new observation. Fertil Steril. 2009;92(2):620–5.
52. Royal College of Obstetricians and Gynaecologists. The management of ovarian hyperstimulation syndrome (Green-top guideline no. 5). London: RCOG Press; 2006. https://www.rcog.org.uk/guidelines.
53. Kearon C, Akl EA, Comerota AJ, Prandoni P, Bounameaux H, Goldhaber SZ, et al. Antithrombotic therapy for VTE Disease. Antithrombotic Therapy and Prevention of Thrombosis, 9th ed: American College of Chest Physicians Evidence-Based Clinical Practice Guidelines. Chest. 2012;141(2 Suppl): e419S–94.
54. Arya R, Shehata HA, Patel RK, Sahu S, Rajasingam D, Harrington KF, Nelson-Piercy C, Parsons JH. Internal jugular vein thrombosis after assisted conception therapy. Br J Haematol. 2001;115(1):153–5.
55. Hignett M, Spence JE, Claman P. Internal jugular vein thrombosis: a late complication of ovarian hyperstimulation syndrome despite mini-dose heparin prophylaxis. Hum Reprod. 1995;10(12):3121–3.
56. McGowan BM, Kay LA, Perry DJ. Deep vein thrombosis followed by internal jugular vein thrombosis as a complication of in vitro fertilization in a woman heterozygous for the prothrombin 30 UTR and factor V Leiden mutations. Am J Hematol. 2003;73(4):276–8.
57. Mathur R, Evbuomwan I, Jenkins J. Prevention and management of ovarian hyperstimulation syndrome. Curr Obstet Gynaecol. 2005;15(2):132–8.
58. Baglin T, Gray E, Greaves M, Hunt BJ, Keeling D, Machin S, British Committee for Standards in Haematology, et al. Clinical guidelines for testing for heritable thrombophilia. Br J Haematol. 2010;149(2): 209–20.
59. Nelson SM. Prophylaxis of VTE in women – during assisted reproductive techniques. Thromb Res. 2009;123 Suppl 3:S8–15.
60. Aurousseau MH, Samama MM, Belhassen A, Herve F, Hugues JN. Risk of thromboembolism in relation to an in-vitro fertilization programme: three case reports. Hum Reprod. 1995;10(1):94–7.
61. Jacobsen AF, Skjeldestad FE, Sandset PM. Ante- and postnatal risk factors of venous thrombosis: a hospital-based case–control study. J Thromb Haemost. 2008;6(6):905–12.
62. Bates SM, Greer IA, Middeldorp S, Veenstra DL, Prabulos AM, Vandvik PO, American College of Chest Physicians. VTE, thrombophilia, antithrombotic therapy, and pregnancy: Antithrombotic Therapy and Prevention of Thrombosis, 9th ed: American College of Chest Physicians Evidence-Based Clinical Practice Guidelines. Chest. 2012;141(2 Suppl): e691S–736.
63. Potdar N, Gelbaya TA, Konje JC, Nardo LG. Adjunct low-molecular-weight heparin to improve live birth rate after recurrent implantation failure: a systematic review and meta-analysis. Hum Reprod Update. 2013;19(6):674–84.
64. Grandone E, Colaizzo D, Lo Bue A, Checola MG, Cittadini E, Margaglione M. Inherited thrombophilia and in vitro fertilization implantation failure. Fertil Steril. 2001;76(1):201–2.
65. Qublan HS, Eid SS, Ababneh HA, Amarin ZO, Smadi AZ, Al-Khafaji FF, Khader YS. Acquired and inherited thrombophilia: implication in recurrent IVF and embryo transfer failure. Hum Reprod. 2006; 21(10):2694–8.
66. Azem F, Many A, Yovel I, Amit A, Lessing JB, Kupferminc MJ. Increased rates of thrombophilia in women with repeated IVF failures. Hum Reprod. 2004;19(2):368–70.
67. Tsantes AE, Nikolopoulos GK, Bagos PG, Rapti E, Mantzios G, Kapsimali V, Travlou A. Association between the plasminogen activator inhibitor-1 4G/5G polymorphism and venous thrombosis. A meta-analysis. Thromb Haemost. 2007;97(6):907–13.
68. Coulam CB, Jeyendran RS, Fishel LA, Roussev R. Multiple thrombophilic gene mutations are risk factors for implantation failure. Reprod Biomed Online. 2006;12(3):322–7.
69. Glueck CJ, Phillips H, Cameron D, Wang P, Fontaine RN, Moore SK. The 4G/4G polymorphism of the hypofibrinolytic plasminogen activator inhibitor type 1 gene: an independent risk factor for serious pregnancy complications. Metabolism. 2000;49(7): 845–52.
70. Su MT, Lin SH, Chen YC, Kuo PL. Genetic association studies of ACE and PAI-1 genes in women with recurrent pregnancy loss: a systematic review and meta-analysis. Thromb Haemost. 2013;109(1):8–15.
71. Balasch J, Fabregues F, Creus M, Reverter JC, Carmona F, Tassies D, et al. Pregnancy: antiphospholipid antibodies and human reproductive failure. Hum Reprod. 1996;11(10):2310–5.
72. Vaquero E, Lazzarin N, Caserta D, Valensise H, Baldi M, Moscarini M, Arduini D. Diagnostic evaluation of women experiencing repeated in vitro fertilization failure. Eur J Obstet Gynecol Reprod Biol. 2006; 125(1):79–84.
73. Miyakis S, Lockshin MD, Atsumi T, Branch DW, Brey RL, Cervera R, et al. International consensus statement on an update of the classification criteria for definite antiphospholipid syndrome (APS). J Thromb Haemost. 2006;4(2):295–306.

74. Buckingham KL, Chamley LW. A critical assessment of the role of antiphospholipid antibodies in infertility. J Reprod Immunol. 2009;80(1–2):132–45.
75. Di Nisio M, Rutjes AW, Ferrante N, Tiboni GM, Cuccurullo F, Porreca E. Thrombophilia and outcomes of assisted reproduction technologies: a systematic review and meta-analysis. Blood. 2011;118(10):2670–8.
76. Seko Y, Fukuda S, Nagai R. Serum levels of endostatin, vascular endothelial growth factor (VEGF) and hepatocyte growth factor (HGF) in patients with acute myocardial infarction undergoing early reperfusion therapy. Clin Sci. 2004;106(5):439–42.
77. Tessler S, Rockwell P, Hicklin D, Cohen T, Levi BZ, Witte L, et al. Heparin modulates the interaction of VEGF165 with soluble and cell associated flk-1 receptors. J Biol Chem. 1994;269(17):12456–61.
78. Di Simone N, Di Nicuolo F, Sanguinetti M, Ferrazzani S, D'Alessio MC, Castellani R, et al. Low-molecular weight heparin induces in vitro trophoblast invasiveness: role of matrix metalloproteinases and tissue inhibitors. Placenta. 2007;28(4):298–304.
79. Chen Y, Wu XX, Tan JP, Liu ML, Liu YL, Zhang JP. Effects of low molecular weight heparin and heparin-binding epidermal growth factor on human trophoblast in first trimester. Fertil Steril. 2012;97(3):764–70.
80. Tersigni C, Marana R, Santamarìa A, Castellani R, Scambia G, Simone ND. In vitro evidences of heparin's effects on embryo implantation and trophoblast development. Reprod Sci. 2012;19(5):454–62.
81. Noci I, Milanini MN, Ruggiero M, Papini F, Fuzzi B, Artini PG. Effect of dalteparin sodium administration on IVF outcome in non-thrombophilic young women: a pilot study. Reprod Biomed Online. 2011;22(6):615–20.
82. Qublan H, Amarin Z, Dabbas M, Farraj AE, Beni-Merei Z, Al-Akash H, et al. Low-molecular weight heparin in the treatment of recurrent IVF-ET failure and thrombophilia: a prospective randomised placebo-controlled trial. Hum Fertil (Camb). 2008;11(4):246–53.
83. Urman B, Ata B, Yakin K, Alatas C, Aksoy S, Mercan R, Balaban B. Luteal phase empirical low molecular weight heparin administration in patients with failed ICSI embryo transfer cycles: a randomized open-labeled pilot trial. Hum Reprod. 2009;24(7):1640–7.
84. Akhtar MA, Sur S, Raine-Fenning N, Jayaprakasan K, Thornton J, Quenby S, Marjoribanks J. Heparin for assisted reproduction: summary of a Cochrane review. Fertil Steril. 2015;103:33–4.
85. Mancini A, Milardi D, Di Pietro ML, Giacchi E, Spagnolo AG, Di Donna V, De Marinis L, Jensen L. A case of forearm amputation after ovarian stimulation for IVF-ET. Fertil Steril. 2001;76(1):198–200.

Index

H. Cohen, P. O'Brien (eds.), *Disorders of Thrombosis and Hemostasis in Pregnancy: A Guide to Management*, DOI 10.1007/978-3-319-15120-5, © Springer-Verlag London 2015

R

S

MIX
Papier aus verantwortungsvollen Quellen
Paper from responsible sources
FSC® C105338
FSC
www.fsc.org

If you have any concerns about our products,
you can contact us on
ProductSafety@springernature.com

In case Publisher is established outside the EU,
the EU authorized representative is:
Springer Nature Customer Service Center GmbH
Europaplatz 3, 69115 Heidelberg, Germany

Printed by Libri Plureos GmbH
in Hamburg, Germany